GERIATRIC HEART DISEASE

Edited by

Eugene L. Coodley, MD, FACP, FACC, FACA
Professor of Medicine
University of California, Irvine California School of Medicine
Chief of Gerontology
Long Beach VA Medical Center
Long Beach, California

PSG PUBLISHING COMPANY, INC.
LITTLETON, MASSACHUSETTS

Library of Congress in Publication Data
Main entry under title:

Geriatric heart disease.

Bibliography: p.
Includes index.
1. Geriatric cardiology. I. Coodley, Eugene L., 1920– . [DNLM: 1. Cardiovascular Diseases--in old age. WG 100 G369]
RC669.G47.1984 618.97′612 84-1074
ISBN 0-88416-468-3

Published by:
PSG PUBLISHING COMPANY, INC.
545 Great Road
Littleton, Massachusetts 01460

Medicine is an ever-changing science. As new research and clinical experience broaden our knowledge, changes in treatment and drug therapy are required. The authors and the publisher of this work have made every effort to ensure that the treatment and drug dosage schedules herein are accurate and in accord with the standards accepted at the time of publication. Readers are advised, however, to check the product information sheet included in the package of each drug they plan to administer to be certain that changes have not been made in the recommended dose or in the indications and contraindications for administration. This recommendation is of particular importance in regard to new or infrequently used drugs.

Printed in the United States of America.

International Standard Book Number: 0-88416-468-3

Library of Congress Catalog Card Number: 84-1074

Contributors

Abdulla M. Abdulla, MD
Associate Professor of Medicine
Section of Cardiology
Medical College of Georgia School of Medicine
Augusta, Georgia

Erik Agner, MD
Senior Registrar
Department of Internal Medicine
Glostrup Hospital
University of Copenhagen
Copenhagen
DENMARK

Colin M. Bloor, MD
Professor of Pathology
Department of Pathology
University of California, San Diego
La Jolla, California

David C. Brewster, MD
Assistant Professor of Surgery
Vascular Surgery Department
Massachusetts General Hospital
Boston, Massachusetts

Bruce H. Brundage, MD
Chief, Section Cardiology
University of Illinois College of Medicine
Associate Professor of Medicine and Radiology
Director, Adult Cardiac Catheterization Laboratories
Chicago, Illinois

F.I. Caird, DM, MRCP, MA, FRCP
Professor of Geriatric Medicine
University of Glasgow
University Department of Geriatric Medicine
Southern General Hospital
Glasgow
SCOTLAND

Alfred Coodley, MD, PhD
Clinical Professor of Psychiatry
University of Southern California School of Medicine
Los Angeles, California

Eugene L. Coodley, MD, FACP, FACC, FACA
Professor of Medicine
University of California, Irvine, California School of Medicine
Chief of Gerontology
Long Beach VA Medical Center
Long Beach, California

Gregg Coodley, BA
University of California, San Diego, School of Medicine
La Jolla, California

Kevin Cullen, MD, FRCP, FRACP
Busselton Population Studies
Raine Medical Statistics Unit
University of Western Australia
Nedlands
WESTERN AUSTRALIA

G.K. David, MD
Cardiologist
Department of Cardiology
Academisch Medisch Centrum
Amsterdam
NETHERLANDS

William J. deGroot, MD
Professor of Medicine
Director, Pulmonary Disease
The University of Texas Medical School at Galveston
Galveston, Texas

T. Anthony Don Michael, MD, FACP, FRCP
Clinical Professor of Medicine
UCLA School of Medicine
Los Angeles, California

Jan I.M. Drayer, MD
Associate Chief
Section of Clinical Pharmacology & Hypertension
Long Beach VA Medical Center
Associate Professor of Medicine
University of California, Irvine, California College of Medicine
Irvine, California

D. Düren, MD
Cardiologist
Department of Cardiology
Academisch Medisch Centrum
Amsterdam
NETHERLANDS

Myrvin H. Ellestad, MD
Chief, Division of Cardiology
Memorial Medical Center of Long Beach
Clinical Professor of Medicine
University of California, Irvine, California College of Medicine
Irvine, California

Jerome L. Fleg, MD
Gerontology Research Center (NIA, NIH)
Associate Professor of Medicine
The Johns Hopkins University School of Medicine
Baltimore, Maryland

Lloyd D. Fisher, PhD
Department of Cardiovascular Disease
Mayo Clinic
Rochester, Minnesota

J. Colin Forfar, BSc, MB, ChB, MRCP
Cardiovascular Research Unit
Edinburgh
SCOTLAND

Martin J. Frank, MD
Professor of Medicine
Chief, Section of Cardiology
Medical College of Georgia School of Medicine
Augusta, Georgia

David Fray, BS
Department of Cardiovascular Diseases
Mayo Clinic
Rochester, Minnesota

Sandor A. Friedman, MD
Professor of Medicine
State University of New York
Downstate Medical Center College of Medicine
Chief, Department of Medicine
Coney Island Hospital
Brooklyn, New York

Vladimir V. Frolkis, MD
Professor of Medicine
Chief, Experimental Department
Institute of Gerontology AMS USSR
Kiev
USSR

Robert L. Frye, MD
Department of Cardiovascular Disease
Mayo Clinic
Rochester, Minnesota

Francisco Fuentes, MD
Associate Professor of Medicine
Department of Medicine
Division of Cardiology
The University of Texas Medical School
Houston, Texas

Julius M. Gardin, MD
Director, Cardiology
Noninvasive Laboratory
University of California, Irvine, California School of Medicine
Chief of Cardiology Section
Long Beach VA Medical Center
Long Beach, California

Bernard J. Gersh, MD
Department of Cardiovascular Disease
Mayo Clinic
Rochester, Minnesota

William M. Girard, MD
Associate Professor of Clinical Medicine
The University of Texas Health Medical School at Houston
Houston, Texas

Paula Bursztyn Goldberg, PhD
Assistant Professor
Department of Pharmacology
The Medical College of Pennsylvania
Philadelphia, Pennsylvania

K. Lance Gould, MD
Professor and Director
Division of Cardiology
The University of Texas Medical School at Houston
Houston, Texas

John Hamer, MD, PhD, FRCP
Consultant Cardiologist
Department of Clinical Pharmacology
St. Bartholomew's Hospital
London
ENGLAND

Elias Hanna, MD, FACS, FACC
Chief, Thoracic Cardiovascular Surgery
St. Mary's Hospital
San Francisco, California

Charles H. Hicks, MD
Assistant Professor of Medicine
Department of Medicine
Division of Cardiology
The University of Texas Medical School at Houston
Houston, Texas

Jack Hirsh, MD
Professor and Chairman
Department of Medicine
McMaster University School of Medicine
Hamilton, Ontario
CANADA

H. Malcolm Hodkinson, DM, FRCP
Professor of Geriatric Medicine
University of London
Royal Postgraduate Medical School
Hammersmith Hospital
London
ENGLAND

David R. Holmes, Jr, MD
Consultant, Division of Cardiovascular Diseases and Internal Medicine
Mayo Clinic
Assistant Professor of Medicine
Mayo Medical School
Rochester, Minnesota

Russell D. Hull, MD, FRCP(C)
Associate Professor of Medicine
Department of Medicine
McMaster University School of Medicine
Chedoke-McMaster Hospital
Hamilton, Ontario
CANADA

David Hunt, MD, FRACP, FACC
Director of Cardiology
Royal Melbourne Hospital
Victoria
AUSTRALIA

Tetsuo Ishimori, MD, FACP, FACC
Clinical Associate Professor of Medicine
University of California, San Francisco, School of Medicine
Central Cardiology Medical Group
Bakersfield, California

Ram Kannan, PhD
Department of Cardiology
Wadsworth VA Hospital
Department of Medicine
UCLA School of Medicine
Los Angeles, California

G. Kan, MD
Cardiologist
Department of Cardiology
Academisch Medisch Centrum
Amsterdam
NETHERLANDS

Angelika Kleinebenne
Research Fellow
Cardiovascular Unit
Royal Postgraduate Medical School
London
ENGLAND

Thomas Killip III, MD
Department of Cardiovascular Disease
Mayo Clinic
Rochester, Minnesota

Albert J. Kolibash, MD
Associate Professor of Medicine
Division of Cardiology
Ohio State University College of Medicine
Columbus, Ohio

Richard A. Kronmal, PhD
Department of Biostatistics
University of Washington
Seattle, Washington

Edward G. Lakatta, MD
Cardiovascular Section (NIA, NIH)
Associate Professor of Medicine
The Johns Hopkins University School of Medicine
Adjunct Associate Professor of Physiology
University of Maryland
Baltimore, Maryland

J.R. Leclerc, MD, FRCP(C)
Research Fellow
Ontario Heart Foundation
Thromboembolic Unit
McMaster University School of Medicine
Hamilton, Ontario
CANADA

James J. Leonard, MD
Professor and Chairman
Department of Medicine
Uniformed Services University of the Health Sciences
School of Medicine
Bethesda, Maryland

K.I. Lie, MD
Professor of Cardiology
Department of Cardiology
University of Groningen
Groningen
NETHERLANDS

James Light, MD
Director, Cardiology Fellowship Training Program
Memorial Hospital
Clinical Professor of Medicine
University of California, Irvine, California School of Medicine
Irvine, California

Richard W. Light, MD, FCCP
Associate Professor of Medicine
University of California, Irvine, California School of Medicine
Chief, Pulmonary Section
Long Beach VA Medical Center
Long Beach, California

Edgar Lichstein, MD
Director of Cardiology
Maimonides Medical Center
Professor of Medicine
State University of New York
Downstate Medical Center College of Medicine
Brooklyn, New York

James R. Licht, MD
Director, Cardiology Fellowship Training Program
Memorial Medical Center of Long Beach
Clinical Assistant Professor of Medicine
University of California, Irvine, California School of Medicine
Irvine, California

Michael Lye, MD
Professor and Head
Department of Geriatric Medicine
University of Manchester
Manchester
ENGLAND

Anthony Martin, MD
The Crawley Research Unit
Crawley Hospital
Sussex
ENGLAND

John H. McAnulty, MD
Associate Professor of Medicine
University of Oregon Health Sciences Center School of Medicine
Portland, Oregon

William J. McKenna, MD
Senior Registrar
Cardiovascular Unit
Royal Postgraduate Medical School
London
ENGLAND

Jawahar Mehta, MD
Associate Professor of Medicine
Department of Medicine
Division of Cardiovascular Medicine
University of Florida College of Medicine
Gainesville, Florida

Marcello Mellino, MD
Senior Clinical Instructor
Case Western Reserve University School of Medicine
Director, Coronary Care
Lutheran Medical Center
Cleveland, Ohio

Michael B. Mock, MD
Department of Cardiovascular Diseases
Mayo Clinic
Rochester, Minnesota

Koonlawee Nademanee, MD
Department of Cardiology
Wadsworth VA Hospital
Department of Medicine
UCLA School of Medicine
Los Angeles, California

Jane F. Potter, MD
Chief, Section of Geriatrics and Gerontology
Department of Internal Medicine
University of Nebraska College of Medicine
Omaha, Nebraska

Shahbudin H. Rahimtoola, MD
Professor of Medicine
Chief, Section of Cardiology
University of Southern California School of Medicine
Los Angeles, California

Jay Roberts, PhD
Professor and Chairman
Department of Pharmacology
The Medical College of Pennsylvania
Philadelphia, Pennsylvania

William J. Rogers, MD
Associate Professor of Medicine
The University of Alabama School of Medicine
Birmingham, Alabama

Warren E. Sanford, MD
Department of Internal Medicine
Naval Regional Medical Center
San Diego, California

Hartzell V. Schaff, MD
Department of Cardiovascular Disease
Mayo Clinic
Rochester, Minnesota

Mohandas Shenoy, MD
Assistant Professor of Clinical Medicine
State University of New York
Downstate Medical Center College of Medicine
Associate Chief, Cardiology Division
Coney Island Hospital
Brooklyn, New York

Bramah N. Singh, MD
Professor of Medicine
UCLA School of Medicine
Director, Cardiovascular Research Laboratory
Wadsworth VA Medical Center
Los Angeles, California

Graeme Sloman, ED, BSc, FRCP, FRACP, FACC
Director of Cardiology
Chairman, Cardiovascular Unit
Epworth Hospital
Richmond, Victoria
AUSTRALIA

Richard W Smalling, MD, PhD
The University of Texas Health Sciences Center
Houston, Texas

N.S. Stenhouse, MSc
Raine Medical Statistics Unit
University of Western Australia
Nedlands
WESTERN AUSTRALIA

John R. Stratton, MD
Assistant Professor of Medicine
Division of Cardiology
University of Washington School of Medicine
Seattle, Washington

Enrique Vargas, MD, PhD, MSc
Research Associate
Department of Geriatric Medicine
University of Manchester
Withington Hospital
Manchester
ENGLAND

Emmanuel C. Vasilomanolakis, MD
Attending Physician
Division of Cardiology
Memorial Medical Center of Long Beach
Long Beach Community Hospital
Long Beach, California

Nagammal Venkatesh, MD
Department of Cardiology
Wadsworth VA Hospital
Department of Medicine
UCLA School of Medicine
Los Angeles, California

W.V.R. Vieweg, MD, FACP, FACC
Department of Behavioral Medicine and Psychiatry
University of Virginia School of Medicine
Charlottesville, Virginia

C.A. Visser, MD
Cardiologist
Department of Cardiology
Academisch Medisch Centrum
Amsterdam
NETHERLANDS

Marge Wanta-Matthews, RN, CVNS
Research Nurse
Department of Medicine
Division of Cardiology
The University of Texas Medical School
Houston, Texas

Sanford E. Warren, MD, CDR, MC, USNR
Department of Medicine
Naval Hospital
Associate, American College of Cardiology
San Diego, California
Presently
Department of Cardiology
Beth Israel Hospital
Boston, Massachusetts

Laurence O. Watkins, MD
Assistant Professor of Medicine
Section of Cardiology
Medical College of Georgia School of Medicine
Augusta, Georgia

David W. Webb, MD
Assistant Chief of Medicine for Clinical Care
Long Beach VA Medical Center
Adjunct Assistant Professor of Medicine
University of California, Irvine, California School of Medicine
Irvine, California

Michael A. Weber, MD
Chief, Section of Clinical Pharmacology and Hypertension
Long Beach VA Medical Center
Associate Professor of Medicine
University of California, Irvine, California School of Medicine
Irvine, California

Asher Woldow, MD
Chief of Cardiology
Department of Medicine
Philadelphia Geriatric Center
Professor of Medicine
The Medical College of Pennsylvania
Philadelphia, Pennsylvania

Charles F. Wooley, MD
Professor of Medicine
Division of Cardiology
Ohio State University College of Medicine
Columbus, Ohio

Frederic A. Wyle, MD
Adjunct Professor of Medicine
Vice Chairman, Department of Medicine
University of California, Irvine, California
School of Medicine
Chief, Medical Service
Long Beach VA Medical Center
Long Beach, California

Diane Zebari, MD
Senior Instructor
University of California, Irvine, California
School of Medicine
Staff Physician
Long Beach VA Medical Center
Long Beach, California

Contents

SECTION III CHARACTERISTICS OF HEART DISEASE

Preface

At the present time, 11% of the population in the United States is over the age of 65 and this is expected to reach 20% before the end of this century. Similar rapid increase in the number of older patients is occurring in other countries. With heart disease representing one of the most common medical conditions seen by physicians, it has become necessary to be very familiar with the differing aspects of cardiac disease in the older patient.

This volume is designed to bring to the practicing physician and academician the newer knowledge about heart disease in the older patient. The book is unique in that it represents a multinational-authored approach to this topic; each chapter is written by an authority on the topic covered, and the latest research on the particular topic is presented. Much of the material is so new that it has not been published elsewhere as yet.

The term *elderly* has been variously defined as falling between the ages of 62 and 70, but is more related to physiologic status than to chronologic number, and the authors in the succeeding chapters have arbitrarily taken age groups within this span.

The book is divided into four basic sections: (1) Physiology and Epidemiology; (2) Diagnostic Technics; (3) Characteristics of Heart Disease; and (4) Therapy.

The first section reviews the physiologic changes that accompany normal aging and includes materials from researchers in almost every aspect of cardiac function. Section II examines the role of commonly used diagnostic parameters in terms of their applicability to the older patient and provides guidelines to the clinician as to the appropriate selection of these studies. Section III is a review of the various types of cardiac disease and abnormalities of blood pressure and vascular diseases that are encountered in older patients. It attempts to provide guidelines for a clear understanding of the pathophysiology, hemodynamics, and evolution of these disease processes. Several chapters are also devoted to a consideration of prognostic factors in the older aged population who are suffering from coronary artery disease. The last section is devoted to consideration of therapeutic modalities, both medical and surgical, with regard to their applicability in the older aged population. While experience with newer technics in the older age groups is still limited, these chapters present recent data from groups who have had wide experience with these technics.

Throughout the book the theme has been an emphasis on differences in various aspects of heart disease between the younger and older patient. Each author has included such comparison in addressing his or her topic.

It is our hope that this comprehensive and timely presentation will serve to assist physicians in dealing with cardiac problems of the older patient, both from a clinical and a research standpoint.

CHAPTER 1
Cardiovascular Aging

John Hamer

Heart disease in elderly patients is often said to be "multifactorial," but this approach is diagnostically unhelpful and tends to diminish the application of specific treatment of correctible factors. The accumulation of problems with increasing age is often associated with a background of hypertension and coronary artery disease to which is added the more specific diseases of the elderly such as calcific valvar degeneration and myocardial amyloid infiltration, together with the effects of age-related arrhythmias such as atrial fibrillation and heart block. The more lethal effects of hypertension and coronary artery disease are most prevalent in the younger elderly as they reduce survival to very old age.[1] Many of these senile conditions in the surviving very old subjects may be related to the collection of autoimmune responses with increasing age; both senile amyloid and heart block are under suspicion of this etiologic basis. Nevertheless, there is no evidence of a specific "presbycardia" producing an inevitable deterioration in cardiac function with age.

VALVE LESIONS IN THE ELDERLY

Systolic murmurs in the elderly are the usual manifestation of senile valve disease, and are often thought to be "benign."[2] Calcific degeneration, a frequent complication of minor valve disease, is common with increasing age and is frequently the basis of the changes in the elderly. The usual calcific form of aortic valve stenosis in middle life probably arises on the basis of minor congenital or rheumatic damage and may affect congenital bicuspid valves in men later in life[3] but in the elderly a similar process does apparently affect previously normal valves,[3,4] especially in elderly women producing a rigid triradiate orifice. If obstruction is not significant the resulting systolic murmur is unimportant except as a basis for infective endocarditis[2] and the lesion is described as "aortic sclerosis."

In contrast to the aortic valve, degenerative calcification of the mitral valve is most frequent in women[5] and may extend from the valve ring to the nearby bundle of His to produce heart block as described by Lev.[6] Heart block is another not uncommon consequence of extension of the adjacent severe aortic ring calcification in calcific aortic stenosis. The mitral lesion is thought to arise from mechanical stress and may produce large calcified masses which distort the valve to produce regurgitation and a systolic murmur, provide a site for infective endocarditis, or ulcerate to allow thrombus formation and an uninfected embolus. Mucoid degeneration of the mitral cusps may produce similar mechanical consequences with a murmur due to mitral valve prolapse or more severe incompetence secondary to chordal rupture.[5]

Infective endocarditis has become increasingly a disease of the elderly in recent years, often in relation to bacteremia following urologic or gynecologic procedures such as urethral catherization or uterine curettage, combined with failure to recognize the presence of a degenerative valve lesion which should lead to appropriate antibiotic prophylaxis. This change in age incidence has been associated with a change from the usual prevalence of infection with oral organisms such as *Streptococcus viridans*, with increasing difficulties of antibiotic cure[7] although this can usually be achieved. Delay in diagnosis is the major factor responsible for the persisting high mortality (20%) of infective endocarditis at any age and is accentuated in the elderly by unusual forms of presentation, such as a confusional state without focal neurologic signs or as progressive renal failure as part of a generalized autoimmune vascular disease[7] or to the onset of congestive heart failure due to progressive valvular damage from the destructive lesion which usually increases regurgitation. Suspicion is raised by any of the classical triad of low-grade fever, changing murmurs, or a systemic embolus, and should lead to diagnosis by early blood culture. Prompt diagnosis in this way brings good rewards in terms of effective cure in close cooperation with bacteriologists. This policy with urgent valve replacement where necessary has reduced the overall mortality at all ages to 10%.[8] Nonbacterial endocarditis may produce an embolus without bacteria in moribund patients and cause diagnostic confusion even at necroscopy.[3,9]

MYOCARDIAL DISEASE IN THE ELDERLY

Ischemic myocardial lesions due to coronary artery disease do not become less common in the elderly,[9] supporting the concept of progressive accumulation of disease, and recent infarction is a common cause of death. The incidence of hypertension continues to increase with age,[9] adding to the causes of left ventricular hypertrophy which easily outruns the limited capacities of the main coronary arteries[10] leading to scattered fibrosis which increases the diastolic stiffness of the hypertrophied ventricles, and further impairs systolic function.

Senile cardiac amyloid with amyloid deposition confined to the heart is very common in the elderly, reaching 10% over the age of 80 years, but is not consistently present even in the very old.[11,12] Two distinct forms of amyloid have recently been recognized in the heart[13]: an isolated atrial form of little functional significance, and a less common generalized form, affecting both atria and ventricles with a different and distinct protein, which may also be found in vessel walls elsewhere. This form of cardiac amyloid is presumably a minor version of the presenile cardiac amyloid which presents as a restrictive cardiomyopathy with biventricular failure.[12] Such a presentation is rare in the senile group[13] but a similar minor effect may add to ventricular problems and to cardiac failure in the elderly. The recent detection of a specific scintigraphic pattern in the amyloid heart[14,15] may lead to easier diagnosis and more information, if the lesser changes of senile amyloid can be detected. Digitalis sensitivity is a feature of amyloid heart in younger patients, but does not seem to play a part in the elderly[16] where increased sensitivity is largely pharmacokinetic due to poor renal function and reduced lean tissue mass[17] low red cell sodium levels may be an indication of a general increase in tissue sensitivity.[18]

CLINICAL FEATURES OF CONGESTIVE HEART FAILURE

Congestive heart failure is common in the elderly as a consequence of ventricular hypertrophy from hypertension, mitral valve disease, previous myocardial infarction, plus senile amyloid, and the adverse effect of the common arrhythmia of the elderly, atrial fibrillation.

Cardiac edema is postural, but affects the ankle only in active ambulant patients. In those confined to bed, edema is best detected over the sacrum, in the genitalia or on the medial aspects of the thighs. It is useful to find clinical elevation of jugular venous pressure or hepatic congestion to confirm the cardiac origin of the edema.

Left heart failure is just as "congestive" as right heart failure but the edema is invisible in the lungs. Basal moist sounds (medium rales) are poor evidence of pulmonary congestion; these are present in many patients in bed and usually clear with a cough or a deep breath. In hospital they are prevented by routine physiotherapy.

The diffuse fine rales (crepitations) of pulmonary edema usually first appear between the scapulae, but are a late event coming just before the patient starts to cough up blood-stained froth. The best early warning is given by the chest x-ray film which shows the prominent symmetrical Y-shaped shadows of the distended upper zone pulmonary veins as pulmonary pressure rises, even before interstitial edema produces the horizontal linear Kerley B lines in the costophrenic angles.

TREATMENT OF CONGESTIVE HEART FAILURE

The main standby in the treatment of congestive heart failure is diuretic therapy[19] and large doses of potent loop diuretics may be needed to counteract the powerful salt-retaining state in some patients. The poor reputation of diuretic therapy in the elderly often relates to the inappropriate use of potent drugs for trivial indications, such as furosemide for minor postural edema or the ankle edema associated with varicose veins, or even as an illogical aid to the correction of obesity. Under these circumstances excessive reduction in circulating blood volume with hemoconcentration can produce postural hypotension and thrombotic accidents such as hemiplegia or cardiac infarction.

The elderly are thought to be particularly liable to potassium (K) depletion perhaps because of a habitual low K diet[20] but reduced K stores secondary to loss of lean tissue may be a factor[21] and can be accentuated by the wasting associated with prolonged survival on diuretic therapy that leads eventually to the appearance of "cardiac cachexia."[22] Mild hypokalemia is asymptomatic and its role as a cause of serious arrhythmias is doubtful. A more serious fall to plasma levels below 3.0 mEq may produce weakness or fatigue and can potentiate digitalis effect.[23] Fortunately the plasma K is labile and relatively easily corrected[24]; the danger is that K supplements in the presence of minor renal impairment may easily lead to dangerous hyperkalemia.[19] In minor degrees of failure, treatment with thiazide diuretics produces little K loss, and any depletion is usually correctible with cautious use of K supplements such as potassium chloride tablets.

The thiazides have a flat dose response curve and more severe failure that does not respond will require the use of the more potent loop diuretics, such as furosemide or ethacrynic acid. The resulting volume depletion provokes hyperaldosteronism[25] and accentuates K loss. On doses of furosemide of 80 mg twice daily, large doses of K supplements would be needed, such as two potassium chloride tablets three times daily. These large tablets are often rejected by the patient and a better alternative may be an aldosterone antagonist such as spironolactone or amiloride hydrochloride. A suitable combination will generally maintain a normal serum K level which can usefully be measured monthly.

A stepped care approach to treatment of heart failure[19] envisages the use of digitalis to control atrial fibrillation, where necessary, followed by the progressive application of diuretic therapy as described above. Geriatricians were early to point out that there was little benefit from digitalis treatment of heart failure in sinus rhythm, and an increased risk of toxic effects in this group suggests that digitalis is best avoided.[26] Unless there are special contraindications giving a specifically high risk, such as chronic lung disease, myocardial infarctions, or heart block,[17] a cautious trial of digitalis is suggested as some patients seem to respond, and may be usefully controlled by aiming for steady plasma levels of digoxin of 1 to 2 ng/ml.

The introduction of alternative myocardial stimulant drugs such as sympathetic agonists or amrinone may produce a temporary hemodynamic advantage at the cost of further myocardial damage which can limit life[19] and probably has little to offer except as a temporary measure in an emergency. Vasodilator therapy may be more useful on the basis of unloading the ventricles. It might be expected to cause problems in the elderly on the same basis as the difficulties found in controlling hypertension, but may justify cautious trial, as tachycardia usually gives warning of an adverse response.[19] That it may be effective is confirmed from the reports of adverse effects on withdrawal in the elderly.[27]

ATRIAL FIBRILLATION

This arrhythmia is the functional disturbance that comes closest to being a specific cardiac disease of old age. It usually arises on a background of chronic pathologic changes in the atrial muscles,[28] presumably resulting in interruption of the normal uniform conduction of atrial activation. The common causes in younger patients, mitral valve disease, thyrotoxicosis, and ischemic heart disease, produce left atrial dilatation and accentuate this process. A striking feature of the natural history of atrial fibrillation in these conditions is the tendency for the arrhythmia to occur in middle age; younger patients usually remain in sinus rhythm until the age of about 45 years. In the elderly apparently trivial disease of these types may be associated with atrial fibrillation and it was found in 10% of fit active elderly subjects.[29] The arrhythmia will accentuate any tendency to congestive heart failure. The age-related tendency is so strong that attempts to revert the patient to sinus rhythm and control it with antiarrhythmic drugs are necessarily doomed to failure in the long run, and lead to recurrent episodes of disturbing or even dangerous arrhythmia. A better policy for recurrent atrial fibrillation is to maintain controlling treatment with, for instance, digitalis, so that the episodes are not associated with any disturbing tachycardia. In the long run permanent atrial fibrillation usually becomes established and is treated by long-term control of the ventricular rate. The days of repeated reversion to sinus rhythm with its embolic risk each time are now over, and this aggressive management is better replaced by the more passive policy of allowing atrial fibrillation to continue and controlling the ventricular rate. The extreme view,[30] that all patients with atrial fibrillation should receive anticoagulant therapy, should be tempered by the possibility that the risks of treatment may outweigh the benefit, and this treatment should be reserved for the patients with mitral stenosis awaiting surgical correction where the dangers of embolus are particularly high.

Lone atrial fibrillation without other evident heart disease accounted for 31% of the total in a recent report from the Framingham study.[31] In the elderly, lone atrial fibrillation may be the result of focal disease of the sinus node as part of the sick sinus syndrome, and in this case represents a reasonably safe and easily managed escape rhythm. This senile atrial fibrillation is not particularly related to atrial amyloid deposits.[16] A strong plea[32] has recently been made for the consideration of occult thyrotoxicosis as a cause of apparently isolated atrial fibrillation. It is important not to overlook this potentially correctible disturbance. Frank thyrotoxicosis may be missed if there is no tachycardia because of poor atrioventricular (AV) conduction of atrial fibrillation. The classical features of thyrotoxicosis may also be masked by the reduction in cardiac output associated with the tendency to heart failure resulting from atrial fibrillation. An apparent difficulty in controlling the ventricular rate with digitalis may be a hint of thyrotoxic cause of atrial fibrillation; this difficulty may be overcome by adding a beta-blocking drug, and is eliminated when the thyrotoxicosis is corrected.

Control of atrial fibrillation usually relies on the proper application of the vagal effect of digitalis.[17] Urgent control is rarely needed, and in view of the risks of a vasoconstrictor response to intravenous injection, oral treatment is generally to be preferred. As the elderly are particularly at risk of digitalis toxicity it may be preferable to avoid an oral loading dose, as maintenance doses of digoxin will produce a therapeutic effect in a day or two. In urgent situations, such as acute myocardial infarction, prompt control can be obtained with an intravenous beta-blocker or verapamil at the same time as the first oral dose of digoxin which will take control as the effect of intravenous treatment fades.

The adverse effect of atrial fibrillation which tends to accentuate congestive heart failure is largely related to the tachycardia produced by continual activation of the atrioventricular (AV) node which leads to a ventricular rate of about 160 beats per minute (bpm) in a normal heart, the rate being limited only by the refractory period of the AV node. The rapid rate shortens the duration of diastole which is important for ventricular filling in most forms of heart disease, classically seen with the obstruction of mitral stenosis, but also a factor in the stiff left ventricles of myocardial hypertrophy or fibrosis, and with amyloid infiltration. The object of digitalis treatment is by judicious vagal AV block to produce a near to normal ventricular rate. The ventricular rate in this situation gives a built-in biological assay of digitalis effect. Proper control of the rate to 70 to 90 bpm at rest will allow better ventricular filling and remove one component of congestive heart failure. The useful nursing rule, that if the rate is below 60 bpm a dose is omitted and the physician informed, has undoubtedly avoided much toxicity, as larger doses can produce excessive slowing with progression to dangerous AV block. All forms of heart block tend to accentuate this effect and make the risks of excessive digitalis effect much greater, so that great caution is needed with digitalis therapy in the presence of minor AV block.

The association of senile atrial fibrillation with sinus node disease is often accompanied by evidence of some degree of AV block as part of the manifestation of a generalized disease of the conducting system.[33] In some patients this results in a natural slow ventricular rate even without digitalis treatment, which is then not only unnecessary but actually dangerous and likely to produce severe bradycardia.

The alternative toxic effect of digitalis is the production of ventricular ectopic beats, which often pass unnoticed in the irregularities of the response to atrial fibrillation. The regular alternating ectopic beats of bigeminy often produce a more regular rhythm, and the rate is slowed as the ectopic beat is ineffectual, giving a pulse rate half the true ventricular rate, seen in the ECG. It was formerly thought that bigeminy at rest was a sign of an adequate degree of digitalization, as the improved AV conduction on exercise usually increased the ventricular rate and abolished the ectopic beats, but it is now generally appreciated as a warning of more serious ventricular arrhythmias, and the situation is best met by a reduction in digitalis dose. If there is undue exercise tachycardia when the resting rate is well controlled, the judicious addition of a small dose of beta-adrenergic blocking drug will prevent the sympathetically mediated improvement in AV node conduction on exercise.

If there are problems with management on digitalis, an alternative approach is to block the

AV node with the calcium antagonist, verapamil, which is effective as the AV nodal cells rely specifically on Ca^{++} ion currents for their action potential, rather than Na^{+} ion currents of other cardiac cells. Verapamil has its pharmacokinetic problems, the large first pass metabolism in the liver making the oral dose (120 to 180 mg), some ten times the intravenous dose (10 mg), with corresponding individual variations and risks of disturbance by interactions with other drugs. In contrast with beta-blockers, verapamil shows a pharmacokinetic interaction with digoxin, and the two drugs probably ought not to be used together in the long term. Although regularization of the ventricular rhythm may be a feature of control of atrial fibrillation with verapamil, this offers no practical advantage, as the irregularity in itself produces no hemodynamic disturbance. In most patients a digitalis glycoside will give satisfactory control on the basis of titrating the ventricular rate as described, and in the senile group it is fortunate if no treatment is needed as the rate is naturally slow.

HEART BLOCK

It is not the slow rate of the ventricular escape rhythm that is the major problem in complete AV block, as an otherwise normal heart will easily correct for this by producing a larger stroke volume to reliably maintain resting cardiac output, although the output response to exercise is necessarily impaired. The main disability arises from the instability of this escape rhythm, which tends to stop transiently producing episodic syncope (Adams-Stokes attacks).

It is useful to distinguish the autonomically mediated block at the AV node, seen with digitalis effect, from the disease of the bundle of His and its branches (His-Purkinje system) which is generally responsible for heart block in the elderly. Although heart block is produced by damage to the bundle branches in anteroseptal myocardial infarction, these patients rarely survive, even with pacing, and, if they do survive with heart block, are generally middle-aged rather than elderly and have severe problems due to myocardial damage and angina with a consequent poor outlook.

The common form of heart block in the elderly arises as a diffuse fibrosis of the conducting system first described by Lenègre[34] with relatively intact working myocardium and coronary arteries accounting for the good hemodynamic adjustment to bradycardia and good prognosis on pacing. The etiology is still obscure; there is no local coronary disease to cause the fibrosis and suspicion is accumulating that it might have an autoimmune basis with Purkinje cell antibodies. In other patients block results from extension of Lev's mitral valve calcification.[6] The good prognosis of British patients, who survive with pacing as long as unaffected subjects of the same age,[35] may relate in part to the cautious British policy of waiting for Adams-Stokes attacks before starting pacing. This automatically selects a fit group who have survived an attack and eliminates many with associated myocardial disease. As the first Adams-Stokes attack may be fatal, it is a reasonable policy to insert a pacemaker prophylactically if serious His-Purkinje disease is detected. As the disease in the His-Purkinje tissue is progressive in a representative fashion in the bundle, bifascicular block, indicating disease of two of the three main branches, it is a useful preliminary warning that block is about to become complete, and a pacemaker may be life saving. Minor syncopal episodes with bifascicular block or minor degrees of AV block in the interval ECG is a useful indication for demand pacemaker insertion. The complexity and expense of modern pacing systems[33] is in many ways a limitation on use, and there would seem to be a case for a simple inexpensive fixed rate system for use in the elderly with established complete block; such a system might have wide application in less developed countries.

In general, pacing is well-accepted by the elderly, and modern systems are reliable, so that little follow-up is needed. As modern systems are set to slow as the battery fades, assessment is reduced to regular measurement of the patient's pulse rate, which can be a nursing procedure, with replacement arranged when the rate falls below 70 bpm. The complete transformation of the patient's life achieved by freedom from Adams-Stokes attacks makes this one of the most satisfactory and effective forms of rehabilitation in the elderly.

SICK SINUS SYNDROME

Perhaps as part of a generalized conductive system disease[33] sinus node disease is being increasingly recognized as a cause of bradycardia and syncope requiring pacing in the elderly.[36] It may present as minor faintness or Adams-Stokes attacks due to asystole or sino-atrial block, alternating with bradycardia due to a slow sinus rate and atrial fibrillation with a slow ventricular response. Some patients also have episodes of tachycardia which are presumably due to re-entry in or around the diseased sinus node. The rate is often 120 to 140 bpm and is rarely as fast as the 180 to 200 bpm of the usual form of AV nodal re-entry tachycardia; attempts to control the tachycardia with antiarrhythmic drugs such as beta-blockers may produce disastrous bradycardia and should not be attempted without a pacemaker in place. The need for pacing in sinus node disease has been questioned[33] as the general course is often benign and sudden death is rare, but frank syncope is certainly an indication and other patients require close observation. Vagal block with atropine produces temporary improvement in a crisis in some patients.

Digitalis is probably contraindicated in sinus node disease, as the vagal action tends to inhibit the node further. The report that the heart rate by Holter monitoring did not change with digitalis in the sick sinus syndrome[37] relied on the appearance of a relatively fast AV nodal escape rhythm when the sinus node was blocked by the vagal effect of digitalis, a disturbance that would generally be regarded as evidence of digitalis toxicity. I doubt if this is a reasonable therapeutic approach. It should rarely be needed.

HYPERTENSION

The progressive increase in systolic blood pressure with age[38] adds another factor to the load on the left ventricle in older patients and may contribute to left ventricular hypertrophy and failure. As most hypertension in the elderly is of mild or moderate degree, it is difficult to demonstrate any prognostic benefit from treatment in terms of stroke prevention, and further trials are in progress.[39] The problem of control of cerebral blood flow in the elderly[40] had led to many difficulties with overenthusiastic treatment with potent drugs which have largely disappeared in recent years with the change to the more gentle "stepped-care" approach.[39] The difficulty in showing benefit of treatment in mild hypertension suggests that we would do well to aim for a reduction of blood pressure to diastolic of 105 mmHg, below which we can show no further benefit, rather than aim for the theoretical ideal of "normalization."[38]

The suggestion that the upper limit of blood pressure in old age was 210/110 mmHg[41] has similar therapeutic implications. The failure of the diastolic blood pressure to rise with age[38] is in keeping with greater rigidity of the aorta. The lack of a fall of diastolic pressure with the increased pulse pressure must imply some increase in peripheral resistance with age, but systolic blood pressure rises steeply with age and may be an independent risk factor related to the rigid aorta[39] with different therapeutic indications.[40]

There have been reports of gross overestimates of blood pressure by the usual cuff method in the elderly, and if suspicion is raised by inconsistencies with other data the pressure may be safely confirmed by continuous aorta-arterial recordings.[39] A careful approach to treatment and the avoidance of drugs producing postural hypotension[39,42] allows us to safely control hypertension when there is a clear indication such as left ventricular hypertrophy[43] and may be appropriate in severe systolic hypertension. Control of the cerebral circulation may adjust[40] and avoid long-term problems with gradual treatment. Although the risk of excessive and rapid reduction of blood pressure is clear,[44] therapeutic timidity may deny the elderly hypertensive the possible benefit of treatment.[43]

REFERENCES

1. WHO and the elderly. *Lancet* 1982;2:8304:909.
2. Systolic murmurs in the elderly. *Br Med J* 1975;4:69–70.
3. Pomerance A: Pathology of heart disease in the elderly. *Br J Hosp Med* 1974;11:245–252.
4. Pomerance A: Pathogenesis of aortic stenosis and its relation to age. *Br Heart J* 1972;34:569–574.
5. Pomerance A: Pathology and valvular heart disease, editorial. *Br Heart J* 1972;34:437–443.
6. Lev M: Anatomic basis for atrioventricular block. *Am J Med* 1964;37:742.
7. Hamer J, O'Grady F: Infective endocarditis, in Hammer J (ed): *Recent Advances in Cardiology.* London, Churchill-Livingstone, 1977, vol 7, pp 425–471.
8. Lowes JA, Hamer J, Williams G, et al: Ten years of infective endocarditis at St. Bartholomew's Hospital: Analysis of clinical features and treatment in relation to prognosis and mortality. *Lancet* 1980;1:133–136.
9. Pomerance A: Pathology of the heart with and without cardiac failure in the aged. *Br Heart J* 1965;27:697–710.
10. Linzbach AJ: Heart failure from the point of view of quantitative anatomy. *Am J Cardiol* 1960;5:370–382.
11. Pomerance A: Senile cardiac amyloidosis. *Br Heart J* 1965;27:711–718.
12. Meaney E, Shabetai R, Bharaava V, et al: Cardiac amyloidosis, constrictive pericarditis and restrictive cardiomyopathy. *Am J Cardiol* 1976;38:547–556.
13. Cornwell GG, Watermark D: Senile amyloidosis: A protean manifestation of the aging process. *J Clin Pathol* 1980;23:1146–1152.
14. Wizenberg TA, Muz J, Soha YH, et al: Value of technetium 99m pyrophosphate scintigraphy in the noninvasive diagnosis of cardiac amyloidosis. *Am Heart J* 1982;103:468–473.
15. Schiff S, Bateman T, Moffatt R, et al: Diagnostic

considerations in cardiomyopathy; Unique scintigraphic pattern of diffuse biventricular technetium 99m pyrophosphate uptake in amyloid heart disease. *Am Heart J* 1982;103:562–563.
16. Hodkinson HM, Pomerance A: The clinical significance of senile cardiac amyloidosis: A prospective clinico-pathological study. *Q J Med* 1977;46: 381–387.
17. Hamer J: Drugs used in cardiac failure: Digitalis and vasodilators. *Recent Advances in Clinical Pharmacology*. London, Churchill-Livingstone, 1980, vol 2, pp 73–100.
18. Cumberbatch M, Morgan DB: Relations between sodium and sodium concentration in human erythrocytes in health and disease. *Clin Sci* 1981;60: 555–564.
19. Hamer J: The modern treatment of congestive heart failure, in *Recent Advances in Cardiology*. London, Churchill-Livingstone, 1984 (in press).
20. Macleod CC, Judge JG, Caird FI: Nutrition of the elderly at home. III. Intake of minerals. *Age and Ageing* 1975;4:49–57.
21. Lye M, Winston B: Whole body potassium and total exchangeable potassium in elderly patients with cardiac failure. *Br Heart J* 1979;42:568–572.
22. Walesby RK, Goode AW, Bentall HH: Nutritional status of patients undergoing valve replacement by open heart surgery. *Lancet* 1978;1:76–77.
23. Steiness E, Olesin KH: Cardiac arrhythmias induced by hypokalaemia and potassium loss during maintenance digoxin therapy. *Br Heart J* 1976;38: 167–172.
24. Nagant de Deuxchaisnes C, Mach R-S: Potassium depletion and potassium supplementation in cardiac failure. *Lancet* 1974;1:517.
25. Knight RK, Miall PA, Hawkins LA, et al: Relation of plasma aldosterone concentration to diuretic treatment in patients with severe heart disease. *Br Heart J* 1979;42:316–325.
26. Hamer J: The paradox of the lack of efficacy of digitalis in congestive heart failure with sinus rhythm. *Br J Clin Pharmacol* 1979;9:109–113.
27. Hanley SP, Cowley A, Hampton JR: Danger of withdrawal of vasodilator therapy in patients with chronic heart failure. *Lancet* 1980;1:735–736.
28. Davies MJ, Pomerance A: Pathology of atrial fibrillation in man. *Br Heart J* 1972;34:520–525.
29. Camm J, Evans KL, Ward DE, et al: The rhythm of the heart in active elderly subjects. *Am Heart J* 1980;99:598–603.
30. Mitchell JRA: The use of long-term oral anticoagulants: A personal view. *Prescribers' Journal* H.M. Stationery Office, London, England, 1982;22:120–129.
31. Kannel WB, Abbott RD, Savage DD, et al: Epidemiologic features of chronic atrial fibrillation. The Framingham Study. *N Engl J Med* 1982;306:1018–1022.
32. Forfar JC, Toft AD: Thyrotoxic atrial fibrillation: An underdiagnosed condition? *Br Med J* 1982;285: 909–910.
33. Parsonnett V: The proliferation of cardiac pacing: Medical, technical and socio-economic dilemmas. *Circulation* 1982;65:841–845.
34. Lenègre J, Moreau P: Lebloc auriculo-ventriculaire chronique. Etude anatomique, clinique et histologique. *Arch Mal Coeur* 1963;56:867–888.
35. Ginks W, Leatham A, Siddons H: Prognosis of patients paced for chronic atrioventricular block. *Br Heart J* 1979;41:633–636.
36. Shaw DB, Kekwick C: Potential candidates for pacemakers. Survey of heart block and sino-atrial disorder (sick sinus syndrome). *Br Heart J* 1978;60: 98–105.
37. Vera Z, Miller RR, McMillin D, et al: Effects of digitalis on sinus node function in patients with sick sinus syndrome. *Am J Cardiol* 1978;41:318.
38. Miall WE, Lovell HG: Relation between change of blood pressure and age. *Br Med J* 1967;3:660–664.
39. Hamer J: The modern treatment of hypertension, in Hamer J, Rowlands DJ (eds): *Recent Advances in Cardiology*. London, Churchill-Livingstone, 1981, vol 8, pp 1–28.
40. Appenzeller O, Descarries L: Circulatory reflexes in patients with cerebrovascular disease. *N Engl J Med* 1964;271:820–823.
41. Caird FJ: Heart disease in old age. *Postgrad Med J* 1963;39:408–420.
42. Simon A Ch, Levenson JA, Safar ME: Systolic hypertension: Differences of mechanism according to age and possible application to treatment. *Eur Heart J* 1982;3(suppl C):65–69.
43 Waldek S: Hypertension in the elderly. *Lancet* 1977;1:1055–1059.
44. Wollner L, McCarthy ST, Soper NDW, et al: Failure of cerebral autoregulation as a cause of brain dysfunction in the elderly. *Br Med J* 1979;1: 1117–1118.

CHAPTER 2
Effects of Aging on Cardiac Measurements

Jane F. Potter

A potential error in any study of the normal aging heart is the likely inclusion of some individuals with ischemic heart disease. Therefore, when it is stated by the author, information on subject selection and exclusion will be included to assist the reader in evaluation of this confounding variable. If subjects could be selected who were completely free of heart disease, then all the observed changes would be attributed to age. Unfortunately, disease becomes increasingly frequent with age which makes selection difficult. The changes in cardiac measurements with age presented in this chapter are similar to but of smaller magnitude to those seen in certain disease states. Although it is problematic to attribute these changes to age rather than occult disease, this attribution is based on the fact that in longitudinal studies the changes are seen to occur in most of the subjects studied. The differentiation of normal from abnormal changes in old age is important in order to set normative standards for laboratory studies and because understanding of such true age-related changes provides insight into the physiology of aging. In spite of the difficulties inherent in the study of older persons, standards of normality for old age can only be set after study of that population.

Most "aging" studies use a cross-sectional design because of constraints of cost and time, and in so doing present a select set of survivors in the older age groups. Only longitudinal studies are able to define true normal aging with certainty. An additional advantage of longitudinal studies is the ability to relate a measured variable prospectively to outcome (death or disease). While cross-sectional studies may suggest that alterations are part of normal aging, they cannot exclude a detrimental effect. Therefore, the final section of this chapter summarizes prospective studies which have related changes in cardiac measurements to survival.

CHEST RADIOGRAPHY

The cardiothoracic ratio (CTR) calculated from radiographic data is an important clinical measure for assessing the heart. The usual standard of normality is a CTR less than 50%, as first suggested by Danzer[1] in a report that does not state the ages of the subjects. Although radiographically measured cardiac diameter adjusted for height and weight is felt to be a more reliable index of heart size,[2-4] the CTR is more widely applied. Although Ungerleider[4] states that, on the basis of his study of insurance applicants, no age adjustment of cardiac diameter is necessary, a number of studies have challenged this assumption. The basis of this debate is in studies of older, compared to younger, people where both cardiac diameter and thoracic diameter are seen to change with age. Initially these changes were noted in cross-sectional studies, but the same phenomenon has recently been noted in longitudinal studies as well.[5,6]

Cardiac Diameter

Six cross-sectional studies published between 1952 and 1982 report observations on differences in cardiac diameter of older as compared to younger people. The results of these studies are summarized in Table 2-1. All studies utilized 6-foot posteroanterior (PA) radiographs and measured cardiac diameter as the sum of the greatest deviation of the heart to the right and left of the midline. The earliest study[7] was a report of 22 older men that noted a tendency toward higher cardiac diameters only in the oldest subjects. The author speculated that either there was little change in the diameter of the heart with age or that, "there may be an aging change which is late in appearing to a significant extent." A few years later, Cowan[8] reported a series of over 6000 subjects from youth through old age. Results for selected age groups from that study are summarized in Table 2-1. Subjects were attendees at regional health clinics and were excluded if disease was recognized, or if chest asymmetry or body weight were more than 25% above ideal. Cowan demonstrated that beginning in childhood, there was an almost regular rise in cardiac diameter that continued past maturity through middle and late life.

A third and much smaller study[9] in which subjects were described as "healthy" apparently did not exclude patients with significant hypertension and reported slightly larger cardiac diameters than Cowan in a somewhat older group. Values nearly identical to those of Cowan's older subjects were reported by Rabushka et al.[10] In this study, subjects with elevated cardiothoracic ratios were evaluated separately. The author rationalized this approach by stating that in all but one case subjects with elevated CTRs were found to have heart disease after scrutiny of their medical record. In this study, values of cardiac diameter for the older group were not significantly different from those of the younger subjects.

Two longitudinal studies also reported cross-sectional results.[11,6] In the first, Milne and Lauder[11] divided subjects into those with definite ischemic heart disease, probable heart disease, and no apparent heart disease. Because no statistical difference in cardiac diameter was found when the various heart disease groups were compared, the authors provide only the mean values of cardiac diameter for all subject groups. These combined values of cardiac diameter are reproduced in Table 2-1 and are the highest values in the table for comparable age groups. This undoubtedly reflects the inclusion of subjects with heart disease.

In analysis of data from the Baltimore Longitudinal Study of Aging,[6] the authors reported data at the time of the subject's last longitudinal visit, which yielded a cross-sectional view of the study population at its oldest age. Subjects underwent extensive examinations at 12- to 24-month intervals which included ECGs and stress testing. These tests served as the basis for classifying subjects as to the presence of heart disease. The data in Table 2-1 are for subjects without heart disease. Cardiac diameters were greater in the older groups than in the young control group for subjects with or without heart disease.

Examination of the collective data from these studies of chest films as summarized in Table 2-1 suggests that cardiac diameter increases with age in subjects without detectable heart disease. Cross-sectional studies, however, have the disadvantage that the older age groups are comprised only of those subjects who have survived to that age and may be misleading if the parameter under study influences mortality. If, for example, there is a selective advantage to having a large heart size, individuals with larger hearts would be overrepresented in the older age groups. Thus, one might incorrectly suggest that cardiac diameter had increased with age. Cross-sectional studies may also be misleading if the parameter under study varies between age cohorts. For example, it is known that the average adult height of individuals born after 1900 has gradually increased. Since height and weight are the major determinants of cardiac diameter measured on chest films[4] the diameter of the heart of individuals born in 1940 will be greater than that of subjects born in 1900. Therefore, cross-sectional comparisons of individuals born in 1900 to those born in 1940 might fail to recognize an increase in cardiac diameter with age.

Only longitudinal studies which perform repeated measures on the same individuals over time can determine true aging changes with certainty. Five-year follow-up by Lauder and Milne[5] of their earlier report from the Edinburgh Study of Aging[11] showed that the mean values of cardiac diameter had increased during the five-year period. In men over 70 years of age there was a significant increase in cardiac diameter. An increase in cardiac diameter in men aged 62 to 69 years did not reach statistical significance. In women, cardiac diameter increased in the over and under 70-year age groups but the increase was significant only in those aged 62 to 69 years. The fact that an increase in cardiac diameter was not seen in the oldest group of female subjects was thought to be due to an excessive death rate among female subjects with the largest hearts. The meaning of these increases in cardiac diameter are somewhat less clear because subjects with known heart disease were included and the relatively short period of follow-up in this study may not have allowed sufficient time for changes to be detected in all age groups.

The Baltimore Longitudinal Study of Aging reported longitudinal findings on 243 subjects in 1982.[6] The characteristics of this population have

Table 2-1
Cardiac Diameter, Thoracic Diameter and Cardiothoracic Ratio

Author	Age Range	No. of Cases		Cardiac Diameter (cm) mean ± SE		Thoracic Diameter (cm) mean ± SE		Cardiothoracic Ratio (%) mean ± SE	
		Male	*Female*	*Male*	*Female*	*Male*	*Female*	*Male*	*Female*
Tirman and Hamilton[7]	20–49	35	NI	12.7 ± 0.23	NI	29.9 ± 0.33	NI	43 ± 0.8	NI
	50–59	11	NI	13.1 ± 0.39	NI	30.2 ± .76	NI	44 ± 0.9	NI
	60–75	11	NI	13.8 ± 0.48	NI	29.6 ± .53	NI	47 ± 1.9	NI
Cowan[8,17]*	20–49	1163	1561	12.2 ± 0.04	11.2 ± 0.02	NR	NR	41 ± 0.1	43 ± 0.1
	60–69	185	124	12.2 ± 0.08	12.0 ± 0.09	28.5 ± 0.2	25.0 ± 0.1	43 ± 0.3	49 ± 0.3
	70–79	139	112	12.8 ± 0.09	12.2 ± 0.08	28.2 ± 0.2	24.1 ± 0.1	45 ± 0.3	51 ± 0.4
	80–89	55	44	13.1 ± 0.15	12.3 ± 0.10	NR	NR	46 ± 0.5	54 ± 0.6
Edge et al[9]*†	20–40	26	44	13.4	11.5	30.5	26.0	44	44
	75–99	47	53	13.6	12.7	28.2	22.7	48	56
Rabushka et al[10]‡	20–45	50	50	13.4 ± 0.2	11.8 ± 0.2	32.1 ± 0.2	26.9 ± 0.2	41	44
	>65	52	68	13.2 ± 0.2	12.2 ± 0.2	30.9 ± 0.3	27.1 ± 0.3	44	46
Edinburgh	62–69	108	132	13.6 ± 0.1	12.8 ± 0.1	30.2 ± 0.2	25.6 ± 0.2	45 ± 0.4	50 ± 0.4
Longitudinal Study	70–79	66	97	13.8 ± 0.2	13.2 ± 0.1	29.4 ± 0.2	25.0 ± 0.2	47 ± 0.6	53 ± 0.4
Milne and Lauder[11]	80–90	17	26	14.4 ± 0.3	13.4 ± 0.3	29.2 ± 0.3	24.0 ± 0.5	49 ± 0.9	56 ± 1.2
Baltimore	32–50	60	NI	12.5 ± 0.2	NI	31.6 ± 0.2	NI	40 ± 0.4	NI
Longitudinal Study§	60–69	32	NI	13.3 ± 0.2	NI	31.8 ± 0.3	NI	42 ± 0.5	NI
	70–79	33	NI	13.4 ± 0.2	NI	31.4 ± 0.3	NI	43 ± 0.6	NI
Potter et al[6]	80–95	29	NI	13.1 ± 0.3	NI	30.2 ± 0.3	NI	43 ± 0.9	NI

*Heart disease excluded by clinical history.
†Standard errors not reported.
‡Patients with CTR over 50% excluded; all but one had clinical histories compatible with heart disease.
§Heart disease excluded by history, physical, ECG, stress test.
NR = data not reported; NI = not included.

been reported previously.[12] Standard 6-foot PA chest radiographs were part of the routine testing between 1958 and 1975. A total of 1124 radiographs were examined, an average of 4.5 per subject. The average time span between first and last examinations was 12.3 years (range 8 to 21 years). Measurements of cardiac diameter and thoracic diameter were made without knowledge of the subject's age or date of the examination. In the longitudinal analysis of chest radiographic measurements, the rate of change with age was computed as the slope of the regression line of age on cardiac diameter for each subject on the basis of three or more data points. The line segments in Figure 2-1 are the average values for each age group. The effect of normal aging, ie, in the absence of detectable heart disease, on these variables is shown in this longitudinal analysis. Changes in cardiac diameter followed the pattern suggested by the cross-sectional results in other[7-10] studies, ie, that the diameter of the heart increases after 50 years of age even in the absence of detectable heart disease (Figure 2-1). Because the slopes of cardiac diameter on age were different from zero, an increase in the diameter of the heart appears to be a true age-related change.

Thoracic Diameter

Several studies[8,9,11] on the cardiothoracic ratio have criticized its use in older people because of the decline in thoracic diameter with age, particularly in women. Narrowing of the lower chest cage can make the heart appear to be enlarged. The cross-sectional studies summarized in Table 2-1 uniformly show a decline in thoracic diameter except for the study of Rabushka et al, which had excluded subjects with elevated CTRs.[10] On the average, the decrease in the diameter of the thorax is small, but of greater magnitude in women than men. While Edge et al[9] described a slightly decreased thoracic size in men and a greater reduction in thoracic diameter with age in women, Cowan[13] demonstrated a significant reduction in the diameter of the thorax only in his female subjects. Milne and Lauder,[11] on the other hand, reported smaller thoracic diameters in both men and women with age.

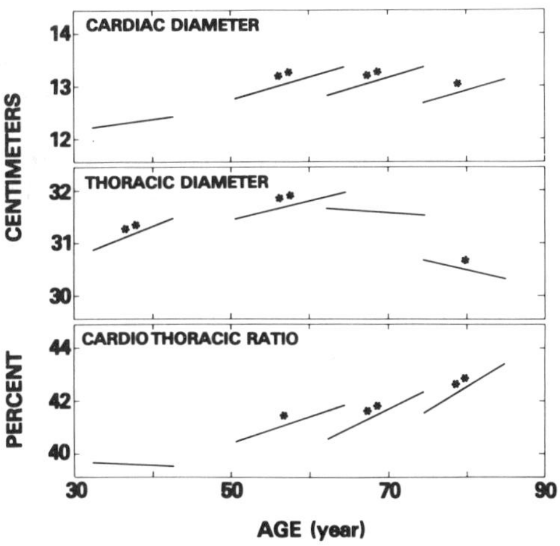

Figure 2-1 Longitudinal analysis of changes in radiographic variables in subjects with no evidence of heart disease. See text for explanation of construction of the line segments. Significances of slope were compared with deviation from zero. (*P <0.025, **P <0.005). (Reproduced with permission from Potter et al.[6])

Longitudinal studies[5,6] have confirmed the changes in thoracic diameter seen in cross-sectional studies. The five-year follow-up of Lauder and Milne[5] reported a decline in thoracic diameter in both men and women over 62 years of age. This decrease was statistically significant in each of the groups studied except for men over 70 years of age. During an average 12-year follow-up, the Baltimore Longitudinal Study[6] reported longitudinal changes in the diameter of the thorax for men aged from 32 to 92 years (Figure 2-1). The line segments in Figure 2-1 represent rates of change in thoracic diameter for various age groups. From age 32 to 62 years thoracic diameter increased, between ages 62 to 72 years there was no detectable change, and after 72 years of age there was a significant decline in thoracic diameter with increasing age. These authors felt that the reduction of thoracic diameter in old age was caused by a change in the mechanical properties of the chest wall. Rizzoto and Marazzini[14] had reported that expansion of the rib cage, measured as change in chest circumference during inspiration, accounted for 39% of the total lung capacity in young subjects, but only 30% in older subjects. This same study showed significantly smaller chest circumferences in subjects of the 70 to 79 and 80 to 95 years age groups than in the young controls. This finding is consistent with the age-related changes in thoracic diameter measured in studies of chest radiographs. Using anthropometrically defined chest circumference, the Veterans Administration cooperative study also showed a negative association between chest expansion and age.[15]

The most extensive study of age-related differences in chest anthropometry was conducted by Takahashi and Atsumi[16] who studied 9369 Japanese aged 0 to 85 years. In subjects over 25 years of age, there was a progressive rounding of the thorax, an increase in chest depth, and decrease in chest breadth. Unfortunately, total chest circumference was not reported.

In the Baltimore Longitudinal Study[6] subjects underwent extensive anthropometric measurements, including chest circumference. Changes in chest circumference measured anthropometrically and thoracic diameter from radiographic studies between the first and last longitudinal visits correlated well ($r = 0.43$, $P < 0.001$). It would thus appear that the reduction in thoracic diameter observed on chest radiographs is simply another measure of the decline in rib-cage mobility with age.[14,15]

Cardiothoracic Ratio

From the foregoing description of changes in cardiac and thoracic diameter with age, it is apparent that both an increase in cardiac diameter and a decrease in thoracic diameter would contribute to a rise in cardiothoracic ratio in old age. In cross-sectional studies (Table 2-1) the average values of cardiothoracic ratio follow this expected trend. In each study, cardiothoracic ratio increases through successive age groups. It is of interest that the mean value of cardiothoracic ratio for women exceeded 50% in three of the four studies in which such data is reported. Table 2-2 presents selected percentile values for cardiothoracic ratio from Cowan[17] by sex and age for subjects 60 years and older. If the central 80% of values is taken as normal, then an upper limit for cardiothoracic ratio of 50% does not apply to men over 80 years of age and is completely inappropriate for women after 60 years of age.

Cross-sectional percentile values of cardiothoracic ratios reported by the Baltimore Longitudinal Study of Aging (BLSA)[6] for subjects with or without heart disease are presented in Figure 2-2. The distribution of cardiothoracic ratio shifted further to the right with each successive age decade. Of subjects without heart disease, none of those under 50 years of age had a ratio exceeding 47%. The 90th percentile values for age groups 60 to 69, 70 to 79, and 80 to 89 years were 45%, 47%, and 49%, values somewhat lower than Cowan's 90th percentile values for men and almost identical to his 75th percentile values. The minor differences between the two studies may be accounted for by differences in sample size (somewhat larger for Cowan), or subject selection (BLSA subjects screened with stress testing) which may have excluded subjects with asymptomatic ischemic heart disease from the BLSA group. Women were added to the BLSA too recently to be included in this report. However, based on the close comparability of data for men in the BLSA and Cowan studies it would appear that an upper limit for cardiothoracic ratio of 50% is not appropriate for women aged over 60 years.

Cross-sectional cardiothoracic ratios from the Baltimore Longitudinal Study were greater in the older groups than in the young controls for subjects with or without heart disease.[6] As expected, greater cardiothoracic ratios were seen in subjects with heart disease in each age group (Figure 2-3). The effect of normal aging, ie, in the absence of detectable heart disease, on cardiothoracic ratio is shown in longitudinal studies. Results from two longitudinal studies of cardiothoracic ratio[5,6] follow the pattern suggested by the cross-sectional results, ie, an increase in cardiothoracic ratio with increasing age. The Edinburgh Longitudinal Study[5] reported significant increases in cardiothoracic ratio for age groups 62 to 69 and over 70 years in both men and women. Increases in cardio-

Table 2-2
Selected Percentile Values for the Cardiothoracic Ratio (percent) Derived from Cumulative Percentage Curves by Sex and Age*

	Men n = 242			Women n = 190		
Percentiles	*60–69 years*	*70–79 years*	*80–89 years*	*60–69 years*	*70–79 years*	*80–89 years*
90	48	50	52	53	56	58
75	46	47	49	52	53	56
50	44	46	47	50	51	54
25	41	44	44	47	49	51
10	40	42	42	45	46	48

*Data from Cowan.[17]

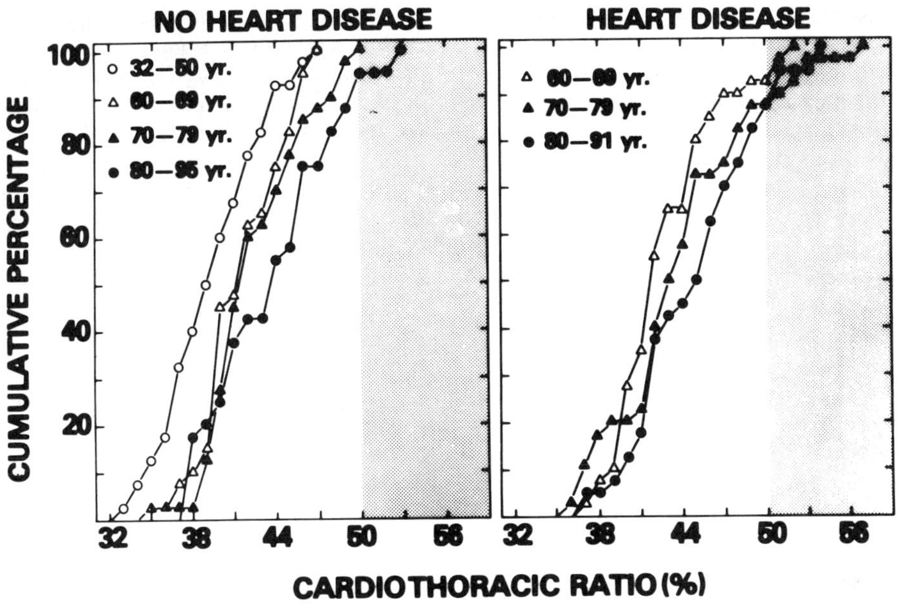

Figure 2-2 Distribution of cardiothoracic ratios in four age groups in subjects with and subjects without heart disease. (Reproduced with permission from Potter et al.[6])

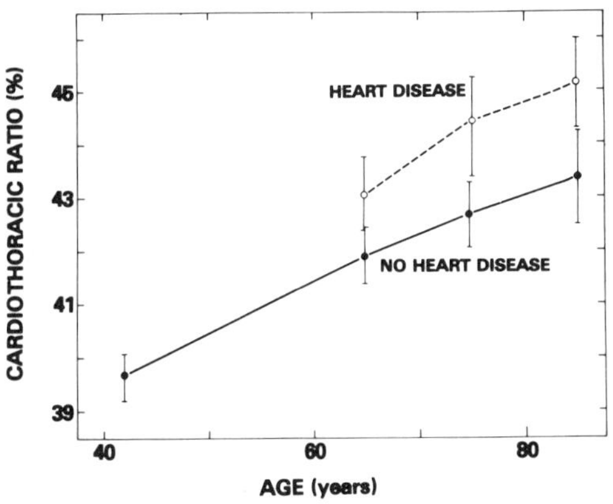

Figure 2-3 Cross-sectional differences (mean ± SE) in cardiothoracic ratio in four age groups of subjects with or without heart disease. Cardiothoracic ratio increases with age to a greater extent in subjects with heart disease. (Unpublished diagram courtesy of Potter et al.[6])

thoracic ratio were due both to a decrease in thoracic diameter and to an increase in cardiac diameter in each age group studied. Comparable results from the Baltimore Longitudinal Study[6] are presented in Figure 2-1. The line segments represent the rate of change in individual age groups. Because the slopes of cardiac diameter were positive for the three oldest age groups and the slope of thoracic diameter was negative in the oldest group, the slopes of cardiothoracic ratio on age were positive in all three of the older age groups.

MYOCARDIAL VOLUME STUDIES

A more accurate determination of cardiac size can be achieved from roentgenographic studies by calculation of the relative heart volume.[18] Although this technic is not in common use in this country, the extensive data on heart volume in the European literature provides additional insight as to the relationship between age and heart size. This technic employs PA and lateral chest films from which volume is calculated using the long and broad areas in the PA film and the longitudinal axes on the lateral film in a formula developed by Jonsell[19] which assumes the heart approximates an ellipse. Christie[20] employed this technic with a series of randomly sampled chest films which were taken as part of the London Civil Service Health Survey. In stepwise multiple regression analysis the relationship between heart volume and other physical characteristics was examined. The important determinants of heart volume were found to be weight, thoracic diameter, systolic blood pressure, heart rate, and age. An additional analysis confirmed the fact that systolic blood pressure and age were independent factors in the determination of heart volume.

The increase in heart volume with age noted by Christie was similar to that found in Norwegian,[21] Swedish,[18,22] and German[23] populations. At variance with these reports are those of Konig et al[24,25] and Kjellberg et al[26] which fail to show a significant association between age and cardiac volume. Erikson and Backlund[18] compared the technic of Jonsell with that of Kjellberg et al and found the later technic, which employed films taken in the upright rather than the supine position, to be less reliable in estimating heart volume. Strandell[27] studied the relationship between heart volume and a number of variables including age. He found a statistically significant relationship between age and relative heart volume of men 30 to 83 years of age. However, age lost its significance when tested together with ECG abnormalities and the correlation between age and heart volume was thus attributed to the increase with age of abnormal ECG findings. An abnormal ECG was that which showed any of the following: ST segment depression, frequent ventricular or supraventricular ectopic beats, two or more ectopic beats in series, or ectopic beats from more than one focus. The presence of supraventricular and ventricular ectopic beats is certainly a strongly age-related phenomenon, but whether or not they are truly abnormal in old age is a matter of some debate.

It thus appears that radiographically measured heart volume increases with age as does the somewhat cruder index of heart size, cardiac diameter.

ECHOCARDIOGRAPHIC MEASURES

Cardiac diameter and heart volume increase in normal aging individuals. The increase in these radiographic measures may be due either to an increase in cardiac chamber size (dilatation) or to an increase in myocardial mass (hypertrophy). M-mode echocardiography is ideally suited to differentiate the two alternatives. Since extensive studies of echocardiographic measurements have been found to correlate with body surface area independent of sex, conclusions from these studies should apply equally well to men and women.

Gerstenblith et al[28] studied 105 male participants of the Baltimore Longitudinal Study of Aging, aged 25 to 84 years who were free of cardiovascular disease. This study failed to show a change in left ventricular (LV) end-systolic or end-diastolic dimension with age. Henry et al[29] in a study of 228 individuals of both sexes aged from 1 month to 97 years, actually observed a slight decline in LV dimensions with age. Safranov et al[30] studied 841 individuals aged from 2 weeks to 70 years and found no difference in right ventricular, left ventricular, or left atrial dimensions when subjects 21 to 44 years of age were compared to those aged 45 to 70 years. From these studies it appears that the increase in heart volume seen in radiographic studies is not accounted for by dilatation of the cardiac chambers.

If the size of the cardiac chambers does not increase with age, then the thickness of the ventricular wall must, in order to account for the increased cardiac volume seen in radiographic studies. Two large studies[28,29] of 105 and 228 subjects up to age 85 and age 97 showed significant increases in the thickness of both the intraventricular septum (IVS) and left ventricular free wall (LVFW) with age.

Although blood pressure tends to increase somewhat with age, neither systolic nor diastolic blood pressure was significantly different among the age groups studied,[28] suggesting that blood pressure was not the driving force behind the increase in myocardial mass with age.

A third study[31] of 300 men aged 20 to 60 years reported a significant increase in LVFW thickness with age but failed to show a similar increase in IVS thickness. At variance with the three abovementioned studies, is that of Safranov et al[30] who could demonstrate no change in either LVFW or IVS thickness when comparing mean values between groups of subjects 21 to 44 years and 45 to 70 years of age.

An accurate method for calculation of LV mass from echocardiographic measures was reported by Devereaux and Reichek[32] based on a study of premortem echocardiograms and postmortem anatomic LV mass. Lakatta[33] used this technic in combination with the Baltimore study data[28] to show that the mass of the heart increases with age in normal man. Therefore, the weight of evidence from echocardiographic studies indicates that myocardial mass increases with age and accounts for the increase in cardiac diameter and heart volume noted in radiographic studies.

The effects of hypertension on the heart reproduce the changes in myocardial mass seen with normal aging. Intraventricular septal thickness of 20-year-old hypertensives was equal to that seen in normal 70-year-old subjects.[34] After adjusting the echocardiographic values for age and body surface area, intraventricular septal and/or ventricular free wall thickness was increased in 61% of hypertensive subjects. These changes occurred prior to ECG or chest film abnormalities.

AUTOPSY STUDIES

The preceding discussion of noninvasive methods presents good evidence for a gradual increase in mass of the heart with age. If this actually occurs, one would also expect to see an increase in the mass of the heart at autopsy. Autopsy studies might also identify asymptomatically diseased hearts, and further elucidate the changes in cardiac mass with normal aging. On the other hand, the postmortem heart is not completely comparable to the heart during life, particularly if death was preceded by a wasting disease. Significant weight loss is known to reduce the mass of many body tissues, including the heart.[35]

The largest study of postmortem hearts[36] examined 7112 cases aged 0 to 109 years. Relative heart weight, calculated as the weight of the heart divided by the weight of the body multiplied by 100, increased from 0.55% in middle age to 0.8% in centenarians. Mean heart weight increased throughout life until the ninth decade and declined only slightly in the 10th and 11th decades. Senile atrophy of the heart, formerly a popular concept, was not seen. Rather, small hearts (200 g or less) were more common in young people. Of some interest is the fact that the variability of the heart weight did not increase with age. As a rule, variability, ie, the difference between maximum and minimum values, is greatest in the older groups in almost all gerontologic studies. This study reported relative heart weight for 67 centenarians. Similar data for an additional 23 centenarians comes from Ishii and Sternby[37] who reported relative heart weight as 0.7%.

In 1928, Smith[38] reported relative heart weight for 1000 autopsies that had been selected from 6000 cases. Cases were excluded if there was systemic disease known to affect the size and weight of the heart, as were cases in which the heart was enlarged without demonstrable cause. In this highly select group there was no increase in heart weight with age. The autopsy series reported by Hegglin[39] reported gross weight rather than relative weight and studied few subjects in the oldest group (n = 9, 80 to 89 years). This author found that when epicardial fat was removed there was no increase in heart weight with age.

A carefully analyzed series of 292 unselected cases aged 21 to 92 years reported by Reiner et al[35] does not report relative heart weight for the series because none of the bodies were weighed at autopsy. No correlation was found between age and either total weight or total muscle mass of the heart. However, the weight of epicardial fat was positively correlated with age.

In a study of 334 patients over 60 years old whose mean age was 81 years, Hodkinson et al[40] found that age and body weight were positively correlated with heart weight. The importance of age was lost, however, when a variety of clinicopathologic factors were taken into account, which led them to conclude that the age correlation related to accumulation of relevant pathology with age rather than an age effect per se. The factors that made a significant contribution to prediction of heart weight were pathologic evidence of ischemia or infarction. Thus, when only an elderly group of subjects is considered, the presence of ischemic disease overrides the effect of age in determination of heart weight.

MORTALITY AND CARDIAC MEASUREMENTS

Studies of aging seek to delineate changes that occur normally with age and also the impact of those changes on survival. While cross-sectional studies may suggest that age-related differences are part of normal aging, they cannot exclude a detrimental effect. Only studies which relate prospective measurements to outcome at a later time can differentiate benign from detrimental changes. If the increase in cardiac diameter and heart volume seen in radiographic studies and the increase in cardiac muscle mass seen on echocardiography are due to asymptomatic heart disease, a detrimental effect on survival should be seen. Studies which relate cardiac mass measured on chest films to survival have been reported in two longitudinal and one prospective insurance study.

A longitudinal study initiated in Edinburgh in 1968[41] was composed of 215 men and 272 women aged 62 years and over who were drawn as a random sample from 27,000 older people living in a defined area in Edinburgh. Subjects underwent examinations at the outset and at one and five years.[5] On the basis of Rose's questionnaire and a 12-lead ECG, subjects were classified as having probable ischemic heart disease, possible ischemic heart disease, or no evidence of such disease. Because cardiac diameter was not significantly different in subjects with or without heart disease at the initial examination, diseased and nondiseased cases were considered together at the five-year follow-up. At the end of five years 102 men and 124 women were dead or lost to follow-up. The entrance cardiac diameter of five-year survivors was compared to the cardiac diameter of nonsurvivors. In men aged 62 to 90 years and women aged 62 to 69 years who died, heart diameter at the beginning of the study was not significantly different from survivors. In women over 70 years of age, cardiac diameter was significantly higher in those who did not survive to the five-year follow-up.

The Baltimore Longitudinal Study of Aging (BLSA) has also analyzed the impact of cardiac diameter measured from chest films on survival.[6] Subjects were divided into those with and those without heart disease as previously described. Of the original 243 subjects, 49 had died by the time the analysis was performed. Each of the 49 deceased subjects was matched with a survivor in the following categories: age, time of last longitudinal visit, and cardiovascular status. When the longitudinal change (ie, the slope of the line segments seen in Figure 2-2) in cardiac diameter and cardiothoracic ratio for the deceased subjects was compared to that of the survivors, the slopes for subjects dying with known heart disease were significantly higher than those of the survivors. However, for subjects who died without known heart disease, the slopes were no different from those of matched survivors. In this analysis, the increase in cardiac diameter with age in the absence of identifiable heart disease does not adversely affect survival.

The life insurance industry has provided a wealth of information on correlations of morbidity and mortality based on experience with insured lives. Singer et al[42] reported the mortality experience with 4143 insured applicants aged 20 to 74 years who had relative heart diameters calculated from chest films. Subjects were screened with ECG, chest films, and history and physical examination, and were rated as standard risk, at risk for cardiovascular reasons, and at risk for noncardiovascular reasons. Cardiac diameter was measured from chest films and expressed as percent predicted heart diameter based on a nomogram for heart diameter developed by Ungerleider,[4] which adjusts the diameter of the heart for height and weight. Subjects were followed for a minimum of one year and standardized mortality ratios (observed deaths/expected deaths) calculated (Table 2-3). No upward trend in mortality ratio was found with increasing cardiac diameter in the

Table 2-3
Comparative Mortality by Relative Heart Diameter

Relative Heart Diameter*	Exposure: *Person-Yrs* E	No. of Deaths: *Observed* d	No. of Deaths: *Expected*† d′	Mortality Ratio 100 d/d′
3054 Standard Issue Cases				
Under 90%	5292	32	39.0	82
90–96%	12674	89	104.2	85
97–104%	14283	91	135.7	67
105% and up	6817	48	72.6	68
269 Cases Rated for Noncardiovascular Risk				
Under 90%	467	4	4.46	90
90–96%	861	5	6.89	73
97–104%	1333	15	12.80	117
105% and up	365	4	4.29	93
440 Cases Aged 20–49, Rated for Cardiovascular Risk				
Under 90%	709	4	3.80	105
90–96%	1342	12	6.97	172
97–104%	1976	13	8.96	145
105% and up	1164	11	5.54	199
380 Cases Aged 50–74, Rated for Cardiovascular Risk				
Under 90%	280	6	4.82	124
90–96%	871	19	13.18	144
97–104%	1631	46	28.20	163
105% and up	1163	32	19.85	161

*Ratio (%) of observed diameter to diameter predicted from Ungerleider.[4]
†Basis of expected deaths: 1965–1970 select and ultimate tables, separate male and female rates.
Adapted from Singer et al.[42]

standard cases or cases rated for noncardiovascular reasons. Mortality ratios were actually higher for the groups with relative heart diameter below the mean. However, among cases rated for cardiovascular risk, a trend for increasing mortality with increasing relative heart diameter was shown both in individuals under 50 years of age and in the age group 59 to 74 years.

The width of the aortic arch on chest film increases both with age and in certain disease states. Just as with cardiac diameter, one could ask what impact such changes have on mortality. The life insurance companies have studied aortic root dimension with this question in mind. Sheridan[43] found that the aortic arch was approximately 46% of the cardiac diameter in persons free of cardiovascular disease and that an age correction was necessary. Based on studies of people up to 65 years of age, age adjustment was accomplished by subtraction of 1 mm for each three years below 43 years of age and addition of 1 mm for each three years above this age. The applicability of this standard (known as the Sheridan index) to persons over 65 years was examined by Rodstein and Wolloch in a study of 150 residents of the Jewish Home and Hospital who were free of detectable cardiovascular disease. The Sheridan index was found to apply equally well to men aged over and under 65 years. However, the average transverse diameter of the aortic arch for females 65 years and over was approximately 37% of the cardiac diameter. The similarity of the Sheridan index in aged males to those under 65 years was felt to reflect the predominately male population of the younger group studied.

Singer et al[42] also examined the influence of aortic root dimension on mortality. Using the Sheridan index[43] for aortic width, aortic root dimensions were rated percent predicted, corrected for age. Aortic root dimension was not predictive of mortality in cases rated as at risk for cardiovascular death or in cases of standard risk.

CONCLUSIONS

The diameter of the heart measured on PA chest films has been shown to increase with age in men and women without identifiable heart disease. Longitudinal studies have confirmed the results seen in earlier cross-sectional studies and have provided evidence that, in the absence of heart disease, there is no detrimental effect from an increase in cardiac diameter with age. The cardiothoracic ratio increases not only because of an increase in cardiac diameter, but also is due to a decline in thoracic diameter with age. While the usual upper limit of normal for cardiothoracic ratio of 50% applies to men of advanced age, the standard does not apply to older women. Because thoracic diameter declines more rapidly with age in women, an upper limit of 55 or 60% seems more appropriate.

Radiographically determined relative heart volume is also seen to increase with age and provides supportive evidence in the form of an independent measurement for the increase in cardiac diameter measured on PA chest films. However, these radiographic technics cannot differentiate muscle hypertrophy from chamber dilatation. Echocardiographic studies on the other hand can. Echocardiography of normal aging populations has shown no increase in ventricular chamber size but rather an increase in both posterior left ventricular wall and intraventricular septal thickness. When ventricular mass is extrapolated from echocardiographic measurements, the mass of the heart is seen to increase significantly with age. Thus, radiography shows an increase in heart size with age which on echocardiography is due to an increase in myocardial muscle mass.

Autopsy studies do not fit this picture quite so neatly and some autopsy studies may be interpreted to be in frank disagreement. Those studies which report relative heart weight and which do not exclude cases solely on the basis of increased mass show a gradual increase in relative heart weight with age. Studies which consider only crude weight of the heart, uncorrected for body weight, are difficult to interpret since body weight increases throughout the middle years and declines somewhat in old age.[45] One study[40] was unable to show an effect of age on heart weight when subjects aged over 60 years (mean age 81 years) were examined. In this age group the most important factor in determining heart weight was the presence of ischemic pathology. If an old group only is studied, it is perhaps not surprising that age is seen to have little effect on the variability of heart weight and that disease becomes the predominant factor. Thus from autopsy studies there appear to be at least three factors at play in determining cardiac mass, ie, body weight, age, and disease of the heart, which is essentially what is also seen in noninvasive studies.

Left ventricular mass increases in radiographic and echocardiographic studies. This change is characteristic of nearly all members of the population of longitudinal studies and is unassociated with an increase in mortality. Therefore, an increase in left ventricular mass appears to be a true age-related change rather than secondary to occult disease. The increase in blood pressure, which is also known to occur with age, does not appear to be the driving force behind the increase in left ventricular mass.[6,28] However, the age-associated increase in size, stiffness, and arteriolar tone of the peripheral vascular bed may result in an increase in total vascular resistance during both rest and exercise.[46] Left ventricular hypertrophy, which would decrease wall stress, may therefore represent an adaptation to a chronic state of increased impedance to left ventricular ejection.[28]

REFERENCES

1. Danzer CS: The cardiothoracic ratio: An index of cardiac enlargement. *Am J Med Sci* 1919;157:513–521.
2. Eyster JAE: Determination of cardiac hypertrophy by roentgenray methods. *Arch Intern Med* 1928;41:667–682.
3. Hodges FJ, Eyster JAE: Estimation of transverse cardiac diameter in man. *Arch Intern Med* 1926;37:707–714.
4. Ungerleider HE: A study of the transverse diameter of the heart silhouette with prediction table based on the teleoroentgenogram. *Assn Life Ins Med Dir Am* 1938;25:84–94.
5. Lauder IJ, Milne JS: Longitudinal study of heart size in older people. *Br Heart J* 1976;38:1286–1290.
6. Potter JF, Elahi D, Tobin JD, et al: Effect of age on the cardiothoracic ratio of men. *J Am Geriatr Soc* 1982;30:404–409.
7. Tirman WS, Hamilton JB: Aging in apparently normal men. IV. The roentgenologic appearance of the thorax and thoracic organs. *J Gerontol* 1952;7:394–398.
8. Cowan NR: The heart-lung coefficient and the transverse diameter of the heart. *Br Heart J* 1964;26:116–120.
9. Edge JR, Millard FJC, Reid L, et al: The radiographic appearances of the chest in persons of advanced age. *Br J Radiol* 1964;37:769–774.
10. Rabushka SE, Melamed JL, Melamed ME: The geriatric chest; A radiographic survey. *Geriatrics* 1968;23(8):136–141.
11. Milne JS, Lauder IJ: Heart size in older people. *Br Heart J* 1974;36:352–356.
12. Stone JL, Norris AH: Activities and attitudes of participants in he Baltimore longitudinal study. *J Gerontol* 1966;21:575–580.
13. Cowan NR: The transverse diameter of the heart in older people. *Br Heart J* 1960;22:391–394.
14. Rizzato G, Marazzini L: Thoracoabdominal mechanics in elderly men. *J Appl Physiol* 1970;28:457–460.
15. Kory RC, Callahan R, Boren HG, et al: The Veterans Administration–army cooperative study of pulmonary function. *Am J Med* 1961;30:243–258.
16. Takahashi E, Atsumi H: Age differences in thoracic form a indicated by thoracic index. *Hum Biol* 1955;27:65–74.
17. Cowan NR: The heart lung coefficient in older people. *Br Heart J* 1958;21:238–242.
18. Erikson U, Backlund L: Heart volume and its relation to age; Aspects of the technique. *Acta Radiol [Diagn]* 1981;22:541–543.
19. Jonsell S: A method for the determination of the heart size by teleroentgenography (a heart volume index). *Acta Radiol [Diagn]* 1939;30:325.
20. Christie D: Physical correlates of radiologic heart volume. *Acta Radiol [Diagn]* 1978;19:732–736.
21. Humerfeldt S: An Epidemiological Study of High Blood Pressure. Bergen, Oslo, Universitets Forlaget, 1963.
22. Braun VH: Das Herzvolumen und seine Beziehung zu den anderen hämodynamischen Faktoren unter Anwendung neuer röntgenologischer Untersuchungsmethoden. *Arch Kreislaufforschung* 1960;32:87–109.
23. Maurea C, Nylin G, Sollberger A: Normal heart volume. *Acta Cardiol* 1955;10:336–361.
24. Konig VK, Reindell H, Roskamm H: Das Herzvolumen und die Leistungsfähigkeit bei: 60–75 jährigen gesunder männern. *Arch Kreislaufforschung* 1962;39:143–181.
25. Konig VK, Reindall H, Musshoff K, et al: Das Herzvolumen und die körperliche leistungsfähigkeit bei: 20–60 jährigen gesunden männern. *Arch Kreislaufforschung* 1960;35:37–67.
26. Kjellberg SR, Lonroth H, Rudhe U, et al: The relationship between the heart volume and the blood volume and its physiological and pathologic variability. *Acta Med Scand* 1951;140:446–453.
27. Strandell T: Heart rate, arterial lactate concentration and oxygen uptake during exercise in old men compared with young men. *Acta Physiol Scand* 1964;60:197–216.
28. Gerstenblith G, Frederiksen J, Yin FCP: Echocardiographic assessment of a normal adult aging population. *Circulation* 1977;56:273–278.
29. Henry WL, Gardin JM, Ware JH: Echocardiographic measurements in normal subjects from infancy to old age. *Circulation* 1980;62:1054–1061.
30. Safronov VV, Kuzmichev YG, Modzgvrishvili RA, et al: Age differences in basic echocardiometric indices. *Fiziol Cheloveka* 1979;6:329–335.
31. Arsenescu GH, Sabau M, Tintoiv I, et al: Effect of age on the heart electrical phenomena, left ventricular wall thickness and blood pressure in men. *Rev Roum Med-Med Int* 1982;20(1):33–38.
32. Devereaux RB, Reichek N: Echocardiographic determination of left ventricular mass in man. *Circ Res* 1977;55:613–618.
33. Lakatta EG: Alterations in the cardiovascular system that occur in advanced age. *Fed Proc* 1979;38:163–167.
34. Savage DD, Drayer JIM, Henry WL, et al: Echocardiographic assessment of cardiac anatomy and function in hypertensive subjects. *Circulation* 1979;59:623–632.
35. Reiner L, Mazzoleni A, Rodriguez FL, et al: The weight of the human heart. *Arch Pathol* 1959;68:68–83.
36. Linzbach AJ, Akuamoa-Boateng E: The alterations of the aging human heart: I. Heart weight with progressive age. *Klin Wochenschr* 1973;51:156–163.
37. Ishii T, Sternby JH: Pathology of centenarians. I.

The cardiovascular system and lungs. *J Am Geriatr Soc* 1978;26:108-115.
38. Smith HL: The relation of the weight of the heart to the weight of the body and of the weight of the heart to age. *Am Heart J* 1928;4:79-83.
39. Hegglin R: Über Organvolumen und Organgewicht. *Konstitutionslehre* 1934;18:110-134.
40. Hodkinson I, Pomerance A, Hodkinson HM: Heart size in the elderly: A clinicopathological study. *J R Soc Med* 1979;72:13-16.
41. Milne JS, Chopin JM: Reviews after one and five years in a longitudinal study of aging persons. *Age Ageing* 1975;4:152-160.
42. Singer RB, Siber FJ, Brown AE, et al: Mortality in 4100 insured applicants with ECG and chest x-ray. *Trans Assoc Life Ins Med Dir Am* 1982;62:180-193.
43. Sheridan JT: The transverse diameter of the cardiac silhouette. *Trans Assoc Life Ins Med Dir Am* 1941; 28:49-73.
44. Rodstein M, Wolloch L: The determination of aortic size by use of the Sheridan index in the elderly – A study of 300 individuals 65 years of age and older. *Trans Assoc Life Ins Med Dir Am* 1967;51:341-349.
45. Rossman I: Anatomic and body composition changes with aging, in Finch CE, Hayflick L (eds): *Handbook of the Biology of Aging.* New York, Van Nostrand Reinhold Press, 1977, pp 193-195.
46. Granath A, Jonsson B, Strandell T: Circulation in healthy old men, studied by right heart catheterization at rest and during exercise in supine position. *Acta Med Scand* 1964;176:425-446.

CHAPTER 3
Cardiac Rhythms in the Healthy Elderly Patient

Anthony Martin

Since the introduction of ambulatory electrocardiographic monitoring, with facilities for high semiautomatic playback and analysis, our knowledge of rhythm abnormalities of the heart has increased greatly. Previous investigators of older populations using simple 12-lead electrocardiograms (ECG) have suggested that there was a high incidence of rhythm abnormalities in this age group.[1-3] However, several workers using dynamic ambulatory electrocardiography (DCG) have been able to document the incidence of arrhythmias in both the elderly[4-6] and younger populations.[7-9] It is now clear that the incidence of cardiac arrhythmias in apparently healthy people increases with advancing age (Table 3-1).

Considerable debate continues as to what constitutes a "normal" elderly population. Our own work was based on the premise that the healthy elderly population consisted of elderly people living at home independently. We excluded any patients who had consulted their doctor for any acute medical condition in the past three months, but not those who were taking medications for any reason, or who, on direct questioning, had symptoms that could have been indicative of cardiovascular disease.

However, these criteria of "normality" have been criticized on the basis that up to one half of our sample could have had evidence of latent ischemic heart disease if noninvasive diagnostic screening, such as treadmill exercise, thallium scanning, or two-dimensional echocardiograms had been used.[6] Since the incidence of ischemic heart disease is so prevalent in the apparently healthy elderly population[10] it seems highly unrealistic to exclude this great majority from a sample of the "normal" healthy elderly population. Indeed, of our original 268 subjects aged 75 years and over who are living independently at home, all but 12 would have been excluded if such strict criteria of normality had been used.[11] Furthermore, symptoms of breathlessness, dizziness, and palpitations are extremely common in the elderly and have a multitude of causes, the vast majority of which have nothing to do with the heart.

The exact diagnostic criteria of "normality" may not be so important, however, since the incidence of rhythm abnormalities in every group of the elderly that have been examined has been found to be extremely high, including those who have apparently no evidence of latent ischemic heart disease.[6] What is of much greater importance is the prognostic significance of the rhythm abnormalities that have been demonstrated in this age group. At the time of writing only one long-term follow-up study has been reported as to the prognostic significance of cardiac arrhythmias in the elderly age group.[11] This study indicates that the finding of ventricular ectopic beats with a frequency of greater than 10 per hour is associated with a significant increase in mortality, whereas supraventricular rhythm abnormalities, such as atrial fibrillation and other features of the "sick sinus syndrome" have no serious implications for mortality. Similarly, the presence of bundle branch block, which is increasingly prevalent with advancing age, does not seem to be a predictor of death. However, the implications of cardiac rhythm abnormalities that are commonly associated with the "sick sinus syndrome" may well be a major cause of morbidity, and thus require treatment with either drugs or pacemaker implantation.

Another area of considerable difficulty involves the correlation of cardiac rhythm abnormalities with clinical symptoms, such as dizziness, palpitation and syncopal episodes. These symptoms are extremely common in the elderly population and the causes are multitudinous and are often due to noncardiac causes. We found that only one third of our original apparently healthy subjects were free from the symptoms of palpitations, dizziness, and syncopal attacks on direct questioning; but in those that admitted to symptoms there was a small, but not significant, increase in the finding of cardiac rhythm disturbance (Table 3-2).

Many patients who have symptoms of a nonfocal neurologic nature often are symptomatic at relatively infrequent intervals, and thus one cannot expect them to be symptomatic during periods of ECG recording. Thus there is a concept that the occurrence of asymptomatic arrhythmias may give some clues to the potential occurrence of major arrhythmias which may be likely to cause symptoms. The experience of De Bono et al[12] agrees with our own work[13] in that it is bradyarrhythmias rather than tachyarrhythmias that are likely to be associated with such symptoms. De Bono et al found that 25 of their 89 patients with transient nonfocal neurologic symptoms had signs on ECG monitoring that contributed to the diagnosis. It is also true, however, that cardiac causes of such transient neurologic problems must be based on a balance of probabilities. In cases where there is difficulty, the working diagnosis may be tested by means of a prophylactic trial of either antiarrhythmic drugs or electrical therapy.

The symptoms of palpitations are also very common in elderly people. The correlation of palpitations and demonstrable cardiac rhythm abnormalities is extremely variable. One of the difficulties is the varied interpretation that the patient puts on palpitations. To some it is merely an awareness of the heart "thumping," others will be aware of the heart "missing a beat," and others are able to describe the occurrence of rapid irregular rhythms. The latter two situations are more likely to be able to be correlated with demonstrable rhythm abnormalities; missed beats perceived by the patient may be due to either atrial or ventricular premature contractions with a compensatory pause. Rapid irregular rhythms are usually due to paroxysmal atrial fibrillation.

Retrosternal chest pain is a common symptom in the elderly and is usually due to true angina pectoris, but it may well be produced by paroxysmal tachycardias, most usually atrial fibrillation. Similarly dyspnea, either at rest or on exertion, is a frequent complaint of elderly people. The most common cause is chronic lung disease, but the sudden onset of dyspnea, especially at night, in a previously healthy person is very likely to be due

Table 3-1
Incidence of Some Common Arrhythmias in Different Age Groups

Author	Southall et al[8]	Bordsky et al	Blake et al	Camm et al[4]
Age range	12½ hr–6 wk	23–27 yr	16–65 yr	75 yr & over
No. studied	80	50	86	106
Occasional VPCs (%)	2.5	50	73	70
Frequent VPCs (%)	1	2	8	12
Ventricular tachycardia (%)	4	2	2	4
SVT (incl. AF) (%)	6	2	5	13

VPC = ventricular premature contractions; SVT = supraventricular tachycardia; AF = atrial fibrillation.

Table 3-2
Incidence of Arrhythmias in 106 Asymptomatic and Symptomatic Subjects

	Normal	Minor Arrhythmias	Major Arrhythmias	Total
Asymptomatic	4	19	14	37
Palpitations	4	12	15	31
Dizziness	14	18	23	55
Syncope	2	9	6	17

Adapted from Camm et al.[4]

to left ventricular failure, and the most frequent cause of this in the elderly is the development of atrial fibrillation with an uncontrolled ventricular rate.

ELECTROPHYSIOLOGIC CONSIDERATIONS

The normal cardiac pacemaker is the sino-atrial node. This node is situated in the upper part of the right atrium and consists of fibers that have the fastest inherent electrical discharge rate (automaticity) of all cardiac tissue. The discharge rate of the sino-atrial node is modified by the autonomic nervous supply, chiefly by the vagus nerve which reduces the rate when stimulated. The discharge rate is also modified by other factors, particularly endocrine secretions such as thyroxine, circulating toxins, and bacterial organisms, and by coronary artery insufficiency. The blood supply to the sino-atrial node arises from the right coronary artery in 60% of people and from the left coronary artery in 40%.

Disturbances of sino-atrial function (sick sinus syndrome) are extremely common in the elderly and are described in more detail below. The main problem is the gradual disappearance of fibers from the node with advancing age and this has been well reviewed by Pomerance and Davies.[14]

From the sino-atrial node electrical impulses pass through the atria to reach the atrioventricular node. This important junction is supplied with blood from the right coronary artery in 90% of cases and from the left circumflex artery in the remaining 10%. It is a major site of degenerative and ischemic disease in the elderly. Certain drugs will also interfere with atrioventricular conduction, digitalis being the most frequent offender.

Calcific degeneration of the mitral valve may also encroach on the AV node (Rytand's syndrome). From the atrioventricular node the electrical impulses pass down the His bundles to the ventricular walls. The left bundle of His divides into two fascicles, the anterior one running superiorly and laterally and the posterior one running inferiorly and medially. It has been recognized in recent years that ischemic or degenerative myocardial disease may destroy the left anterior branch (left anterior hemiblock) much more commonly than the left posterior branch and that block of either fascicle may be combined with right bundle-branch block, a condition known as bifascicular block in which the two fascicles of the left bundle and the right bundle are regarded as part of a three-part conducting system.

CELLULAR MECHANISMS OF ARRHYTHMIAS

In the last few years there have been major changes in our understanding of the cellular electrophysiologic mechanisms that are involved in arrhythmias. Currently it is thought that there are three main mechanisms involved in arrhythmias: abnormal automaticity, reflection, and re-entry.

The normal sinus rhythm of the heart is maintained by the rate of spontaneous depolarization and threshold potential of the sinus node which is sufficiently faster than the rate of other potential pacemakers in cardiac tissue. Any damage to cardiac tissue at any site may give that tissue the property of spontaneous rhythmicity and if the discharge rate of this abnormal "pacemaker" exceeds that of the sinus node it may take over the cardiac rhythm. The action potential may be altered by an increase in the slope of the diastolic depolarization or by lowering of the threshold potential. In addition the repolarization phase may be altered in certain circumstances, eg, with digitalis, by increased electrical activity ("after potentials"), which may be great enough to exceed the threshold potential and trigger automatic tachycardias.

The phenomenon of reflection is caused by the delayed recovery of damaged tissue immediately adjacent to normally recovering tissue. The prolonged action potentials of the abnormal cells may lead to re-excitation of the adjacent normal cells thus producing return extrasystoles or "echo beats."[15] An example of reflection is the chaotic ventricular rhythm that is associated with the long QT syndrome.

Re-entry rhythms are caused by the reactivation of electrically excitable tissue by a continuously circulating impulse. In this situation the electrical impulses are blocked by refractory tissue (anterograde block) which then recovers and allows retrograde conduction back into the original antegrade pathway. Usually re-entrant tachycardias are both easily precipitated and terminated by premature stimuli, but in certain circumstances, if the balance of refractoriness and conduction velocity is such that the refractoriness does not exceed the cycle length of circus movement, sustained tachycardias may result. There are many sites in the normal heart in which the requirements for slow conduction and re-entry are fulfilled, and this mechanism may occur both in large anatomical circuits and within very small groups of cells. The classical example of a re-entrant tachycardia is the paroxysmal "supraventricular" tachycardia associated with the Wolff-Parkinson-White syndrome, but many paroxysmal arrhythmias such as atrial fibrillation and ventricular tachycardia have a reentrant basis.

SINUS NODE ABNORMALITIES

The sino-atrial node is composed of muscle cells with an inherent automaticity that is greater than any other cardiac tissue and thus acts as the pacemaker of the heart rhythm under normal circumstances. As a result of the degenerative processes of aging the number of these muscle cells diminishes. At an unspecified level of cell reduction the dominant control of the sinus node is lost and gives rise to the spectrum of clinical entities that comprise the sick sinus syndrome. These include sinus bradycardia, sino-atrial block, sinus arrest, atrial fibrillation and flutter, and reciprocating episodes of bradycardia and tachycardia. While it is true that sinus node disease does not appear to confer a major risk to death[16] the symptoms that it may produce in the elderly are often extremely severe and are a common cause of morbidity. Generally the bradycardias produce fainting episodes, falls, giddiness, and confusion, and the tachycardia gives rise to symptoms of left ventricular failure and angina.[13]

Sinus bradycardia, defined as a heart rate of 50 beats/min or less during waking hours, is known to occur with increasing frequency as age advances. In a very large population survey in Belgium using a resting 12-lead ECG, Kulbertus et al[17] found that just over 3% of almost 2000 people aged over 75 years had a heart rate of 55 beats per minute (bpm) or less. This corresponds with our own work using ambulatory electrocardiography; we found just over 4% of subjects in the same age range had heart rates that fell below 50 bpm during waking hours, although this figure rose to 11% if sleeping recordings were included. Although sinus bradycardia is one of the signs of sinus node disease it frequently does not give rise to symptoms and, therefore, requires no treatment. However, in some cases the bradycardia may be profound and the author knows of one case where sinus rhythm persisted at a rate of only 16 bpm and was accompanied by severe symptoms of dizziness and syncope. In symptomatic people the correct treatment is with a permanent on-demand pacemaker. Sinus bradycardia may be simulated by nonconducted atrial bigeminy.

Sinus Arrhythmia

Sinus arrhythmia, defined as a beat-to-beat P-P interval variation of greater than 10%, is not a feature of sinus node disease. It is common in infants and young people but does not appear to be very prevalent at the older extremes of life.[4] There have not been many large studies of elderly people using ambulatory ECG monitoring and our study showed that 15% of healthy elderly people had sinus arrhythmia which is still a much higher incidence than shown by conventional resting ECGs.[18] Of greater interest is the finding of severe restriction in the dynamic range of heart rates in over 30% of our subjects. The relative rarity of sinus arrhythmia and the apparent inability of the sinus node to vary its rate of discharge in the elderly probably reflects reduced sinus node reactivity to autonomic influences. This "lazy sinus" response has previously been reported as a feature of the sick sinus syndrome[19,20] and occurs in nonbradycardic elderly people.[21]

Sinus Pauses

Sinus pauses may be caused by either sinus node arrest or sino-atrial block. The differentiation between these two phenomena is sometimes difficult, but the exercise is usually academic since both reflect a significant degree of sinus node disease. Sinus arrest often results in a long period of asystole (Figure 3-1) and the cardiac cycle is restarted by an escape beat which may arise from any part of the conducting system. In general the escape beat arises from the atria or the AV junction, but the longest pauses are followed by a sinus escape beat. Sino-atrial block of the second degree type shows a pause that is twice as long as the normal sinus cycle and during the pause there are no P waves or QRS complexes. Any sinus pause in the elderly that exceeds 2 seconds usually gives rise to symptoms of severe dizziness or syncope. Symptomatic patients should be treated, whatever their age, with permanent pacing.

Sinus Tachycardia

Sinus tachycardia is not a feature of sinus node disease. It is commonly seen in elderly people, and is a manifestation of exercise, fever, anxiety, or left ventricular failure. It may also be seen in elderly people with thyrotoxicosis, although these patients almost always have either paroxysmal or established atrial fibrillation.

The management of sinus tachycardia is that of the underlying cause and is virtually never a condition that requires treatment symptomatically.

Atrial Fibrillation

Atrial fibrillation is one of the most common and most important arrhythmias in the elderly. It

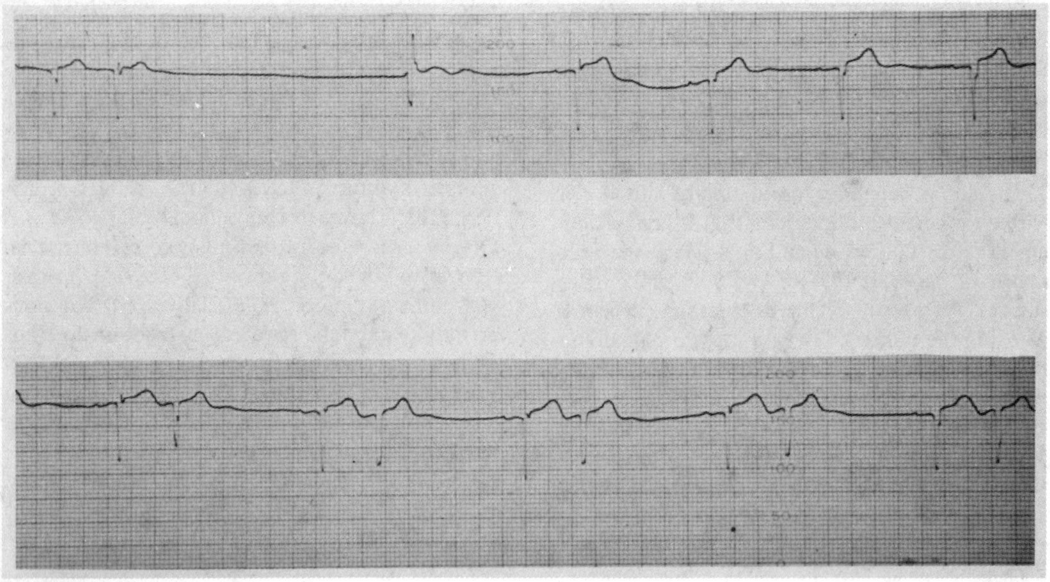

Figure 3-1 Sinus node arrest. *Note*: Long pause following second beat in upper tracing. The heart beat is re-started by a junctional escape beat.

is a feature of sinus node disease where the dominant sinus pacemaker is failing. Histopathologic studies have shown that patients with atrial fibrillation show a considerable reduction in the muscle cell content of the sinus node. Studies using resting 12-lead ECGs have shown that the incidence of atrial fibrillation in the aged is between 3% and 8%.[2,22,3,17] It should be noted that some of these studies have involved people in hospitals and homes for the aged, without including people from the community. The more general use of long-term ambulatory cardiac monitoring has revealed a rather different pattern of incidence, presumably due to the previously unrecognized frequency of paroxysmal atrial fibrillation. A study of 106 apparently healthy people aged 75 years and over living in their own homes in the United Kingdom using ambulatory monitoring, showed that the incidence of atrial fibrillation, both established and paroxysmal, was 11%. However, when a slightly younger group of people (aged over 60 years) are examined, and those with overt heart disease excluded, atrial fibrillation is rarely found,[6,23] although Fleg and Kennedy found that paroxysmal benign slow atrial tachycardia occurred in 28% of their group.[6]

Paroxysmal atrial fibrillation has been recognized for a long time[24] and the apparently higher prevalence at the present time is undoubtedly due to more sophisticated methods of cardiac monitoring, and the greater interest that is now shown in our ever-increasing elderly population. It is likely that all cases of atrial fibrillation due to degenerative heart disease start off by being paroxysmal before becoming established. This is well illustrated by the coexistence of atrial fibrillation with thyrotoxicosis. It has long been recognized that the incidence of atrial fibrillation in hyperthyroid patients rises with age.[25,26] Hamilton showed that by the seventh decade 83% of hyperthyroid patients had established atrial fibrillation, and after the age of 70 years it is probable that all hyperthyroid patients have either established or paroxysmal atrial fibrillation. It is also unusual for these elderly patients to revert to sinus rhythm when their thyrotoxic state has been adequately controlled by either drugs or radioactive iodine treatment. It is also worth remembering that the classical form of Graves' disease[27] is not very common in the elderly, and that many of the very old patients may have a "masked" form of hyperthyroidism where the main features are weight loss and atrial fibrillation.[28,29] Thus, all patients with atrial fibrillation should have thyroid function tests performed.

The other important feature of paroxysmal atrial fibrillation is that during the paroxysms the ventricular rate may be very rapid (Figure 3-2). These rates are an important cause of left ventricular failure. Indeed, in contrast to younger patients, the two most common causes of left ventricular failure in the elderly are myocardial infarction and atrial fibrillation with an uncontrolled ventricular rate; hypertension is a very rare cause of heart failure in the elderly.

The treatment of atrial fibrillation is with digoxin if the ventricular rate is rapid. There is probably one quarter of elderly patients with atrial fibrillation who have well-controlled ventricular rates without treatment with digitalis, and this is presumably because these patients also have widespread conduction system disease with built-in atrioventricular block. There are also some patients who are euthyroid and in whom the ventricular rate is difficult to control with digitalis alone. These patients can be usefully controlled with a small dose of digitalis with the addition of a beta-blocking agent such as pindolol which has some intrinsic sympathomimetic action.[30] The dosage of digoxin in the elderly needs to be carefully reviewed, especially if there is any evidence of renal impairment. Even if renal function tests are apparently normal the progressive nephron loss in the elderly[31] does compromise the handling of digitalis and toxic effects are common. The toxic effects of digitalis in the elderly are especially severe, since nausea and other gastrointestinal side-effects are not prominent and the major effects are directly on the heart, producing severe ventricular slowing, paroxysmal atrial tachycardia with atrioventricular block, ventricular premature beats, ventricular tachycardia, and fibrillation.

It is now possible with some antiarrhythmic drugs to control paroxysmal atrial fibrillation and maintain sinus rhythm for long periods. Amiodarone is probably the best drug in this condition,[32,33] but care must be taken to control the blood levels since this drug has a very long half-life and has a cumulative action. It is a class 3 antiarrhythmic drug.[34] Verapamil in large doses may also be effective, but unlike amiodarone has a negative inotropic action. Disopyramide may also be effective in controlling paroxysmal atrial fibrillation, but has the disadvantage of causing urinary retention in older men, and also has a marked negative inotropic effect.

Atrial Flutter

Atrial flutter is a condition that is not often seen in the healthy elderly patient, but presents considerable problem when it does occur in the sick elderly. Atrial flutter is almost always associated with some degree of atrioventricular block (Figure 3-3). Since the flutter rate is usually about 300 bpm the detection of a heart rate of 150 bpm should always alert the physician to the possibility of atrial flutter with 2:1 block. At this rate of heart action there will almost always be symptoms of either angina or heart failure if it is sustained. Some patients may have chronic atrial flutter with either 3:1 or 4:1 block and hence their heart rates will be slow enough to produce no symptoms. Sometimes atrial flutter, like atrial fibrillation, may be associated with a high degree of atrioventricular block and result in a very slow ventricular rate. This may occur with digitalis toxicity but most frequently is due to degenerative conduction system disease.

Atrial flutter is an extremely difficult condition to treat satisfactorily. If the ventricular rate is fast, treatment becomes something of an emergency, since heart failure may be present or will shortly occur if the rapid ventricular rate is

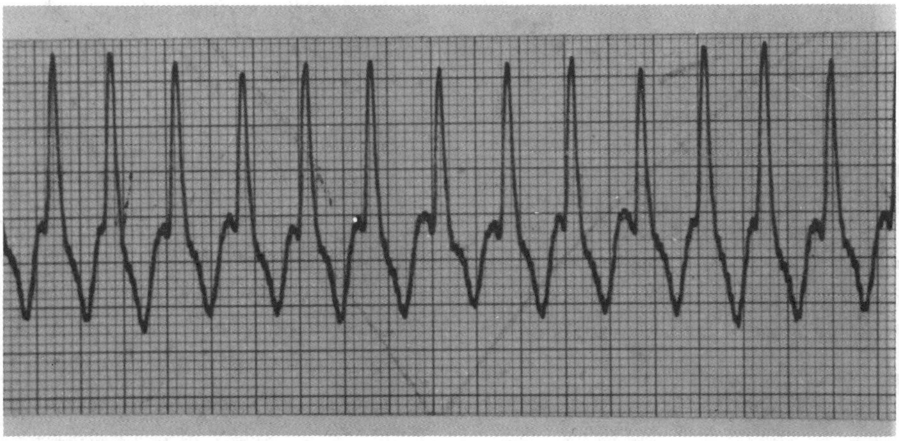

Figure 3-2 Atrial fibrillation with rapid ventricular rate. *Note*: Absence of P waves and irregular ventricular rhythm.

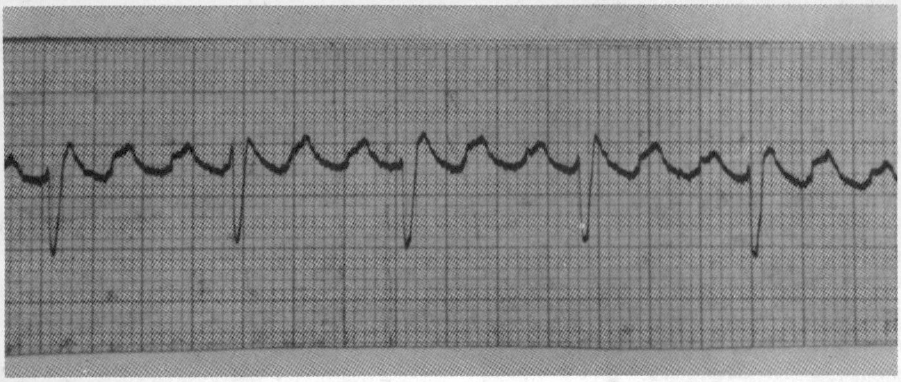

Figure 3-3 Atrial flutter with 3:1 atrioventricular block.

sustained. Intravenous amiodarone, verapamil or disopyramide may be successful in converting the rhythm to sinus, but on occasion direct current countershock may be necessary. Digoxin will increase the degree of atrioventricular block and slow the ventricular rate, but if it is unsuccessful electrical cardioversion may be dangerous.

Chronic atrial flutter may be paroxysmal and is usually associated with a low degree of atrioventricular block so that the ventricular rate is fast. Management is often difficult. Amiodarone is probably the single best antiarrhythmic agent in this condition, but verapamil and disopyramide may also be satisfactory; sometimes a combination of amiodarone and disopyramide may be successful if one or the other have failed to control the arrhythmia on their own.

The use of anticoagulant drugs in paroxysmal atrial fibrillation and flutter has been the subject of controversy for some time. Certainly there are slight risks of embolization immediately after cardioversion,[35,36] but the vast majority of patients with paroxysmal atrial fibrillation go in and out of sinus rhythm frequently, for many years, without sustaining systemic emboli.[3] It is possible that degenerative atrial fibrillation without mitral valvular disease and its consequently enlarged left atrium, behaves in a very different way from those patients with chronic rheumatic heart disease. The sheer logistics of treating all elderly patients with atrial fibrillation with anticoagulant therapy are staggering, and my own practice is to only anticoagulate those who have one clear episode of pulmonary or systemic embolization.

PRE-EXCITATION SYNDROMES

The discovery of abnormal bypass tracts of the atrioventricular node as in the Wolff-Parkinson-White[37] and in the Lown-Ganong-Levine[38] syndromes has led to our greater understanding of re-entry supraventricular tachycardias. These conditions are not uncommon in the elderly and may result in rather resistant paroxysmal tachycardias (Figure 3-4).

Treatment of these tachycardias is often satisfactorily with amiodarone.[33,38,39] Disopyramide and verapamil may also be of benefit in these cases. There are other methods for controlling supraventricular tachycardias, which at present do not have a significant place in elderly patients. These include overdrive pacing[40] and, more recently, surgical excision of the accessory pathway.[41] The problems of ventricular tachycardia associated with these accessory pathway syndromes are discussed below.

ECTOPIC BEATS

Supraventricular Premature Beats

Narrow complex premature beats arising from the atria or the upper part of the atrioventricular node are extremely common in elderly people and occur in over 20%. Their significance is not known but it is likely that they are of no serious consequence.[11] Perhaps this could have been predicted from the fact that they appear to occur as frequently during sleeping as waking hours and appear to be as common in healthy as in the less healthy elderly population. Atrial premature beats may be both normally and aberrantly conducted, and may precipitate runs of atrial fibrillation.

Ventricular Premature Beats

Ventricular premature beats (Figure 3-5) are known to be common in all age groups and rise in frequency with increasing age.[9,17] In the elderly they may be found in about half the population.

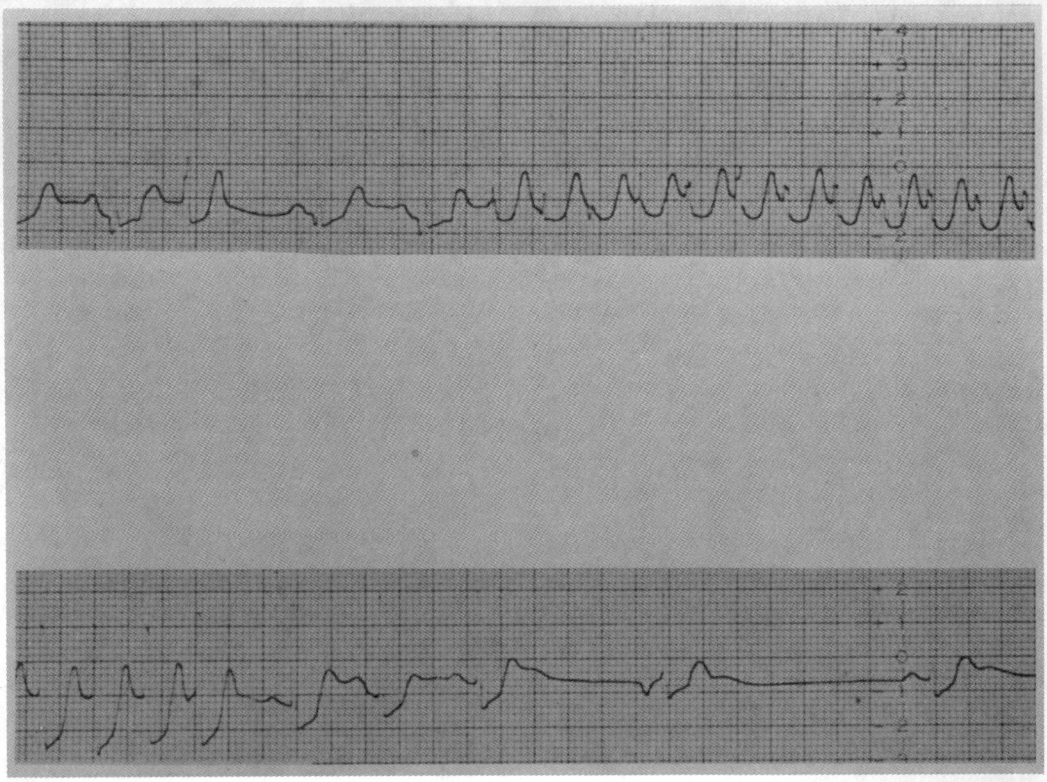

Figure 3-4 Paroxysmal supraventricular tachycardia.

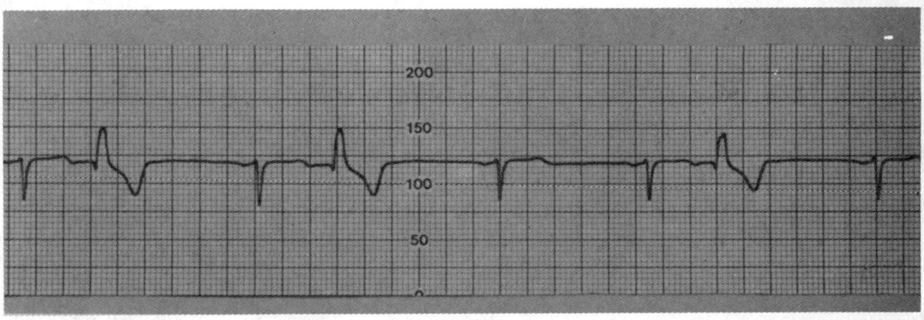

Figure 3-5 Ventricular premature beats.

Ventricular arrhythmias have been classified into minor and major types according to Lown and Wolff's criteria.[42] Isolated ventricular premature beats (10/h) are the most frequently found and moderately frequent (10 to 99/h) and frequent ventricular premature beats occur equally in about 13% of the elderly. About a quarter of the elderly population have other features of major ventricular arrhythmias such as paired and multiform beats, ventricular bigeminy, and salvos of ventricular beats.

Despite their frequent occurrence ventricular premature beats are often completely unnoticed by the patient and occur much more frequently during waking hours. However, the prognostic significance of ventricular premature beats is extremely important. It is known that there is an increased risk of serious ventricular arrhythmias and sudden death in patients with stable coronary artery disease who have ventricular premature beats.[43] A similar situation exists in patients with acute coronary heart disease[44] and even in middle-aged people without obvious heart disease.[45,46]

Since the occurrence of ventricular premature beats in the elderly is so high, the question of possible treatment remains one of considerable concern to physicians. The only large study aimed at elucidating this problem is our own,[4] and we found that there was a significantly higher risk of death in those people who had more than 10 ventricular premature beats per hour. It can, of course, be argued that many of our patients had associated coronary artery disease, but they do represent a typical cross section of the elderly population living independently at home. Clearly more extensive long-term follow-up studies are required to either support or refute our thesis, before large scale long-term antiarrhythmic treatment is given to a potentially sizeable number of people throughout the world, who have asymptomatic ventricular premature beats.

Treatment of ventricular ectopy is readily available with a large number of effective drugs. These include disopyramide, mexiletine, verapamil, amiodarone, quinidine, and tocainide. The relevant advantages of these agents are discussed elsewhere in this volume. For the ventricular ectopy that occurs after acute myocardial infarction the intravenous use of lidocaine is still the most effective method of control.

Other Arrhythmias

Ventricular tachycardia occurs paroxysmally in 4% of healthy elderly people. The paroxysms are usually short-lived and may not give rise to symptoms. The ventricular rate during these attacks is usually about 150 bpm. According to Lown and Wolff's criteria ventricular tachycardia is a major arrhythmia and therefore should probably be treated, whether symptomatic or not. The symptoms are more likely to be dyspnea and angina rather than seizures of syncopal episodes.

Ventricular fibrillation and flutter are usually terminal events and are most commonly seen in the intensive care unit in a patient following acute myocardial infarction. These serious arrhythmias may, however, on occasion be seen as a self-limiting phenomenon in patients on ambulatory heart monitoring. Ventricular fibrillation is often precipitated by a ventricular premature beat falling on the upstroke of the preceding T wave, the so-called R on T phenomenon (Figure 3-6). Clearly the acute appearance of ventricular fibrillation should be treated with DC countershock, and thereafter prophylactic antiarrhythmic treatment commenced.

Escape Beats

Escape beats are ectopic beats occurring from a site anywhere in the heart following a cardiac pause. An escape beat is, therefore, a late phenomenon and becomes manifest when the sinus pacemaker fails to dominate the heart rhythm (Figure 3-7). Escape beats usually arise from the atria, the atrioventricular junction, and the ventricles. The lower down in the conducting system the shorter the pause and sinus escape beats have the longest pauses. An escape beat may develop into an escape rhythm when there is severe conduction system disease.

SUMMARY

Many cardiac arrhythmias are extremely common in the elderly and become more frequent as

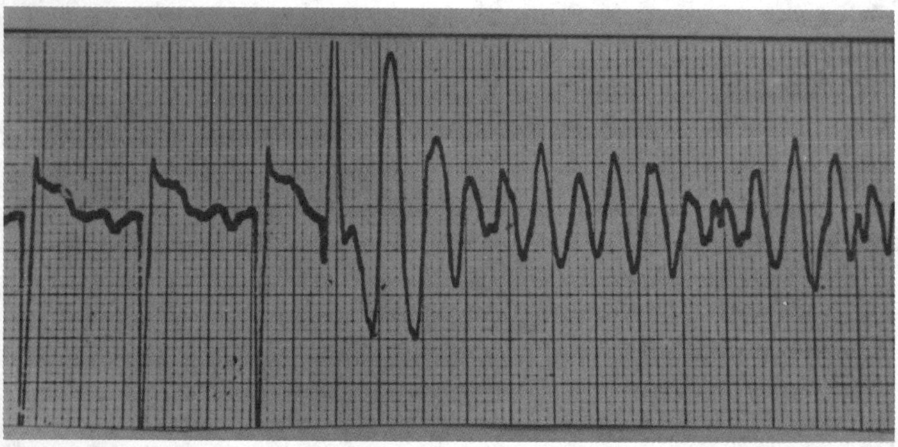

Figure 3-6 Ventricular fibrillation initiated by ventricular premature beat occurring on preceding T wave (R on T phenomenon).

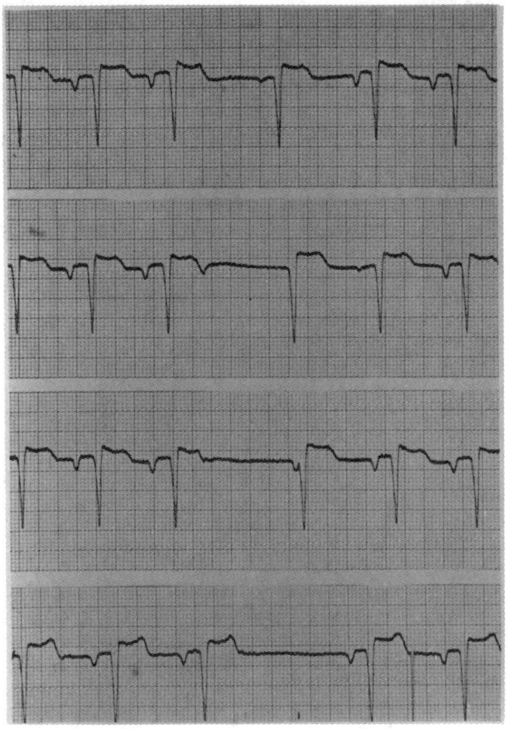

Figure 3-7 Escape beats of various types. 1st tracing: atrial escape beat; 2nd tracing: junctional escape beat; 3rd tracing: atrial/junctional escape beat; 4th tracing: sinus escape beat.

age advances. In many patients symptoms may not be associated even with serious disorders of rhythm. In general bradycardias produces dizziness and syncope, and tachycardias give rise to angina and symptoms of left ventricular failure.

Sinus node degeneration may produce a wide spectrum of rhythm disorders of which severe sinus bradycardia, sinus arrest, and atrial fibrillation are the most important. Although the sick sinus syndrome is usually regarded as posing little threat to life, this condition usually has a marked effect on morbidity and treatment is required either with drugs or permanent cardiac pacing.

Ventricular ectopy is extremely common, even in asymptomatic patients. Although more long-term follow-up research is required, it does appear that simple ventricular ectopic beats occurring at rates of more than 10 per hour may have a significant effect on mortality even in asymptomatic people and thus require treatment. Ventricular ectopy occurring in the presence of acute coronary artery disease in both young and old patients alike may lead to sudden death and require treatment.

REFERENCES

1. Gavey CJ: The cardiology of old age. *Lancet* 1946;2:725–736.
2. Mihalick MJ, Fisch C: Electrocardiographic findings in the aged. *Am Heart J* 1974;87:117–128.
3. Martin A: The Natural History of Atrial Fibrillation in the Elderly, thesis. Loyola University, 1974.
4. Camm AJ, Evans KE, Ward DE, et al: The rhythm of the heart in active elderly subjects. *Am Heart J* 1980;99:598.
5. Rai GS: Cardiac arrhythmias in the elderly. *Age and Ageing* 1982;11:113.
6. Fleg JL, Kennedy HL: Cardiac arrhythmias in a healthy elderly population. *Chest* 1982;81:302–307.
7. Raftery EB, Cashman PM: Long-term recording of the electrocardiogram in a normal population. *Postgrad Med J* (Suppl)1976;52:32–38.
8. Southall DP, Orrell MJ, Talbot JF, et al: Study of cardiac arrhythmias and other forms of conduction abnormality in newborn infants. *Br Med J* 1977; 2:597.
9. Verbaan CJ, Poole J: Incidence of cardiac arrhythmias in a presumed healthy population. *Proceedings of the 2nd International Symposium on Ambulatory Monitoring.* London, Academic Press, 1978.
10. Gerstenblith G, Fleg JL, VanTosh A, et al: Stress testing redefines the prevalence of coronary artery disease in epidemiologic studies. *Circulation* 1980; 62:69–75.
11. Martin A, Benbow LJ, Butrous G, et al: Five year followup of 106 elderly subjects by means of long-term ambulatory cardiac monitoring, in press.
12. De Bono DP, Warlow CP, Hyman NM: Cardiac rhythmias abnormalities in patients presenting with transient non-focal neurological symptoms: A diagnostic grey area? *Br Med J* 1982;284:1437.
13. Martin A, Camm AJ: Transient cardiac arrhythmias and fractures of the femur. *Br Med J* 1981;1: 400.
14. Davies MJ: Pathology of the conducting system, in Pomerance A, Davies MJ (eds): *The Pathology of the Heart.* Oxford, Blackwell, 1975.
15. Cranefield PF: *The Slow Response and Cardiac Arrhythmias.* Mt Kisco, New York, Futura Press, 1975.
16. Shaw DB, Holman RR, Gowers JI: Survival in sinoatrial disorder (sick sinus syndrome). *Br Med J* 1980;1:139.
17. Kulbertus HE, De Leval-Rutten F, Albert A, et al: Electrocardiographic changes occurring with advancing age, in Wellens HJJ, Kulbertus HE (eds): *What's New in Electrocardiography.* The Hague, Martinus Nijhoff, 1981.
18. McNamara RJ: A study of the electrocardiogram in persons over seventy. *Geriatrics* 1949;4:140.
19. Dighton DH: Sinus bradycardia. Autonomic influences and clinical assessment. *Br Heart J* 1974; 36:791.
20. Friedman G: Sinus bradycardia in the aged. *J Am Geriatr Soc* 1978;26:289.
21. Agruss NS, Rosin EY, Adolf RJ, et al: Significance of chronic sinus bradycardia in elderly people. *Circulation* 1972;46:924.
22. Wosika PH, Feldman E, Chesrow EJ, et al: Uni-

polar precordial and limb lead electrocardiograms in the aged. *Geriatrics* 1950;5:130.
23. Clee MD, Smith N, McNeill GP, et al: Dysrhythmias in apparently healthy elderly subjects. *Age and Ageing* 1979;8:173.
24. Cushny AR, Edmunds CW: Paroxysmal irregularity of the heart and auricular fibrillation. *Am J Sci* 1907;133:66.
25. Hamilton BN: The heart in toxic thyroid states. *Surg Clin North Am* 1924;4:1411.
26. Sandler G, Wison GM: The nature and prognosis of heart disease in thyrotoxicosis. *Q J Med* 1959; 111:347.
27. Graves RJ: Adam Waldie clinical lectures delivered during sessions of 1834–1835 and 1836–1837. Philadelphia, 1838.
28. Likoff WB, Levine SA: Thyrotoxicosis as the sole cause of heart failure. *Am J Med Sci* 1943;206:425.
29. Jeffreys PM: The prevalence of thyroid disease in patients admitted to a geriatric department. *Age and Ageing* 1972;1:33.
30. Wang R, Camm J, Ward D, et al: Treatment of chronic atrial fibrillation in the elderly, assessed by ambulatory electrocardiographic monitoring. *J Am Geriatr Soc* 1980;28:529.
31. Papper S: The effects of age in reducing renal function. *Geriatrics* 1973;28:83.
32. Rosenbaum MO, Chiale PA, Halpern MS, et al: Clinical efficacy of amiodarone as an antiarrhythmic agent. *Am J Cardiol* 1976;38:934.
33. Ward DE, Camm AJ, Spurrell RAJ: Clinical antiarrhythmic effects of amiodarone in patients with resistant tachycardias. *Br Heart J* 1980;44:91.
34. Singh BN, Vaughan-Williams EM: A third class of anti-arrhythmic action. Effects on atrial and ventricular intracellular potentials, and other pharmacological actions on cardiac muscle, of MJ1999 and AH3474. *Br J Pharmacol* 1970;39:675.
35. Resnekov L, McDonald L: Complications in 220 patients with cardiac dysrhythmias treated by phased direct current shock, and indications for electroconversion. *Br Heart J* 1967;29:926.
36. McCarthy C, Varghese PJ, Barritt DW: Prognosis of atrial arrhythmias treated by electrical counter shock therapy. *Br Heart J* 1969;31:496.
37. Wolff L, Parkinson S, White PD: Bundle branch block with short P-R interval in healthy young people prone to paroxysmal tachycardia. *Am Heart J* 1930;5:685.
38. Lown B, Ganong WF, Levine SA: The syndrome of short P-R interval, normal QRS complex and paroxysmal rapid heart action. *Circulation* 1952;5: 693.
39. Hollman A, Holt PM: Effectiveness of amiodarone in resistant arrhythmias. *J Roy Soc Med* 1980;73: 842.
40. Wellens HJJ: Contribution of cardiac pacing to our understanding of the Wolff-Parkinson-White syndrome. *Br Heart J* 1975;37:231.
41. Sealy WC, Gallagher JJ, Pritchett ELC: The surgical anatomy of Kent bundles based on electrophysiological mapping and surgical exploration. *J Thorac Cardiovasc Surg* 1978;76:804.
42. Lown B, Wolff M: Approaches to sudden death from coronary heart disease. *Circulation* 1971;44: 130.
43. Vismara LA, Pratt C, Price JE, et al: Correlation of the standard electrocardiogram and continuous ambulatory monitoring in the detection of ventricular arrhythmias in coronary patients. *J Electrocardiol* 1977;10:299.
44. Kotler MN, Tabatznik B, Maver MM, et al: Prognostic significance of ventricular ectopic beats with respect to sudden death in the late post infarction period. *Circulation* 1973;47:959.
45. Hinkle LE, Carver ST, Stevens M: The frequency of asymptomatic disturbances of cardiac rhythm and conduction in middle-aged men. *Am J Cardiol* 1969;24:629.
46. Rabkin SW, Mathewson FAL, Tate RB: Relationship of ventricular ectopy in men without apparent heart disease to occurrence of ischemic heart disease and sudden death. *Am Heart J* 1981;101: 135.

CHAPTER 4
Left Ventricular Wall Motion and Function in Elderly Patients

S. E. Warren
W. V. R. Vieweg

There are two contradictory hypotheses of longevity that divine the future of an American population whose average life expectancy increased from 47 years in 1900 to about 73 years today: one is a vision of life in which the individual is ever more aged, more infirm, and who requires an increasingly weighty share of goods and services to sustain a life low in vigor and prospects; the other hypothesis is that since *maximum* life expectancy has probably not changed over the years,[1] it will be possible to live longer on average, to be more vigorous till a greater fraction of maximum expectancy has been achieved. The populace will get slightly older for a time, then plateau; but the opportunity for continued vitality to a late age will expand, compressing morbidity to a short space.

Whether the first or second hypothesis is correct, the physician will increasingly be confronted with a complex array of cardiovascular problems in the elderly. Some of these may, as in the first example, be solved without result greater than the maintenance of tenuous infirmity; on the other hand, the physician will certainly have to deal with potentially robust older individuals who deserve medical care that comprehends their special needs. This chapter has been written with the latter patients in mind and will focus on left ventricular wall motion and function in the elderly.

The opinions and assertions contained herein are solely those of the authors and do not necessarily reflect those of the U.S. Navy.

GENERAL CONCEPTS OF AGING

With aging, cells that have a finite life span or a finite number of cell doublings enter a phase of dysfunction that leads to their death. If enough cells in any organ become sick, that organ will fail first by losing its reserve—a process likely to be detected only when the organism is stressed or exercised. Later, the dysfunction occurs at rest. Underlying this functional decline are such cellular impairments as a reduction in oxidative phosphorylation,[2] in adrenergic responsiveness,[3] and in DNA[4] and RNA[5] synthesis. We do not know, in the case of the myocardium, whether such impairments are environmentally determined or part of some lifelong genetic message that summons the organ to obsolescence.[6] Fortunately, the reserve of cardiac function is great—output may increase many times with need. The task is now to define how this reserve is dissipated; to define and examine the characteristics of "presbycardia," to differentiate them from the narrower concept of "disease."

CARDIAC PATHOLOGY OF AGING

The pathologist may find almost any cardiac condition in the elderly patient that he might encounter in the younger individual.[7] This includes even such congenital diseases as atrial septal defect, bicuspid aortic valve, and, rarely, tetralogy of Fallot, Ebstein's anomaly, patent ductus arteriosus, or coarctation of the aorta.[7,8] Findings from a geriatric autopsy series previously reported by Pomerance[7] are tabulated in Table 4-1, showing that only ischemic heart disease, senile cardiac amyloidosis, and hypertensive heart disease are both (1) common in the elderly and (2) pathologic processes capable of altering myocardial function and wall motion. Cardiac amyloidosis has elsewhere been reported in the hearts of 30% to 69% of people over the age of 60 years at autopsy.[9-12] The deposits are usually small and incidental: uncommonly do they produce the clinical syndrome of congestive heart failure, low ECG voltage, left axis deviation, pseudoinfarction ECG pattern, and systolic murmur.[9] This leaves, for practical purposes, ischemic heart disease and hypertension as disease states common enough to influence any generalizations one might make about geriatric myocardial function and wall motion. Excluding these entities, which will be discussed later, one may say that structurally the senescent myocardium undergoes relatively few normal aging changes.[7]

Some few changes have been noted, however. There may be diminished heart muscle bulk, a function of reduced body weight and lean muscle mass;[13-15] conversely, an age-related increase in relative heart weight[16] and myocardial hypertrophy[17] have been reported, perhaps related to age-dependent increases in systolic blood pressure[16] or to ischemia.[18] It should be underscored that aging and hypertrophy are not synonymous and need not coexist. Both, however, are associated experimentally with an increased presence of connective tissue precursors.[19-24] In aged man collagen increases in the interventricular septum,[25] collagen and elastic tissue increase in the atria,[26] and fat accumulates in the interatrial septum.[27] The factors commonly altering heart weight in advanced age are summarized in Table 4-2. In general, those favoring an increase in myocardial bulk usually predominate, though they may not all be considered aging changes per se. Where pronounced, increased myocardial bulk and replacement with noncontractile tissue may lead to a stiffened muscle of diminished diastolic compliance.

Table 4-1
Cardiac Pathology in the Elderly

Findings in 240 Patients	Incidence (%)
Ischemic heart disease	29
Aortic calcification	26
Senile cardiac amyloidosis	25
Hypertensive heart disease	18
Mitral ring calcification	18
Mitral scarring	12
Aortic stenosis	9
Mitral mucoid degeneration	7
Mitral stenosis	3
Nonbacterial endocarditis	3
Bacterial endocarditis	1
Cor pulmonale	1
Miscellaneous (cardiomyopathy, myocarditis, functional aortic insufficiency, congenital heart disease, syphilis, rheumatoid heart disease, carcinoid, neoplasm)	<1

Pathologic findings of general hospital geriatric autopsies: Nortwick Park Hospital 1971–1974, England. Adapted from Pomerance.[7]

MYOCARDIAL FUNCTION

Heart Rate

Having noted that gross pathologic changes of the aged heart are small in the absence of hypertension or coronary artery disease, one may turn to the voluminous data on cardiac function, summarized as follows: aging is associated with reduced demand, normal myocardial function at rest, and diminished maximum function with exercise. Basal oxygen uptake is reduced.[28] Resting heart rate is unchanged,[29] but maximum exercise heart rate (HR_{max}) declines both in aging athletes and in the untrained population.[30] For cross-sectional data the reduction in HR_{max} is about 1 bpm per year from middle age; for longitudinal data the decline is 0.4 to 0.7 bpm per year.[30] The variation around the data points for HR_{max} is wide, however, and the standard deviation is 10 bpm or more.[30] A further reduction in HR_{max} may occur after myocardial infarction. Other reported ECG changes of aging include lower wave ampli-

Table 4-2
Factors Which Determine Heart Weight in the Elderly

Decreased heart weight
1. Diminished body muscle mass
2. Deconditioning

Increased heart weight
1. Increased systolic blood pressure
2. Ischemia
3. Replacement of heart muscle with fat and connective tissue

Factors favoring increased heart bulk usually predominate; this may lead to diminished diastolic compliance.

tudes, leftward axis shift, longer PR and QT intervals, and shorter QRS interval.[31]

What is the explanation for this reduction in HR_{max} from middle to advanced age? Some possible explanations for geriatric HR_{max} decrements include (1) structural or chemical changes in the pacer tissue, (2) decreased responsiveness of autonomic reflexes, (3) diminished adrenergic responsiveness, and (4) deconditioning; the elderly have a normal intrinsic heart rate but steeper increments with exercise to a point short of HR_{max} in youth.[32]

The significance of these changes in exercise heart rate centers on the existence of wide individual differences. If an exercise stress test (EST) is taken to a predicted heart rate short of the true HR_{max}, short of fatigue, there is great error in interpreting both oxygen uptake and the results of the test itself.[30] Therefore, ESTs should terminate at fatigue rather than predicted HR_{max}. Secondly, though resting heart rate may be normal in the elderly and HR_{max} less, the rapid ascent of heart rate and blood pressure at the start of exercise in the deconditioned may provoke angina or cardiac arrhythmias. Exercise for health maintenance in this age group should be gradual and should include a warm-up period.

Cardiac Output

Decreases in maximum stroke volume, maximum cardiac output, and maximum oxygen uptake occur with aging in both animals and man.[33-37] Radionuclide angiography in healthy adults has disclosed the following effects of advanced age: normal resting left ventricular ejection fraction, end-diastolic volume, and regional wall motion; with exercise, absolute ejection fraction and its degree of change from resting values were reduced in older subjects.[38] Wall motion abnormalities during exercise occurred with increasing frequency in patients aged 50 years and older (Table 4-3).[38] These abnormalities occurred in the absence of age-related differences in end-diastolic volume or blood pressure. Moreover, heart rate at peak exercise did not correlate with ejection fraction. These observations tend to discount the notion that diminished exercise performance in elderly subjects was due to aberrations of heart rate or loading conditions; rather, there appears to exist an old age (not disease)-dependent diminished contractile reserve.[38] Echocardiography in the normal elderly has revealed increased left ventricular (LV) wall thickness, decreased mitral e-to-f slope, and increased aortic root diameter.[34] These findings suggest that altered diastolic filling is also

Table 4-3
Prevalence of Exercise Left Ventricular Dysfunction by Decade in 77 Healthy Volunteers Aged 20 to 95 Years

	Subjects with Abnormal	
Decade	*Ejection Fraction (%)*	*Wall Motion (%)*
3	2	2
4	2	2
5	10	2
6	30	11
7	55	33
8–10	95	44

Adapted from Port et al.[38] Results were obtained by nuclear angiocardiography.

a characteristic of the aging process.[34] A summary of the factors discussed so far that may be contributory to LV dysfunction and wall motion abnormalities in the elderly appears in Figure 4-1.

PATHOPHYSIOLOGY OF ALTERED SENESCENT MYOCARDIAL FUNCTION

At this time it may be fair to make the generalization that in the normal elderly, ventricular wall motion abnormalities will occur more as a result of age-dependent decreased contractile reserve, and then only with exercise; in the older patient with hypertension and/or ischemic heart disease the severity of the pathologic process will influence pump function via effects on loading conditions, compliance, or anoxia. Lakatta and Yin[39] have elegantly dissected the functional and cellular mechanisms of myocardial aging based on animal and human data, including contractility, excitation-contraction coupling, myocardial hypertrophy, and energy production and delivery. This is important, not only to better understand the possible cellular basis for diminished contractile reserve, but to discriminate that process from disease hypertrophy. Their preliminary findings are summarized as follows: the predominant functional and cellular abnormalities that underlie diminished cardiac function in the aged are (1) selective (and not global) decrements in the contractile response to certain stimuli, including drugs and catecholamines; (2) more diffuse, multistep abnormalities of excitation-contraction coupling; and (3) diminished energy production and delivery, including decreased small coronary blood flow.[39] There appear to be no abnormal intrinsic myofilament properties, and maximum force

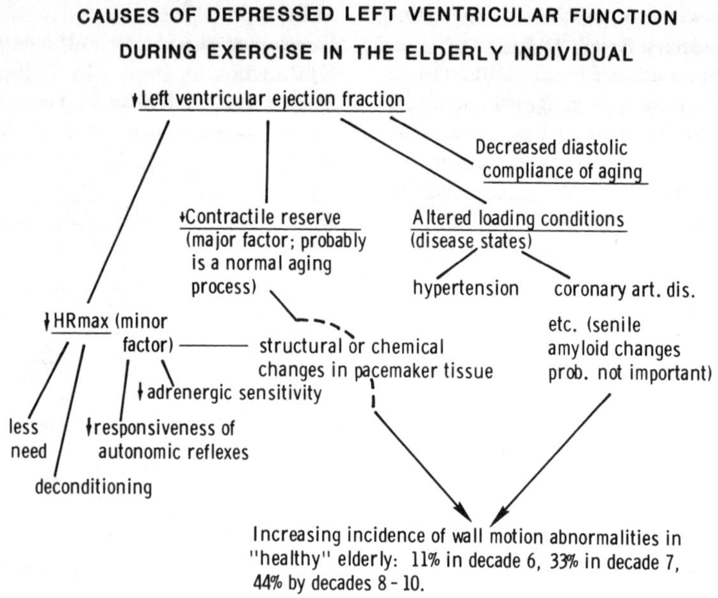

Figure 4-1 Causes of abnormal ventricular function during exercise.

developed is normal. This would place the burden of diminished exercise performance more on the diastolic properties of the aging heart. Hypertrophy, if present, is mild and does not explain the previously mentioned changes of senescence. It is noteworthy that certain of the old-age abnormalities are reversible to an extent by regular exercise: prolonged isometric myocardial contraction, decreased microsomal calcium sequestration, and diminished capillary density (Table 4-4).

We have now seen that decreased exercise myocardial function occurs in normal senescent myocardium, leading to a high age-dependent incidence of systolic and diastolic wall motion dysfunction. This reduction of myocardial reserve is due to ultrastructural, biochemical, and physiologic changes.[38,39]

Because of the high incidence of coronary artery disease and hypertension in the elderly, it is necessary to include a discussion of these pathologic processes in any analysis of geriatric left ventricular function.

ISCHEMIC HEART DISEASE

The incidence of atherosclerotic coronary artery disease (CAD) increases with age and has been estimated to be as high as 65% in the elderly.[40,41] A classic history of angina pectoris may be difficult to elicit, however, due to reduced physical activity or other medical problems.[42] Independent risk factors for CAD in patients over 60 years of age include only age itself and hypertension.[43] If a clinical diagnosis of CAD is made and the patient taken to angiography, there will be greater prevalence of confirmatory findings at catheterization in the geriatric than in the young population.[44-46] Noninvasive tests, such as the exercise stress test or exercise radionuclide scan, are harder to interpret in the elderly because of deconditioning, submaximal effort, underestimation of the true maximum heart rate, and the diminished myocardial function of aging already noted.[30,38]

Of the patients who were studied invasively by us for previous myocardial infarction,[47] those under 35 years of age presented a heterogeneous etiologic picture of atherosclerosis/obstruction (82%), normal coronary arteries (13%), and congenital coronary artery anomalies (4%). The findings in the middle-aged and in the elderly patient, usually studied for ischemic symptoms, show an overwhelming preponderance of atherosclerotic heart disease.[48] Thus it makes sense to study *all* young patients with prior myocardial infarction for reasons of etiology (about 20% do not have atherosclerosis) and prognosis (prognosis is better with normal coronary arteries or single vessel disease)[47,49]; the older patient, and particularly the elderly one, is studied more on the basis of refractory symptoms and surgical candidacy.

Table 4-4
Symptomatic Coronary Artery Disease Differences: Young vs Elderly

	Young	Elderly
Incidence	Low	High
Symptoms	Classic	Variable
Risk factors	Usually present in patients >30 years of age	Only hypertension and age are independent risk factors in patients 60 years of age and older
Diagnosis	Conventional approach	Decreased exercise capacity and HRmax limit interpretation of the exercise stress test; do not perform invasive diagnostic tests only on the basis of an abnormal ejection fraction response to exercise; contrast dye may worsen renal function in the elderly with depressed glomerular filtration rate
Distribution of coronary artery disease (CAD)	Atherosclerotic: Young patients may have a higher incidence of normal coronary arteries or anomalies	No difference
Left ventricular dyssenergy pattern	Similar distribution in 3rd through 8th decades	No age difference; greater incidence in elderly
Mortality rate and prognosis	Determined by extent of CAD and left ventricular function	Elderly have higher mortality after myocardial infarction (MI); MI is leading cause of death in patient >80 undergoing general surgery
Treatment	Age per se is not a contraindication to coronary surgery, young or elderly adulthood	Elderly are more likely to have drug-induced myocardial depression (beta-blockers, thiopental sodium, etc), and orthostatic hypotension (limit use of nitrates); elderly may not understand or take medicine properly

The distribution of CAD is not affected by age in patients with *angina.*[48] About 80% of such cases have multivessel disease. The CAD seems to be a diffuse process: patients with CAD have smaller coronary arteries generally than those without disease.[48] Single-vessel disease in over-30 age groups tends to have the following descending frequency of involvement: left anterior descending coronary artery > right coronary artery > circumflex/marginal coronary artery.[50] For two-vessel disease the order is left anterior descending and right coronary artery > combinations involving the circumflex/marginal coronary artery.[51] Thus, in the elderly patient the circumflex/marginal system contributes least to symptomatic CAD.

In patients with CAD studied because of angina pectoris the left ventricular dyssynergy pattern is similar from the third through the eighth decade.[52] The dyssynergy is anterior in one third of cases, posterior in one third, and both anterior and posterior in one third. Hypokinesis was the most common wall motion abnormality except at the apex, where dyskinesis was the most common expression of dyssynergy. Left ventricular dyssynergy was not altered by coronary arterial pattern (dominance).[53] It took a 90% reduction in cross-sectional coronary luminal diameter to produce these wall motion disturbances.[53] Since it is unlikely that most ambulatory elderly patients are asymptomatic with 90% coronary artery stenoses, the high incidence of wall motion abnormalities found in the exercised elderly normal population by noninvasive methods[38] must probably be attributed to aging changes per se, rather than "silent" CAD.

As for prognosis of coronary atherosclerosis, the main negative determinants are anatomic severity and poor left ventricular function,[54,55] followed by older age.[56,57] Given that the elderly have a greater incidence (though not necessarily greater severity of symptoms) of CAD, greater decrements in myocardial reserve as a function of aging, and advanced age itself, it is easy to understand their more guarded long-term prognosis. Since risk factors for coronary ischemia play a smaller role here than in the middle years, there is potentially less to reverse, less environmentally to modify and treat in old people with CAD. Moreover, beta-blockers and nitrates must be used with caution in the elderly, due to the risk of myocardial depression in the first instance and orthostatic hypotension in the second. Myocardial infarction may be the leading cause of death in patients over the age of 80 years who undergo surgery,[58] so that careful assessment of this group of patients with diminished cardiac reserve must be done preoperatively. A grouping of CAD considerations in the elderly is found in Table 4-4.

HYPERTENSION AND IMPEDANCE

Although not strictly considered a normal aging change, hypertension in the elderly contributes to CAD, increased myocardial work, left ventricular hypertrophy, and decreased ventricular compliance. Though it is generally recognized that arterial blood pressure increases with age, systolic blood pressure actually increases in the adult to a greater degree than the diastolic pressure.[43] After the age of 80, however, Master et al report that systolic blood pressure (sBP) remains stationary in men and may fall in women. Diastolic arterial pressure (dBP) tends to fall after age 80 in both men and women.[59] Kamel reports that there is no rise in sBP in men after age 68; dBP tends to fall after age 60.[60] Thus, many of the extreme elderly do not have hypertension, or may in fact have very labile[61] arterial blood pressures that render them sensitive to medications.

A second consideration involves the indirect measurement of arterial pressure. Berliner et al[62] find that for patients under age 70, indirect blood pressure (iBP) exceeds that measured directly by arterial transducer (tBP); for patients over 70, however, the situation is often reversed: tBP > iBP. Thus, the cuff may on occasion underestimate arterial blood pressure in the elderly; unless the cuff is narrow and the patient's arm large, one should certainly not assume that pseudohypertension is present.

A detailed discussion of the pathogenesis of hypertension in the elderly is beyond the scope of this paper. The main findings are as follows: (1) high peripheral resistance—the salient systemic and renal vascular hemodynamic abnormality[63]; (2) age-related decreased plasma renin activity[64,65] without plasma volume expansion; (3) increased plasma norepinephrine levels with decreased beta-adrenergic sensitivity[43,66]—the elderly may thus be more dependent on alpha than beta tone to regulate peripheral flow.[66] These considerations would make diuretics (especially the vasodilatory thiazides), sympatholytics that do not depress myocardial function (such as clonidine), and vasodilators (such as hydralazine) ideal for a stepped-care therapeutic approach.

In conclusion, it is hoped that a thorough understanding of myocardial wall motion and left ventricular function—the variables that pertain in healthful aging and in disease—will be used to promote continued vigor throughout a maximum quantum of the biologically finite human life span.

REFERENCES

1. Fries JF: Aging, natural death, and the compression of morbidity. *New Engl J Med* 1980;303:130–135.
2. Brouwer A, Van Bezooijen C, Knook DC: Respiratory activities of hepatocytes isolated from rats of various ages—A brief note. *Mech Aging Develop* 1977;6:265–269.
3. Lakatta EG: Age-related alterations in the cardiovascular response to adrenergic mediated stress. *Fed Proc* 1980;39:2173–2177.
4. Cristofalo VJ, Sharf BB: Cellular senescence and DNA synthesis. *Exp Cell Res* 1973;76:419–427.
5. Macierira-Coelha A, Ponten J, Philipson L: The division cycle and RNA synthesis in diploid human cells at different passage levels in vitro. *Exp Cell Res* 1966;42:673–684.
6. Scoggin CH: The cellular basis of aging. *West J Med* 1981;135:521–525.
7. Pomerance A: Cardiac pathology in the elderly, in Noble RJ, Rothbaum DA (eds): *Geriatric Cardiology*. Philadelphia, FA Davis, 1981, pp 9–54.
8. Perloff JK: Postpediatric congenital heart disease: Natural survival patterns. *Cardiovasc Clin* 1979; 10(1):27.
9. Buja LM, Khoi NB, Roberts WC: Clinically significant cardiac amyloidosis. Clinicopathologic findings in 15 patients. *Am J Cardiol* 1970;26:394–405.
10. Schwartz P, Kurucz J: Amyloid deposits in the hearts of aged persons. New aspects of cardiovascular disease. *J Am Geriatr Soc* 1965;13:718–722.
11. Wright JH, Calkins E, Breen WJ, et al: Relationship of amyloid to aging. Review of the literature and systematic study of 83 patients derived from a general hospital population. *Medicine (Baltimore)* 1969;48:39–60.
12. Pomerance A: Senile cardiac amyloidosis. *Br Heart J* 1965;27:711–718.
13. Bowles LT, Portnoi V, Kenney R: Wear and tear:

Common biologic changes of aging. *Geriatrics* 1981; 36(4):77–93.
14. Reiner L, Mazzoleni A, Rodriguez FL, et al: The weight of the human heart. I. "Normal" cases. *Arch Pathol* 1959;65:58–62.
15. Reiner L: in Gould SE (ed): *Pathology of the Heart*. Springfield, Ill, Charles C Thomas, 1960.
16. Linzback AJ, Akuamoa-Boateng E: The alterations of the aging human heart. I. Heart weight with progressing age. *Klin Wochenschr* 1973;51:156–159.
17. Lakatta EG: Alterations in the cardiovascular system that occur in advanced age. *Fed Proc* 1979;38: 163–167.
18. Hodkinson I, Pomerance A, Hodksinson HM: Heart size in the elderly: A clinicopathological study. *J R Soc Med* 1979;72:13–16.
19. Bing OHL, Fanburg BL, Brooks WW, et al: The effect of the lathyrogen beta-amino proprionitrile (BAPN) on the mechanical properties of experimentally hypertrophied rat muscle. *Circ Res* 1978; 43:632–637.
20. Buccino R, Harris AE, Spann JF Jr, et al: Response of myocardial connective tissue to development of experimental hypertrophy. *Am J Physiol* 1969;216: 425–428.
21. Hickson RC, Hammons GT, Holloszy JO: Development and regression of exercise-induced cardiac hypertrophy in rats. *Am J Physiol* (Heart Circ Physiol 5) 1979;236:H268–H272.
22. Lindy S, Turto H, Uitto J: Protocollagen proline hydroxylase activity in rat heart during experimental cardiac hypertrophy. *Circ Res* 1972;30:205–209.
23. Schaub MC: The aging of collagen in the heart muscle. *Gerontologia* 1964/1965;10:38–41.
24. Weisfeldt ML, Loeven WA, Shock NW: Resting and active mechanical properties of trabeculae carnae from aged male rats. *Am J Physiol* 1971;220: 1921–1927.
25. Lenkiewicz JE, Davies MJ, Rosen D: Collagen in human myocardium as a function of age. *Cardiovasc Res* 1972;6:549–552.
26. Davies MJ, Pomerance A: Quantitative study of aging changes in the human sinoatrial node and internodal tracts. *Br Heart J* 1972;34:150–155.
27. Page DL: Lipomatous hypertrophy of the cardiac interatrial septum: Its development and probable clinical significance. *Hum Pathol* 1970;1:151–156.
28. Keys A, Taylor HL, Grande F: Basal metabolism and age of adult man. *Metabolism* 1973;22:579–582.
29. Amery A, Wasir H, Bulpitt C, et al: Aging and the cardiovascular system. *Acta Cardiol* 1978;33: 443–447.
30. Wilmore JH: Applied physiologic concerns and benefits in cardiovascular rehabilitation, in Pollock ML, Schmidt DH (eds): *Heart Disease and Rehabilitation*. New York, John Wiley and Sons, 1979, pp 678–680.
31. Bachman S, Sparrow D, Smith LK: Effect of aging on the electrocardiogram. *Am J Cardiol* 1981; 48:513–516.
32. Kostis JB, Moreyra AE, Amendo MT, et al: The effect of age on heart rate in subjects free of heart disease. *Circulation* 1982;65:141–145.
33. Templeton GH, Platt MR, Willerson JT, et al: Influence of aging on left ventricular hemodynamics and stiffness of beagles. *Circ Res* 1979;44:189–194.
34. Gerstenblith G, Fredericksen J, Yin FCP, et al: Echocardiographic assessment of a normal adult aging population. *Circulation* 1977;56:273–278.
35. Yin FCP, Raizes GS, Guarneri T, et al: Age-associated decrease in ventricular response to a hemodynamic stress during beta adrenergic blockade. *Br Heart J* 1978;40:1349–1355.
36. Lakatta EG, Gerstenblith G, Angell CS, et al: Diminished inotropic response of aged myocardium to catecholamines. *Circ Res* 1975;36:262–269.
37. Yin FCP, Spurgeon HA, Greene HL, et al: Age-associated decrease in heart rate response to isoproterenol in dogs. *Mech Aging Dev* 1979;10:17–25.
38. Port S, Cobb FR, Coleman RE, et al: Effect of age on the response of the left ventricular ejection to exercise. *New Engl J Med* 1980;303:1133–1137.
39. Lakatta EG, Yin FCP: Myocardial Aging: Functional alterations and related cellular mechanisms. *Heart Circ Physiol* 1982;11:H927–H941.
40. Tejada C, Strong JP, Montenegro MR, et al: Distribution of coronary and aortic atherosclerosis by geographic location, race, and sex. *Lab Invest* 1968;18:509–526.
41. White NK, Edwards JE, Dry TJ: The relationship of the degree of coronary atherosclerosis with age, in men. *Circulation* 1950;1:645–654.
42. Rothbaum DA: Coronary artery disease, in Noble PJ, Rothbaum DA (eds): *Geriatric Cardiology*. Philadelphia, FA Davis Co, 1981, pp 105–118.
43. Amery A, Hansson L, Andren L, et al: Hypertension in the elderly. *Acta Med Scand* 1981;210: 221–229.
44. Proudfit WL, Shirey EK, Sones FM Jr: Selective cine coronary arteriography. Correlation with clinical findings in 1000 patients. *Circulation* 1966; 33: 901–910.
45. Proudfit WL, Shirey EK, Sheldon WC, et al: Certain clinical characteristics correlated with extent of obstructive lesions demonstrated by selective cine-coronary angiography. *Circulation* 1968;38:947–954.
46. Proudfit WL, Welch CC, Siqueira C, et al: Prognosis of 1000 young women studied by coronary angiography. *Circulation* 1981;64:1185–1190.
47. Warren SE, Thompson SI, Vieweg WVR: Historic and angiographic features of young adults surviving myocardial infarction. *Chest* 1979;75:667–670.
48. Vieweg WVR, Warren SE, Alpert JS, et al: Comparison of coronary arteriographic and left ventriculographic findings in patients with single, double, and triple vessel disease and angina pectoris. *Cathet Cardiovasc Diagn* 1981;7:155–164.
49. Glover MU, Kuber MT, Warren SE, et al: Myocardial infarction before age 36: Risk factor and arteriographic analysis. *Am J Cardiol* 1982;49: 1600–1603.
50. Vieweg WVR, Warren SE, Alpert JS, et al: The distribution and severity of coronary artery disease and left ventricular dysfunction among patients with single coronary disease and angina pectoris. *Clin Cardiol* 1980;3:241–245.
51. Vieweg WVR, Warren SE, Alpert JS, et al: Coronary arterial and left ventriculographic findings in patients with double vessel disease and angina pectoris. *Clin Cardiol* 1980;3:246–251.
52. Vieweg WVR, Alpert JS, Johnson AD, et al: Distribution and severity of left ventricular wall motion abnormalities according to age and coronary artery

disease and angina pectoris. *Am Heart J* 1980;99: 707–713.
53. Vieweg WVR, Alpert JS, Johnson AD, et al: Coronary artery disease and ventricular function in angina. *South Med J* 1981;74:1079–1083.
54. Ross RS: Ischemic heart disease: An overview. *Am J Cardiol* 1975;36:496–505.
55. Bruschke AVG, Proudfit WL, Sones FM Jr: Progress study of 590 consecutive nonsurgical cases of coronary artery disease followed 5–9 years. *Circulation* 1973;47:1147–1153.
56. Bruschke AVG, Proudfit WL, Sones FM Jr: Clinical course of patients with normal and slightly or moderately abnormal coronary arteriograms. *Circulation* 1973;47:936–945.
57. Bruschke AVG, Proudfit WL, Sones FM Jr: Progress study of 590 consecutive nonsurgical cases of coronary artery disease followed 5–9 years. *Circulation* 1973;47:1154–1163.
58. Djokovic JL, Hedley-Whyte J: Prediction of outcome of surgery and anesthesia in patients over 80. *JAMA* 1979;242:2301–2306.
59. Master AM, Lasser RP, Jaffe HL: Blood pressure in white people over 65 years of age. *Ann Intern Med* 1958;48:284–287.
60. Kamel WB: Blood pressure and the development of cardiovascular disease in the aged, in Chaird FI, Dall J, Kennedy RD (eds): *Cardiology and Old Age*. New York, Plenum Press, 1976, pp 143–176.
61. Colandrea MA, Friedman GD, Nichaman MZ, et al: Systolic hypertension in the elderly. An epidemiologic assessment. *Circulation* 1970;41: 239–242.
62. Berliner K, Fujry H, Lee DH, et al: Blood pressure measurements in obese persons. *Am J Cardiol* 1961;8:10–14.
63. Warren SE, O'Connor DT, Cohen IM, et al: Renal hemodynamic changes during chronic antihypertensive therapy. *Clin Pharmacol Ther* 1981;29: 310–317.
64. Sambhi M, Crane MG, Genest J: Essential hypertension: New concepts and mechanisms. *Ann Intern Med* 1973;79:411–424.
65. Weidman P, de Myttenaere-Bursztein S, Maxwell MH, et al: Effect of aging on plasma renin and aldosterone in normal man. *Kidney Int* 1975;8:325–333.
66. Van Brummelen P, Buhler FR, Kiowski W, et al: Age related decrease in cardiac and peripheral vascular responsiveness to isoprenaline: Studies in normal subjects. *Clin Sci* 1981;60:571–577.

CHAPTER 5
Aging of the Normal Cardiovascular System

Jerome L. Fleg
Edward G. Lakatta

The interval of time between maturation and senescence is host to two distinct but closely interacting processes—"normal" aging and the development of disease. The fact that about two thirds of the deaths past the age of 65 years in America are attributable to cardiovascular disease[1] highlights the difficulty in separating these processes. Aging per se and its attendant changes in life style alter the substrate upon which specific cardiovascular disorders are superimposed. This chapter will focus upon those changes in the heart and peripheral vasculature thought to represent "normal" aging. An understanding of these physiologic aging changes should provide a useful framework for recognizing the various manifestations of cardiac disease peculiar to the elderly.

EFFECTS OF LATENT CARDIOVASCULAR DISEASE AND LIFE STYLE VARIATIONS

A major obstacle that has retarded a true understanding of the effect of aging on the heart is the high prevalence of coronary artery disease (CAD) in the elderly. Autopsy studies in subjects dying from random causes have disclosed significant narrowing of at least one major coronary artery in over 60% of men who survived the sixth decade.[2] In women a similar age-related increase in CAD prevalence is found, but the peak is delayed by two decades.[3] In a more recent postmortem study, 46% of unselected white New Orleans men ages 55 to 64 years of age had significant coronary stenosis.[4] Thus, at least half of a typical American community must be excluded from studies of cardiovascular aging, solely due to the presence of CAD. An even greater obstacle to such studies is the fact that in approximately half of these individuals, the disease is occult.

In epidemiologic studies utilizing a history of angina pectoris or myocardial infarction plus resting electrocardiography (ECG), the prevalence of CAD ranges from 2% to 30% depending on the age bracketing employed. The highest prevalence of CAD found in an elderly community dwelling population older than 75 years is about 30%.[5,6] This is well below the 50% to 60% prevalence found in necropsy studies, again emphasizing the high prevalence of undetected or latent CAD in the general population. It therefore seems likely that many studies which have purported to characterize the effect of age on the cardiovascular system have not studied aging per se but rather aging as modified by occult CAD.

During life, occult CAD can be diagnosed by applying a stress to the cardiovascular system. Such an approach, employing graded treadmill exercise with thallium radionuclide imaging, has been taken in 189 consecutive volunteers from the Baltimore Longitudinal Study on Aging (BLSA), an active community dwelling population.[7] In this technic, 1 to 2 mCi of thallium 201, a potassium analog, is injected into a peripheral vein at the peak of treadmill exercise. Immediately postexercise, the heart is imaged in multiple views with a gamma camera. Because the myocardium takes up thallium in proportion to the blood flow it receives, a significant coronary arterial stenosis will reduce the amount of thallium reaching the myocardium it supplies, thus creating a defect on the image. In 189 consecutive BLSA volunteers in the sixth to ninth decades, the prevalence of CAD by the usual resting criteria (history of angina pectoris or myocardial infarction or abnormalities on the resting ECG suggesting ischemia or prior infarction) ranged between 13% and 22%. When stress criteria were added (either an ischemic ECG response to treadmill exercise or an abnormal exercise thallium scan), the CAD prevalence was doubled,[8] and agreed more closely with autopsy estimates. It is apparent then that cardiovascular stress testing is imperative when selecting a population subset free from CAD for studies of cardiovascular aging.

Additional factors such as the blood pressure level used to define hypertension at a given age, nutritional status, social habits and level of physical fitness may also modify the results of investigation of the "normal" cardiovascular aging process. For example, the physical deconditioning commonly accompanying senescence will accentuate age-related decreases in maximal cardiovascular performance. Thus, in elderly subjects maximal oxygen consumption (VO_{2max}) is not fixed but increases with aerobic training.[9] Similarly, the age-related decline in VO_{2max} in such physically conditioned older persons is only about half of that observed in sedentary individuals of similar age.[10]

CARDIOVASCULAR ANATOMY

Contrary to the once widely held impression that cardiac atrophy occurs with aging, the consensus of recent studies in both animals and man supports the opposite conclusion—a modest age-related hypertrophy of the left ventricular (LV) myocardium. From autopsy data in 7112 human hearts, Linzbach and Akuamoa-Boateng[11] found that between the ages of 30 and 90 years, heart weight increased an average of 1 to 1.5 g per year. Since this study included hearts from individuals with cardiovascular disease as well as normals, some of the age-related increase in cardiac mass may merely reflect a higher prevalence of disease in the older hearts. In the male Wistar rat, Yin et al[12] demonstrated a 14% increase in LV weight but no change in right ventricular weight between middle age and senescence.

Echocardiography has enabled investigators to make accurate noninvasive determinations of cardiac wall thickness and chamber size in living subjects. In 100 healthy men and women, Sjogren[13] demonstrated a progressive increase in LV posterior wall thickness between the ages of 15 and 65 years. The age-related increase in LV posterior wall thickness corrected for body surface area (BSA) in 62 screened healthy men aged 25 to 80 years from the BLSA, all of whom had resting blood pressure less than 140/90 mmHg is shown in Figure 5-1 (A and B).[14] This increase in LV wall thickness, which is seen in both diastole and systole, approximates 30% between ages 25 and 80 years and is similar whether or not measurements are corrected for BSA. No age-related changes in LV diastolic or systolic cavity dimensions were noted in these subjects.

An obvious question, then, is what constitutes the stimulus for this age-associated LV hypertrophy? Such hypertrophy usually occurs in response to a chronic pressure or volume overload such as occurs in valvular disease or hypertension. As wall thickness increases, the abnormally elevated LV wall stress (systolic pressure × radius/wall thickness) returns toward normal. This enhances shortening of each cardiac muscle cell and allows normal ejection of blood during systole. Since neither resting LV dimension nor stroke volume increases substantially with age, volume overload would seem an unlikely cause of this LV hypertrophy. Systolic blood pressure increases with age at rest and at submaximal workloads, even when persons with hypertension are excluded.

Thus, the moderate increase in LV wall thickness that occurs with advancing age may be considered an adaptive mechanism to the increased myocardial workload imposed by a higher systolic blood pressure. The mild age-related dilatation of the ascending aorta may be an additional stimulus for hypertrophy since this augmented volume of blood must be accelerated by the heart for ejection to occur. It should be emphasized that the degree of LV hypertrophy found with aging is mild relative to that seen in most pathologic conditions.

In addition to the changes in LV wall thickness just discussed, echocardiography has elicited additional aging changes. The age-related dilatation of the aortic root alluded to above averaged 6% between the fourth and eighth decades in BLSA men.[14] The similar mild enlargement of the left atrium (LA) which occurs with advancing age is often found in conditions associated with LV hypertrophy, suggesting diminished LV compliance as an etiologic factor. The early diastolic closure rate (E-F slope) of the mitral valve has consistently been found to decrease with age. Such a decrease may reflect impaired early diastolic LV filling secondary to decreased LV compliance or may reflect a primary stiffening of the valve itself. Indeed, the endocardium and its specialized extension, the cardiac valves, have generally been found to thicken with age in pathologic studies. In the Framingham population, the prevalence of a posterior echo-free space[15] (usually indicative of a pericardial effusion) and mitral subvalvular calcification[16] both increased significantly with advancing age. The frequent association of these echocardiographic findings with organic heart disease suggests that they are probably not manifestations of normal aging. Although autopsy studies have commonly shown modest deposition of amyloid and adipose

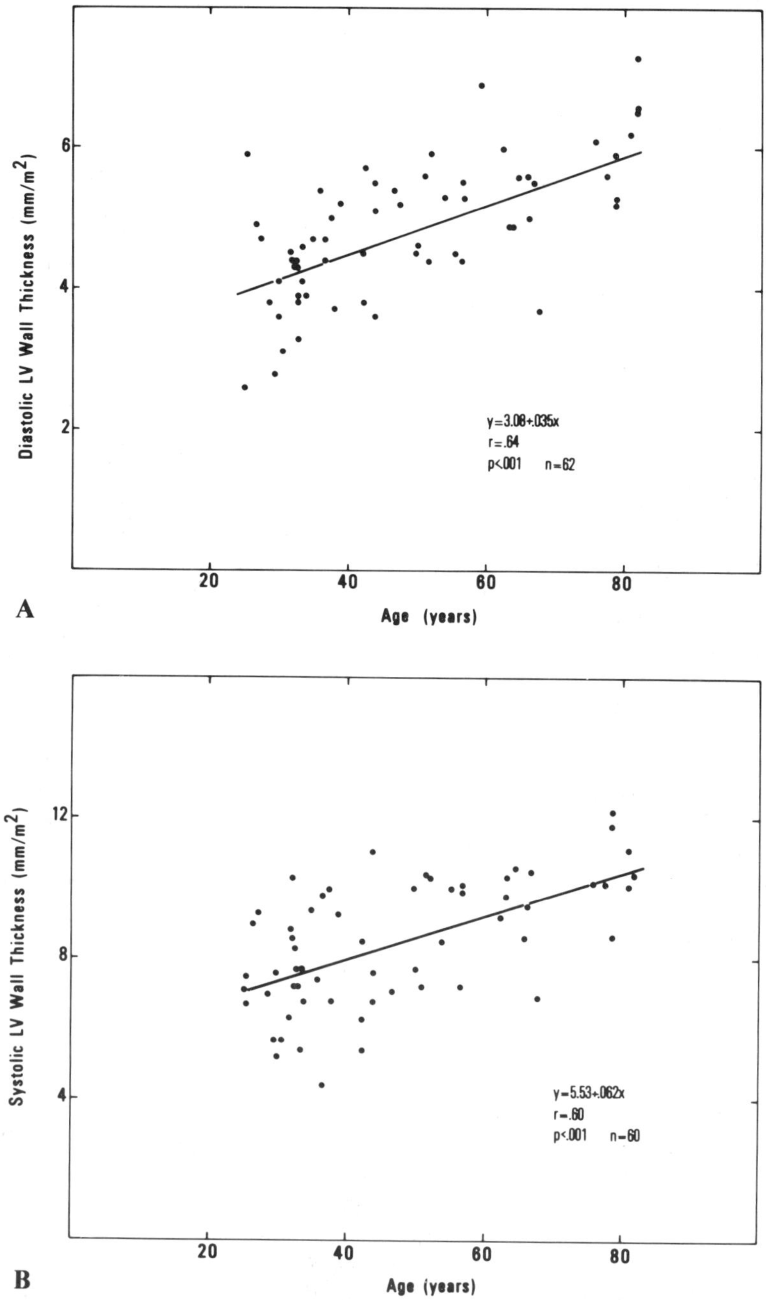

Figure 5-1 The effect of age on the left ventricular posterior wall thickness in diastole **(A)** and systole **(B)**, determined by echocardiography in 62 healthy normotensive men. The wall thickness has been normalized for body surface area to correct for differences in body size. (Reprinted with permission from Gerstenblith et al.[14])

in the myocardium as well as a brownish lipid-laden substance called lipofuchsin, the functional significance of these depositions is uncertain.

Chest Roentgenology

Certain age-related changes are demonstrable in the standard chest roentgenogram. Chest deformities caused by kyphoscoliosis and emphysema frequently alter the normal relationship between the heart and chest cavity and may cause factitious cardiomegaly. In 66 rigorously screened healthy men from the BLSA whose initial mean age was 48 years, a longitudinal increment of cardiothoracic ratio (CTR) from .405 to .427 was found over a 17-year follow-up.[16a] The modest increment in CTR is caused by a small increase in cardiac diameter and a diminution in chest diameter with advancing age. CTR did not exceed .51 in any man, thus supporting the specificity of a CTR greater than 50% for cardiac pathology in senescence as in younger subjects, so long as major chest deformities are absent. There was an age-related increase in aortic dimension over time, confirming the dilatation noted in cross-sectional echocardiographic studies. Aortic knob calcification and aortic tortuosity develop commonly in older men and therefore do not by themselves indicate cardiovascular disease. On the other hand, intracardiac calcification is rarely detected; such calcification may arise from the aortic valve, mitral annulus, pericardium, coronary arterial tree, or a ventricular aneurysm and should nearly always be considered pathologic.

Conduction System and Electrophysiology

With advancing age, histologic changes appear throughout most of the conduction system. Elastic and collagenous tissue increases throughout the system. Fat envelopes the sino-atrial (SA) node and may produce a partial or complete separation of the node from the atrial musculature; in extreme cases this may contribute to the development of sick sinus syndrome. A progressive decrease in the number of pacemaker cells in the SA node begins by 60 years of age, such that only about 10% of the number found in young adults remain by age 75. In the bundle of His, aging is associated with a loss of cells, an increase in fibrous and adipose tissue, and amyloid infiltration. A variable degree of fibrosis of the left side of the cardiac skeleton, which includes the mitral and aortic anuli, the central fibrous body, and the proximal interventricular septum, occurs in senescence. Due to their proximity to these structures, the atrioventricular (AV) node, His bundle, and proximal left and right bundle-branches may be involved in this process. The resultant "idiopathic" or "primary" block is the most common cause of chronic AV block in the elderly. Frequently, however, such conduction disturbances in the aged accompany arteriosclerotic, hypertensive, and amyloid disease.

Perhaps related to these histologic changes, several aspects of the ECG are altered by aging. Although the resting heart rate is not substantially age-related, the intrinsic sinus node rate defined in the presence of sympathetic and parasympathetic blockade decreases from 104 bpm at age 20 years to 92 bpm by age 45 to 55.[17] Respiratory variation in resting sinus rate (sinus arrhythmia) diminishes with aging. Minor age-related prolongations of the PR, QRS, and QT intervals are present in healthy men. In BLSA subjects undergoing high-resolution surface electrocardiography, the increase in PR interval was due to conduction delay proximal to the His bundle; conduction time from the bundle of His to the ventricle was not affected.[18]

A leftward shift of the QRS axis occurs with advancing age, perhaps secondary to some fibrosis in the anterior fascicle of the left bundle-branch plus mild LV hypertrophy. Such axis deviation, even when leftward of −30 degrees or −45 degrees, is not associated with increased cardiac morbidity or mortality when an isolated finding.[19] Complete right bundle-branch block (RBBB) not infrequently occurs in elderly men with no apparent cardiac disease. Twenty-four such individuals, whose mean age was 64 years, experienced no increase in cardiovascular events or decline in aerobic performance over an 8.4-year follow-up when compared to age-matched controls.[20] These men comprised 2.1% of the BLSA male population.

Although LV mass appears to be increased in elderly subjects, the QRS voltage actually diminishes with age. This apparent paradox may be explained by extracardiac factors such as senile emphysema or chest wall deformities which increase the distance between the heart and the exploring electrodes. The most readily observed ECG changes caused by aging involve repolarization: flattening of the ST segment and diminution of T wave amplitude.

Physical Findings

Based on the structural changes in the heart and vasculature, several physical findings which might be considered pathologic in younger individuals are "normal" in the elderly. The most prominent such example is an S4 gallop, an indicator of diminished LV compliance, which is heard in as many as 73% of normal geriatric subjects.[21] Perhaps due to a decrease in pulmonary vascular compliance, inspiratory splitting of the second heart sound is audible in only 30% to 40% of subjects older than 60 years.[22] A soft basal systolic ejection murmur, probably arising from age-related dilatation and stiffening of the proximal aorta, can be heard in 30% to 60% of such subjects. The age-related increased stiffness of the peripheral vasculature causes the carotid upstroke to appear brisk in the elderly, possibly masking significant aortic stenosis.

Arrhythmias

The presence of cardiac arrhythmias, both at rest and during normal activity, has been found to increase with age. Although ectopic beats are sometimes present on a resting 12-lead ECG, prolonged ambulatory monitoring—usually for 24 hours—is a much more sensitive technic for detecting arrhythmias. Studies of clinically healthy subjects investigated by this technic have shown that both supraventricular (SVEB) and ventricular ectopic beats (VEB) vary directly with age, although the number of subjects older than 60 years has been small.[23,24] In 98 BLSA subjects 60 to 85 years old, carefully screened to exclude CAD, 24-hour ambulatory ECG recordings detected isolated SVEB and VEB respectively in 88% and 78% of subjects[25] (Table 5-1). More than 100 SVEB in 24 hours were found in 26% and more than 100 VEB in 17%. Supraventricular tachyarrhythmias, found in a third of subjects, were most often of the benign slow atrial tachycardia variety, though standard supraventricular tachycardia was also common. Ventricular couplets were detected in 11% and short runs of ventricular tachycardia in 4%. The prevalence of each of these arrhythmias was much greater than in healthy young subjects studied by other investigators.[26] In contrast, atrial flutter and fibrillation as well as sinus bradycardia less than 40 bpm, sinus pauses exceeding 2.0 seconds and high degree AV block were extremely uncommon or nonexistent in these carefully screened elderly subjects.

In summary, structural alterations in the cardiovascular system occur with advancing age, the most significant of which is a mild but definite LV hypertrophy which probably arises due to age-related stiffening of the arterial tree. A variable degree of fibrosis of the left side of the cardiac skeleton may explain the small increase in PR and QRS intervals and leftward shift of the QRS axis seen with aging. The prevalence and frequency of both supraventricular and ventricular arrhythmias increase with age. Small age-related increases in the CTR and aortic knob diameter are found on chest roentgenogram, although a CTR greater than .50 remains uncommon in the absence of organic heart disease. The frequent presence of an S4 gallop, basal systolic ejection murmur, and brisk carotid arterial upstroke in elderly subjects may be explained on the basis of age-related structural alterations of the cardiovascular system.

Table 5-1
Supraventricular and Ventricular Arrhythmias Observed in 98 Healthy Elderly Subjects

	No. Subjects (%)
Supraventricular	
Any	86 (88)
Isolated ectopic beats	86 (88)
≥30 beats in any hour	22 (22)
≥100 beats in 24 h	25 (26)
Benign slow atrial tachycardia	27 (28)
Paroxysmal atrial tachycardia	13 (13)
Atrial flutter	1 (1)
Accelerated junctional rhythm	1 (1)
Ventricular	
Any	78 (80)
Isolated ectopic beats	76 (78)
≥5 in any hour	37 (38)
≥30 in any hour	12 (12)
≥60 in any hour	7 (7)
≥100 in 24 h	17 (17)
Multiform	34 (35)
Ventricular couplets	11 (11)
Ventricular tachycardia	4 (4)
R on T phenomena	1 (1)
Accelerated idioventricular rhythm	1 (1)

Data from Fleg and Kennedy.[25]

CARDIAC PERFORMANCE AT REST

Cardiac output, the product of heart rate and stroke volume, indicates the amount of blood pumped by the heart per minute and is probably the most important measure of cardiac performance because it represents the ability of the heart to meet the oxygen requirements of the entire body. Several cross-sectional studies over the past five decades have found the resting cardiac output to decline with age.[27,28] In a group of 67 hospitalized men without obvious cardiovascular disease, cardiac output determined by indicator dilution fell from 6.5 L/min in the third decade to

3.9 L/min in the ninth—an average decline of 1% per year.[27] Stroke volume decreased from 85 ml to 60 ml over this age span. Even after correction for a small age-related diminution of BSA, these age differences remained highly significant. In this and other studies showing similar results, a significant proportion of elderly subjects with latent CAD were likely included.

Strikingly different results regarding the effect of age on resting cardiac output have been found in healthy BLSA subjects (47 men and 14 women) studied by gated radionuclide angiography (Figure 5-2B).[29] This subset consisted of consecutive active community dwelling volunteers in whom angina and symptoms of cardiovascular disease were absent and in whom ECGs at rest and during maximal exercise were normal. In addition, all subjects aged 40 and older had undergone exercise thallium scintigraphy and demonstrated no myocardial perfusion defects. In these individuals, varying in age from 30 to 80 years, resting cardiac output was not age-related. It should be noted that even in these carefully screened subjects, daily activity cardiac expenditure declined with age, indicating that the elderly participants did not represent an atypical, highly conditioned subgroup.

It can therefore be seen that the effect of age on cardiac output in cross-sectional studies is significantly influenced by differences in the study populations. A comparison of resting hemodynamic variables in the two studies above is shown in Table 5-2. Although slight age-related decreases in heart rate and increases in systolic blood pressure occurred in both populations, a decrease in stroke volume and increase in systemic vascular resistance was seen only in the earlier study. The age-related decline in cardiac output and stroke volume found in prior studies may be attributable to the effects of undetected CAD, significant deconditioning and/or other changes in life style not defined.

Ventricular Function at Rest

The pump performance of the left ventricle is a function of the preload or filling volume, the contractile state of the ventricular myocardium, and the afterload or impedance to ventricular ejection. Each of these parameters, of course, can be influenced by disease. Technical advances over the past decade allow relatively noninvasive assessment of cardiac pump performance.

Preload At rest, the LV end-diastolic dimension,[14] area,[30] and volume[29] as assessed respectively

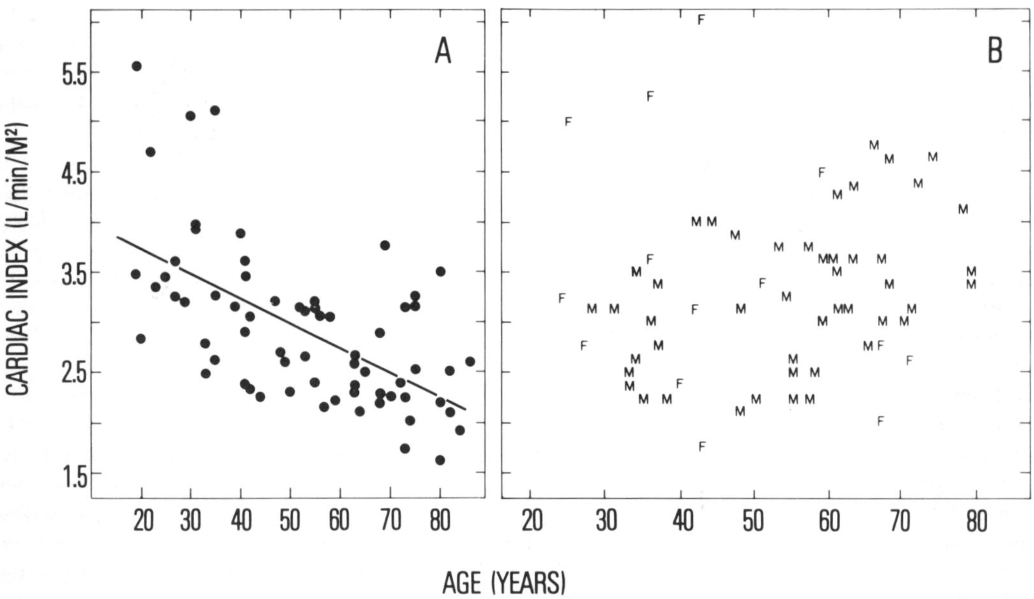

Figure 5-2 **A**. Resting cardiac index as a function of age in two types of "normal" populations. In 67 hospitalized men (**A**) without apparent circulatory disorders, a striking age-related decline in Fick determined cardiac index was observed, approximately 1% per year. (Reproduced with permission from Brandfonbrener et al.[27]) **B**. In contrast to the results in **A**, resting cardiac index was not related to age in 61 active community dwelling men (M) and women (F) carefully screened to exclude latent coronary artery disease. (Reproduced with permission from Rodeheffer et al.[27])

Table 5-2
Effect of Adult Age on Resting Cardiac Function

	Population A* Institutionalized, Unscreened for Occult CAD (2nd–9th Decade)	Population B† Active in Community Life Screened for Occult CAD with Cardiovascular Stress (3rd–8th Decade)
Heart rate	Slight decrease	Slight decrease
Systolic blood pressure	Increase	Increase
Stroke volume	Decrease	Slight increase
Diastolic pressure	No effect	No effect
Cardiac output	Decrease	No effect
Cardiac index	Decrease	No effect
Peripheral vascular resistance	Increase	No effect

*From Brandfonbrener et al.[27]
†From Rodeheffer et al.[29]

by M-mode echocardiography, two-dimensional echocardiography, and gated blood pool scintigraphy are not age-related in healthy BLSA subjects. However, the rate of early diastolic filling, as indexed by the early diastolic closure rate (E-F slope) of the anterior mitral valve leaflet on M-mode echocardiography, declines significantly with advancing age. The E-F slope in 65 to 84-year-old men was approximately half of that observed in those 25 to 44 years old. This impairment of LV filling has several possible contributors. First of all, it may derive in part from the previously mentioned age-related increase in LV wall thickness which would decrease LV diastolic compliance. Animal studies in both intact hearts and isolated cardiac muscle have demonstrated an augmentation of myocardial stiffness in senescence, thus supporting this hypothesis.[31] The mitral valve becomes thickened and sclerotic with age. Finally, a prolongation of isometric relaxation has been shown in man and many animal models.[32] At the cellular level, myocardial relaxation is accomplished by the removal of Ca^{++} from the contractile proteins by the sarcoplasmic reticulum. The rate of Ca^{++} accumulation in sarcoplasmic reticulum isolated from senescent rat hearts was about 50% less than in those of young adult rats. Although the diminished filling rate of the senescent heart may not impair cardiac performance at rest, the impairment of LV compliance might cause an exaggerated increase in LV diastolic pressure during tachycardia in the elderly and thus lead to a lower threshold for dyspnea than in the young adult.

Afterload Afterload or impedance to LV emptying appears to be modestly increased at rest in senescent man. Mild LV hypertrophy occurs as an adaptive mechanism to maintain normal LV wall stress. Although the expected rise in resting systolic blood pressure occurred with aging in BLSA subjects studied by gated blood pool scintigraphy, the calculated peripheral vascular resistance was not age-related (Table 5-2). The increase in afterload with age is found mainly in the harmonic components of impedance and in an animal model becomes more pronounced during exercise.

Contractility The "contractile state" of the myocardium is difficult to assess in the intact organism due to the complex interactions of the various modulators of cardiac performance. Our knowledge of how aging affects intrinsic muscle performance must therefore derive from studies of isolated hearts or cardiac muscle preparations obtained from various animal species.

Studies in isolated cardiac muscle have indicated no age-related compromise in the ability to generate force. However, a 15% to 20% prolongation of contraction duration accompanies senescence in numerous species, including man. Studies in isometric muscle preparations suggest that the extent of sarcomere shortening during a contraction is not age-related.

The development of echocardiography and radionuclide blood pool scanning in recent years allows accurate direct, yet relatively noninvasive assessment of cardiac performance in man. The most widely employed index of overall cardiac pump function is the ejection fraction (EF), defined by stroke volume divided by end-diastolic volume. In the same carefully selected BLSA subjects studied by radionuclide angiography, resting EF was not age-related (Figure 5-3).[29] This confirms prior M-mode echocardiographic investigations in BLSA and other apparently healthy populations in whom shortening fraction, a one-

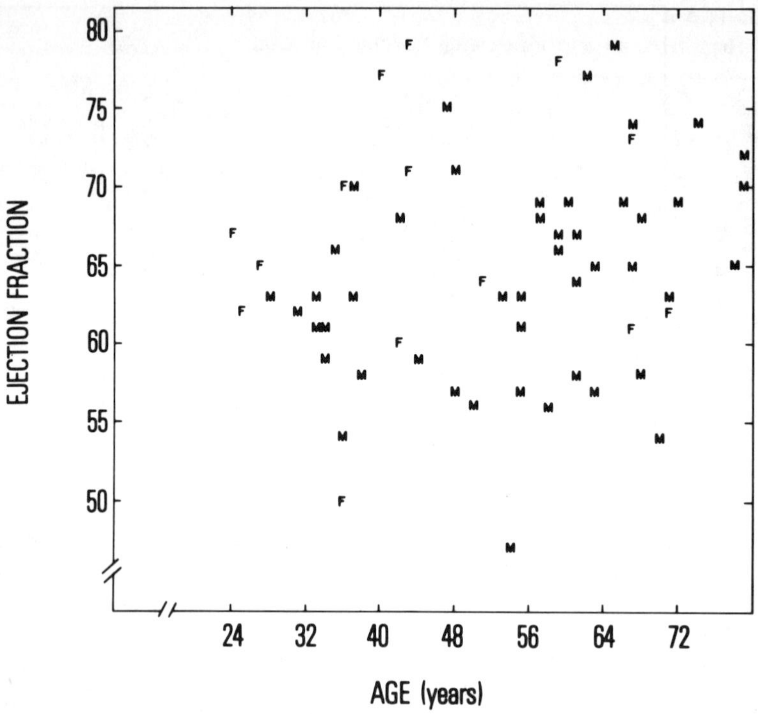

Figure 5-3 Resting ejection fraction, determined by radionuclide angiography, as a function of age in 61 healthy men (M) and women (F). There was no significant relationship to age. (Reproduced with permission from Rodeheffer et al.[29])

dimensional representation of EF, was independent of age.[14] An intrinsic decline in contractility could be masked by an increase in preload, ie, the Frank-Starling mechanism, resulting in an unchanged EF; the previously noted similarity in LV end-diastolic volume between young and old subjects[29] would make this possibility unlikely. From a given end-diastolic volume, an age-related diminution in afterload could also mask a decrease in contractile function. As has been previously discussed, afterload, as measured by vascular impedance, appears to increase rather than decline with advancing years.

Perhaps a "purer" index of cardiac muscle function than EF is the velocity of fiber shortening (Vcf), defined echocardiographically as the shortening fraction divided by ejection time. Although Vcf is thought to be relatively independent of preload, it varies directly with heart rate and inversely with afterload. In BLSA subjects[14] resting Vcf was unaffected by age (Figure 5-4). Since resting heart rate in man does not increase with age and afterload does not decrease, the maintenance of Vcf with advancing age cannot be explained by alterations in these variables. Thus, notwithstanding the difficulty of measuring intrinsic muscle performance or contractility in man, there is no evidence for an age-related change in resting cardiac function in healthy individuals.

To summarize, resting cardiac output does not appear to decline with advancing age in active community dwellers who are free of CAD. Resting heart rate, LV end-diastolic volume, and contractility are similarly unaffected by aging per se in man. Although afterload increases modestly with age, the compensatory LV hypertrophy allows maintenance of normal wall stress and normal systolic function. A significant age-related retardation of LV filling rate and prolongation of isometric relaxation do not impair resting cardiac performance.

CARDIOVASCULAR PERFORMANCE DURING STRESS

In many organ systems functional derangements only become manifest under conditions which tax the capabilities of the system, ie, stress. Thus, the well-maintained resting cardiovascular function in elderly subjects by no means implies

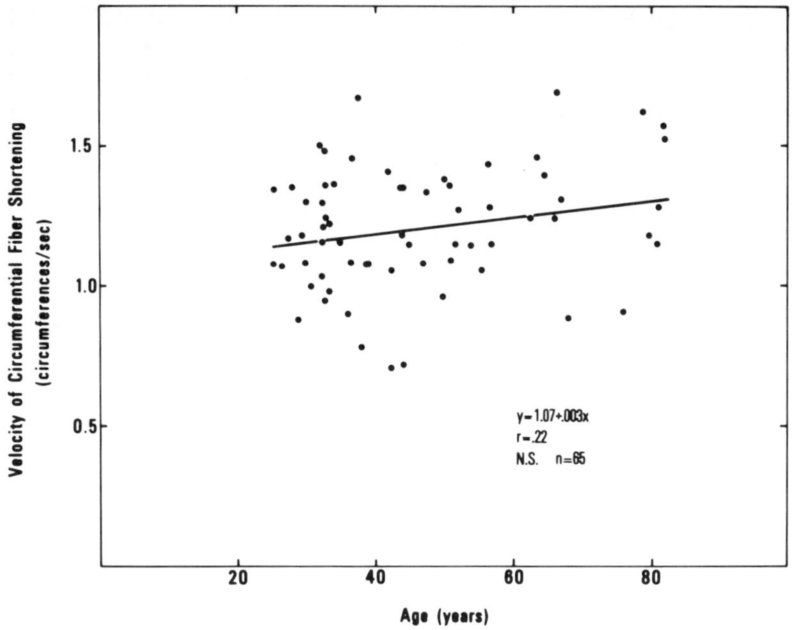

Figure 5-4 The relationship between age and velocity of circumferential fiber shortening, measured by echocardiography in 47 healthy men. Age has no significant effect on this variable. (Adapted from Gerstenblith et al.[14])

that similar findings pertain during stress. This section will discuss the age-related changes in cardiovascular performance in response to the most widely studied stress involving this system—aerobic exercise.

Because the maximal capabilities of an organ are more sensitive to the effects of disease than is resting function, consideration of the effects of undetected CAD on cardiovascular function is even more critical in aging studies during exercise than at rest. Several studies of apparently healthy individuals have demonstrated an age-related increase in the prevalence of ECG changes during exercise highly suggestive of CAD.[8,28] Inclusion of such individuals in exercise studies of "normal" aging may cause spurious results. Furthermore, the status of physical conditioning has a profound influence on aerobic performance and its hemodynamic components. Additional factors such as smoking habits and degree of obesity may likewise affect cardiovascular function during exercise. Finally, the "natural selection" bias of any cross-sectional study in which the elderly survivors represent a more highly select group than the young, may confound the results of such exercise studies.

Even the casual spectator recognizes that athletic performance for most aerobic sports peaks in the 20s and declines significantly by the mid-30s. An early quantitation of this decline in a heterogeneous population was reported in 1929 by Master and Oppenheimer[33] who found that work performance during their two-step test reached a maximal value of 3795 ft-lb at age 27 years and declined to 2250 ft-lb by age 74 in men; in women the corresponding values at these ages were 2950 and 1700 ft-lb respectively.

In the modern laboratory, maximal exercise performance is usually assessed by means of a multistage continuous treadmill or bicycle test, each stage requiring greater cardiovascular effort than the preceding one. During such efforts, the cardiovascular system meets the increasing metabolic requirements of the exercising muscles by delivering larger amounts of oxygen-rich blood to them. The muscles and other peripheral tissues extract sufficient oxygen from this blood to maintain the aerobic effort. This maximal integrated ability of the cardiovascular system to deliver oxygenated blood to the periphery and the latter's ability to extract oxygen from the delivered blood is termed VO_{2max} and is the product of maximal cardiac output and maximal systemic arteriovenous oxygen (A-VO_2) difference. For a given individual, this value is not affected by increasing the percentage of inspired oxygen or involving additional muscles, once 50% to 60% of the muscle mass is being exercised.[34] VO_{2max} is therefore considered the best overall measurement of cardiovascular fitness.

A consistent finding over nearly half a century is an age-related diminution in VO_{2max} which averages 5% to 10% per decade between ages 25 and 75 years (Figure 5-5).[9,10,35,36] Since this decline in VO_{2max} with age parallels the decline in work capacity, it does not arise from greater metabolic efficiency in the elderly. At a given workload, in fact, elderly subjects may demonstrate a slightly higher VO_2 than younger ones, perhaps due to decreased efficiency of walking.[37] The magnitude of the age-related decline of VO_{2max} is affected by numerous factors such as the degree of physical activity or conditioning, smoking, and obesity. For example, in one longitudinal study, a 25% decline in VO_{2max} occurred over the ensuing 22 years in men initially 18 to 22 years old.[9] By entrance into long-term physical conditioning programs, cessation or reduction of cigarette smoking and reduction of body weight, a subgroup of these men actually increased their VO_{2max} an average of 11% over the following five years. Nevertheless, even champion athletes who continue training after retirement from competition experience an age-associated decline in VO_{2max}, although this decline appears to be closer to 5% per decade than the 10% figure found in sedentary individuals.[10]

VO_{2max}, although an excellent measure of overall cardiorespiratory performance, has certain limitations which must be recognized. Exercise capacity may be limited by noncardiac factors such as ventilatory capacity, peripheral blood flow, or motivational factors. The age-related increase in minute ventilation at submaximal workload suggests that ventilation is not limiting in elderly subjects.[37] The age-related diminution in maximal A-VO_2 difference suggests that a relative inefficiency in diversion of blood to the exercising muscle or in the ability of the muscles to extract and utilize oxygen exists in elderly subjects. The absence of a plateau in the VO_{2max} curves in many aging studies raises the question of whether maximal cardiac performance was truly achieved in the elderly or was instead limited by noncardiac factors. Furthermore, it should be emphasized that the VO_{2max} tells nothing about cardiac pump function per se.

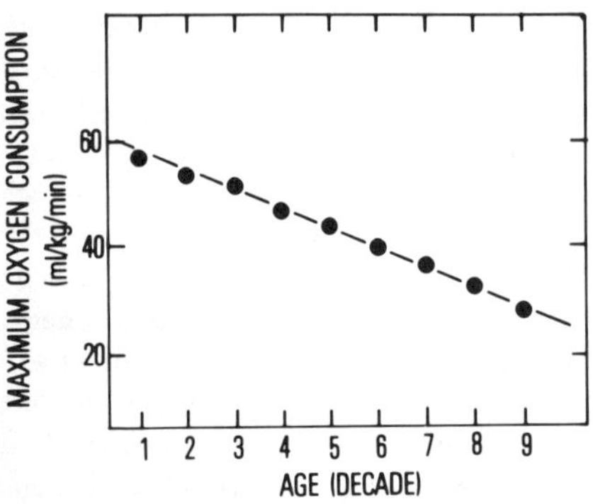

Figure 5-5 The effect of age on VO_{2max}. The points represent 700 observations obtained from 17 studies in the literature. An age-related reduction in VO_{2max}, normalized for body weight, begins in childhood and continues throughout life. (Adapted from Dehn and Bruce.[36])

A more direct measure of exercise cardiovascular performance than VO_{2max} is the maximal cardiac output, determined by the product of heart rate and stroke volume at peak exercise. As with resting cardiac output, several studies have demonstrated significant declines in maximal cardiac output with age. However, the possible inclusion of individuals with occult CAD as well as the invasive methodology employed may limit the general applicability of these studies. In the previously described group of 61 BLSA subjects carefully screened to exclude CAD, maximal work load achieved during upright bicycle ergometry declined with age, but this decline was relatively modest, approximating 17% between ages 30 and 75 years. Despite an age-related decline in maximal heart rate from 183 bpm at age 30 to 137 bpm at age 75, the maximal cardiac output did not decline with age, the result of a compensatory increase in maximal stroke volume (Table 5-3). These results suggest that a decline in maximal aerobic performance and in maximal heart rate are indeed "aging" changes whereas the diminution of cardiac output and stroke volume during maximal exercise reported by others may reflect previously "nonaging" changes such as undetected CAD or deconditioning.

Ventricular Function During Exercise

The pump function of the exercising left ventricle is characterized by the same parameters as in the resting LV: preload, contractility, and afterload. Only in the last few years, since the advent of exercise radionuclide angiography, has accurate and relatively noninvasive assessment of ventricular size and function during vigorous upright exercise been possible. The effect of age on these parameters, drawn largely from the BLSA experience, is discussed below.

Preload A major mechanism by which cardiac output during exercise can be augmented in nor-

Table 5-3
Effect of Age on Hemodynamic Performance During Maximum Upright Bicycle Exercise in BLSA Subjects (n = 61)

Parameter	Linear Regression	*r*	*p*
Heart rate (bpm)	208.19 − .94 (age)	−.66	<.001
Systolic blood pressure (mmHg)	175.31 + .33 (age)	.17	<.19
End-diastolic volume (CC)	107.56 + .86 (age)	.28	<.03
End-systolic volume (CC)	6.51 − .51 (age)	.41	<.001
Ejection fraction	89.5 − .21 (age)	−.37	<.003
Stroke volume (CC)	101.6 + .34 (age)	.14	<.25
Cardiac output (L/min)	20.36 + .05 (age)	−.14	<.26
Total peripheral vascular resistance	5.84 − .04 (age)	−.24	<.06

Data from Rodeheffer et al.[27] Values for $p < .05$ are statistically significant.

mal man involves an increase in venous return which enhances cardiac filling, thus allowing a greater stroke volume to be ejected.[38] This is known as the Frank-Starling mechanism. One might hypothesize that the age-related reduction in early diastolic filling rate and prolongation of isovolumetric relaxation previously demonstrated at rest might limit diastolic filling during exercise. In the BLSA study, however, quite the opposite occurred—end-diastolic volume increased with age (Table 5-3).[27] This age-related cardiac dilatation was statistically evident by intermediate bicycle workloads (75 W) and became progressively more striking with increasing loads. As a result of this enhanced preload, stroke volume increased with age in a parallel fashion, offsetting the age-related decline in heart rate which was observed at each exercise stage. Thus cardiac output was well maintained in the older subject at every stage. A similar age-related reliance on the Frank-Starling mechanism was found in another subset of BLSA subjects studied by two-dimensional echocardiography during semisupine bicycle exercise.[30] In this study, the LV end-diastolic area at a common heart rate of 120 bpm was larger in an elderly subset averaging 64 years than in a younger group whose mean age was 31 years. The fact that this greater end-diastolic area in the elderly occurred at a common heart rate suggests that it is not merely a function of increased filling time due to a lower heart rate in the elderly. Enhanced reliance upon the Frank-Starling mechanism may therefore be construed as an adaptive mechanism by which the older subject maintains cardiac output during exercise.

Afterload Afterload or resistance to LV emptying consists of two vascular components—a static component termed peripheral vascular resistance (PVR) and a pulsatile component termed characteristic impedance. The former term, calculated from the quotient of mean arterial pressure divided by cardiac output, has been found to increase with age during maximal exercise by some investigators. In contrast, the PVR in BLSA subjects at maximal effort was not age-related (Table 5-3). This raises the possibility that the augmentation of PVR with age seen in these earlier studies reflected subclinical peripheral vascular disease or a more rapid progression of the age-related structural changes in the arterial tree than that seen in the BLSA participants, perhaps related to differences in life style.

Contractility The EF response to exercise, despite its partial dependence on exercise-induced changes in preload and afterload, is a valuable index of myocardial function in the intact animal. In 1977, Borer et al[39] demonstrated with radionuclide angiography that normal individuals responded to maximal bicycle exercise with an increase in EF of at least five points from the resting value whereas patients with CAD usually responded with a decrease or no change. In a large percentage of such CAD patients, this abnormal EF response is associated with the development of a wall motion abnormality indicating regional ischemia. Port et al[40] found that in 72% of apparently healthy volunteers aged 60 years or older, maximal exercise was similarly accompanied by a fall in EF below resting levels; wall motion abnormalities developed in 44% of those subjects older than 70 years.

By contrast, in the previously described BLSA population screened by prior treadmill ECGs and thallium scintigraphy, neither a drop in EF from resting level nor regional wall motion abnormalities were observed during maximal bicycle exercise.[29] In these BLSA subjects it was found, however, that the absolute EF at maximal effort declined with age secondary to an age-related increase in the end-systolic volume (Table 5-3). Given the greater exercise-induced augmentation of end-diastolic volume with advancing age, the lesser augmentation of EF implies that some additional factors serve to compromise the ejection of blood in elderly subjects. Because PVR was not related to age in these subjects, it is tempting to implicate a decreased catecholamine-stimulated contractility as the mechanism for the age-associated decline in maximal EF. The more striking limitation of EF and the development of wall motion abnormalities in the elderly subjects of Port et al,[40] suggest that many of these individuals had latent CAD.

Autonomic Modulation

At high exercise levels, complete withdrawal of vagal tone occurs and the sympathetic nervous system becomes the exclusive autonomic modulator. An age-related diminution of sympathetic function could explain all of the aging changes in cardiovascular performance during exercise: the decrease in maximal heart rate, the increase in characteristic impedance, the impaired EF response, the greater reliance upon the Frank-Starling mechanism, and the diminution of maximal A-VO_2 difference. Further understanding of the effects of age on cardiovascular function during exercise may be obtained by looking directly at the effects of pharmacologic manipulation of this system either by the direct infusion of catecholamines or by beta-adrenergic blockade.

Bolus infusion of isoproterenol elicited a smaller increment in heart rate in healthy men aged 62 to 80 years than in men 18 to 34 years old (Figure 5-6).[41,42] Although the results of these studies could be explained by either a decreased response to catecholamines or an enhancement of vagal tone, a similar age-related decrease in maximal heart rate during isoproterenol infusion was observed in beagle dogs even after complete vagal blockade with atropine,[43] suggesting that aging changes in cholinergic modulation were not involved.

A second approach toward isolating the adrenergic component of cardiovascular performance during exercise utilizes beta-adrenergic blockade. In the presence of such blockade, the age-associated decrease in maximal cardiac output is significantly attenuated. This suggests that the efficiency of beta-adrenergic stimulation whether on the heart, peripheral vasculature, or central nervous system, is greater in the young than in the elderly during maximal exercise, thereby permitting a greater increase in cardiac output.

The age-related decrease in the effectiveness of catecholamines during exercise could be due to a decrease in their elaboration or to a reduced end-organ responsiveness to their effects. In a carefully screened subset of nonsmoking BLSA men, plasma epinephrine and norepinephrine actually demonstrated a striking increase with age both at submaximal and at maximal treadmill workloads (Figure 5-7).[44] Young et al[45] have shown that such increased blood levels of catecholamines during stress in elderly subjects are secondary to enhanced secretion rather than decreased degradation. Taken together, then, these studies support animal data demonstrating a diminished responsiveness to catecholamines with advancing age.

In summary, several changes in the cardiovascular response to aerobic exercise occur with advancing age. Age-associated decreases in maximal work capacity, VO_{2max}, and maximal heart rate have been universally found although the magnitude of these decreases is highly dependent upon the subject selection criteria employed. Maximal A-VO_2 difference appears to fall with advancing age, due to either a failure to effectively divert blood to exercising muscles or a diminished capacity of those muscles to utilize oxygen. Although many studies in apparently healthy populations have demonstrated age-related declines in cardiac output during maximal aerobic exercise, recent data in more rigorously chosen subjects suggest that this parameter does not undergo a significant change between ages 30 and 80 years. In these subjects, maximal cardiac output was preserved in the elderly by a greater reliance on the Frank-Starling mechanism than seen in younger subjects. The age-associated increase in end-diastolic volume allowed stroke volume to increase with age, even though the ab-

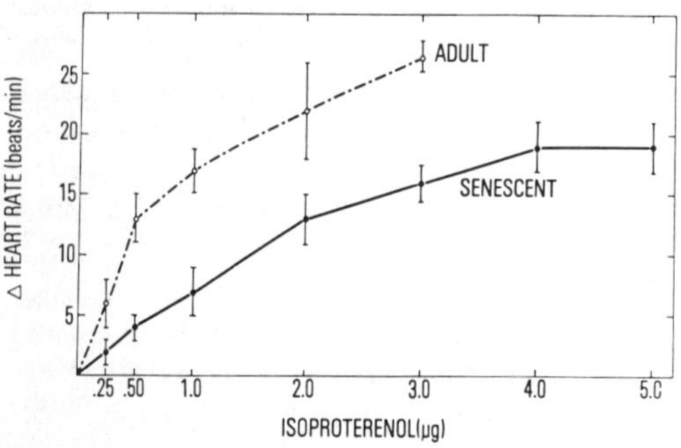

Figure 5-6 The acceleration of heart rate induced by incremental intravenous boluses of isoproterenol in healthy adult (aged 18 to 34 years) and senescent (aged 62 to 80 years) men. At all isoproterenol doses exceeding 0.25 μg, a significantly greater increment in heart rate is observed in the younger men. (Reproduced with permission from Lakatta.[32])

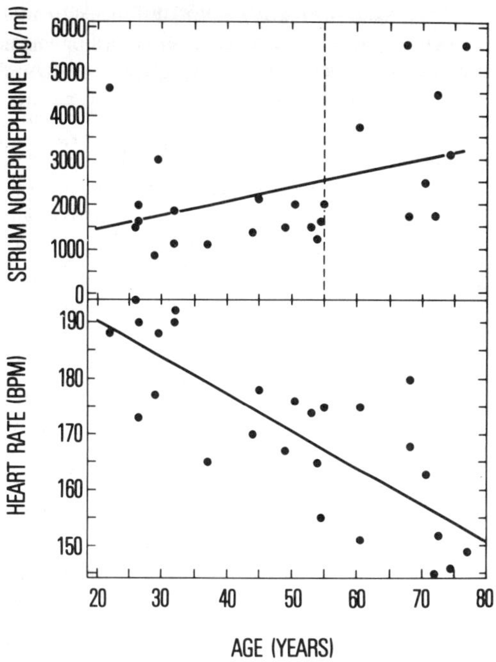

Figure 5-7 The contrasting effects of age on serum norepinephrine (above) and heart rate (below) in 26 healthy men during maximal treadmill effort. The vertical dashed line indicates that only above the age of 55 years was the difference in serum epinephrine significant. A lower heart rate in the face of higher norepinephrine concentrations suggests an age-related reduction in sensitivity to catecholamines. (Reproduced with permission from Tzankoff et at.[44])

solute increase in EF at maximal exercise declined with age. Studies in both animals and man suggest that these age-dependent changes in the cardiovascular response to exercise may be explained by a decreased sensitivity of the senescent heart and vasculature to the chronotropic, inotropic, and vasoregulatory effects of catecholamines.

REFERENCES

1. World Health Organization: *World Health Statistics Annual.* Geneva, 1979.
2. White NK, Edwards JE, Dry TJ: The relationship of the degree of coronary atherosclerosis with age, in men. *Circulation* 1950;1:645–654.
3. Ackerman RF, Dry TJ, Edwards JE: Relationship of various factors to the degree of coronary atherosclerosis in women. *Circulation* 1950;1:1345–1354.
4. Tejada C, Strong JP, Montenegro MR, et al: Distribution of coronary and aortic atherosclerosis by geographic location, race and sex. *Lab Invest* 1968; 18:49–66.
5. Kannel WB, Gordon T, Offutt D: Left ventricular hypertrophy by electrocardiogram. Prevalence, incidence, and mortality in the Framingham study. *Ann Intern Med* 1969;71:89–105.
6. Kennedy RD, Andrews GR, Caird FI: Ischemic heart disease in the elderly. *Br Heart J* 1977;39: 1121–1127.
7. Stone JL, Norris AH: Activities and attitudes of participants of the Baltimore Longitudinal Study. *J Gerontol* 1966;21:575–580.
8. Gerstenblith G, Fleg JL, Vantosh A, et al: Stress testing redefines the prevalence of coronary artery disease in epidemiologic studies. *Circulation* 1980; 62(parts 2, 3):308.
9. Robinson S, Dill DB, Ross JC, et al: Training and physiological aging in man. *Fed Proc* 1973;32: 1628–1634.
10. Heath GW, Hagberg JM, Ehsani AA, et al: A physiological comparison of young and older endurance athletes. *J Appl Physiol* 1981;51:634–640.
11. Linzbach AJ, Akuamoa-Boateng E: Die Alernsversanderungen des menschlichen Herzens. I. Das Herzgewicht im Alter. *Klin Wochenschr* 1973;51: 156–163.
12. Yin FCP, Spurgeon HA, Weisfeldt ML, et al: Mechanical properties of myocardium from hypertrophied rat hearts. A comparison between hypertrophy induced senescence and by aortic banding. *Circ Res* 1980;46:292–300.
13. Sjogren AL: Left ventricular wall thickness in patients with circulatory overload of the left ventricle. *Ann Clin Res* 1972;4:310–318.
14. Gerstenblith G, Frederiksen J, Yin FCP, et al: Echocardiographic assessment of a normal adult aging population. *Circulation* 1977;56:273–278.
15. Savage DD, Garrison RJ, Brand F, et al: Prevalence and correlates of posterior extro-echocardiographic spaces in a free-living population–based sample: The Framingham Study. *Am J Cardiol* 1983;51:1207–1212.
16. Savage DD, Garrioson RJ, Castelli WP, et al: Prevalence of submitral (annular) calcium and its correlates in a general population–based sample (The Framingham Study). *Am J Cardiol* 1983;51:1375–1378.

16a. Ensor RE, Fleg JL, Kim YC, et al: Longitudinal x-ray changes in normal men. *J Gerontol* 1983;38: 307–314.

17. José AD: Effect of combined sympathetic and parasympathetic blockade on heart rate and cardiac function in man. *Am J Cardiol* 1966;18:476–478.
18. Das DN, Fleg JL, Lakatta EG: Effect of age on the components of atrioventricular conduction in normal man. *Am J Cardiol* 1982;49:1031.
19. Ostrander LD: Left axis deviation: Prevalence, associated conditions and prognosis. *Ann Intern Med* 1971;75:23–28.
20. Fleg JL, Das DN, Lakatta EG: Right bundle branch block: Long-term prognosis in apparently healthy men. *J Am Coll Cardiol* 1983;1:887–892.
21. Spodick DH, Quarry VM: Prevalence of the fourth heart sound by phonocardiography in the absence of cardiac disease. *Am Heart J* 1974;87:11.
22. Slodki SJ, Hussain AT, Luisada AA: The Q-H interval III. A study of the second heart sound in old age. *J Am Geriatr Soc* 1969;17:673–679.
23. Raftery EB, Cashmann PMM: Long-term recording of the electrocardiogram in a normal population. *Postgrad Med J* 1976;52(suppl 7):32–37.
24. Clarke JM, Shelton JR, Nawer J, et al: The rhythm

of the normal human heart. *Lancet* 1976;2:508–512.
25. Fleg JL, Kennedy HL: Cardiac arrhythmias in a healthy elderly population: Detection by 24 hour ambulatory monitoring. *Chest* 1982;81:302–307.
26. Brodsky M, Wu D, Denes P, et al: Arrhythmias documented by 24 hour continuous electrocardiographic monitoring in 50 male medical students without apparent heart disease. *Am J Cardiol* 1977;39: 390–395.
27. Brandfonbrener M, Landowne M, Shock NW: Changes in cardiac output with age. *Circulation* 1955;12:557–566.
28. Strandell T: Circulatory studies on healthy old men. *Acta Med Scand* 1964;176:205–218.
29. Rodeheffer RJ, Gerstenblith G, Becker LC, et al: Exercise cardiac output is maintained with advancing age in healthy human subjects: Cardiac dilatation and increased stroke volume compensate for a diminished heart rate. *Circulation* 1984;69:203–213.
30. VanTosh A, Lakatta EG, Fleg JL, et al: Ventricular dimensional changes during submaximal exercise: Effect of aging in normal man. *Circulation* 1980; 62(part 3):129.
31. Templeton GH, Platt MR, Willerson JT, et al: Influence of aging on left ventricular stiffness. *Clin Res* 1975;23:210A.
32. Lakatta EG: Alterations in the cardiovascular system that occur in advanced age. *Fed Proc* 1979; 38:163–167.
33. Master AM, Oppenheimer ET: A simple exercise tolerance test for circulatory efficiency with standard tables for normal individuals. *Am J Med Sci* 1929;177:223–243.
34. Rowell LB: Human cardiovascular adjustments to exercise and thermal stress. *Physiol Rev* 1974; 54:75–159.
35. Astrand I: Aerobic work capacity in men and women with special reference to age. *Acta Physiol Scand* (suppl 169) 1960;49:1–92.
36. Dehn MM, Bruce RA: Longitudinal variations in maximal oxygen intake with age and activity. *J Appl Physiol* 1972;33:805–807.
37. Montoye HJ: Age and oxygen utilization during submaximal treadmill exercise in males. *J Gerontol* 1982;37:396–402.
38. Poliner LR, Dehmer GJ, Lewis SE, et al: Left ventricular performance in normal subjects: A comparison of the response to exercise in the upright and supine positions. *Circulation* 1980;62:528–534.
39. Borer J, Bachrach S, Green M, et al: Real time radionuclide cineaugiography in the noninvasive evaluation of global and regional left ventricular function at rest and during exercise in patients with coronary artery disease. *N Engl J Med* 1977;296: 839–845.
40. Port E, Cobb FR, Coleman RE, et al: Effect of age on the response of the left ventricular ejection fraction to exercise. *N Engl J Med* 1980;303:1133–1137.
41. Yin FCP, Spurgeon HA, Raizes GS, et al: Age-associated decrease in chronotropic response to isoproterenol. *Circulation* 1976;54(suppl 2):167.
42. Vestal RE, Wood, AJJ, Shand DG: Reduced β-adrenoceptor sensitivity in the elderly. *Clin Pharmacol Ther* 1979;26:181–186.
43. Yin FCP, Spurgeon HA, Greene HL, et al: Age-associated decrease in heart rate response to isoproterenol in dogs. *Mech Ageing Dev* 1979; 10:17–25.
44. Tzankoff ST, Fleg JL, Norris AH, et al: Age-related increase in serum catecholamine levels during exercise in healthy adult men. *Physiologist* 1980;23:50.
45. Young JB, Rowe JW, Palotta JA, et al: Enhanced plasma norepinephrine response to upright posture and oral glucose administration in elderly human subjects. *Metabolism* 1980;29:532–539.

CHAPTER 6
Neurohumoral Regulation of Cardiovascular Function in Aging

Vladimir V. Frolkis

Cardiovascular function is self-regulated by two processes which provide for its adaptation to the organism's demands: the intrasystemic regulation (the Frank-Starling mechanism, the cardiac work/vascular tone ratio, interrelationships between the automation nodes within the heart, etc), and the hemodynamic regulation of the cardiovascular system. To characterize the peculiarities of neurohumoral regulation an analysis will be made of the changes that ensue along the various links of the self-regulatory process: (*a*) age changes in the central regulatory mechanisms (hemodynamic center); (*b*) shifts at the stage of direct links (extracardial neural and hormonal influences); (*c*) changes in cardiac and vascular reactivity to regulatory effects; (*d*) local mechanisms of regulation; (*e*) changes in feedback control (reflexes from cardiac and vascular receptors). This chapter will present data on the role of changes of neurohumoral regulation in the development of age-associated circulatory pathology.

The data available suggest that the shifts in neurohumoral regulation, modify, first, the response of the cardiovascular system in old age and limit its adaptive capacities and, second, lead to metabolic, structural, and functional disturbances in heart and vessels.

CENTRAL MECHANISMS OF REGULATION OF THE CARDIOVASCULAR SYSTEM

The hemodynamic center is a combination of central neurons, providing for the regulation of an optimal level of overall circulatory function.[1] Each level of the hemodynamic center regulates, to a greater or lesser degree, these cardiovascular functions. Thus, the brain stem structures are responsible for the maintenance of the basal level of hemodynamics, the structure of the limbic system for the coordination of the organism's autonomic and emotional-behavioral reactions, and the cortical level for coordination of autonomic and higher brain functions.

During aging, significant changes occur in the function of the hemodynamic center and it is these changes that largely determine the age-related shifts in cardiovascular reactions and the restriction of the adaptive capacities of the circulatory system. This can be substantiated, first, by the shifts in reflex reactions, which proceed with the participation of the center and, second, by the peculiarities of hemodynamic effects induced by direct stimulation of CNS structures.

The influences of conditioned reflexes upon the cardiovascular system are attenuated in old age. A great number of combinations are required to produce conditioned reflex reactions in aged subjects. The shifts induced by conditioned reflexes in arterial blood pressure, heart rate, and cardiac output diminish as well. Mankovsky and Mints[2] observed inertness of unconditioned reflex vascular reactions along with prolonged latency of their development in elderly and old subjects. Persistent vascular reactions can be produced by thermal and tactile stimuli. The elderly subjects more rarely develop a positive oculocardiac (Aschner) reflex.

The cardiovascular response to physical loads is of complex reflex character. At small loads, many hemodynamic and respiratory shifts (arterial blood pressure, heart rate, cardiac output, total peripheral resistance, lung ventilation, oxygen consumption, expiration of carbon dioxide) were found to be more pronounced in male subjects aged 60 to 65, whereas at large loads these shifts were strongly marked in males aged 25 to 30.[3] In other words, the range of stable cardiovascular activity narrows in old age. At moderate loads, the age-related differences level off. The response of the elderly to physical load is characterized by increased latency, and an extended wavelike alteration of the hemodynamics, with delayed restoration of initial levels. The weakening of the reflex component (from cardiac and vascular mechanoreceptors) determines more marked hemodynamic shifts with change of the elderly subject's body position.

In old age, the reliability of reflex regulation of blood circulation is attenuated. Thus, repeated severe painful stimulation of old rabbits results in earlier hemodynamic shifts (fall of arterial blood pressure and cardiac output).

The development of circulatory shifts in response to muscular activity is linked to motor cortical activity. Experiments on rabbits showed significant increase of thresholds of stimulation of the sensorimotor area of the cerebral cortex, which produce shifts in arterial blood pressure (Figure 6-1).

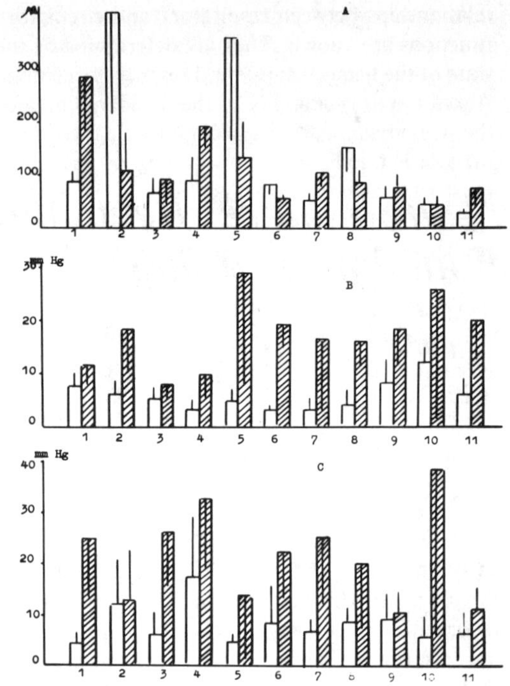

Figure 6-1 Thresholds of pressor influences of various parts of the brain (A) and pressor reactions of arterial blood pressure following intracerebral microinjection of epinephrine (B) and acetylcholine (C) to mature (white columns) and old (shaded columns) rabbits. 1, 2: sensorimotor and pyriform regions of the cerebral cortex; 3: dorsal hippocampus; 4, 5: medial and central nuclei of the amygdala; 6–8: anterior, lateral, and posterior parts of the hypothalamus; 9, 10: reticular nuclei of the pons and tegmentum of the mesencephalon; 11: medulla oblongata (the fundus of the IV ventricle in the region of the calamus scriptorius).

The hypothalamus is an important part of the hemodynamic center. The hypothalamic structures regulate the adaptive reactions of the cardiovascular system, and its participation in varied emotional and behavioral reactions. The hypothalamic structures are the effector link in the realization of systemic reactions induced by other parts of the limbic system (amygdaloid nuclei, hippocampus, etc). Changes occur in old age in the excitability of the hemodynamically active hypothalamic elements, in their sensitivity to physiologically active substances, in the hemodynamic content of cardiovascular reaction induced by hypothalamic stimulation, as well as in the reliability of the hypothalamic regulation of blood circulation. Some hypothalamic nuclei become less excitable in old age (lateral hypothalamus), others become more excitable (anterior hypothalamic nucleus, rostral part of the supraoptic nucleus, medial and lateral mamillary nuclei), while the excitability of others remains unchanged (medial preoptic area, caudal part of the supraoptic nucleus). Threshold stimulations were determined according to shifts of arterial blood pressure. Such shifts lead first to irregular age-related cardiovascular disturbances induced by various emotional and behavioral reactions and, second, predispose to the development of inadequate circulatory reactions.

Shifts in arterial blood pressure of old animals in response to hypothalamic stimulation are mainly determined by changes in cardiac output, whereas adult animals demonstrated more variable interrelationships between cardiac output and total peripheral resistance. An increase of intensity of hypothalamic stimulation leads to greater changes in arterial blood pressure and total peripheral resistance in adult rabbits, whereas reactions in old animals are more persistent.

The basal level of circulatory regulation and its reliability depend on the bulbar part of the hemodynamic center. As is seen in Figure 6-1, the excitability of medullary structures falls in old age. This may account in part for the age-related weakening of many cardiovascular reflexes, which are essential in circulatory self-regulation. The relationships between respiratory and circulatory functions are known. They are determined by the state of the hemodynamic and respiratory centers. Alteration of excitability of the medullary area of the hemodynamic center facilitates the disruption of coordination of the functioning of these two most vital centers.

Figure 6-1 presents data on diversely oriented changes in excitability of various brain structures resulting from complex redistribution of brain activity rather than simple diminution of function. All these shifts result in a leveling off of the differences in excitability of various parts of the hemodynamic center in old age and in the development of its characteristic isoexcitability.

The functional state of the hemodynamic center is determined by the effect of physiologically active substances. Firstly, the transmitters determine the interneuronal information transfer; secondly, the center's tone depends greatly on the blood circulation of hormones.

Bezrukov[4] reported shifts in brain electrical activity and arterial blood pressure of old animals in response to small intraventricular doses of epinephrine and acetylcholine. It is of interest, that in old animals the shifts in brain electrical activity often were not accompanied by the corresponding peripheral effect, ie, by shifts in the peripheral blood pressure.

Substances administered intraventricularly affect many nervous structures simultaneously. Figure 6-1 presents data on changes in the arterial blood pressure in response to epinephrine and acetylcholine administered to particular brain structures. In most cases, the more marked changes of arterial blood pressure occur in old animals. The tone of neurons of the hemodynamic center is maintained owing to the information entering along the afferent nervous pathways as well as by the effect of physiologically active substances. The latter pathway acquires special importance in old age. The increase of neuronal sensitivity to transmitters is an important adaptive mechanism in conditions of altered synthesis.

The reliability of central, including hypothalamic, mechanisms of cardiovascular regulation diminishes in old age. The disruption of hypothalamic mechanisms is assumed to be an essential cause in the development of age-related pathology.[5,6]

Figure 6-1 presents data on changes in arterial blood pressure in response to long-term daily stimulation of zones of the hypothalamus productive of emotional disturbances. Old rabbits more often developed marked arterial hypertension. Some of the animals die as a result of increased diminution of myocardial contractility following daily stimulation. Rushkevich[7] reported significant structural changes within the old-animal myocardium in response to long-term stimulation of these hypothalamic zones. Old animals more frequently displayed more extensive cardiac necrosis, protein and basophilic dystrophy, homogenization of mitochondrial matrix, disturbances of microcirculation, etc. The increase of vasopressin and epinephrine concentrations induced by daily hypothalamic stimulation plays an important role in the development of structural and functional disturbances within the heart. The stimulation of the negative hypothalamic zones leads to an increase in myocardial free fatty acids and lysophospholipids, and to a decrease in phosphatidylcholine, phosphatidylethanolamine, and cardiolipin, as well as to the activation of peroxide oxidation. All these shifts promote cardiac cell damage.

EFFERENT NERVOUS REGULATION

The regulatory effects of the hemodynamic center upon heart and vessels are achieved via adrenergic and cholinergic neural pathways. Experiments on rats, rabbits, and dogs showed a weakening of the neural control over cardiac activity with aging.[7,8] As is seen in Figure 6-2, the thresholds of stimulation of sympathetic and parasympathetic nerves, which induce hemo- and cardiodynamic changes, are increased. It was found that the changes in arterial blood pressure, cardiac output, cardiac index, left ventricular (LV) pressure, maximal rate of shortening and relaxation of myocardial fibers, contractility index, etc occur in old rats, rabbits, and dogs at higher stimulation of extracardial nerves, as compared with young animals. Stimulation of vagal nerve produced more marked effect upon the atrioventricular (AV) node of old animals, ie, they more frequently developed neurogenic AV blockade, and single and multiple extrasystoles.

In old age, the effect of extracardial nerves upon human heart is weakened as well. It is known that the higher the tonic effect of sympathetic and vagal nerves upon the heart, the more significant are the changes in its activity following blockade of cholinergic (atropine) and adrenergic (propranolol) effects. It was found that after atropine administration (1.0 ml 0.1%), the heart rate of men aged 20 to 25 increased by 36.4 ± 2.8 bpm, while propranolol hydrochloride (1.0 ml 0.1%) induced fall of the heart rate by 24.5 ± 6.8 bpm. In

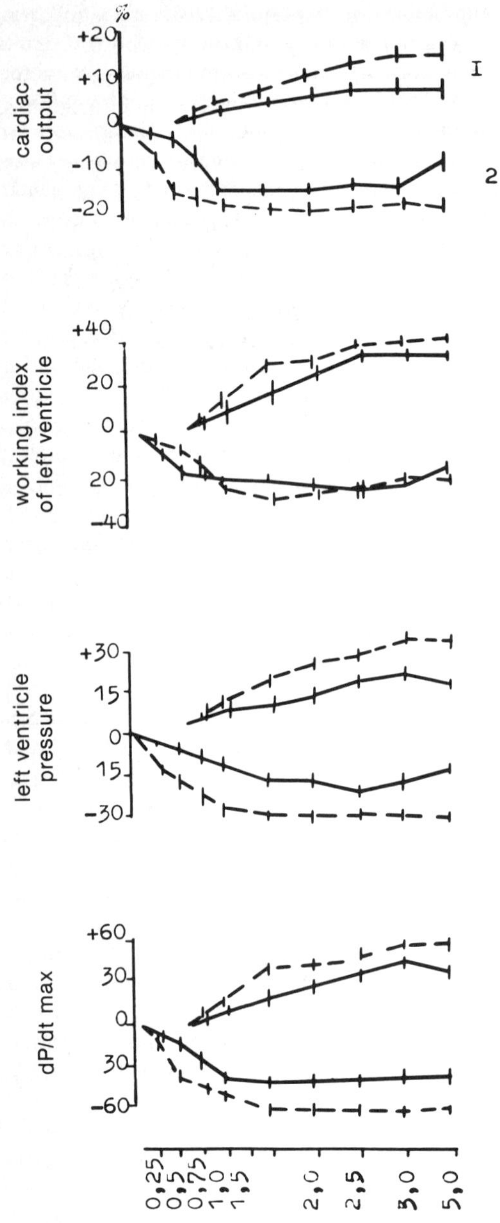

Figure 6-2 Changes in hemodynamics and myocardial contractility following stimulation of sympathetic and vagal nerves of animals of different age. I: sympathetic nerve: 2: vagal nerve. Broken line: mature rabbits; solid line: old rabbits.

men aged 60 to 70 years the corresponding changes were $+16.7 \pm 1.8$ and -12.8 ± 3.4 bpm.

In old age, the changes in sympathetic nervous control vary from one vascular area to another (Figure 6-3). Thus, the threshold of sympathetic effects upon the tone of old rat hind vessels, intestine, and kidneys increase, decrease, and remain unchanged, respectively. As a result, the generalized sympathetic reactions produce in old animals a different spectrum of changes of vascular tone; the increase of arterial blood pressure by reflex action can be attained at the expense of differing blood supply to organs.

In old age there is a loss of lability of stellate ganglia and vagal nerve ganglia in the myocardium. The same occurs with the intensity of acetylcholine synthesis in sympathetic ganglia and with hydrolysis of acetylcholine, while the sensitivity of ganglia to ganglion blockers increases.[9]

According to Shvalev et al[10] the ultrastructural disturbances in sympathetic ganglia were more pronounced than in intracardial parasympathetic ganglia. In the nonsympathetic zone, the sensitivity of cardiac cells to catecholamines is increased. Thus, the weakening of extracardial neural control is related to age-related changes in the ganglionic apparatus.

Shifts in postganglionic nerve endings, as well as structural changes and decreased transmitter synthesis, play an important role in regulatory changes. According to Verkhratsky[11] the content of norepinephrine in an old heart, and especially in its atria, is decreased. The study of H^3-norepinephrine distribution at the subcellular level revealed a decreased capacity of an old rat heart granule to retain norepinephrine. The amount of norepinephrine is also affected by the decreased capacity of sympathetic terminals for re-uptake of norepinephrine, and by weakened transport of

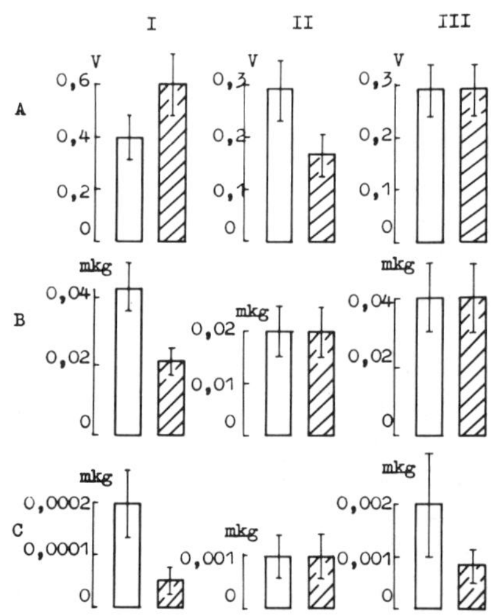

Figure 6-3 Age peculiarities of vascular response of extremity (I), small intestine (II), and kidneys (III) to stimulation of sympathetic nerve (A), intravenous epinephrine (B), and intra-arterial acetylcholine (C). White columns: adult rats; hatched columns: old rats.

norepinephrine-containing vesicles along sympathetic axons. At similar intensity and duration of stimulation of the stellate ganglion, a smaller amount of catecholamines was found in canine blood flowing from old hearts, as compared to young hearts.

The data on reserpine-induced sympathetic block indicate age-related changes in adrenergic nervous effects upon the heart. Reserpine is known to deplete norepinephrine stores in the sympathetic terminals, and for this reason is widely used in clinical practice. More marked hemodynamic shifts in elderly subjects are produced by smaller doses of adrenolytics. The more marked shifts induced in old age by pharmacologic sympathetic block may be explained by the smaller catecholamine stores in sympathetic terminals, which are depleted by reserpine more readily.[12]

The weakening of cholinergic neural effects upon the heart is also linked to the destruction of parasympathetic ganglia, postganglionic nervous fibers, and the decrease of neurotransmitter (acetylcholine) synthesis,[11] the latter being determined in the atria by the fall in CoA concentration and in choline acetyltransferase activity.

A significant influence upon extracardial nervous regulation of the heart is produced by age-related changes in transmitter breakdown, in the state of postsynaptic membrane, in the number and properties of receptors, and in changes of cell reaction to transmitters.

Changes occur with aging in the response of the cardiovascular system to catecholamines. Tuttle,[13] Pandya,[14] and Parker et al,[15] showed a reduced catecholamine effect upon rat aortic strip with aging. According to Strozzi et al[16] the administration of adrenomimetic metaproterenol to elderly subjects induced more marked hypotension and tachycardia.

According to Hruza,[17] smaller doses of catecholamines produce threshold cardiovascular reactions in old animals. In elucidating the causes of these discrepancies, a differentiation should be made between the concept of sensitivity (threshold reaction–inducing concentrations of reagents) and reaction capacity (maximal reaction to the reagent's effect). In old age, the reaction capacity is decreased, ie, the maximal reaction of the cardiovascular system to catecholamines is higher in young and adult animals than in old. The pattern of changes of sensitivity in the various links of the blood circulatory system is irregular. As is seen in Figure 6-3, in old rats the sensitivity of vessels of skeletal muscles to epinephrine is increased, while that of intestine and kidneys remains unchanged. Hemodynamic shifts in old rats are induced by smaller doses of norepinephrine.

Changes in arterial blood pressure occur in old rabbits after intravenous (IV) administration of 1.4 ± 0.5 μg/kg acetylcholine, as compared with 9.4 ± 1.7 μg/kg in adult rabbits. In subjects aged 20 to 29 years, the changes in arterial blood pressure, deceleration of cardiac rhythm, and fall in cardiac output were produced by a dose three times higher than that needed to produce the same effects in subjects aged 60 to 69 years.[18,19]

The increase of sensitivity of some elements of the cardiovascular system to transmitters in old age is an important adaptive mechanism aimed at maintaining an adequate level of regulation in conditions of destruction of nerve endings and decrease in the amount of transmitter released by them.

Shifts in the metabolism of transmitters play an important role in the mechanism of changes in sensitivity to them. During aging, cholinesterase activity in the heart is decreased, thus promoting the effects of acetylcholine. In old age, irregular changes evolve in different pathways of catecholamine catabolism in the heart, ie, the activity of monoamine oxidase is increased, and the role of the catecholomethyl transferase pathway is decreased. The weakening of norepinephrine reuptake by sympathetic terminals results in the longer presence of norepinephrine in the zone of its action, ie, in the synaptic junction, thus promoting the rise of sensitivity to the transmitter.

The transmitter, released into the synaptic junction, reacts with corresponding receptors on postsynaptic membrane. The cardiovascular reaction depends greatly on the number, state, and transmitter-binding capacity of the receptors. According to Zitnik and Roth[20] and Narayanan and Derby[21] the number of myocardial beta-adrenoreceptors does not decrease in old age, but their properties alter. They reported a 10- to 20-fold decrease in β-receptor affinity to catecholamines in old rats, whereas sensitivity to β-blockers remained unchanged.

Binding with adrenergic and cholinergic receptors is the first link in the molecular mechanism of transmitter effect upon the cell. The subsequent activation of adenylate or guanylate cyclase leads to the synthesis of cyclic nucleotides, which are the second transmitter of reaction. Figure 6-4 presents the data of Kulchitsky[22] which show that small doses of norepinephrine and acetylcholine produce more pronounced shifts of cAMP and cGMP in aged animal hearts. These shifts may account for the increase in myocardial sensitivity to

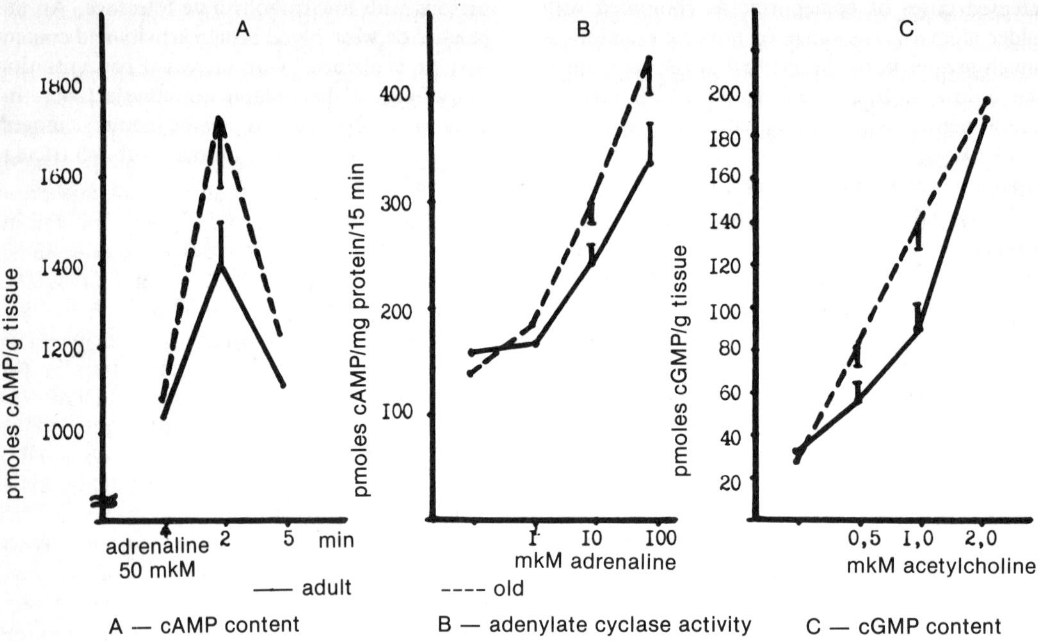

Figure 6-4 The cyclase system of the rat myocardium in aging.

small doses of transmitters in old age.[23] Altura and Altura[24] concluded that larger doses of catecholamines are necessary to stimulate smooth muscle cells of the mesenteric arterioles of old animals.

Extracardial nerves are responsible for the control of cardiac metabolism. The diminution of neural control promotes disturbances in myocardial trophicity. In conditions of reduced neural control over cardiovascular activity, the regulatory role of humoral factors becomes more significant.

HORMONAL REGULATION

Hormonal regulation alters during aging with changes in hormonal synthesis, secretion, and degradation, and changes of cell receptors. This influences significantly the cardiovascular system since hormones are known to alter circulation and control metabolism within the heart and vessels.

The cardiovascular system is greatly affected by vasopressin, which is released by the neuronal cells of the supraoptic nuclei of the hypothalamus into the posterior lobe of the pituitary. As an active pressor substance of pituitary extracts, vasopressin had been discovered by Oliver and Schäfer[25] as early as 1895. However, the discovery of vasopressin's antidiuretic activity diminished the interest in the effect it produced upon the cardiovascular system. The data obtained during recent decades strongly suggest that vasopressin is capable of not only altering circulatory function, but also of producing pathologic changes. The concentration of blood vasopressin varies with different physiologic reactions of an organism. In stress it increases tenfold.[26] In aged animals and humans blood vasopressin is increased. The increase is especially marked in hypertensive and ischemic heart diseases.[27]

The pressor effect of vasopressin is associated with constriction arterial smooth muscle, and the increase in total peripheral resistance. Still, cardiac output decreases under the effects of vasopressin.[28] This decrease can be attributed to the diminished venous return, the weakening of myocardial contractility conditioned by coronary constriction, and to the reflex bradycardia.

The sensitivity of the cardiovascular system to vasopressin increases with age. In aged rats and rabbits, signs of coronary insufficiency can be produced by smaller vasopressin doses. The increased cardiovascular response to vasopressin, its increase in the blood, and the decreasing response to tachyphylaxis enhance its effect upon the cardiovascular system in old age and its role in the development of coronary insufficiency.

In old age, the reactivity of cardiovascular system to epinephrine alters. The increased hemodynamic effects and myocardial contractility of adult animals are more pronounced following increased doses of epinephrine as compared with older animals. The range of possible reactions is much greater in the latter, and at the same time, small doses of hormone (0.05 μg/100 g) induce a more marked increase of cardiac output and stroke volume, arterial blood pressure, and contractility index. Extrasystoles, fibrillation, and pulmonary edema are more common in old rats after large doses of epinephrine. According to Korkushko,[29] administration of 0.5 ml of 0.1% solution produced no changes in arterial blood pressure in 20 to 29-year-old subjects, whereas in persons aged 80 to 89 years it increased from 117.9 ± 3.5 to 138.8 ± 6.3 mmHg. Under stress, significant amounts of vasopressin and epinephrine are released in the blood. Epinephrine activates mechanisms of vasopressin secretion and increases vascular sensitivity to it. The combination of these factors may induce substantial changes in cardiac function, especially in aging.

Thyroxine is capable of changing cardiovascular function by increasing the heart rate, arterial blood pressure, and the maximal rate of increase of intraventricular pressure.[30,31] The thyroxine-induced hyperfunction and direct activation of protein biosynthesis result in the development of cardiac hypertrophy. According to Florini et al[32] thyroxine (100 mg/animal every second day) produced cardiac hypertrophy after 9 days in old rats and after 6 days in adult rats. Frolkis et al[33] showed age-related cardiovascular differences after thyroxine administration by comparing the changes that ensued on the fourth and 14th days after daily administration (10.0 μg/100 g, intraperitoneally). As is seen in Figure 6-5, the hemo-and cardiodynamic shifts reached a peak on the fourth day in old rats, but were still on the increase on the 14th day in adult rats.

The increase of cardiac sensitivity to thyroxine in old age cannot be accounted for only by the fall of the blood concentration of the thyroid hormones. First, the level of free thyroxine in the blood remains unchanged in old age. Second, in experiments with thyroidectomy, ie, in conditions of leveling off the age-related changes in thyroxine content, old animals also display increased hormonal sensitivity. The production of an iodine-free state is essential in the mechanism of tissue response to thyroid hormones. Valueva[34] reported increased deiodinating activity of a hormone in the older heart, which may be a cause for the increased sensitivity to its effect.

During aging, there is a decrease in the insulin provision of the organism, and in blood insulin activity, despite the rise of insulin content in some persons with low carbohydrate tolerance. An imbalance between blood insulin activity and content may be explained by an increased concentration of substances that inhibit hormone activity. Insulin produces marked hemodynamic changes: a decrease of cardiac output, left ventricular

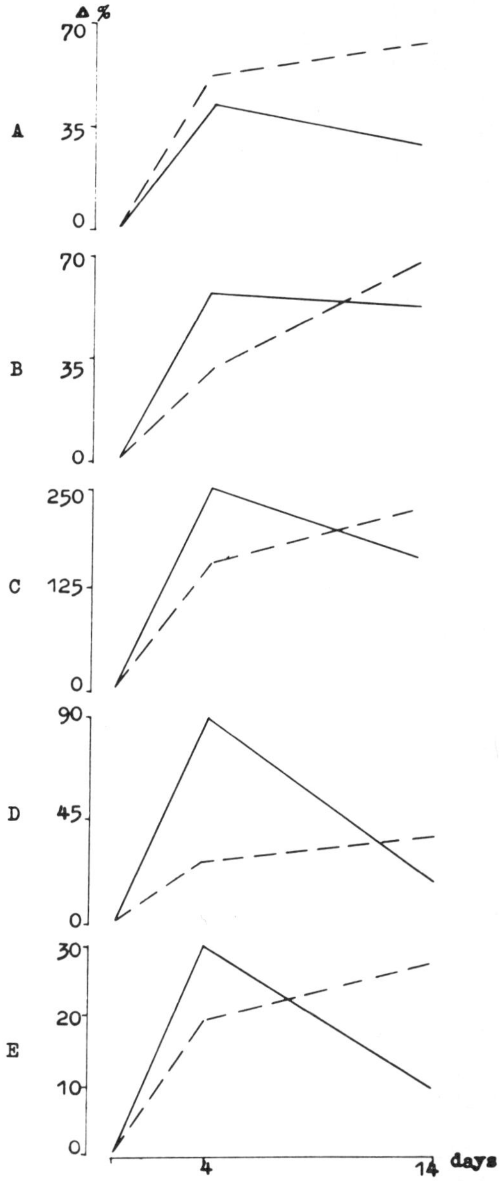

Figure 6-5 Changes in hemodynamics and myocardial contractility following short-term (4 days) and long-term (14 days) administration of thyroxine (10.0 μg/100 g body weight) to adult (broken line) and old (solid line) rats. Ordinate: A: systemic arterial blood pressure; B: cardiac rhythm; C: cardiac output; D: maximal rate of increase of intraventricular pressure; E: contractility index. Abscissa: days of thyroxine administration.

working index, arterial blood pressure, etc. The threshold hemodynamic shifts appear in aged rats and rabbits at smaller doses. The hemodynamic shifts are believed to be linked to the direct effect of insulin, rather than mediated by the hypoglycemia. This is substantiated by the fact that the hemodynamic effects persist after simultaneous administration of insulin and glucose. Age-related changes in response to the various links of the cardiovascular system to insulin are diverse. According to I. Frolkis[35] the sensitivity of vascular smooth muscular cells to insulin decreases with age. Large concentrations of insulin produce less marked relaxation and hyperpolarization of old animal smooth muscular cells.

In summary, the cardiovascular response to hormonal effects alters significantly during aging. This occurs in conditions of altered secretion of hormones, and their blood concentration. The diminished circulatory response to hormonal effects limits the capacity of the cardiovascular system to adapt to conditions of the organism's existence. The increase in sensitivity to some hormones under conditions of their decreased blood concentration has adaptive value. Noteworthy is the fact that owing to uneven changes of blood concentrations of some hormones, and of the cardiovascular response to their effect, there are qualitative changes in hormonal regulation of metabolism and cardiovascular function in old age.

REGULATION OF CORONARY BLOOD FLOW

The discrepancy between oxygen demand and blood supply of the myocardium in old age may often limit not only cardiac activity, but also the adaptive capacities of the whole organism. This is especially evident in humans due to the high incidence of coronary atherosclerosis.

In old age, the heart becomes more sensitive to the restriction of coronary perfusion. Old dogs develop more significant changes in myocardial contractility in response to the restriction of perfusion.

The prevalence of coronary insufficiency in old age is also related to the peculiarities of neurohumoral regulation of coronary vascular tone. The peculiarities of response of cardiac vessels to regulatory effects have been studied in experiments on dogs with catheterization of coronary vessels and extracorporal perfusion of coronary vessels, and in experiments with direct measurements of volume blood flow in the circumflex branch of the left coronary artery. The thresholds of stimulation of the vagal nerve and the subclavian loop of sympathetic nerve, which induce dilatation of coronary vessels, were found to increase from 0.4 ± 0.02 V in to 0.9 ± 0.03 V, and from 0.55 ± 0.03 V to 1.2 ± 0.02 V in adult and aged dogs, respectively. In different situations, activated via adrenergic pathways, there occurs significant enhancement of metabolism and contractility of the myocardium. The increase of coronary blood flow in these conditions has great adaptive significance. The weakening of neural effects on coronary vessels and less pronounced dilatation of coronary vessels will promote the development of myocardial ischemia. Still, it was found that smaller intracoronary doses of norepinephrine and acetylcholine induce dilatation of coronary vessels in old dogs.

It is important that the paradoxical responses to the effects of regulatory factors occur in old age. Thus, it was found that in 45% of old dogs certain doses of epinephrine may produce constriction, rather than dilatation, of coronary vessels. The combination of epinephrine-induced activation of metabolism with constriction of coronary vessels may result in significant damage to the myocardium.

Most physiologically active substances are capable of dilating coronary vessels. Marked constriction of coronary vessels can be produced by vasopressin. It has already been pointed out that the sensitivity of coronary vessels to vasopressin is increased in old age. In old rabbits and dogs, smaller doses of the hormone induce a fall of coronary blood flow, an increase in vascular resistance, and the development of coronary insufficiency. Vasopressin, like epinephrine, is released in large quantities in stressful situations. Epinephrine sharply increases the sensitivity of vessels to vasopressin, and this becomes an important mechanism in the development of vasoconstriction. Vasopressin affects the coronary vessels via special cell receptors. The use of vasopressin competitors in preventing the coronary constriction shows promise, but more promising may be the use of derivatives of the vasopressin molecule. Vasopressin has been shown to prevent the development of vasopressin-induced coronary insufficiency.[36] Competing for vasopressin receptors, this reagent does not produce its physiologic effects. Thus, uneven changes in the sensitivity of heart and coronary vessels may promote the development of coronary insufficiency in old age.

LOCAL MECHANISMS OF NEUROHUMORAL REGULATION

In the complicated hierarchy of neurohumoral regulation of the cardiovascular system, the local, intraorganic regulatory mechanisms are of special importance. These include local reflexes, pacemaker function, and production of local hormones within the heart. Local reflexes are activated with the participation of the intracardiac nervous system. Both local cholinergic and adrenergic reflexes can be activated via cardiac ganglia. This is linked, in large measure, to structural and metabolic changes in cardiac ganglia. With aging, there occurs increase in the size of ganglion cells, emergence of irregularly shaped cells, thickening of neuronal capsules, decrease in density of localization of nervous elements, and proliferation of connective tissue in nodal stroma. In old age, the nervous cells of cardiac ganglia demonstrate fragmentation, swelling of mitochondria, clarification of mitochondrial matrix, and decrease in the number of mitochondria per volume unit of cytoplasm.

All these structural shifts are combined with age-related metabolic changes in cardiac ganglia. Histochemical analysis reveals a decrease in cholinesterase activity, redistribution of localization of monoamine oxidase, and a decrease in glycogen content, etc. In addition, in old animals the lability of intracardic ganglia is decreased. The weakening of local, peripheral reflexes in old age may limit participation of essential intraorganic regulatory mechanisms in the adaptation of the cardiovascular system.

The decrease of spontaneous activity of the sino-atrial (SA) node is an important link in the mechanism of intracardiac regulation. In experiments on isolated strips of atria (zone of location of sinus node) the frequency of pacemaker activity was found to be 187.8 ± 8.5 impulses/min in adult rats, and 136.1 ± 10.2 impulses/min in aged rats.

The decrease in intensity of acetylcholine synthesis, and the reduction of potassium conductivity play an important role in the mechanism of the decrease in sinus nodal lability. The fall of spontaneous activity of the SA node in combination with disturbed conductivity promote the development in old age of ectopic foci of excitation, ie, extrasystoles. The frequency of the SA node-generated cardiac rhythm determines the intensity of many metabolic cycles within the heart. In the myocardial cells, the phosphorylation of adenosine monophosphate (AMP), which is catalyzed by 5′-nucleotidase, results in the formation of adenosine. Adenosine, formed on the outer membrane, is released into extracellular space.[37] Adenosine metabolism and the rate of its release from the myocardium are closely linked to oxygen balance within the heart. Adenosine produces marked coronary dilatation, and is capable of influencing glucose metabolism and its transport into the cell. The activity of 5′-nucleotidase is increased in the blood of old rabbits and myocardial tissue (Figure 6-6). The increased activity of adenosine deaminase in old age is less marked. Correlations of the activity of the adenosine catalysts suggest enhancement of adenosine formation in old age. However, in old age, the capacities of the adenosine-forming system are exhausted and cannot

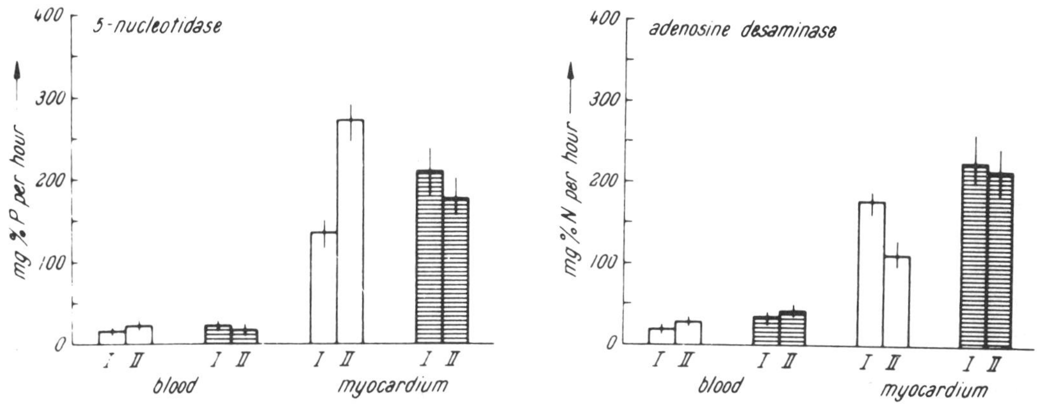

Figure 6-6 Effect of long-term vasopressin administration upon the activity of enzymes of adenosine metabolism in the blood and myocardium of adult (while columns) and old (hatched columns) rabbits. I: control; II: long-term administration of vasopressin.

respond to hypoxia with significant activation. In experiments on rabbits, coronary insufficiency and the oxygen deficit in the heart were simulated by daily administration of vasopressin. In adult rabbits the activity of 5′-nucleotidase increased and that of adenosine deaminase decreased. In old animals, no such changes occurred despite marked hypoxic shifts in the heart.[38]

Among the local humoral regulatory mechanisms of the cardiovascular system, much attention has been attributed in recent years to the kallikrein-kinin system. Bradykinin is capable of increasing coronary blood flow, venous return, and cardiac output, while decreasing the tone of coronary vessels, etc. Definite activation occurs in the kallikrein-kinin system during aging: the content of the kallikrein precursor kallikreinogen increases; the antitryptic and kininase activities decrease. The attenuated enzymatic degradation of kinins leads to a more prolonged effect of peptides. This may explain the fact that small doses of bradykinin (0.25 μg/kg) produced more marked hemodynamic changes in old rabbits than in adult ones. During aging, significant changes evolve in the microcirculation: the number of capillaries is decreased, the diffusion area increases. A decrease under these conditions of kinin degradation may promote the maintenance of a certain level of microcirculation. However, in vasopressin-induced hypoxia, the activation of the kallikrein-kinin system is more marked in adult rabbits.

Prostaglandins play an important role in the mechanisms of local regulation of cardiac metabolism and function. The basal level of prostaglandins E and A in the myocardium remains unchanged with age. However, vasopressin (0.5 U/kg) produced no changes in prostaglandin levels in adult rats, whereas in old rats it increased remarkably (from 14.8 ± 1.5 to 29.3 ± 3.1 ng/kg tissue). This increase in prostaglandins in the myocardium of old rats is of adaptive value, being related to more marked myocardial hypoxia. Prostaglandins are capable of altering the state of cardiac adrenergic receptors. By inhibiting adenylate cyclase, the prostaglandins limit the effect of catecholamines. Epinephrine (30 μg/100 g, intraperitoneally) produced no changes in the myocardial prostaglandins of adult rats, and increased their level from 16.6 ± 1.4 to 31.5 ± 4.2 ng/g in old rats. Such marked activation of prostaglandin synthesis may represent a mechanism aimed at limiting adrenergic reactions.

Serotonin has a significant hemodynamic effect. It is capable of changing vascular tone, cardiac output, and of inducing reflexes from the chemoreceptors of heart and vessels. The content of serotonin in the heart does not alter with age. However, hemodynamic shifts are produced by doses of 0.01 μg/kg in old rabbits, and by 0.15 μg/kg in adult rabbits. With increase in dose the hemodynamic shifts in old animals become smaller than in adult animals. Thus, many local humoral mechanisms of regulation are activated in old age under conditions of weakened neural control over the activity of cardiovascular system.

FEEDBACK CONTROL IN MECHANISMS OF NEUROHUMORAL REGULATION

The reliability of neurohumoral regulation of the cardiovascular system and its adaptation to the organism's demands are attained through feedback control mechanisms. In their achievement great importance is attributed to reflexes from the mechano- and chemoreceptors of heart and vessels. Moreover, the disturbance of feedback control and the change of character of reflexes from the receptive vascular zones promote the development of pathologic cardiovascular states, including hypertension. The hemodynamic center may affect cardiovascular receptors, modify their activity, and trigger special activation or inhibitory mechanism.[39]

With aging, reflexes from the pressoreceptors of the carotid sinus and the aortic arch, and from cardiac receptors are diminished. Thus, the depressor reflex from isolated carotid sinus in old rabbits occurs at much higher perfusion pressure than in young rabbits. In old animals, the pressor reflex from the carotid sinus, which can be reproduced with fall of pressure in the latter, is also diminished. The diminution of the carotid sinus reflex has also been reported in elderly subjects.[40,41] Reflexes from baroreceptors are aimed at restoring arterial blood pressure with orthostatic changes of body position. In elderly subjects, the occurrence of decrease of arterial blood pressure on orthostatic testing is more than threefold higher than in young subjects.

In old animals, the reflexes from atrial mechanoreceptors are attenuated. Thus, similar distention of the right atrium of old animals causes less marked deceleration of heart rate, fall of arterial blood pressure, change of intraventricular pressure and contractility index, etc.

In adapting the cardiovascular system to the state of the organism's milieu interieur, the reflexes from chemoreceptors of heart and vessels are significant. The sensitivity of carotid sinus receptors and intestinal vessels to hypoxia and cholinomimetics increases with age. As is evident from Figure 6-7, in old animals smaller doses of some substances induce cardiovascular and respiratory reflexes. It is noteworthy that with age there are changes in the response of vascular receptors to hormones.

The diminution of reflexes from cardiovascular mechanoreceptors and the substantial decrease in reflexes from chemoreceptors lead to fundamental age-related changes in feedback control of neurohumoral regulation of blood circulation. This results in the development of long-term stagnant hemodynamic shifts with changes in load, and to hypertensive reactions. Prompt adaptation of reflexes from mechanoreceptors in old age, ie, their switching-off with long-term increase of arterial blood pressure, promotes the development of arterial hypertension. The destruction of cardiac receptors and diminution of reflexes from this receptive zone are assumed to explain the occurrence of painless myocardial infarctions in old age.

There are two feedback control channels in the regulation of the cardiovascular system. The first, which has been analyzed above, is linked to data on changes in cardiovascular activity and metabolism; the second, with data on the blood content of hormonal substances, is capable of inducing cardiovascular reactions. These are epinephrine, vasopressin, insulin, among others, which influence both heart, vessels, and the corresponding nervous centers. This may lead in turn to changes in secretion and cardiovascular function. As was emphasized above, the sensitivity of the hemodynamic center to some hormones and transmitters changes significantly in old age. This may result in an inadequate response to changes in the organism's milieu interieur.

NEUROHUMORAL MECHANISMS OF DEVELOPMENT OF AGE-RELATED PATHOLOGIC CONDITIONS

Age-related changes in neurohumoral regulation appear to play a significant role is shaping cardiovascular pathology in old age. The attenuation of neural control over heart and vessels, and the shifts in their reactivity to hormones, transmitters, and other physiologically active substances largely determine the specificity of age-related pathologic changes. The prevalence of arterial hypertension in old age and the role played by disturbances in the neurohumoral regulation of vascular tone and cardiac activity are well known.

Figure 6-8 illustrates data on the development of arterial hypertension, induced by the disturbance of different regulatory mechanisms.

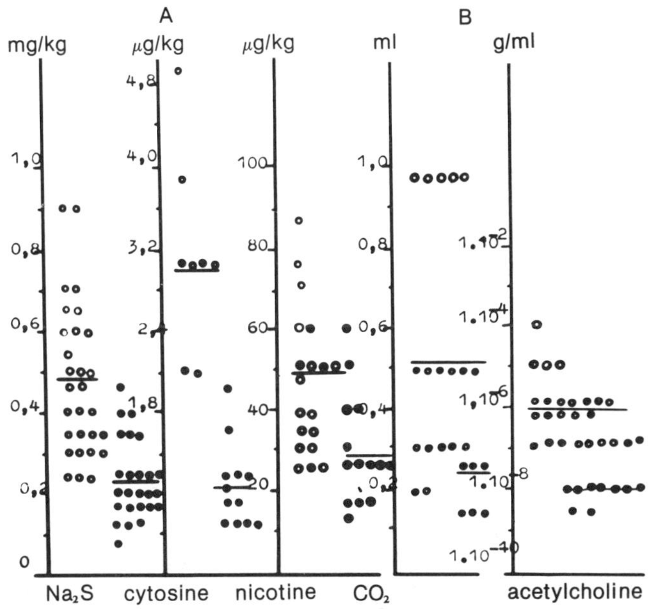

Figure 6-7 Threshold doses of various substances which cause reflexes from chemoreceptors of the carotid sinus in rabbits (A) and from chemoreceptors of the intestine vessels in cats (B). White circles: adult animals; dark circles: old animals.

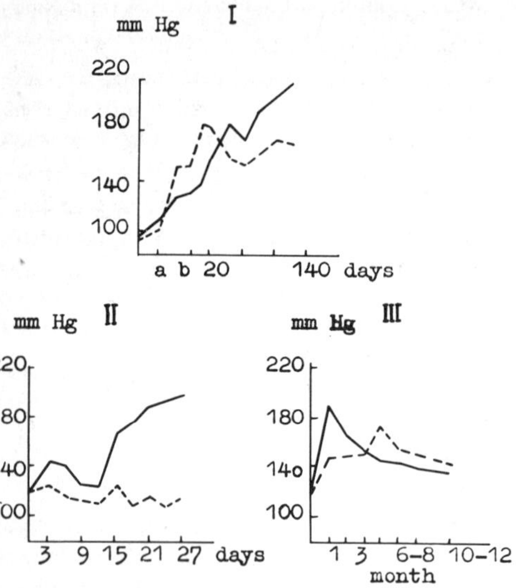

Figure 6-8 Age differences in changes of arterial blood pressure in various forms of experimental hypertension. I: reflexogenic hypertension; II: vasopressin-induced hypertension; III: renal hypertension. Broken line: adult rabbits; Solid line: old rabbits. Abscissa: period after reproduction of experimental hypertension. Abscissa I: sections of aortic and carotid nerves on left (a) and on right (b). (Data on renal hypertension were obtained by N.P. Stroganova, 1965.)

Changes also occur in old age in the hemodynamic pattern of arterial hypertension. Thus, with development of vasopressin-induced and renal hypertension, cardiac output is increased, as a result of the high initial level of total peripheral resistance and vascular tone.

The role of powerful reflexogenic depressor zones of vessels in maintaining arterial blood pressure levels is known. In aging, the reflexes from vascular mechanoreceptors are attenuated, thus reducing the reliability of depressor mechanisms and enhancing the development of hypertensive reactions.

Vasopressin plays an important role in the development of cardiovascular pathology in old age. The concentration of blood vasopressin and the sensitivity of heart and vessels to it are increased. In addition, there is direct evidence for an increase of vasopressin concentration in arterial hypertension.

The increase of aldosterone content in conditions of reduced activity of membrane K^+-Na^+ adenosine triphosphatase (ATPase) will promote more marked accumulation of intracellular Na^+ and increase of vascular tone, accumulation of intracellular Ca^{++}, and increase of cardiac output. Thus, the weakening of reflexes from vascular mechanoreceptors, activation of the vasopressin-aldosterone mechanism, and the change in the state of the juxtaglomerular apparatus promote the development of arterial hypertension.

Catecholamines are known to cause the development of myocardial hypoxia. In old animals, smaller doses of catecholamines were found to produce ECG manifestations of myocardial hypoxia and disturbances of myocardial contractility. The changes of neurohumoral regulation in old age promote the development of disturbances of cardiac rhythm. Thus, vasopressin-/and epinephrine-induced arrhythmias are more prolonged in old age. In old rats, smaller doses of catecholamines induce fibrillation and pulmonary edema. All these factors further the development of cardiac insufficiency in old age.

ACKNOWLEDGEMENT

Alex A. Volkov translated the original Russian text into English.

REFERENCES

1. Frolkis VV: *Reflex Regulation of the Activity of the Cardiovascular System*. Kiev, Gosmedizdat, 1959, p 285 (in Russian).
2. Mankovsky NB, Mints A Ya: *Aging and the Nervous System*. Kiev, Zdorovja Publications, 1972, p 278 (in Russian).
3. Frolkis VV: Regulation, Adaptation and Aging. Leningrad, Nauka, 1970, p 432 (in Russian).
4. Bezrukov VV: Age specificity of the EEG changes following intravenous and intraperitoneal administration of adrenaline, noradrenaline and acetylcholine. Proceedings of the 8th Scientific Conference on Age Morphology, Physiology and Biochemistry. Moscow, Institute of Age Physiology, part 2, 1967, pp 44–45 (in Russian).
5. Dilman VM: The hypothalamic control of aging and age-associated pathology: The elevation mechanism of aging, in Everitt AV (ed): *Hypothalamus, Pituitary and Aging*. Springfield, CC Thomas, 1976, pp 634–667.
6. Everitt AV: Conclusion: Aging and its hypothalamic-pituitary. *Hypothalamus, Pituitary and Aging*. Springfield, CC Thomas, 1976, pp 676–702.
7. Rushkevich Yu E: Structural disturbances of the myocardium following many-day stimulation of the hypothalamus in animals of different age. *Actual Problems of Modern Pathophysiology*. Kiev, Naukova Dumka, 1981, pp 305–307 (in Russian).
8. Lakiza T Yu: Analysis of the age specificity of the adrenergic regulation of the cardiovascular system. *Biochemical and Physiological Mechanisms of Aging*. Minsk, Nauka i Tekhnika, 1980, pp 121–128 (in Russian).
9. Shevchuk VG: Influence of acetylcholine and catecholamines on hemodynamics at various stages of ontogenesis. USSR, Vestnik AMN, 1973, N12, pp 52–55.

10. Shvalev VN, Vikhert AM, Stropus RA, et al: New developments in the reconstruction of neurohumoral regulation of human heart in the gerontological aspect. Proceedings of 4th All-Union Congress of Gerontology and Geriatrics. Kiev, Institute of Gerontology, 1982, pp 430 (in Russian).
11. Verkhratsky NS: Characteristics of catecholamine metabolism during aging. Proceedings of 9th International Congress of Gerontology. Kiev, Institute of Gerontology, 1972, vol 1, pp 106–110.
12. Zhubrikova LA: Ontogenetic differences in the concentration of catecholamines and activity of monamine oxidase in the organs of albino rats. Vestnik Kharkovskogo Universiteta, 1978, N164, pp 19–22 (in Russian).
13. Tuttle RS: Age-related changes in the sensitivity of rat aortic strips to norepinephrine and associated chemical and structural alteration. *J Gerontol* 1966;21:510–516.
14. Pandya KH: Postnatal developmental changes in adrenergic receptor responses of the dog tracheal muscle. *Arch Int Pharmacodyn Ther* 1977;4:(N230)53–64.
15. Parker RJ, Berkowitz BA, Lee Ch-ho, et al: Vascular relaxation, aging and thyroid hormones. *Mech Ageing Develop* 1978;8:(N6)397–405.
16. Strozzi C, Morsiani M, Paresche P: Risposta al betastimoto dell coccolo peruferico del soggento anziano. *G Gerontol* 1975;23:(N7)553–557.
17. Hruza Z, Zweifach B: Effect of age on vascular reactivity to catecholamines in rats. *J Gerontol* 1967;22:1469–1472.
18. Chebotarev DF, Korkushko OV: Cardiovascular system in elderly and old age. *Problems of Age, Physiology and Pathophysiology of the Cardiovascular System.* Moscow, *Institute of Gerontology*, 1966; pp 147–149 (in Russian).
19. Korkushko OV, Ivanov LA: *Hypoxia and Aging.* Kiev, Institute of Physiology 1980, p 274 (in Russian).
20. Zitnik G, Roth RS: Effects of thyroid hormones on cardiac hypertrophy and beta-adrenergic receptors during aging. *Mech Ageing Develop* 1981;15:19–28.
21. Narayanan N, Derby JA: Alterations in the properties of beta-adrenergic receptors of myocardial membranes in aging: Impairments in agonist-receptor interactions and guanine nucleotide regulation accompany diminished catecholamine-responsiveness of adenylate cyclase. *Mech Ageing Develop* 1982;19:127–139.
22. Kulchitsky OK: Effect of acetylcholine on the content of myocardial cyclic guanosine monophosphate in rats of different age. *Bull Exp Biol Med* 1981;N9:318–319.
23. Frolkis IV: Functional and ultrastructural specificity of the smooth muscle cells of the portal vein of animals of different age, author's abstract of the dissertation for a candidate's degree (medicine). Kiev, Institute of Physiology, 1978 (in Russian).
24. Altura BM, Altura BJ: Pharmacologic studies on aging microvessels. *Vascular Neuroeffector Mechanisms.* New York, Raven Press, 1980, pp 338–341.
25. Oliver G, Schäffer EA: On the physiological action of extracts of pituitary body and certain other glandular organs. *J Physiol* 1895;18:277–279.
26. Saito T, Jochida S: Levels of antidiuretic hormone in plasma after hemorrhage and infusion of hypertonic saline in dogs. *Endocrinology* 1971;88(N6):1511–1513.
27. Golovchenko SF: Concentration of vasopressin in the blood of hypertensive persons of different age. *Probl Endocrinol (Mosk)* 1979;N4:31–35.
28. Nakano J: Studies on the cardiovascular effects of synthetic vasopressin. *J Pharmacol Exp Ther* 1967;157(N1):19–31.
29. Korkushko OV: *Clinical Cardiology and Geriatrics.* Moscow, Meditsina, 1980, p 288 (in Russian).
30. Chakravarty J, Guansing AR, Chakravarty S, et al: Systolic time intervals as indicators of myocardial thyroid hormone effect. *Acta Endocrinol* 1978;67:(N3)507–515.
31. Conri C, Emeriau JP, Emeriau F, et al: Insuffisance thyroidieme et maladie arterielle coronaire. *Bordeaux Med* 1978;11(N8):619–624.
32. Florini JR, Saito V, Manowitz EJ: Effect of age on thyroxine-induced cardiac hypertrophy in mice. *J Gerontol* 1973;28:(N3)293–297.
33. Frolkis VV, Verzhikovskaya NV, Valueva GV: The thyroid and age. *Exp Gerontol* 1973;8:(N5) 255–296.
34. Valueva GV: The role of extra- and intracellular factors in the age changes of the metabolism of thyroid hormones. *Fiziologicheski zhurnal* 1978;N4:18–23.
35. Frolkis VV: Age peculiarities of the effect of insulin upon vascular smooth muscles. Proceedings of 4th All-Union Congress of Gerontology and Geriatrics. Kiev, Institute of Gerontology, 1982, p 401 (in Russian).
36. Frolkis VV: Neurohumoral mechanisms of development of cardiovascular pathology during aging. *Vestnik AMN SSSR* 1980;N3:16–22.
37. Rubio R, Berne RM, Dobson J: Sites of adenosine production in cardiac and skeletal muscle. *Am J Physiol* 1973;225(N8):938–953.
38. Frolkis VV, Golovchenko SF, Medved VI, et al: Vasopressin and cardiovascular system in aging. *Gerontology* 1982;28(N5):920–1302.
39. Korner PI: Integrative neural cardiovascular control. *Physiol Rev* 1971;51:312–367.
40. Lindblad LE: Influence of age on sensitivity and effector mechanisms of the carotid baroreflex. *Acta Physiol Scand* 1977;101:43–49.
41. Winson M, Heath D, Smith P: Extensibility of the human carotid sinus. *Cardiovasc Res* 1974;8(N1):58–64.

CHAPTER 7
Auscultatory Findings in the Elderly

Martin J. Frank
Abdulla M. Abdulla
Laurence O. Watkins

Auscultatory findings in the elderly patient cannot be interpreted without an understanding of the pathophysiology of aging. In the absence of cardiovascular disease, the heart of the geriatric patient is normal in size. Likewise, resting heart rate, ejection fraction, and end-diastolic volume do not differ from the normal values found in younger patients.[1,2] However, the prevalence of hypertension, defined as a systolic blood pressure greater than 160 mmHg and/or a diastolic pressure greater than 95 mmHg, is about 40% to 50% in the population over age 65, while it is only about 16% in the younger adult population.[3] Isolated systolic hypertension is responsible for a major part of this difference, and like systolic/diastolic hypertension is more prevalent in the black population. The higher prevalence of systolic hypertension in older individuals is most likely due to reduced compliance in capacitance arteries and resistance arterioles. The cardiac hypertrophy caused by hypertension results in a progressive increase in heart weight up to the ninth decade of life.[4] There are age-dependent changes in the myocardium independent of blood pressure. These include thickening of the endocardium, including the mitral and aortic leaflets, and an increase in collagen, fat, and elastic tissue throughout the heart including the conduction system. Genetic factors and other cardiovascular diseases may also contribute to the development of cardiac hypertrophy. In addition, myocardial amyloidosis is a degenerative change of old age. Amyloid deposits have been found in 10% of patients between 80 and 90 years of age and in up to 50% of patients dying at 90 years of age and older.[5] In view of all of these factors, it is not surprising that left ventricular function declines with age. The ejection fraction at peak exercise and peak heart rate show a significant decline with increase in age and the increment in ejection fraction from rest to peak exercise is also reduced.[2] These changes are probably due to a decreased responsiveness to catecholamines and an increased afterload. Pathologic changes in the myocardium are responsible for subtle changes in systolic time intervals: mild but progressive prolongation of the preejection phase and left ventricular ejection time, accompanied by significant prolongation of the Q–S_2 interval,[6] and 15% to 20% prolongation in isovolumic relaxation time are found in subjects 62 to 84 years of age when compared to younger adults.[7]

It is also important to appreciate that the geriatric patient rarely has a single disease. The evaluation of the patient should therefore begin with a detailed medical history, which will include the chief complaint, history of present illness, past medical history, social and occupational data, and a review of systems. Interpretation of auscultatory findings is also critically dependent upon observations made during careful examination of the optical fundi, cervical venous and arterial pulses, auscultation of the lungs, inspection and palpation of the precordium, and evaluation of the peripheral pulses.

HEART SOUNDS

First Sound

The intensity of the first heart sound is determined by the position of the mitral valve leaflets at the onset of left ventricular systole and the contractile state of the left ventricle (LV). The former determines the extent of the mitral valve leaflet motion prior to closure, and the latter, the rate of closure. Therefore, prolonged atrioventricular conduction and LV dysfunction result in softening of S_1 because the mitral valve has moved to a more closed position before the onset of systole and the rate of subsequent closure is reduced. Shorter conduction times and more vigorous contraction increase the intensity of S_1 because the leaflets are more separated and closure rate more rapid. These relationships are altered by pathologic changes in isovolumic systole, eg, aortic regurgitation which produces early closure, and changes in the physical characteristics of the mitral apparatus, eg, calcification of the mitral annulus which reduces closure rate. Regardless of the above, alterations in the physical characteristics of the thorax by emphysema, senile osteoporotic kyphosis, heavy musculature, or large breasts tend to reduce the intensity of S_1 as appreciated by the examiner. Since emphysema, first degree heart block, and left bundle-branch block are more common in the elderly, there is a general tendency for S_1 to be soft. In addition, prolongation of the preejection period, along with the tendency toward softening, reduces the likelihood that splitting of S_1 will be appreciated.

Second Sound

Sequential closure of the aortic and pulmonic valves occurs silently. However, motion of the aortic and pulmonic leaflets toward their respective ventricles induces pressure changes and vibration of the valves and contiguous structures, which are transmitted to the chest wall in the form of closure sounds. Since hypertension and atherosclerosis are common in the elderly, the aortic closure sound (A_2) is often accentuated. Senile ectasia of the ascending aorta may impart a drumlike quality to A_2. These structural and physiologic abnormalities are more common than fibrosis and calcification of the aortic valve, which reduce valve mobility and the intensity of A_2. The intensity of the pulmonic closure sound (P_2) is more likely to be reduced because of the presence of pulmonary emphysema than are the intensity of S_1 and A_2. Therefore, S_2 is often appreciated as a single sound. A second factor contributing to the perception of S_2 as single is a reduction in the A_2–P_2 interval, which is a common occurrence with advancing age, probably due to reduced pulmonary compliance and shortening of the right-sided hangout interval. Wide inspiratory splitting of the S_2 is uncommon in the geriatric patient and persistent expiratory splitting in the recumbent position is not a normal finding in older patients. In these circumstances, P_2 is usually accentuated, and the combination of findings suggests pulmonary hypertension. Occasionally, fixed splitting of S_2, indicative of a previously undetected atrial septal defect, will be heard in an older patient, who may have become symptomatic because of the onset of atrial fibrillation or flutter. The single S_2 is particularly common after age 50, but is not due to a significant delay in A_2. However, when A_2 is delayed sufficiently, S_2 may be split paradoxically. The split then narrows or disappears during inspiration, because the timing of P_2 varies normally with respiration, while the delay in the occurrence of A_2 results in expiratory splitting. The most common cause of reversed splitting of S_2 is complete left bundle-branch block (CLBBB). Therefore, reversed splitting may also be appreciated after insertion of a transvenous pacemaker, since right ventricular pacing results in a pattern of electrical activation of the ventricles identical to that produced by CLBBB. Reversed splitting will rarely be caused by prolonged LV ejection in the absence of CLBBB. Moreover, though LV ejection is prolonged in hemodynamically significant aortic stenosis, reversed splitting of S_2 on this basis is rarely detected in the geriatric patient, since fibrosis and calcification of the aortic valve usually result in an inaudible A_2.

Fourth Sound

The fourth sound (S_4) is related to augmentation of ventricular filling by atrial systole. It is an audible, low-pitched vibration occurring more than 70 ms after the electrocardiographic P-wave and preceding the QRS. Because of prior diastolic filling, the ventricle is close to its limits of compliance. As a result, the rapid ventricular filling produced by atrial contraction results in rapid acceleration of the ventricle and sudden deceleration of the blood mass, which causes vibration of the LV walls and mitral apparatus. Coupling of the ventricle with the chest wall also contributes to the genesis of the S_4, since the intensity of S_4 is greater over the chest wall than within the ventricle. The phonocardiogram often records two sets of vibrations. The first set is of very low frequency and is generally inaudible with a stethoscope, while the second set, higher in frequency and intensity, is most likely responsible for the audible S_4. A physiologic S_4 may be heard in infants, small children and adults over the age of 50, but is almost invariably pathologic between these age groups and is then referred to as an atrial gallop or S_4 gallop sound (S_4G). Some authors have maintained that since the S_4 is such a common finding in the elderly, it has little diagnostic value.[8] However, it is our view that the presence of an S_4 in patients over 50 most likely indicates a noncompliant, distended, or ischemic ventricle. This view is shared by others.[9,10] The multiple factors contributing to increased stiffness of the ventricle and thus to the relatively high prevalence of the S_4G in the elderly have been discussed in the introduction to this chapter. A few additional comments are required concerning hypertension. Normal levels for blood pressure in the geriatric patient are not generally established or accepted. Some clinicians consider a pressure as high as 170/100 mmHg as a normal value in a patient aged 70 years. However, this is not a reasonable assumption, since chronic elevation of the blood pressure to this level results in myocardial hypertrophy sufficient to cause an S_4. For interpreting the findings of physical assessment, 150/90 mmHg should be considered the upper limits of normal and an S_4 heard in a patient with blood pressures above this level may be attributable to the effect of elevated pressure on ventricular mass and distensibility. The incidence of ischemic heart disease also increases with age, and coronary atherosclerosis is rarely absent at autopsy in patients over age 70. However, exertional angina is frequently absent, because peripheral vascular disease, peripheral muscle weakness, and a natural tendency toward a more sedentary life style limit physical activity in the elderly. In these circumstances an S_4G may be the only evidence of the acute or chronic effects of myocardial ischemia. Other causes of an S_4G include anemia, thyrotoxicosis, cardiomyopathy, aortic regurgitation, acute mitral regurgitation, aortic stenosis, arteriovenous fistula and chronic sinus tachycardia. A right-sided S_4G may be found with chronic cor pulmonale resulting from senile kyphosis, emphysema, pulmonary fibrosis, chronic bronchitis (particularly in the smoker), previous infection, and occupational exposure to pulmonary irritants. Inspection of the chest and back and auscultation of the lungs may reveal signs of chronic pulmonary disease and provide valuable clues to explain the presence of an S_4G. Other causes include pulmonary hypertension of any origin, acute pulmonary emboli, and cardiomyopathy. Since the geriatric patient rarely presents with a single disease, the S_4G is often multifactoral. One should always make an attempt to identify its cause(s).

The left-sided S_4G is heard best with the patient in the left semilateral position and the bell of the stethoscope applied at the apex beat with just enough pressure to ensure a seal with the skin. Firmer pressure may eliminate the sound. The S_4G is appreciated as a low-pitched sound preceeding S_1. It is often "felt" by the tympanic membranes rather than "heard" at the chest wall. The pathologic nature of the S_4 is unquestionable when a visible or palpable S_4 shock is identified. This will be appreciated as a double impulse consisting of presystolic expansion (recorded as the A wave in the apexcardiogram) followed by the usual systolic thrust. When pulmonary emphysema or a thick chest wall prevents palpation of the apex beat, transmission of an S_4G to the primary aortic area and the suprasternal notch strongly suggests a pathologic sound. The right-sided S_4G is usually best heard at the lower left sternal border or, in patients with significant pulmonary emphysema, below the xiphoid process. The bell of the stethoscope must be applied with a degree of care similar to that for the identification of the left-sided S_4G. The right-sided S_4G is often well-heard at the right side of the neck and may be identified in this location even when inaudible over the chest. The patient's chin must be turned up and to the left while one listens at the base of the neck, between the insertions of the sternocleidomastoid muscle (over the internal jugular vein). This sound is often accentuated by deep inspiration and is commonly associated with a prominent A-wave in the jugular venous pulse.

Regardless of the origin of an S_4G, its loudness may be increased following exercise, isometric hand grip, raising of the legs, or the injection of phenylephrine hydrochloride. Its audibility may be decreased by maneuvers which diminish venous return such as quiet standing or the application of tourniquets, and by carotid sinus massage.

Third Sound

The third heart sound (S_3) is related to augmentation of ventricular filling during early diastole. It is an audible, low-pitched vibration occurring 100 to 200 ms after closure of the semilunar valve of the ventricle involved. The S_3 is generated at the moment of abrupt transition between rapid ventricular filling (active ventricular relaxation) and the slower filling of elastic distention. This transition produces sudden deceleration of the blood mass, which causes vibration of the ventricular walls and valvular apparatus. Coupling of the ventricle with the chest wall also contributes to the genesis of the S_3, since the intensity of S_3 is greater over the chest than within the ventricle. A physiologic S_3 is commonly heard in healthy children and young adults, particularly those with rapid filling rates and large flow volumes. It is infrequent after 30 years of age, and very rare after the age of 35. Therefore, an S_3G is never a normal finding in the geriatric population. However, the prognostic importance of an S_3G depends upon its cause. A third heart sound is a common finding in hyperdynamic circulatory states, eg, those produced by severe anemia or thyrotoxicosis. Since these conditions are completely correctable when identified, the S_3G should disappear following therapy. However, the hyperthyroid state in the elderly may be missed, because it is more likely to present as apathetic thyrotoxicosis; often with depression or a confusional state, while younger patients are most often clearly hypermetabolic.[11] Examination of the thyroid gland of the elderly patient most commonly reveals a moderately enlarged, multinodular gland. The fine rales of pulmonary congestion are common as are peripheral edema and muscle wasting. Examination of the heart reveals some degree of cardiomegaly, an irregularly irregular rhythm (atrial fibrillation), and a relatively loud S_3G, often accompanied by an S_4G (with sinus rhythym) and a systolic murmur. Atrial fibrillation usually converts spontaneously to sinus rhythm, and the S_3G disappears following proper management, unless other forms of organic heart disease are also present.[12]

The S_3G is far more often associated with heart failure than is the S_4G. It reflects an important degree of ventricular dysfunction and can be used as a prognostic indicator when subjected to serial evaluation during therapy. In general, the louder the intensity of the S_3G, the greater its clinical significance, and persistence after adequate treatment, particularly when there is associated tachycardia, implies a poor prognosis.

An apical S_3G is commonly found in hemodynamically significant mitral regurgitation or aortic regurgitation, and in these circumstances, does not necessarily signify clinical heart failure. However, the presence of an S_3G is important in the assessment of left ventricular performance in chronic aortic regurgitation. Its presence indicates an expanded end-systolic volume (diminished contractile reserve), rather than severe regurgitation per se.

The S_3G is a dull, low-pitched sound occurring 100 to 200 ms after S_2. The LV S_3G is best heard at the cardiac apex, whereas the right ventricular (RV) S_3G is usually best heard at the lower left sternal border or below the xiphoid. The RV S_3G is usually well transmitted to the internal jugular vein (see the atrial gallop section for method of auscultation). Identification of the sound in this location may be the only sign of RV involvement in a patient with a loud LV S_3G. The S_3G is most often heard *only* with the bell chest piece of the stethoscope, and with the patient in the left semilateral position. As with the S_4G, the bell should be applied with just enough force to provide skin closure. Maneuvers that tend to exaggerate the S_4G will also tend to accentuate the S_3G, but significant softening of the pathologic S_3 upon standing is uncommon.

Systolic Sounds

Ejection sounds Ejection sounds occur as a result of vibrations in either of the great vessels (aorta or pulmonary artery) and the associated semilunar valve at the instant of maximal valve leaflet opening. The presence of an ejection sound in association with evidence of left or right ventricular outflow tract obstruction indicates that the lesion is valvular in location. However, a much higher prevalence of fibrosis and calcification of the valves of the elderly patient as compared with younger patients and consequent loss of valve mobility makes this cause of an ejection sound uncommon in patients over the age of 65 years. Most ejection sounds heard in the elderly arise in the aortic root coincident with the onset of pressure rise in the central aorta. These are commonly observed in high output states, hypertensive cardiovascular disease, and in patients having a sclerotic, tortuous aorta. The ejection sound of valvular aortic stenosis is loudest at the cardiac apex, but is commonly heard in all auscultatory areas; whereas left-sided vascular ejection sounds are invariably loudest in the aortic area and are relatively poorly transmitted. The aortic ejection sound is a high-pitched extra sound heard in early systole, shortly after S_1. It is best heard with the diaphragm chest piece of the stethoscope pressed firmly against the chest wall. It does not change significantly with normal respiration or when the patient sits or stands. The pulmonic ejection sound heard in the elderly patient is most commonly due to dilatation of the pulmonary artery caused by pulmonary hypertension. In these circumstances it will be associated with abnormal splitting of S_2 and an accentuated P_2.

An ejection sound should be considered to be of aortic origin when there is apparent wide splitting of S_1 in the primary aortic area in the presence of evidence for increased LV systolic pressure or stroke output; or when there is roentgenographic evidence of a sclerotic, tortuous thoracic aorta. Apparent wide splitting of S_1 or an unusually loud S_1 in the pulmonic area should make one think of a pulmonic ejection sound, when there is evidence of increased RV systolic pressure or stroke output. At times the ejection sound may be confused with a loud S_4G. Remember that the ejection sound is better heard with the diaphragm chest piece, whereas an S_4G is better heard with the bell of the stethoscope. The S_4G is heard prior to S_1, whereas the ejection sound follows S_1. Pulmonic ejection sounds will increase in intensity during forced expiration, while an RV S_4G will soften. Also remember that an S_4G of left-sided origin is very often associated with a palpable S_4 shock and is widely transmitted, whereas the ejection sound is unassociated with palpable precordial activity and is relatively well localized to an auscultatory area assigned to one or the other of the great vessels.

Nonejection systolic clicks It is now recognized that the vast majority of mid- to late-systolic clicks are related to prolapse of the posterior or both mitral leaflets, or much less commonly, the tricuspid valve leaflets. The most common cause of the nonejection click is idiopathic myxomatous degeneration of the fibrosa layer of the mitral leaflet. In these patients, associated musculoskeletal abnormalities, such as a narrow anteroposterior (AP) diameter of the chest (straight back syndrome), pectus excavatum, kyphoscoliosis, and hypermobility of the joints are quite common.[13] The true prevalence of idiopathic prolapse is unknown. It has been assessed mostly in younger patients, the vast majority of whom are asymptomatic.[14] However, since mitral regurgitation due to myomatous degeneration of the mitral valve may be progressive, elderly patients are apparently more likely to present with congestive heart failure due to progressive mitral regurgitation. Another important life-threatening complication is infective endocarditis. Not surprisingly, however, most elderly patients with a prolapsed mitral leaflet will be unaware of having a cardiac abnormality until the diagnosis is made following a complication. The prognosis for the idiopathic form continues to be benign in most patients. Secondary causes of mitral valve prolapse of importance in the elderly include papillary muscle dysfunction due to ischemic heart disease, congestive and hypertrophic cardiomyopathies, and trauma. However, it may be difficult in any individual case to be sure that a nonejection click did not exist prior to identification of a possible secondary cause.[15]

Accurate assessment of the timing of the nonejection click is the sine qua non for distinguishing it from the ejection sound. Both are high frequency, sharp sounds heard best with the diaphragm chest piece. However, the ejection sound occurs immediately after S_1, whereas the midsystolic click occurs in mid- or late systole. Some patients will have multiple audible nonejection clicks. Those arising from the mitral valve are usually best heard at the cardiac apex, although they may be heard over the entire left precordium. The right-sided click is best heard at the lower left sternal margin. In most elderly patients the nonejection click will be followed by a systolic murmur. If mitral regurgitation has become hemodynamically important, the click will occur earlier and the murmur will be prolonged. In some cases the murmur will be holosystolic, and no click will be appreciated. In these patients the origin of the murmur may not be readily apparent by physical assessment, and the diagnosis will be made only by echocardiography or left ventricular angiography.

SYSTOLIC MURMURS

Innocent Murmurs

Innocent ejection murmurs are common in the first and late decades of life and are detected by auscultation in about two thirds of children and elderly hypertensive patients, and about half of geriatric subjects without overt evidence of heart disease.[16] It is believed that these murmurs are caused by exaggeration of the normal turbulence of the ejected blood mass.[17] In elderly subjects, degenerative fibrotic changes at the base of the aortic cusps, near their attachment to the sinuses of Valvalva, cause some stiffening of the cusps. This, coupled with dilatation of the aortic root, causes the maximal turbulence to be transmitted several diameters away from the valve, and the murmur is often heard best in the region of the second right intercostal space. The innocent murmur of the elderly subject may be heard best in the primary or secondary aortic area or occasionally at the apex, while the physiologic murmur of the child or adolescent is identified best at the left upper sternal border. The former is most often an impure and sometimes harsh murmur; the latter usually has pure, medium frequency vibrations and is occasionally musical. In the elderly patient, innocent murmurs are seldom greater than grade 2/6 in intensity when the patient is supine, and become even softer when the patient stands, because venous return and, hence stroke volume, are decreased. Therefore, they are rarely accompanied by palpable thrills. The murmur is usually short (occurring during the first half of systole), peaks early, and unlike the murmur of valvular aortic stenosis, is not well transmitted to the suprasternal notch or the carotids. However, con usion may arise when an elderly patient with an innocent murmur has coexisting occlusive carotid artery disease, because a carotid bruit may be mistaken for a transmitted murmur. In such a case, careful attention to differences in the character, duration, point of peak intensity, and location of *maximal* audibility of the carotid bruits may help the examiner to arrive at the correct diagnosis. Noninvasive tests (oculoplethysmography and carotid phonoangiography) and even cardiac catheterization may be needed in some patients.

Aortic Stenosis

Isolated valvular aortic stenosis (AS) identified during childhood and early adulthood is usually congenital and results in a delayed carotid upstroke, an ejection sound which is loudest at the apex, and a systolic ejection murmur. The latter is heard best at the base and is transmitted to the suprasternal notch and the neck. The usual physical findings may be lacking or misleading in geriatric patients.

First, palpation of the carotid pulse for estimation of the severity of obstruction may prove highly deceptive in elderly patients. For example, occlusive disease of the carotid arteries in a patient with an innocent murmur may reduce the volume and rate of rise of the carotid pulse and create bruits which may be mistaken for the transmitted murmur of significant AS. Conversely, sclerotic changes in the aging arterial vasculature may make vessels less compliant and more resistant to volume change when the left ventricle ejects blood into it. The systemic systolic pressure is increased and even in patients with significant AS, the upstroke velocity and volume of the carotid pulse is greater than might be anticipated. Thus, the severity of stenosis may be grossly underestimated by the unsuspecting physician.

Second, the intensity, character, and location of the murmur may differ in the elderly patient when compared to younger patients with AS. For example, hyperinflation of the lungs and reduced transmission of audible intracardiac vibrations to the chest wall can diminish the intensity of murmurs, make P_2 inaudible, and render S_2 single. In addition, diminution in its intensity may cause the murmur of significant AS to be mistaken for an innocent murmur, particularly when transvalvular flow is reduced because of left ventricular dysfunction. On the other hand, a single S_2 may be mistakenly considered to be a sign of significant AS in patients with an innocent murmur and bilateral carotid artery disease. The murmur of elderly patients with calcific AS often has a musical or cooing quality and is of maximal intensity at the apex.[18] The same vibrations are heard less well at the right upper sternal border, as a lower pitched murmur.

Finally, the apical systolic murmur of calcific AS in geriatric patients may create other problems in diagnosis. It may be mistaken for mitral regurgitation (MR), particularly when S_2 is inaudible at the apex and the murmur appears to occupy all of systole. This error in interpretation may be avoided, if the examiner recognizes other features such as a silent interval between S_1 and the onset of the murmur and transmission of the murmur to the neck. If the early diastolic murmur of aortic regurgitation (AR) can be heard at the left sternal border, this strongly suggests that the aortic valve is the source of hemodynamic disturbance, but if confusion still exists, one can utilize vasoactive maneuvers to narrow the differential diagnosis. The murmur of AS is augmented during amyl nitrite inhalation and is unchanged during isometric handgrip exercise and phenylephrine infusion, while the murmur of MR is diminished during inhalation of amyl nitrite and enhanced during isometric exercise and phenylephrine infusion. In addition, in patients with atrial fibrillation or premature beats, the murmur of AS tends to become louder during the contraction of the ventricle that follows a longer pause, while the murmur of MR remains unchanged.

Hypertrophic Cardiomyopathy

It has been our observation that hypertrophic cardiomyopathy (HCM) in an elderly subject is frequently mistaken for other conditions. For example, the ECG pattern may be ascribed to a healed myocardial infarction, the chest pain to ischemic heart disease, the murmur and S_4G to papillary muscle dysfunction or aortic stenosis, the brisk carotid pulse to arteriosclerotic changes of the aorta, the dyspnea to congestive heart failure, and the syncope to cerebral vascular disease. The high prevalence of arteriosclerotic disease in the elderly makes the physician less likely to suspect HCM. It has been our experience that a meticulous bedside examination and performance of simple maneuvers, such as auscultation with the patient supine, standing, and after prompt squatting are invaluable in establishing the diagnosis of HCM. When the patient stands, the murmur almost always becomes louder than it was with the patient supine, and it becomes softer when the patient squats promptly. The standing position reduces venous return to the heart, and decreases the volume of the left ventricle, while prompt squatting increases both. When the left ventricular volume is reduced, turbulence across the outflow tract in HCM is increased, and the murmur becomes louder, whereas prompt squatting produces the opposite effects. Sublingual nitroglycerin also augments the murmur of HCM because it is a venodilator which reduces left ventricular volume and increases turbulence of flow across the outflow tract. Patients with HCM are also found to have an apical holosystolic murmur in about 50% of cases. This is usually due to asymmetrical hypertrophy of the left ventricle. A holosystolic murmur is present in elderly patients with HCM more often than in younger subjects, because associated mitral annular calcification is not uncommon in such patients and also results in mild mitral regurgitation.[19]

Mitral Annular Calcification

This is a disease of the elderly and is most common after age 65 years, especially in women.[20]

Systolic murmurs associated with mitral annular calcification may range in character from early systolic to holosystolic, and are heard best at the apex. Although this murmur may occasionally be confused with an innocent murmur, a distinction can be made easily by listening to the murmur while the patient inhales amyl nitrite. Since the drug is an arteriolar dilator, it reduces peripheral vascular resistance, promotes forward flow and reduces the degree of mitral regurgitation. Thus, the systolic murmur of mitral annular calcification decreases in intensity. Amyl nitrite, unlike all other nitrates, is also a venoconstrictor. Therefore it promotes venous return, and increases ventricular stroke volumes causing innocent, and other ejection murmurs to become louder. The murmur of mitral annular calcification is augmented by maneuvers which by increasing peripheral vascular resistance (phenylephrine infusion or isometric handgrip exercise) also increase regurgitation across the incompetent mitral valve. In contrast, innocent and other ejection murmurs are usually unchanged or become softer with these maneuvers.

Papillary Muscle Dysfunction

Papillary muscle dysfunction (PMD) may occur transiently during angina pectoris or chronically following myocardial infarction and is invariably associated with segmental dysfunction of the left ventricle. It is common in patients with ischemic heart disease, since fibrosis and atrophy of one or both papillary muscles are reported in as many as 80% of autopsied hearts.[21] Contrary to popular belief, the murmur of PMD is usually not late systolic or pansystolic. Indeed, the murmur of PMD may have almost any imaginable characteristics with regard to timing, intensity, and quality, and is often accompanied by an accentuated first heart sound and an S_4 gallop.[22] It may or may not be associated with a midsystolic click. The gallop may increase in intensity during inspiration.[22] Although the murmur is heard best at the apex, it may be transmitted to the left sternal border and therefore may be confused with a functional murmur or the murmur of aortic stenosis. Identification of a late, palpable impulse distinct from the apical impulse should make one suspect the presence of previous myocardial infarction with a ventricular aneurysm and PMD as the cause of a murmur located at the apex. However, in some cases, the previously discussed vasoactive maneuvers may be needed to allow the examiner to distinguish this form of mitral regurgitation from aortic stenosis or a functional murmur.

Mitral Valve Prolapse

The exact prevalence of mitral valve prolapse (MVP) in geriatric patients is unknown. However, the presence of myxomatous transformation in the valves of about 7% of autopsied men and women over the age of 70 years[23] suggests that the prevalence of MVP may be of similar magnitude. The elderly patient with MVP may present with chest pain, palpitations, ventricular arrhythmias, congestive heart failure (due to progressive mitral regurgitation), infective endocarditis, transient ischemic attacks, or completed embolic strokes.[24] However, since the elderly patient is unlikely to present with *new* chest pain due to MVP, ischemic heart disease is much more likely. The diagnosis of MVP is most often an incidental finding in an asymptomatic subject. The auscultatory phenomena in this condition have been discussed, in part, earlier in this chapter.

Rheumatic Mitral Regurgitation and Congestive Cardiomyopathy

Because the incidence of acute rheumatic fever has been declining since the beginning of this century, the prevalence of rheumatic heart disease (RHD) is greater among elderly patients than younger ones. About two thirds of elderly patients with RHD have predominant mitral regurgitation (MR). Most elderly patients with hemodynamically important MR will present with physical findings similar to those found in younger patients: an apical holosystolic murmur of grade 3 or more in intensity, an S_3 gallop and a middiastolic flow rumble. A grade 1 or 2/6 murmur accompanied by an S_3 gallop and significant cardiomegaly should make one also consider trivial mitral regurgitation due to congestive cardiomyopathy. Patients with rheumatic MR usually give a history of exertional dyspnea, orthopnea, or paroxysmal dyspnea which has been present for many years prior to the onset of right ventricular failure, whereas those with congestive cardiomyopathy usually develop symptoms of biventricular failure almost simultaneously.

Acute Mitral Regurgitation

Acute MR may occur as a result of rupture of a papillary muscle (about 1% of cases of acute myocardial infarction), as a result of ruptured chordae tendineae in patients with MVP and Marfan's syndrome, or as a result of valvular disruption in infective endocarditis. The clinical picture of acute MR is similar in older and younger age groups, except when the aging process alters the auscultatory events, as described above. Acute MR should be suspected whenever an S_4G accompanies classic signs of significant MR. An S_4G *is not* generated by the dilated atrium of chronic MR.

Acute MR may also differ from its chronic counterpart in the following ways: First, the presentation of significant acute MR is often catastrophic; acute pulmonary congestion or edema accompany the onset of a new murmur. Second, in acute MR cardiac chamber size on the x-ray film is usually normal and there is usually no ECG evidence of left atrial abnormality. Also, sinus rhythm is preserved because the left atrium has not become dilated to the point that atrial fibrillation might occur. Third, unlike the murmur of chronic MR, which is heard best at the apex and is transmitted to the left axilla, the murmur of acute MR may be heard best at the left sternal border and may even be transmitted to the neck, simulating the murmur of aortic stenosis. An incompetent posterior mitral leaflet directs the regurgitant jet against the interatrial septum, while the anterior leaflet diverts the jet to the posterior left atrial wall, Finally, the murmur of acute MR is not holosystolic, but is decrescendo or crescendo-decrescendo in character and stops in mid- to late systole.[25]

Tricuspid Regurgitation

Tricuspid regurgitation (TR) in the geriatric patient may occur as a result of infective endocarditis. It may also occur when the right ventricle dilates because of primary pulmonary hypertension or hypertension due to mitral valve disease, or in congestive cardiomyopathy. Atrial fibrillation develops in more than 85% of cases.[26] Tricuspid regurgitation classically presents with a holosystolic murmur that is best heard at the lower left sternal border. An S_3G and a short diastolic rumble may also be heard in the same area when the regurgitation is hemodynamically significant. The S_3G may also be appreciated over the right internal jugular vein at the base of the neck. The murmur is usually less than grade 3/6, is rarely associated with a thrill, and may occasionally be absent even when the lesion is demonstrable by other means. It may be augmented during deep inspiration (Carvallo's sign), Mueller maneuver (attempted inspiration with the mouth closed and nostrils pinched shut), and following inhalation of amyl nitrite. Also, the murmur tends to regain its original intensity within four to eight beats after the release of the Valsalva maneuver. There may be a prominent V-wave, or a single systolic pulsation ("regurgitant wave") in the jugular veins. The liver is often pulsatile and peripheral edema is common.

Ventricular Septal Defect

A large congenital ventricular septal defect (VSD) may result in heart failure in early life, or pulmonary hypertension (Eisenmenger's syndrome) in later years if it is not surgically corrected. Since neither of these complications is consistent with prolonged survival, elderly patients with an uncorrected congenital VSD usually have a small left-to-right shunt which is well tolerated except for an increased risk of infective endocarditis. The clinical findings of a small VSD are similar to those encountered in young patients. There is a holosystolic murmur that is best heard at the left lower sternal border and is transmitted all over the precordium. It is usually grade 3/6, or greater, in intensity and is frequently associated with a thrill. The history of a murmur dates back to infancy.

Ventricular septal defects may also be acquired as a result of rupture of the ventricular septum during acute myocardial infarction (AMI), a rare complication (less than 1%). This complication should always be suspected whenever a new holosystolic murmur is heard in a patient with AMI. The differential diagnosis includes dysfunction or rupture of a papillary muscle. Acquired VSD is often associated with acute heart failure, and its distinction from acute MR, due to a ruptured papillary muscle, may not be possible without insertion of a balloon flotation pulmonary artery catheter to look for a left-to-right shunt and evaluate the contour of the V-wave of the pulmonary capillary wedge pressure.

Atrial Septal Defect

Atrial septal defects result in a grade 2 to 3/6 systolic ejection murmur, wide, fixed splitting of S_2, an incomplete right bundle-branch block (rsr′ pattern) on ECG and "shunt vascularity" on the chest film. An S_3 gallop and a short diastolic rumble may also be heard at the left lower sternal border when the left-to-right shunt exceeds 3:1. Despite this classic constellation of findings, some subjects with this congenital heart disease escape diagnosis until old age and present with congestive heart failure (CHF), usually because of the development of atrial fibrillation. Attention to the clinical findings listed above may be instrumental in diagnosing the presence of an atrial septal defect in elderly patients with otherwise unexplained CHF or atrial fibrillation.

DIASTOLIC MURMURS

Aortic Regurgitation

Like mitral regurgitation (including papillary muscle dysfunction and MVP), chronic aortic regurgitation (AR) is one of the most common valvular lesions in the geriatric patient. Although there are numerous causes of AR, the more common ones include calcification of the aortic valve (calcification of a congenital bicuspid valve or Monckeberg's degenerative calcification of a normal tricuspid valve), rheumatic heart disease, hypertensive cardiovascular disease, chronic renal disease, and "isolated nonsyphilitic" or idiopathic AR. The bedside findings in an elderly patient with AR are similar to those found in younger subjects. Two major exceptions are the intensity and location of the murmur. In the elderly patient, the murmur of AR may be very soft due to the previously discussed changes associated with aging. Also, the murmur may be heard best at the right upper sternal border rather than at the left upper or midsternal border. The murmur is early diastolic, and has a high frequency character and a decrescendo configuration. It is heard best with the diaphragm of the stethoscope firmly applied to the chest, and the patient sitting up and leaning forward with the breath held in expiration. Isometric handgrip exercise or prompt squatting may make the murmur louder. There is usually an associated ejection murmur at the base of the heart, which may be transmitted to the carotid arteries. With significant AR, the carotid pulse may be bounding and have a bisferious contour. There may also be alternating flushing and blanching of the capillaries in the nailbeds synchronous with the heart beat (Quincke's pulse).

In the absence of significant peripheral vascular disease, aortic stenosis and aortic aneurysm, the presence of significant AR may be identified by simultaneous measurement of the systolic blood pressure (BP) in the arms and legs with properly fitting cuffs. If the systolic BP in the leg exceeds that in the arm by more than 20 mmHg, hemodynamically significant AR should be suspected, while a difference greater than 60 mmHg signifies severe AR.[27] The presence of an S_3 gallop in patients with chronic AR is indicative of left ventricular dysfunction,[28] even if left ventricular dimensions and function are normal by M-mode echocardiography.

Acute AR can occur as a result of blunt trauma to the chest, infective endocarditis, or aortic dissection. The onset is sudden, and pulmonary congestion or edema are common when AR is significant.[29] Typically, S_1 is muffled or absent because the mitral valve closes prematurely due to the precipitous rise in ventricular diastolic pressure. Also, unlike chronic AR, in which there is a long, high-frequency, diastolic murmur, the acute condition is often associated with a medium frequency, soft murmur which is confined to early diastole because of early equilibration of the aortic and left ventricular diastolic pressures. The peripheral arterial signs typical of chronic AR are less marked or absent and the patients may demonstrate signs of low cardiac output (altered sensorium, cyanosis, cool clammy skin, and oliguria).

Pulmonic Regurgitation

Mitral stenosis and pulmonary emboli are the most common causes of pulmonic regurgitation (PR) in the geriatric age group. The murmur is similar in character, location, and configuration to the AR murmur, but unlike it, has associated clinical signs of right ventricular overload, including a left parasternal heave, increased retrosternal dullness, and persistent expiratory splitting of S_2 with a loud pulmonic component. The murmur may rarely become louder during inspiration (Carvallo's sign) and will regain its original intensity within four to eight beats after the release of the straining phase of Valsalva maneuver. Radiologic signs of right ventricular enlargement and dilated central pulmonary arteries with rapid tapering ("pruned tree" appearance), and ECG signs of right ventricular hypertrophy are common.

Mitral Stenosis

The classic signs of mitral stenosis (loud S_1, opening snap, middiastolic rumble, and presystolic accentuation) may be missed by the unsuspecting physician, and patients with this form of rheumatic heart disease may survive into the geriatric age group without diagnosis. With aging, the murmur may become even more difficult to hear due to factors that have been discussed previously. Also, the decreased cardiac output associated with mitral stenosis (MS) may further attenuate the intensity of the murmur, while accentuation of S_1 and the opening snap may be absent in patients with calcified and poorly mobile mitral leaflets. MS should be suspected in every patient with otherwise unexplained atrial fibrillation, particularly when the fibrillation waves are coarse and when the history is one of slowly progressive exertional dyspnea, orthopnea, and paroxysmal nocturnal dyspnea. Auscultation at the right upper parasternal area may reveal that S_1 is louder than S_2 (even when the former is not loud in absolute terms), while careful auscultation over the apex, in the left lateral position, with the bell chest piece of the stethoscope applied lightly may reveal the low frequency, rumbling diastolic murmur. A presystolic, crescendo component may also be heard when sinus rhythm is preserved. A left atrial myxoma should be suspected when the patient complains of syncope, has constitutional symptoms, an elevated erythrocyte sedimentation rate and a diastolic murmur that varies or disappears during different examinations. Echocardiography is extremely useful in confirming or ruling out mitral stenosis and left atrial myxoma.[30]

REFERENCES

1. Luchi RJ, Snow E, Luchi JM, et al: Left ventricular function in hospitalized geriatric patients. *J Am Geriatr Soc* 1982;30:700–705.
2. Port S, Cobb FR, Coleman RE, et al: Effect of age on the response of the left ventricular ejection fraction to exercise. *N Engl J Med* 1980;303:1133–1137.
3. National Center for Health Statistics, Rowland M, Roberts J: Blood pressure levels and hypertension in persons ages 6–74 years: United States, 1976–80. Advance Data from Vital and Health Statistics, No. DHHS Pub. No. (PHS)82-1250.
4. Linzback AL, Akuamoa-Boateng EY: Altersveränderungen des menschlichen Herzens. *Klin Wschr* 1973;51:156–163.
5. Pomerance A: Senile cardiac amyloidosis. *Br Heart J* 1965;27:711–718.
6. Weissler AM, Garrard CL: Systolic time intervals in cardiac disease (II). *Mod Conc Cardiovas Dis* 1971;40:5–8.
7. Harrison TR, Dixon K, Russell RO, et al: The relation of age to the duration of contraction, ejection and relaxation of the normal human heart. *Am Heart J* 1964;67:189–199.
8. Spodick DH, Quarry VM: Prevalence of the fourth heart sound by phonocardiography in the absence of cardiac disease. *Am Heart J* 1974;87:11–14.
9. Abrams J: Current concepts of the genesis of heart sounds: II. Third and fourth sounds. *JAMA* 1978; 239:2029–2030.
10. Craige E: The fourth heart sound, in Leon DF, Shaver JA (eds): *Physiologic Principles of Heart Sounds and Murmurs.* Monograph 46. New York, American Heart Association, 1975, pp 74–78.
11. Thomas FB, Mazzaferri EL, Skillman TG: Apathetic thyrotoxicosis: A distinctive clinical and laboratory entity. *Ann Intern Med* 1970;72:679–685.
12. Nakazawa HK, Sakurai K, Hamada N, et al: Management of atrial fibrillation in the post-thyrotoxic state. *Am J Med* 1982;72:903–906.
13. Schutte JE, Gaffney FA, Blend L, et al: Distinctive anthropometric characteristics of women with mitral valve prolapse. *Am J Med* 1981;71:533–538.
14. Darsee JR, Mikolich JR, Nicoloff NB, et al: Prevalence of mitral valve prolapse in presumably healthy young men. *Circulation* 1979;59:619–622.
15. Barlow JB, Pocock WA, Promund Obel IW: Mitral valve prolapse: Primary, secondary, both or neither? *Am Heart J* 1981;102:140–143.
16. Caceres CA, Perry LW: *The Innocent Murmur: A Problem in Clinical Practice*, ed 1. Boston, Little, Brown and Co, 1967, p 79.
17. Legal BL, Norack P, Kasparian H: Intracardiac phonocardiography. *Am J Cardiol* 1964;13:188.
18. Roberts WC, Perloff JK, Costantino T: Severe valvular aortic stenosis in patients over 65 years of age. *Am J Cardiol* 1971;27:497–506.
19. Kronzon I, Glassman E: Mitral ring calcification in idiopathic hypertrophic subaortic stenosis. *Am J Cardiol* 1978;42:60–66.
20. Korn D, DeSanctis RW, Sells: Massive calcification of the mitral annulus. *N Engl J Med* 1962;267:900–909.
21. Brand FR, Brown AL, Berge G: Histology of papillary muscles of the left ventricle in myocardial infarction. *Am Heart J* 1969;77:26–32.
22. Cheng TO: Some new observations on the syndrome of papillary muscle dysfunction. *Am J Med* 1969; 47:924–945.
23. Pomerance A: Aging changes in human heart valves. *Br Heart J* 1967;29:222–231.
24. Steele P, Weily H, Rainwater J, et al: Platelet survival time and thromboembolism in patients with mitral valve prolapse. *Circulation* 1979;60:43–45.
25. Antman EM, Angoff GH, Sloss LJ: Demonstration of the mechanism by which mitral regurgitation

mimics aortic stenosis. *Am J Cardiol* 1978;42: 1044–1048.
26. Sopulveda G, Lukas DS: The diagnosis of tricuspid insufficiency: Clinical features in 60 cases with associated mitral valve disease. *Circulation* 1955; 11:552–563.
27. Frank MJ, Casanegra P, Migliori AJ, et al: The clinical evaluation of aortic regurgitation with special reference to a neglected sign: The Popliteal-brachial pressure gradient. *Arch Intern Med* 1967; 116:357–365.
28. Abdulla AM, Frank MJ, Erdin RA Jr, et al: Clinical significance and hemodynamic correlates of the third heart sound gallop in aortic regurgitation: A potential guide to the optimal timing of cardiac catheterization. *Circulation* 1981;64:464–471.
29. Morganroth J, Perloff JK, Zeldis SM, et al: Acute severe aortic regurgitation. Pathophysiology, clinical recognition and management. *Ann Intern Med* 1977;87:223–232.
30. Abdulla AM, Stefadouros MA, Mucha E, et al: Left atrial myxoma: Echocardiographic diagnosis and determination of size. *JAMA* 1977;238:510–511.

CHAPTER 8
Platelet Function in Cardiac Disease

Jawahar Mehta

It is now recognized that platelets play an important role in the genesis and manifestations of atherosclerosis. Platelet function is also very important in the formation of thrombus on artificial surfaces like prosthetic cardiac valves and vascular grafts. The growing information on the contribution of platelets in the evolution of tissue ischemia and thromboembolic events has led to platelet-suppressive drug trials in patients with coronary artery disease, cerebrovascular ischemia, coronary and noncoronary bypass grafts, and others with tissue or prosthetic cardiac valves. The purpose of this paper is to review the role of platelets in health and in their contribution to atherogenesis and thrombus formation. The mechanism of action of commonly used platelet-suppressive drugs will also be discussed to understand the differences between different drugs.

PLATELETS AND HEMOSTASIS

Platelets, small disklike cells circulating in the blood, have a primary role in hemostasis. Upon stress to the endothelium and its disruption, platelets adhere to the subendothelial collagen. Other circulating platelets are attracted to the adhering platelets resulting in platelet aggregation and formation of a platelet thrombus. Red blood cells, leukocytes, and other blood components are incorporated in the platelet thrombus with the formation of an occlusive clot. Coagulation cascade is also activated at this stage. Platelets upon activation release potent hormones, prostaglandins, polypeptides, and other vasoactive substances some of which promote platelet aggregation (adenosine diphosphate and serotonin), vasoconstriction (thromboxane A_2), and vascular permeability (Figure 8-1). In older individuals, platelet sensitivity to aggregating stimuli has been reported to be increased. Following the endothelial reparative process, platelet clumps disaggregate and the vascular lumen becomes recanalized. This, in brief, is a major mechanism by which extravasation of blood following vascular injury is stopped. Indeed, in conditions associated with thrombocytopenia or platelet "hypofunction," bleeding and petechiae are commonly seen.

Platelets also play an important role in nurturing vascular endothelium and maintaining its continuity. In experimental animals with thrombocytopenia or decreased platelet function, fenestrations appear in the endothelium. Correction of platelet number or the functional defect results in prompt repair of the endothelial injury.[1]

ATHEROSCLEROSIS

The deposition of cholesterol and other fatty materials in the atherosclerotic plaques has long been observed. Atherosclerosis is more often seen at the branch sites of major arteries, presumably due to the hemodynamic stress at branch points. It has long been believed that vascular injury at points of stress leads to deposition of fatty materials.

In the past, there have been two major hypotheses for the pathogenesis of atherosclerosis: (a) the "incrustation" theory,[2,3] which involves intimal thickening due to fibrin deposition with subsequent organization of fibroblasts and accumulation of lipids; and (b) the "imbibition" hypothesis[4] which implies that lipids in the arterial wall represent a transudation of blood lipids that subsequently form complexes with acid mucopolysaccharides. The arterial accumulation occurs

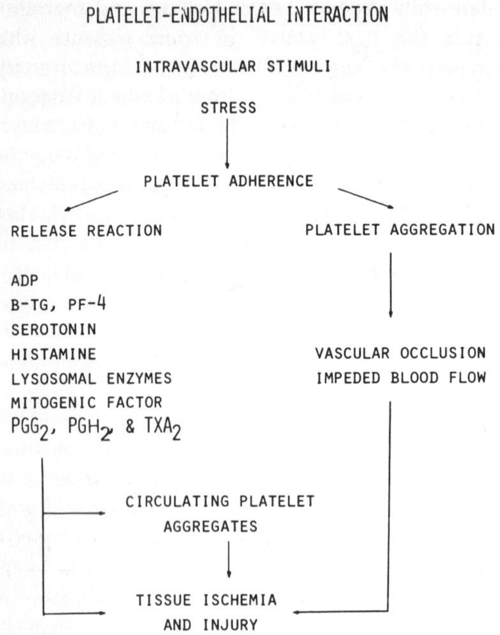

Figure 8-1 Normal platelet function is essential in hemostasis. Persistent platelet activation may lead to tissue ischemia and atherosclerosis.

because of deficiency in the lipid removal mechanism. Recent evidence suggests that hemodynamic stress is an important factor in initiating endothelial injury.[5,6]

Evidence that platelets may be involved in primary injury to the vascular endothelium in regions of blood turbulence has been presented. A number of platelet-derived substances including adenosine diphosphate (ADP), serotonin, histamine, β-thromboglobulin (a cationic protein that increases vascular permeability)[7] and platelet factor 4[8] can injure the vessel wall. Platelet-generated thromboxane A_2 can cause vasospasm and perhaps vascular damage. In experimental atherosclerosis induced by endothelial injury, platelets adhere to the subendothelial denuded areas.[9] This event precedes the migration and proliferation of smooth muscle cells.[10] A platelet-derived growth factor responsible for the proliferation of smooth muscle cells has also been identified.[11] Platelet-derived growth factor, along with platelet factor 4 and β-thromboglobulin, are all released from platelet alpha granules on activation. Sequential studies in atherosclerotic pigeons show a persistent increase in platelet factor 4 activity[12] implying an important association of platelet activation with atherosclerosis. Evidence supporting such a role also comes from studies demonstrating resistance to the development of atherosclerosis in animals with suppressed platelet function.[13-15] Support for this theory is also given in studies by Fuster et al[15] in pigs with von Willebrand's disease, a condition with marked impairment of platelet adhesion, demonstrating resistance to the initiation and progression of atherosclerosis. It should be recognized that atherogenesis is a complex multifactorial process. A variety of plasma proteins such as pituitary hormones and insulin are also mitogens. Multiple episodes of injury,[16] perhaps coupled with lipid abnormalities, are needed to produce atherosclerosis. Nonetheless, observations mentioned above indicate a link between platelets and atherosclerosis.

PLATELET FUNCTION IN CORONARY "RISK FACTORS"

It has been proposed that so-called risk factors for atherosclerosis, eg, hypertension, diabetes mellitus, hyperlipidemia, and smoking, participate in the pathogenesis of atherosclerosis through an abnormal platelet-endothelial interaction.[17] Platelet dysfunction has been identified in smokers. Patients with hypertension have increased platelet adhesion and increased levels of platelet-released protein, β-thromboglobulin, indicating in vivo activation.[18] There is evidence for "hyperactive" platelets in diabetic subjects with vascular injury.[19] Hyperlipidemia is also associated with increased platelet activity and decreased platelet survival.[20] Treatment of hypertension, diabetes mellitus, and hyperlipidemia has been shown to result in reversal of platelet hyperactivity.[18-20]

PLATELETS IN CORONARY ARTERY DISEASE

Animal Data

In several animal models of coronary artery narrowing with evidence of myocardial ischemia and infarction, formation of platelet aggregates in the coronary vasculature occurs. These aggregates formed at the site of coronary narrowing may reduce blood flow to the already ischemic tissue. Disruption of these aggregates may result in distal "embolization" in small arterioles resulting in extension of myocardial ischemia/infarction. Pretreatment of animals with platelet-suppressive drugs has been shown to result in decrease in infarct size and improvement in blood flow to the ischemic tissue.[21,22]

With critical coronary narrowing in the dog, phasic decrease and increase in blood flow are seen, which relate to spontaneous platelet aggregation and disaggregation, respectively.[23] Intracoronary or intravenous administration of platelet aggregants may provoke these phasic changes in coronary blood flow (Figure 8-2). In vivo platelet aggregation and associated release of vasoconstrictor stimuli such as thromboxane A_2 may result in dynamic reduction in blood flow. Episodic decrease in coronary blood flow and vasoconstriction may cause changes similar to coronary artery spasm in man. These phasic changes in blood flow in animals can be ameliorated with aspirin, prostacyclin, and other platelet-inhibitory agents. However, trials of the platelet-inhibitory drugs aspirin and indomethacin in patients with coronary artery spasm have not yielded evidence of benefit.[24,25]

Human Data

Several studies have shown "abnormal" platelet function in patients with stable angina pectoris, vasospastic angina, and myocardial infarction. Some investigators have reported increased platelet aggregation in vitro in response to aggregating stimuli[26] but others failed to identify increased aggregability.[27] Increased circulating platelet aggregates have been identified in patients with acute myocardial infarction with a decline in association with their recovery.[28] Platelet-release products such as β-thromboglobulin and platelet factor 4 are increased in most patients in the active stage of ischemic heart disease. In some studies, enhanced platelet-release reaction has been shown to correlate with patients' hospital course and mortality over the next year.[29] In some patients with vasospastic angina, formation of intracoronary platelet aggregates and release of potent vasoconstrictor prostaglandin thromboxane A_2 have been speculated to have roles in transient and dynamic coronary narrowing.[24] Exercise-induced platelet activation has been clearly shown by several other investigators including us.[30] There is absence of similar platelet activation in patients with coronary disease but a negative exercise stress test. These data suggest a possible involvement of platelets in certain patients with exercise-induced angina.

In most studies, only peripheral venous blood has been examined to measure platelet function. This does not necessarily reflect the changes in platelet function in the atherosclerotic coronary vascular bed. Examination of blood from aorta and coronary sinus shows passage of fewer platelets in the coronary venous compared to the aortic blood in patients with coronary disease. In addition, platelets in the coronary venous blood have decreased aggregation function.[31,32] These differences between aortic and coronary venous platelets can be eliminated with administration of the platelet inhibitors, aspirin and dipyridamole.[33,34] Furthermore, tachycardia stress induced by atrial pacing causes marked activation of platelets in the coronary venous blood associated with ECG evidence of myocardial ischemia.[32,33] Aspirin also blunts this tachycardia-associated platelet activation.[33]

These studies imply an important role for platelets in the genesis and/or propagation of

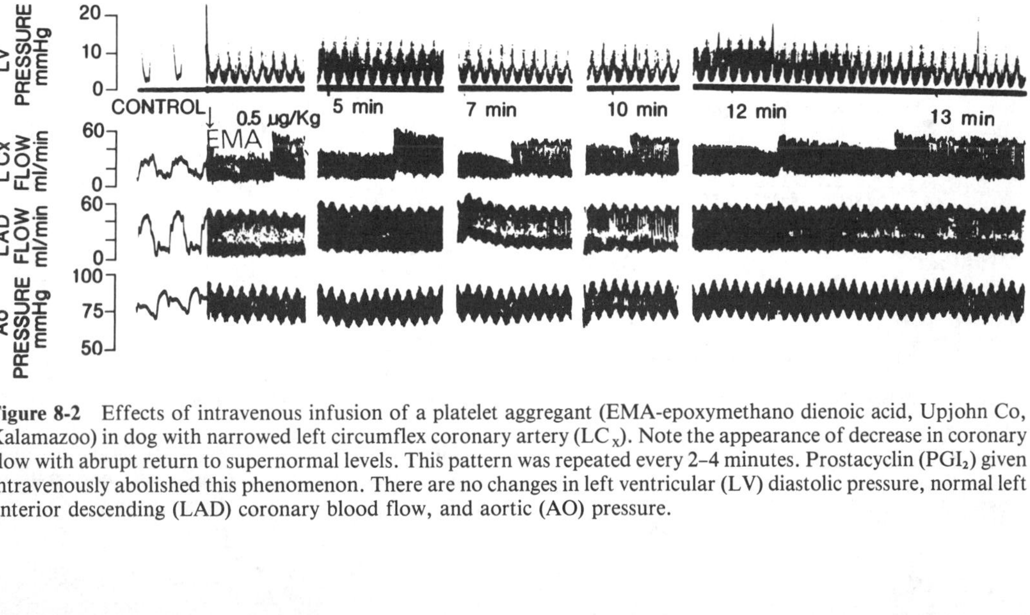

Figure 8-2 Effects of intravenous infusion of a platelet aggregant (EMA-epoxymethano dienoic acid, Upjohn Co, Kalamazoo) in dog with narrowed left circumflex coronary artery (LC_X). Note the appearance of decrease in coronary flow with abrupt return to supernormal levels. This pattern was repeated every 2–4 minutes. Prostacyclin (PGI_2) given intravenously abolished this phenomenon. There are no changes in left ventricular (LV) diastolic pressure, normal left anterior descending (LAD) coronary blood flow, and aortic (AO) pressure.

myocardial ischemia. Whether platelet "hyperactivity" precedes myocardial ischemia or occurs after the acute event has begun is still not resolved. Whatever the precise sequence of events, formation of platelet aggregates in the coronary vessels could limit blood flow and either cause the ischemic event or result in deterioration of already compromised blood flow to the myocardium.

PROSTAGLANDINS IN CORONARY ARTERY DISEASE

Prostaglandins are derived from essential fatty acids obtained from diet or synthesized in the human body. These fatty acids are incorporated in the phospholipids of cell membrane. Arachidonic acid is the precursor of major prostaglandins in man. There are several metabolic pathways, which are crucial to the understanding of platelet-vessel wall interaction as it relates to coronary artery disease.[17]

By action of the enzyme cyclooxygenase, arachidonic acid is transformed to cyclic endoperoxides, PGG_2 and PGH_2, which are further metabolized to vasoactive prostaglandins (Figure 8-3). Platelets upon activation generate thromboxane A_2 which is a very potent vasoconstrictor and proaggregatory agent. Its actions are balanced by vessel-wall generated prostacyclin, a very potent vasodilator and antiaggregatory agent. In the state of health, equilibrium between thromboxane A_2 and prostacyclin is essential in the regulation of vascular tone and platelet homeostasis. Other prostaglandins of the D, E, and F series have been considered important in the past in the regulation of vasomotor tone and platelet homeostasis, but

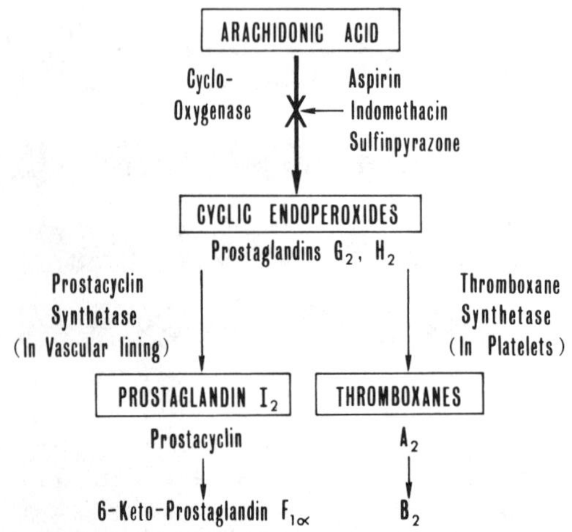

Figure 8-3 Arachidonic acid metabolism in man.

these are considerably weaker in potency than thromboxane A_2 and prostacyclin. Currently, thromboxane A_2 and prostacyclin are thought to have a major role in maintaining blood flow.[35] Recent information suggests that leukocytes and blood vessels are also important sources of thromboxane A_2.[36] Abnormalities in thromboxane A_2 and prostacyclin equilibrium in coronary artery disease are summarized in Table 8-1.

It has been speculated that thromboxane A_2 released from activated platelets may be responsible for localized vasospasm. Several studies, indeed, have shown enhanced thromboxane A_2 synthesis in patients with unstable angina, vasospasm, and myocardial infarction.[37,38] Platelets from patients with acute myocardial ischemia are very sensitive to proaggregatory actions of thromboxane A_2.[38] During exercise, platelets from patients with stable angina generate inappropriately large amounts of thromboxane A_2.[39] In contrast, decreased prostacyclin generation has been identified in human atherosclerotic plaques.[40] Patients with coronary heart disease produce markedly reduced amounts of prostacyclin at rest[41] and during stress[39] compared to normal subjects. Furthermore, platelets from patients with unstable angina are less responsive to the antiaggregatory properties of prostacyclin.[38] Thus, there is some evidence of imbalance in thromboxane A_2-prostacyclin equilibrium in certain patients with coronary disease which could account for vasoconstriction and in vivo platelet aggregation. This imbalance could also relate to the development and progression of atherosclerosis in general.

The other pathways in arachidonic acid metabolism involve leukotriene synthesis and other lipoxygenase reactions. Leukotrienes are bronchoconstrictors and mediators of allergic reactions, and may be involved in inflammatory response during an acute event such as myocardial infarction. The precise role of products of lipoxygenase reactions in myocardial ischemia is not known. These substances involved in leukocyte chemotaxis and vasoconstriction may influence prostacyclin synthesis, and thereby could have a role in acute myocardial infarction.[17]

PLATELETS, PROSTAGLANDINS, AND MYOCARDIAL ISCHEMIA

Thus far, evidence has been presented for platelet function and prostaglandin abnormalities in patients with coronary heart disease. It can be

Table 8-1
Abnormalities in Thromboxane A_2 and Prostacyclin Equilibrium in Coronary Artery Disease

1. Increased thromboxane A_2 production in acute spontaneous ischemia.
2. Increased thromboxane A_2 synthesis with exercise and pacing-induced ischemia.
3. Decreased prostacyclin production by atheromatous vessels.
4. Decreased prostacyclin release with stress.
5. Increased platelet sensitivity to thromboxane A_2.
6. Decreased platelet sensitivity to prostacyclin.

postulated that platelet hyperactivity, either primary or secondary to pre-existing atherosclerosis, could limit coronary blood flow by formation of intravascular platelet aggregates. Increased thromboxane A_2 synthesis alone or in combination with decreased prostacyclin generation may result in the manifestations of coronary artery disease and may perpetuate the atherosclerotic process (Figure 8-4).

PLATELET FUNCTION AND PROSTHETIC SURFACES

Thrombosis and thromboembolism are the major deterrents to the use of arterial grafts and cardiac valves. When the grafts and artificial valves (both tissue and mechanical) are placed in the arterial system, platelets have a predominant role in the development of a thrombus (white thrombus) with its subsequent disintegration resulting in embolism to distal organs. In contrast, fibrin and red cell deposition (red thrombus) predominate in the process of venous thrombosis.

On the arterial side, the evolution of a thrombus at the site of anastomosis involves attachment of platelets to the subendothelial collagen as the initial step. Further aggregation of platelets and incorporation of other blood elements leads to formation of a firm thrombus. This thrombus may dislodge or disintegrate and result in thromboembolism. With time (1 to 3 months), the endothelial lining grows and covers the thrombus. Since the Dacron graft is impervious to cellular ingrowth, the endothelial cells lie directly on an amorphous base consisting of plasma components.[42] The fact that therapy with anticoagulants has not completely eliminated thromboembolic episodes suggests that platelets are important contributors in the formation of thrombus.

Arterial Grafts

In elegant studies by Harker et al in patients (aged 47–70 years, mean age 63 years) receiving aortoiliac, aortofemoral, or both aortofemoral and femoropopliteal grafts,[43] an almost 50% decrease in platelet survival was observed. Shortest platelet survival occurred in patients with both aortofemoral and femoropopliteal grafts. Platelet turnover was reciprocally increased twofold. The results of fibrinogen and plasminogen survival did not show any change compared to controls. Other in vitro platelet function tests such as platelet aggregation to ADP, epinephrine, or collagen, and glass bead retention were normal. These in vivo abnormalities in platelet function reflect platelet sequestration in the thrombus formed soon after the surgery. The magnitude of platelet sequestration decreases with time, and by 6 to 9 months platelet survival returns to base line. This is believed to reflect endothelialization at the graft site. It has been suggested that a reduction in platelet survival may be a useful in vivo indicator of nonendothelialized thrombogenic surface exposed to the circulating blood.[43]

Newer technics using indium 111–labeled platelets have also shown sequestration of a large number of platelets at the site of graft anastomosis.[44]

Other evidence in favor of platelet consumption comes from platelet-inhibitory drug trials. Drugs like dipyridamole (100 mg four times daily) or a combination of dipyridamole (75 mg three times

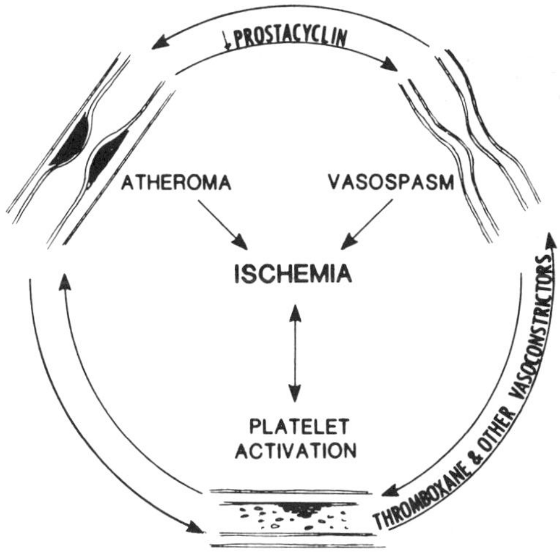

Figure 8-4 A proposed interrelationship between atherosclerosis, platelet activation, vasospasm, and myocardial ischemia. Alterations in prostacyclin and thromboxane may play a key role in this interrelationship.

daily) and aspirin (330 mg three times daily) administered 2 days before surgery and continued in the postoperative phase results in marked improvement in platelet survival.[43] Dipyridamole alone does not affect platelet aggregation, but normalizes platelet survival.

Porcine and Mechanical Valves

A large number of elderly patients are currently undergoing valve replacements for either congenital, eg, bicuspid aortic valves, or acquired, eg, mitral stenosis, aortic regurgitation, etc, valvular diseases. As with the arterial prosthesis, there is major risk of thromboembolic events. Mechanical valves have, generally speaking, a longer life than the porcine heterografts, although mechanical valves are associated with a significantly greater incidence of thromboembolic episodes.

It has been observed that patients with prosthetic valves and thromboembolic events have an increased incidence of decreased platelet survival as compared to those with prosthetic valves without thromboembolism.[45] The lower incidence of thromboembolism in patients with porcine heterografts is thought to be related to early endothelialization of the heterograft and improved platelet survival.[46] In one study,[47] however, similar reductions in platelet survival were observed in patients with porcine or mechanical valves at an average of 19 and 49 months after graft placement. Further evidence of in vivo platelet activation is the finding of elevated levels of platelet factor 4 which persists for a longer period of time in recipients of prosthetic as opposed to porcine valves. It should be mentioned that reduced platelet survival may predate valve replacement.[48]

Administration of platelet inhibitory agents like dipyridamole and sulfinpyrazone has been shown to improve platelet survival in patients with prosthetic valves.[45–49] In conjunction with improvement in platelet survival, incidence of thromboembolism also appears to be decreased when platelet-inhibitory drugs are combined with anticoagulants.[50–52] In patients with porcine heterograft, the need for platelet-suppressive and/or anticoagulants is also decreased at two to three months after surgery as the valve surface is reendothelialized.

The precise selection of therapy (anticoagulants vs platelet-inhibitory drugs) in different kinds of valves and the overall outcome is not clear. Nevertheless, the important role of platelets in formation of a nidus for thrombus on foreign surfaces in the arterial system is generally accepted. Prevention of platelet adhesion and sequestration at the time of surgery may be necessary to avoid formation of this nidus. Thus, a case can be made for institution of therapy directed at preventing or decreasing platelet adhesion at the graft or valve anastomotic site well in advance of surgery.

PLATELET-SUPPRESSIVE DRUGS

New information on the mechanism of action of several drugs has become available in the last decade. Several new drugs are being synthesized and studied based on the understanding of platelet-endothelial interaction and arachidonic acid metabolism. These drugs can be divided into several categories. Actions of commonly used agents are shown in Table 8-2.

Cyclooxygenase Inhibitors

These agents inhibit synthesis of cyclic endoperoxides and thromboxane A_2, and inhibit platelet activity for their entire life span; certainly a desired effect. Since prostacyclin generation also requires cyclic endoperoxides, these drugs decrease prostacyclin synthesis as well. The inhibition of prostacyclin may negate the benefits derived from inhibition of thromboxane A_2. Relative

Table 8-2
Commonly Used Platelet-Suppressive Drugs in Coronary Artery Disease

Aspirin	Inhibits formation of labile endoperoxides and subsequent synthesis of thromboxane A_2 and prostacyclin. Inhibits secondary wave of platelet aggregation and release of platelet-proteins. No effect on platelet adhesion.
Dipyridamole	Inhibits enzyme phosphodiesterase and increases platelet cAMP. Potentiates action of prostacyclin, inhibits thromboxane A_2 synthesis, and stimulates prostacyclin release. Prolongs platelet survival, if shortened.
Sulfinpyrazone	Inhibits formation of endoperoxides. Inhibits platelet adhesion. Reduces thromboxane A_2 synthesis more than prostacyclin generation. Prolongs platelet survival, if shortened.

magnitude of inhibition of thromboxane A_2 and prostacyclin is an area of intense investigation. It has been suggested that small doses of aspirin (325 mg every 3 or 4 days) may selectively inhibit thromboxane A_2 while sparing prostacyclin synthesis.[53] Aspirin, sulfinpyrazone, and ibuprofen also possess cardioprotective and antiarrhythmic properties unrelated to their effects on platelets, although the mechanism is not well understood.

Prostacyclin Stimulants

Phosphodiesterase inhibitors, eg, dipyridamole, potentiate endogenous prostacyclin activity, and stimulate prostacyclin release from blood vessels.[54] Dipyridamole also inhibits thromboxane A_2 generation by platelets[55] and improves platelet survival.[56] Recent studies suggest that simultaneous use of aspirin and dipyridamole may have additive antiplatelet effects, but aspirin may negate potentially beneficial effects of dipyridamole on vascular prostacyclin synthesis.[54]

Newer compounds like Bay G6575 (nafazatrom) prevent degradation of prostacyclin in plasma[57] and prevent thrombus formation in vivo. Blood vessels upon treatment with plasma from subjects administered this compound show potentiation of prostacyclin release.[58]

Another compound, ticlopidine hydrochloride, which inhibits platelet aggregation ex vivo by enhancing actions of prostacyclin and PGE_1, has shown promise in initial studies in patients with myocardial ischemia.[59]

Selective Thromboxane A_2 Blockers

A host of compounds which inhibit thromboxane A_2 synthetase enzyme have been developed.[60,61] Some of these compounds stimulate prostacyclin synthesis while decreasing thromboxane A_2 generation, probably by diverting endoperoxides to the prostacyclin pathway.[60] Clinical trials with these drugs in patients with myocardial ischemia are underway. If thromboxane A_2 inhibition relieves symptoms and objective evidence of myocardial ischemia, these drugs would offer a rational approach to therapy of patients with coronary heart disease.

Other Drugs

Clofibrate, used in the therapy of hyperlipidemias, also improves platelet function.[20]

Beta-adrenergic blockers suppress resting and exercise-induced platelet aggregation, improve exercise tolerance, and enhance survival after myocardial infarction. Beta-blockers also inhibit platelet thromboxane A_2 synthesis by direct action on the platelet membrane, possibly by interfering with calcium availability.[62] Since all beta-blockers improve survival after myocardial infarction, it is possible that inhibition of platelet function is the common underlying mechanism.

Calcium-blockers like verapamil, nifedipine, and diltiazem exert potent antiplatelet effects and decrease thromboxane A_2 synthesis.[63,64] Interference with calcium availability within the platelets is the underlying mechanism. Some calcium-blockers like verapamil also potentiate the actions of prostacyclin[64] and perhaps stimulate prostacyclin release from blood vessels. In recent reports, calcium-blockers have also been shown to limit atherosclerosis in experimental animals.[65]

TRIALS OF PLATELET-SUPPRESSIVE DRUGS

Based on observations of platelet "hyperactivity" in coronary artery disease, several platelet-suppressive drugs have been evaluated in patients with myocardial infarction (Table 8-3). Unfortunately, these drug trials have created more controversy rather than providing a definite answer. Major drugs used have been aspirin, sulfinpyrazone and dipyridamole either alone or in combination. The results of some of the published major trials have been recently reviewed.[66] These trials have provided variable results. Although mortality during the follow-up period in patients with myocardial infarction given antiplatelet drugs appears to be reduced, the data in any single study (except in the Anturane Reinfarction Trial) were not significant. In all studies, except the Aspirin Myocardial Infarction Study, there was a definite suggestion of beneficial effect. The reasons for lack of more significant improvement are numerous, eg, patients were started on antiplatelet drugs at variable intervals from the event, the dose of aspirin used was variable, the impact of other concurrent therapy was not evaluated, etc. Perhaps the most important factor is the dose of aspirin used. As discussed earlier, high dose of aspirin may theoretically negate the beneficial effects derived from suppression of thromboxane A_2 synthesis. Aspirin used in conjunction with dipyridamole may not make prostacyclin precursor available for actions of the latter agent. This became evident in a recent study from the Mayo Clinic group who used dipyridamole alone for two days before bypass surgery to prevent intraoperative platelet adhesion to exposed subendothelial layers of the graft. Postoperative simultaneous

Table 8-3
Effects of Platelet-Suppressive Agents on Secondary Mortality After Initial Myocardial Infarction in Some Studies

Study Trial	Agent	Total No. of Patients	% Reduction (Treated vs Control)			Conclusion
			Mortality	*Sudden Death*	*MI (Nonfatal)*	
Elwood et al, 1974	Aspirin 300 mg/day	1239	24	–	–	Mortality rate reduced, but statistically inconclusive.
German-Austrian, 1980	Aspirin 1.5 g/day	1060	18	36	27	Mortality rate reduced, but statistically inconclusive.
Coronary Drug Project, 1976	Aspirin 972 mg/day	1529	30	19	5	Apparent improvement with aspirin.
Aspirin Myocardial Infarction Study (AMIS), 1980	Aspirin 1 g/day	4524	+11	+35	22*	Aspirin not recommended for routine use.
Persantin-Aspirin Reinfarction Study (PARIS), 1980	Aspirin 972 mg/day or dipyridamole 225 mg/day + aspirin 972 mg/day	2026	18 16	+27 16	29 19	Mortality improved in both groups. Improvement with dipyridamole + aspirin significantly less than aspirin.
Anturane Reinfarction Trial (ART), 1980	Sulfinpyrazone 200 mg qid	1629	30	43*	25	Reduction in mortality statistically significant.

*Significant reduction.
MI = myocardial infarction.

use of aspirin and dipyridamole suppressed platelet "hyperactivity," which may have accounted for reduced incidence of graft closure.

In patients with prosthetic heart valves, antiplatelet drugs, dipyridamole (400 mg daily) dipyridamole (100 to 300 mg daily) plus aspirin, and sulfinpyrazone (800 mg daily), correct shortened survival time. Several studies have shown improved results when antiplatelet drugs are used in combination with anticoagulants. Aspirin alone does not protect against thromboembolism. Dipyridamole plus warfarin has been found to be more effective than warfarin alone in reducing thromboembolic episodes but not mortality.[51] A regimen of warfarin sodium plus daily administration of both dipyridamole and aspirin has also been recommended.[52]

Although both dipyridamole and sulfinpyrazone have been shown to reduce platelet turnover and improve platelet survival, there are no data on clinical efficacy in patients with arterial prosthesis.

RECOMMENDATIONS

It is now obvious that platelets play either a primary role in the genesis of thrombosis and myocardial ischemia, or at least participate in the perpetuation of the thombotic process. Although results of usual therapy aimed at platelet inhibition have failed to give definite information, some general recommendations can be made based on the present knowledge despite some gaps:

1. Patients at high risk of reinfarction may be given aspirin, sulfinpyrazone, or dipyridamole.
2. The dose of aspirin should be kept small, ie, 325 mg every one to three days.
3. Therapy should be initiated soon after myocardial infarction.
4. Patients may be given dipyridamole 75 mg three times daily two days before coronary bypass surgery. Postoperatively, aspirin may be added to dipyridamole.
5. In patients with prosthetic valves, warfarin sodium may be combined with dipyridamole or dipyridamole plus aspirin. This may also be useful in reducing the dose of anticoagulants.
6. Patients with prosthetic valves who cannot tolerate the usual anticoagulants may be given dipyridamole plus aspirin.
7. Patients with arterial grafts could be maintained on antiplatelet drugs, but convincing data are not available.

With increasing knowledge and the development of new drugs acting at selected sites on the arachidonic acid pathway, a wider choice of platelet-suppressive agents should become available to the clinician to treat cardiac patients.

ACKNOWLEDGMENT

Susan Ternet Teets assisted in the preparation of this manuscript.

REFERENCES

1. Kitchens CS: Amelioration of endothelial abnormalities by prednisone in experimental thrombocytopenia in the rabbit. *J Clin Invest* 1977;60:1129–1134.
2. von Rokitansky C: A Manual of Pathological Anatomy. London, Sydenham Society, 1859, vol 4, pp 261–269.
3. Duguid JB, Robertson WB: Mechanical factors in atherosclerosis. *Lancet* 1957;1:1205–1207.
4. Virchow R: Cellular Pathology: As Based Upon Physiological and Pathological Histology. New York, Dover Publications, 1971.
5. Reidy MA, Bowyer DE: Scanning electromicroscopy of arteries. The morphology of aortic endothelium in hemodynamically stressed areas associated with branches. *Atherosclerosis* 1977;26: 181–194.
6. Glagov S: Mechanical stresses on vessels and the nonuniform distribution of atherosclerosis. *Med Clin North Am* 1973;57:63–77.
7. Nachman RL, Weksler B, Ferris B: Increased vascular permeability produced by human platelet granule cationic extract. *J Clin Invest* 1970;49: 274–280.
8. Goldberg ID, Stemerman MB, Handin RI: Vascular permeation of platelet factor-4 after endothelial injury. *Science* 1980;209:611–612.
9. Harker LA, Ross R, Slichter SJ, Scott CR: Homocystine-induced arteriosclerosis: The role of endothelial cell injury and platelet response in its genesis. *J Clin Invest* 1976;58:731–741.
10. Spaet TH, Stemerman MB, Veith FJ, et al: Intimal injury and regrowth in the rabbit aorta: Medial smooth muscle cells as a source of neo-intima. *Circ Res* 1975;36:58–70.
11. Ross R, Glomset J, Kazlya B, et al: A platelet dependent serum factor that stimulates the proliferation of arterial smooth muscle cells in vitro. *Proc Natl Acad Sci USA* 1974;71:1207–1210.
12. Fuster V, Lewis JC, Kottke BA, et al: Platelet factor 4-like activity in the initial stages of atherosclerosis in pigeons. *Thromb Res* 1977;10:169–172.
13. Cohen P, McCombs HL: Platelets and atherogenesis. Part 2. Amelioration of cholesterol atherogenesis in rabbits with reduced platelet counts as a result of ^{32}p administration. *J Atheroscler Res* 1968;8: 389–393.
14. Friedman RJ, Stemerman MB, Wenz B, et al: The effect of thrombocytopenia on experimental atherosclerotic lesion formation in rabbits. *J Clin Invest* 1977;60:1191–1201.

15. Fuster V, Bowie EJW, Fass DN, et al: Arteriosclerosis in von Willebrand and normal pigs: Spontaneous and high cholesterol diet-induced. *J Clin Invest* 1978;61:722–730.
16. Gertz SD, Uretsky G, Wajnberg RS, et al: Endothelial cell damage and thrombus formation after partial arterial constriction: Relevance to the role of coronary artery spasm in the pathogenesis of myocardial infarction. *Circulation* 1981;63:476–486.
17. Mehta J, Mehta P: Role of blood platelets and prostaglandins in coronary artery disease. *Am J Cardiol* 1981;48:366–373.
18. Mehta J, Mehta P: Platelet function in hypertension and effect of therapy. *Am J Cardiol* 1981;47:231–234.
19. Preston FE, Ward JD, Marcola BM, et al: Elevated β-thromboglobulin levels and circulating platelet aggregates in diabetic microangiopathy. *Lancet* 1978;1:238–240.
20. Carvalho AC, Colman RW, Lees RS: Platelet function in hyperlipoproteinemia. *N Engl J Med* 1974; 290:434–438.
21. Capurro NL, Marr KC, Aamodt R, et al: Aspirin-induced increase in collateral flow after acute coronary occlusion in dogs. *Circulation* 1979;59: 744–747.
22. Jugdutt BI, Hutchins GM, Bulkley BH, et al: Salvage of ischemic myocardium by ibuprofen during infarction in the conscious dog. *Am J Cardiol* 1980;46:74–82.
23. Folts JD, Crowell EB, Rowe GG: Platelet aggregation in partially obstructed vessels and its elimination with aspirin. *Circulation* 1976;54:365–370.
24. Robertson RM, Robertson D, Roberts LJ, et al: Thromboxane A_2 in vasotonic angina pectoris: Evidence from direct measurements and inhibitory trials. *N Engl J Med* 1981;304:998–1003.
25. Chierchia S, de Caterina R, Crea F, et al: Failure of thromboxane A_2 blockade to prevent attacks of vasospastic angina. *Circulation* 1982;66:702–705.
26. Dreyfuss F, Zahavi J: Adenosine diphosphate-induced platelet aggregation in myocardial infarction and ischemic heart disease. *Atherosclerosis* 1973; 17:107–120.
27. O'Brien JR, Heywood JB, Heedy JA: The quantitation of platelet aggregation induced by four compounds: A study in relation to myocardial infarction. *Thromb Diath Haemorrh* 1966;16:752–767.
28. Mehta P, Mehta J: Platelet function studies in coronary artery disease. V. Evidence for enhanced platelet micro-thrombus formation activity in acute myocardial infarction. *Am J Cardiol* 1979;43:757–760.
29. Heptinstall S, Mulley GP, Taylor P, et al: Platelet release reaction in myocardial infarction. *Br Med J* 1980;1:80–81.
30. Mehta J, Mehta P: Comparison of platelet function during exercise in normal subjects and coronary artery disease patients: Potential role of platelet activation in myocardial ischemia. *Am Heart J* 1982;103:49–53.
31. Mehta P, Mehta J, Pepine CJ: Platelet aggregation across the myocardial vascular bed in man. *Thromb Res* 1979;14:623–632.
32. Mehta J, Mehta P, Pepine CJ: Platelet aggregation in aortic and coronary venous blood in patients with and without coronary artery disease. III. Role of tachycardia stress and propranolol. *Circulation* 1978;58:881–886.
33. Mehta J, Mehta P, Pepine CJ, et al: Platelet function studies in coronary artery disease. VII. Effect of aspirin and tachycardia stress on aortic and coronary venous blood. *Am J Cardiol* 1980;45:945–951.
34. Mehta J, Mehta P, Pepine CJ, et al: Platelet function studies in coronary heart disease. X. Effect of dipyridamole. *Am J Cardiol* 1981;47:1111–1114.
35. Needleman P, Kaley G: Cardiac and coronary prostaglandin synthesis and function. *N Engl J Med* 1979;298:1122–1128.
36. Mehta P, Mehta J, Crews F, et al: Human vascular tissues produce TXA_2 as well as PGI_2. *Circulation* 1982;66:II–59.
37. Szczeklik A, Gryglewski RJ, Musial J, et al: Thromboxane generation and platelet aggregation in survivals of myocardial infarction. *Thromb Haemost* 1978;40:66–74.
38. Mehta J, Mehta P, Conti CR: Platelet function studies in coronary heart disease. IX. Increased platelet prostaglandin generation and abnormal platelet sensitivity to prostacyclin and endoperoxide analog in angina pectoris. *Am J Cardiol* 1980; 46:943–947.
39. Mehta J, Mehta P, Horalek C, et al: The significance of platelet-vessel wall prostaglandin equilibrium during exercise-induced stress, abstracted. *Am J Cardiol* 1982;49:926.
40. D'Angelo V, Villa S, Mysliewiec M, et al: Defective fibrinolytic and prostacyclin-like activity in human atherosclerotic plaques. *Thromb Haemost* 1978;39: 535–536.
41. Neri Serneri GG, Poggesi L, Galanti G, et al: Reduced prostacyclin production in patients with different manifestations of ischemic heart disease. *Am J Cardiol* 1982;49:1146–1151.
42. Salzman EW: The limitations of heparin therapy after arterial reconstruction. *Surgery* 1965;57:131–138.
43. Harker LA, Slichter SJ, Saurage LF: Platelet consumption by arterial prostheses. *Ann Surg* 1977; 186:594–601.
44. Stratton JR, Thiele BL, Ritchie JL: Platelet deposition on dacron aortic bifurcation grafts in man: Quantitation with Indium-111 platelet imaging. *Circulation* 1982;66:1287–1293.
45. Weily HS, Steele PP, Davies H, et al: Platelet survival in patients with substitute heart valves. *N Engl J Med* 1974;290:534–537.
46. Manohitrajah SM, Rahman AN, Donnelly RJ, et al: Platelet survival in patients with homograft and prosthetic heart valves. *Thorax* 1974;29:639–642.
47. Lee G, Joye JA, Rose A, et al: Evaluation of platelet kinetics following porcine and mechanical valve replacement. *Clin Cardiol* 1981;4:11–14.
48. Steele PP, Weily HS, Davies H, et al: Platelet survival in patients with rheumatic heart disease. *N Engl J Med* 1974;57:537–539.
49. Harker LA, Slichter SJ: Studies of platelet and fibrinogen kinetics in patients with prosthetic heart valves. *N Engl J Med* 1970;283:1302–1305.
50. Altman R, Boullon F, Ronvier J, et al: Aspirin and prophylaxis of thrombo-embolic complications in patients with prosthetic heart valves. *Thromb Haemost* 1976;72:127–129.

51. Sullivan JM, Harker DE, Gorlin R: Pharmacologic control of thrombo-embolic complications of cardiac valve replacement. *N Engl J Med* 1971;286: 1291–1294.
52. Weiss HJ: Anti-platelet therapy. *N Engl J Med* 1978;298:1344–1347.
53. Massotti G, Galanti G, Poggesi L, et al: Differential inhibition of prostacyclin production and platelet aggregation by aspirin. *Lancet* 1979;2: 1213–1216.
54. Mehta J, Mehta P: Dipyridamole and aspirin in relation to platelet aggregation and vessel wall prostaglandin generation. *J Cardiovasc Pharm* 1982;4: 688–693.
55. Mehta P, Mehta J, Horalek C: Dipyridamole inhibits thromboxane generation and promotes prostacyclin release, abstracted. *Circulation* 1981;64:IV–284.
56. Fuster V, Cheesbro JH: Anti-thrombotic therapy: Role of platelet inhibitor drugs. II. Pharmacologic effects of platelet-inhibitor drugs. *Mayo Clin Proc* 1981;56:185–195.
57. Mehta P, Mehta J, Roy L, et al: Effects of nafazatrom on platelet TXA_2 generation, and PGI_2 degradation, abstracted. *Clin Res* 1982;30:839A.
58. Vermylen J, Charmone DAF, Verstraete M: Stimulation of prostacyclin release from vessel wall by Bay G6575, an antithrombotic compound. *Lancet* 1979;1:518–520.
59. Fox LK, Jonathan A, Selwyn AP: Effects of platelet inhibition on myocardial ischemia. *Lancet* 1982; 2:727–730.
60. Parry MJ, Randall MJ, Tyler HM, et al: Selective inhibition of thromboxane synthetase by dazoxiben increases prostacyclin production by leukocytes in angina patients and healthy volunteers, letter. *Lancet* 1982;2:164.
61. Smith JB, Jubiz W: OKY-1581: A selective inhibitor of thromboxane synthesis in vivo and in vitro. *Prostaglandins* 1981;22:353–362.
62. Mehta J, Mehta P: Effects of propranolol therapy on platelet release and prostaglandin generation in patients with coronary heart disease. *Circulation* 1982;66:1294–1299.
63. Johnsson H: Effects of nifedipine (Adalat) on platelet function in vitro and in vivo. *Thromb Res* 1981;21:523–528.
64. Ikeda V, Kikuchi M, Toyama K, et al: Inhibition of human platelet functions by verapamil. *Thromb Haemost* 1981;45:158–161.
65. Henry PD, Bentley KI: Suppression of atherogenesis in cholesterol-fed rabbit treated with nifedipine. *J Clin Invest* 1981;68:1366–1369.
66. Mehta J, Mehta P, Conti CR: Platelets and prostaglandins in coronary heart disease. Rationale for use of platelet-suppressive drugs. *JAMA* in press.

CHAPTER 9
The Interface Between Psychiatry and Cardiology in the Elderly

Alfred Coodley

In 1980 there were 25 million persons in the United States over the age of 65. They constituted 11% of the population and it has been estimated this figure will double in the next 50 years. Thirteen percent of the general elderly population in the United States manifest depression with a very significant percentage of such individuals using medications including psychotropics. As many as 30% or more of the elderly population experience transient depressions without suicidal risk. It is also relevant that some form of ischemic heart disease is present in most persons who are 70 years or older. The importance of the type A personality in coronary heart disease and the impact of psychological stress on sudden death were described some years ago. There is, therefore, a constant interface between psychiatric and cardiovascular problems as well as between psychiatric and cardiovascular drugs which reaches its maximum in elderly persons.

Pain, regardless of its location, is one of the most common reasons for seeking medical care in our society. As Wise wrote: "Pain, no matter how vague, is often the ticket of admission to a physician's office."[1] Because pain is such a subjective experience, it may be secondary to an acute myocardial infarction and/or the reaction to a major emotional conflict. Wise pointed out that:

> Psychogenic pain often has organic concomitants. Similarly, organic pain is never without an emotional reaction. An individual's cultural background, the society in which he resides, the interpersonal relationships he possesses, the intrapsychic meaning of a pain stimulus and the real impersonal organic problems, all color one's response to pain.

Some individuals seek medical assistance as soon as any discomfort is felt; others "stoically tolerate substantial discomfort," and others bemoan their fate.

Pain can occur when a real or fantasied loss occurs such as in heartaches or broken hearts. Family losses and anniversaries of deaths or separations can also produce pain. As Kimball said, "Only when the physician takes a full history in an open-ended manner will he often perceive the specific social or personal nuances which occur in the setting of the specific complaint."[2]

Chest pain can certainly stem from a wide range of conditions such as coronary heart disease, mitral valve prolapse, ventricular arrhythmia, chest wall syndrome, pericarditis, hypertrophic obstructive cardiomyopathy, alcoholic cardiomyopathy, costochondral neuralgia, pleurisy, herpes zoster, chronic mastitis, splenic flexure syndrome, reflux esophagitis, as well as hyperventilation, cardiac neurosis, and pseudoangina. Primary or secondary psychological factors can be involved in all of the above causes of chest pain.

As Jarvik noted:

> . . . although much has been written about the losses of old age, the pain accompanying these losses has not been addressed. The expression of pain is generally not tolerated as a form of human behavior, or is tolerated only for short periods . . . those who after the first outcry stoically bear their pain in silence are the ones who are admired and respected; those who continue to cry out in pain make others feel helpless, impotent witnesses to their agony. An observer in a hospital soon notes that action centers not around the alleviation of suffering, but around the elimination of its expression.[3]

NONCARDIAC SOURCES OF CHEST PAIN

In discussing pseudoangina, Garner and Falk[4] emphasized such may occur in patients concerned over impending death, an event reflecting their guilt over their own hostile and aggressive feelings or actions. Others manifest such pain in order to be protected by others, and chest pain in elderly patients frequently reflects an underlying depression with a sense of hopelessness and helplessness transferred from painful life experiences and situations to the heart.

Flinn described functional chest pain as either reflecting psychogenic pain or conversion hysteria in which the pain appears to "represent a misperception of an emotional state" with metamorphic references such as "it feels like my head is being squeezed in a vise," or referring to a psychophysiologic or psychosomatic process in which the emotional component is "mediated through autonomic innervations and produces muscle or blood vessel spasm."[5] Flinn also commented on the hyperventilation syndrome in which the aerophagia can produce sharp pains in the precordium or rib margin and a persistent aching discomfort can follow the muscle fatigue. Gas can also become trapped in the splenic flexure due to the high bend and left chest pain may be felt along with palpitations and shortness of breath.

Weiss[6] found the following electrocardiographic changes in patients with emotional tension, anxiety and stress: (1) increased P wave amplitude; (2) depression, inversion, or distortion of the T wave; (3) ST segment deviation. Tracings obtained from patients exercised during a period of emotional stress showed marked ST-T changes whereas the same exercise on a day of emotional relaxation produced less change or none at all in studies by Stevenson et al.[7]

CARDIAC SOURCES OF CHEST PAIN: PSYCHOSOMATIC AND SOMATOPSYCHIC

In the differential diagnosis of anxiety, Rakel[8] emphasized the need to consider all the organic diseases resembling anxiety (Table 9-1).

In discussing coronary artery spasm, Braunwald said, "Circumstantial evidence is very powerful that psychological experiences can trigger a spasm."[9] He added:

> Nerve impulses from the brain that cause blood vessels to constrict may be one reason why approximately 400,000 Americans die suddenly each year, some of whom at autopsy show no evidence of blood clots or a serious degree of artery clogging by fatty deposits. There are two possible explanations for coronary spasm. The first has to do with stress and emotions and the second with a chemical, thromboxane, which is released when platelets aggregate.[9]

Eliot and Todd reported, "Sustained emotional stress can elevate catecholamines and increase their urinary excretion. Recent evidence links such catecholamine elevations to myocardial necrosis by increasing peripheral resistance and producing hypertension, hyperlipidemia and hyperglycemia."[10]

Table 9-1
Organic Diseases Whose Signs and Symptoms Mimic Those of Anxiety

Organic Disease	Selected Differential Features
Cardiovascular	
Angina arrhythmias	While severe anxiety may cause true tachycardia—up to 120 bpm—it rarely lasts longer than 10 min. More frequently, anxiety causes palpitations—the sensation of heavy heartbeats.
Costal chondritis	Heart patients are more likely to have rapid shallow respirations.
Congestive heart failure	Anxious patients are more likely to have deep, sighing respirations and sensation of inadequate air supply.
Mitral valve prolapse syndrome	Panic attacks, palpitations, chest pain, and dizziness may be due to mitral valve prolapse syndrome. Echocardiography, electrocardiography and stress testing are diagnostically useful.

Reproduced with permission from Rakel.[8]

Myers and Dewar[11] utilizing coroner's necropsies evaluated the circumstances attending 100 sudden deaths from coronary artery disease. They found that the most significant immediate antecedent to sudden death was acute psychological stress. The reactions of patients in an intensive care coronary unit who observed other patients dying was reported by Wolf et al[12] and by Bruhn et al.[13] They reported an increased risk of lethal arrhythmias during emotional disturbances including events involving patient or staff interactions, visitors, problems with mechanical devices, and especially the activity surrounding cardiac catastrophes on the unit. They indicated that patients with ischemic heart disease had fewer arrhythmias during sleep transitions when monitored in the quiet of the laboratory as compared to the turmoil and confusion of the coronary care unit. Intense emotional arousal necessitating physical action at a time when such action is impossible or fruitless is especially likely to produce dangerous reactions. Whether ventricular fibrillation and death can be induced by neurogenic influences alone in the absence of cardiac abnormality remains a moot point.[12]

In a study of correlates of angina pectoris, Jenkins et al[14] concluded that more attention to the effect of sleep disturbance in fostering myocardial ischemia and/or angina was necessary. Such a study might include how the treatment of sleep problems would minimize anginal episodes in such patients. They felt the role of chronic dissatisfaction and hostility should also be evaluated with regard to angina while at rest or while sleeping. Forty-four percent of the total group indicated their angina was produced by emotional factors. It was found that those with the highest level of exertional angina also reported frequent emotionally precipitated angina, in fact, twice as often as those who had a greater tolerance for exercise. Jenkins et al concluded, "The stronger predictors of angina varied by type of angina, and were primarily behavioral and psychological . . . ."

PSYCHOLOGICAL REACTIONS TO CARDIAC DISEASE

The emotional reactions of patients to myocardial infarction were described by Cassem and Hackett:

> The typical patient, a few hours removed from his life-threatening experience with crushing chest pain, is anxious when he is admitted to the CCU [coronary care unit]. He is preoccupied with death, or its possibility is signalled by recurrence of pain or shortness of breath, a sense of imminent danger or doom, or simply the intimidation of the unknown. As the patient feels better, denial is mobilized. He may find it hard to believe that he had a heart attack and may protest his detention and insist on going back to important business obligations. The 3rd or 4th day, the implications of his cardiac injury begin to take the form of despondency and the more devastating the effects of the infarct, the more profound the depression. Premorbid abrasive personality traits may set in with provocative behavior beginning around the 4th day. Hostile, disruptive behavior on the first day is almost always due to anxiety and subsides as the sense of security increases. Patients who become difficult after the threat is over usually remain so, reverting to life patterns characterizing behavior styles prior to admission to the CCU.[15]

The same authors[15] suggested the routine prescription of mild sedation round-the-clock utilizing a benzodiazepine for its high efficacy, low toxicity, and to preclude the harmful effects of untreated anxiety. Haloperidol was advised if a patient appears panicky or unresponsive or if rationality and judgment seem impaired. Progressive mobilization is effective in reducing both anxiety and depression. In the CCU, the first major threat is death; the second is that of a major blow to self-esteem.[15] The patient may begin to ruminate about what his heart attack has done to him, how he might lose his job and have no money, and that he is getting old and falling apart. Such patients may anticipate not being able to drive, exercise, have sexual relations adequately, and that smoking, drinking, and eating habits will be forbidden. Basically, the patient is beginning to experience a "homecoming depression."

Shine[16] described the value of an early explanation to a patient admitted to a CCU. On the first day, patients are given instructions on the nature and future of a heart attack using printed material and audio tapes. "The more the patients knew about their condition, and the earlier they knew, the less anxious they appeared and the more they participated in their own care with some control over their lives and bodily functions." In patients so reliant on technologic devices for their survival, some degree of autonomy was felt to be essential and access is given to radio and television with control over program selection in order to cope with the sense of isolation and the disorientation secondary to drug use. Access to family, staff, and other patients minimized the isolation and beds were placed to achieve minimal noise and to avoid looking directly at fluorescent lights. Shine found that sleep is enhanced and delirium is less likely if windows are present in the CCU, if drugs are chosen on a one-to-one basis, and if clocks, calendars, and newspapers are made available to foster time and sleep orientation.

CASE MATERIAL FROM PATIENTS ON INTENSIVE CARE

The following cases represent an unselected group of patients seen in a university hospital. All had complained of chest pain and cardiovascular disease was found. Each case is condensed and attention is given to the psychological factors felt to be relevant in contributing to the cardiovascular disease present.

1. An 83-year-old woman with a prior history of myocardial infarction and angina was admitted after experiencing severe substernal pain relieved only with morphine sulfate. She first experienced the pain when it awakened her from sleep in a hospital she had entered for eye transplant surgery. She experienced a great deal of stress while waiting all day for different doctors to examine her. She also felt tired and reluctant when she entered the hospital. She added, "They were interested in only the good feelings I had." When I suggested she may have felt resentful, she agreed adding she had been angry all day because of the frequent examinations coupled with her concern about the surgery. In the past, she felt her anginal attacks had been secondary to stress and that she had always been an emotional person who worried about something negative happening. She also worries about her family and spoke of losing one child 8 years ago and how her other son can never talk about it. When it was suggested she may have anticipated a bad result from surgery, she replied, "I thought I was going to die from it." Frustrated anger coupled with marked anxiety and identification with her dead child were contributory factors in her current myocardial infarction.

2. A 62-year-old man was admitted because of dull, substernal chest pain relieved by morphine. Prior episodes of chest pain brought on by anger or exercise were relieved by nitroglycerine. When asked what had changed just prior to onset of his current chest pain, he said, "I took over an apartment house, but the building was in bad shape. I couldn't understand how people could live under those conditions. I felt intense frustration at the previous owners. If I walk after breakfast and also during, before, or after I vent my spleen, I get chest pain. I guess I have a type A personality with competitive feelings with my son and I also need to overcome my decreased semen I've had since I was struck by lightning when I was 10." The psychological components in this patient's chest pain are apparent.

3. Depression and anticipation of disaster and death were prominent in a 74-year-old woman who was diagnosed as having a tachybradycardia syndrome due to mild digoxin toxicity coupled with ischemic heart disease with mitral regurgitation. She experienced substernal chest pain prior to hospitalization. When it was suggested she seemed tense and unhappy, she then told of how her daughter had been widowed twice, how her son had cancer of the thyroid and was operated on, how her husband died of cancer of the pancreas, and how her grandson had taken her husband's death very badly and was receiving psychiatric care. The patient began crying at this time and admitted feeling very depressed much of the time. Basically, this woman's anticipation of tragedy to herself and her ambivalent identification with the sick or dead key members of her family was part of her depression and represented a significant factor in her present myocardial infarction.

4. The next patient fit the type A personality very well. He was a 61-year-old married man with an acute inferolateral myocardial infarction. He had come to Los Angeles to attend a wedding though he had been absolutely opposed to doing so. He added, "I always took my life seriously and I worked 25 hours a day. Stupidity gives me a headache. That asshole doctor is responsible for my being here and I blame him for not treating my blood pressure adequately. I'm also angry at my wife." It was clear that this patient expressed intense bitter resentment and frustration at those around him following his unwanted trip to Los Angeles and, in that setting, developed his heart attack.

STRESS, PERSONALITY TYPES, AND DEFENSE MECHANISMS

Lutz commenting on stress stated:

> It is capable of producing hypercholesterolemia, of increasing nonesterified fatty acid, catecholamine, and corticosteroid levels and of modifying blood clotting mechanisms. Stress contributes to exercise deprivation by inducing fatigue and decreasing motivation. Stress also fuels compulsive eating, drinking and smoking. The direct and indirect effects of emotional stress should elevate this factor to a position of considerable importance in the complex etiologic picture of cardiovascular disease.[17]

Stress has been defined in many different ways. It is generally used to refer to those psychological factors arousing the body in such a way that no healthy release occurs. But, stress is not always harmful. Some studies have shown that fast-paced and hard-driven executives experienced less cardiovascular disease than lower echelon workers.

Rahe[18] discussed the stress and strain in coronary heart disease and he determined that the death of a spouse, divorce, marital separation, death of a close family member, a major personal injury or illness, sexual difficulties, and trouble with the boss are all potential stressful life events and, if too many such events occur in a year, one can predict illness such as an acute myocardial infarction.

Mayou[19] studied 100 patients at two months and one year after a myocardial infarction. One third of the patients reported psychological symptoms comparable in severity to those of psychiatric patients such as anxiety, depression, fatigue, and poor concentration. He found there was a continuity of response so that measures of mental state at the 2-month phase were highly predictable of long-term prognosis. He suggested that rehabilitation should be routinely started in the hospital for a period of six to eight weeks. He emphasized the importance of consistent precise advice during rehabilitation, involvement with close relatives, and the systematic assessment of the patient's psychological status as well as the cardiac state.

PSYCHIATRIC PROBLEMS AND POLYPHARMACY

Salzman and van der Kolk[20] commented on the aphorism that polypharmacy is an "obligatory curse of the geriatric patient." They surveyed all elderly patients in a Boston medical-surgical teaching hospital one day. No psychiatric or diabetic patients were included and no pediatric or obstetrical patients were in this hospital. All drugs besides electrolytes, fluids and cytotoxic substances were included. Sixty-two elderly patients were taking at least one psychotropic drug in combination with at least two other drugs, the mean number of drugs for the entire sample being eight. As Table 9-2 indicates, 100% of elderly patients who received tricyclic antidepressants were also taking at least one laxative and one cardiovascular drug. The authors noted that constipation frequently follows the use of anticholinergic drugs and some patients were taking several laxatives simultaneously with the result that the absorption of oral medications and food may be impaired. Diazepam was given to nearly nine of ten patients receiving a narcotic. Because diazepam and its active metabolite are long-acting, augmentation of the central nervous system–depressing effects of narcotics, sedatives, and anesthetics can occur, resulting at times in confusion, agitation, disorientation, amnesia, hallucinations, and combative behavior.

Table 9-2
Percentage of Patients Who Received Psychotropic-Medical Drug Combinations

	Flurazepam	Diazepam	Neuroleptics	Antiemetics	Tricyclic Antidepressants	Other Sleep Medications
Laxatives	67	56	62	73	100	80
Cardiovascular drugs	56	44	69	55	100	40
Nonnarcotic analgesics	74	67	62	82	71	40
Narcotics	13	89	46	36	71	40
Vitamins, etc*	15	11	31	36	0	40
Antibiotics	26	28	31	45	0	40
Antihistamines	5	28	38	27	29	20
Steroids, hormones	13	11	8	9	14	0
Antacids	4	11	0	9	0	0
Atropine-containing medications	5	11	8	9	0	20

*Other nutritional supplements such as ferrous sulfate.
Reproduced with permission from Salzman and van der Kolk.[20]

PSYCHOLOGICAL REACTIONS IN CARDIAC DISEASE AND DRUG INTERACTIONS

Older patients taking antihypertensive drugs, particularly the sympatholytics such as reserpine, methyldopa, clonidine, guanethidine, and propranolol, are likely to show sedation and periods of depression. Hammond and Kirkendall[21] reported that propranolol may cause insomnia and hallucinations despite its anti-anxiety effects.

Propranolol may control hypertension or angina in those patients who are also taking tricyclic antidepressants with minimal orthostatic problems as compared to other medications, and with the added benefit of reducing the tachycardia secondary to tricyclic antidepressants.

Glassman and Bigger[22] described the quinidine-like antiarrhythmic effect of tricyclics resulting in the disappearance of premature atrial and ventricular contractions which were present before the medication was started. However, if ventricular arrhythmia occurs during antidepressant medication, the dose must be reduced immediately or a change to a different antidepressant drug made prior to the utilization of antiarrhythmic drugs. Ventricular tachycardia, flutter, or fibrillation require prompt antiarrhythmic medication with a type II drug such as lidocaine or phenytoin, not the type I quinidine-like drugs. Ventricular and atrial premature contractions (PVCs and PACs) usually do not require a change in medication or treatment.

Of all the tricyclic or tetracyclic antidepressants, it is felt that doxepin has the lowest incidence of cardiovascular toxicity when used with elderly patients. Gerner et al[23] indicated that trazodone, an antidepressant of different chemical structure, seems to have minimal cardiovascular toxicity and low anticholinergic effects. Snyder and Yamamura[24] noted that the monoamine oxidase inhibitors have a low anticholinergic activity, but that their cardiac toxicity has not been clearly established in elderly populations although their antihypertensive effect is definite. Neuroleptic drugs have been used in low doses in elderly patients, but they are generally avoided because of the degree of sedation, cardiotoxicity, high anticholinergic activity, and orthostatic hypotension, according to Davis.[25] Lithium is seen as relatively appropriate in elderly patients so far as its cardiovascular effects[26,27] although ECG studies are needed in the presence of cardiac disease. Jefferson and Kalin[28] and Macfie[29] reported that diuretics, especially thiazides, may cause rapidly increasing lithium serum levels. They recommend that hypertension or congestive heart failure be managed, if possible, without diuretics.

Greenblatt[30] discussed delirium as well as visual and gastrointestinal problems secondary to digitalis when given to elderly patients. The impaired renal function of elderly patients can result in an increased half-life of digoxin causing delirium of several days' duration after medication is stopped.[31]

TREATMENT OF PSYCHIATRIC DEPRESSION IN A CCU

A serious depression in an elderly patient with an acute myocardial infarction cannot be treated with tricyclic antidepressants because of possible tachycardia and arrhythmia and electroconvulsive therapy (ECT) has been recommended for those patients with a suicidal depression and/or acute mania. A cardiologist should be present during ECT in case an arrhythmia develops.

PHARMACOLOGIC AND CARDIOVASCULAR EFFECTS OF PSYCHOTROPIC DRUGS

Lower doses of tri- and tetracyclics with the least anticholinergic effects are indicated for the treatment of unipolar major depressive reactions in elderly persons. The cardiac effects of the drugs listed in Table 9-3 makes it advisable to have regular checks of standing and sitting blood pressure, pulse rate, and ECGs. Trazodone appears to have considerably fewer cardiotoxic effects though bradycardia and hypotension may be anticipated. The absence of anticholinergic effects coupled with the capacity to increase coronary flow and relieve anginal pain makes a monoamine oxidase inhibitor acceptable in an elderly patient with coexisting depression and heart disease if there has been no response to tricyclic antidepressants. Finally, ECT can be used in such patients if carefully monitored. Patients with a bipolar major affective disorder and in a chronic manic state are not suited for lithium medication, particularly if preexisting neurologic disease complicates the situation. For the depressed phase of such patients, however, imipramine or a monoamine oxidase inhibitor, tranylcypromine, has been recommended.

Table 9-3
Characteristics of Tricyclic Antidepressants

	Dose Level	
Effects	*Low*	*Therapeutic*
Vascular	Elevations in blood pressure	Postural hypotension
Cardiac	Anticholinergic effects predominant; tachycardia	1. Increase in PR, QRS and QT intervals 2. Increase in AV and IV conduction times 3. Prolonged HV intervals 4. Direct negative inotropic effect

Reproduced with permission from Himmelhoch JM, Auchenbach R, Fuchs CZ: The dilemma of depression in the elderly. *J Clin Psychiatry* 1982;43:26–32.

STEPS IN TREATING ELDERLY PATIENTS WITH PSYCHOTROPIC DRUGS

Dellefield and Miller[32] recommended the following procedures prior to starting medication: (1) Record an accurate and detailed base line of behavior and symptoms over at least 24 hours before initiating nonemergency drug treatment. (2) Understand the disease state or cause of a presenting problem before treating with a medication. Agitation can be caused by depression, schizophrenia, lack of sleep, a drug response, or dehydration. (3) Before prescribing, take or review an accurate and thorough drug history including present drugs to avoid overlapping, mixing contraindicated medication, and to identify prior effective and ineffective drugs. (4) Start low and increase slowly and unless you know the patient's experience with a prescribed drug, start the first dosage at one half to one third of the normal adult dose. (5) Try to avoid giving more than one drug of the same type. Select one drug for its primary effects and those side-effects that are clinically useful for the particular case. (6) Since few physicians know all medications of value in elderly patients with psychiatric and physical illness, it is well to concentrate on a few drugs in each class so that dosages, side-effects, indications, and limitations are well known.

SIDE-EFFECTS OF TRICYCLIC ANTIDEPRESSANTS

Anticholinergic potency varies with amitriptyline being the most parasympatholytic, imipramine slightly less so, nortriptyline and doxepin even less so,[33] and desipramine being the least anticholinergic of those tested by Kantor and Glassman[34] and Sutherland.[35] The anticholinergic, psychiatric, and cardiovascular side-effects are shown in Table 9-4.[32]

Davidson and Wenger[36] also discussed the modus operandi of using antidepressant drugs in patients with cardiovascular disease and prepared the following guidelines:

1. Avoid the use of antidepressants for borderline indications.
2. When an antidepressant is clearly needed, use the lowest effective dose.
3. Minimize potential drug interactions by avoiding use of other drugs or by reducing the dose of antidepressant and/or other drugs.
4. Obtain a careful cardiovascular history, and perform a complete physical examination with ECG before beginning antidepressant therapy. Check for a history of stroke, heart attack, evidence of heart failure, arrhythmias, or syncope during the predrug evaluation. Record lying and standing heart rate and blood pressure values before beginning therapy. Check the pretreatment ECG for evidence of conduction system disease, prolongation of the QT interval, or arrhythmias.
5. Avoid using antidepressants in patients with bradyarrhythmias, heart block, or very long QT intervals; monitor with cardiology backup if treatment is imperative.
6. When using antidepressants in patients with stable arrhythmias, determine whether the drug is having an adverse or beneficial effect on the arrhythmia; be alert for interactions with antiarrhythmic drugs (worsening anticholinergic effects, change in arrhythmia, conduction disturbances, precipitation of congestive heart failure, fall in blood pressure).
7. In patients with stable coronary artery disease, start with small doses and monitor frequently for orthostatic hypotension. Of tricyclics presently available, nortriptyline may be the least likely to cause tachycardia or orthostatic hypotension. Consider using a monoamine oxidase inhibitor.
8. In cases of chronic congestive heart failure, assess for worsening failure or hypotension; watch for increased fluid intake secondary to dry mouth. Consider using a monoamine oxidase inhibitor.

9. In patients with acute myocardial infarction, severe or decompensated angina, or decompensated congestive failure, withhold antidepressant during acute period; when the condition has stabilized, proceed as recommended above if the need for antidepressant therapy is clear-cut.

10. Many depressed patients with cardiovascular disease show psychological improvement with carefully supervised exercise rehabilitation; this removes the need for antidepressant pharmacotherapy.

Vieth et al treated 24 depressed patients with heart disease for 4 weeks in a double-blind trial of imipramine, doxepin, or placebo to evaluate the effects of tricyclic antidepressants (TCAs) on ventricular function and rhythm. They concluded that the TCAs

> . . . had no effect on left ventricular ejection fraction at rest or during maximal exercise as measured by radionuclide ventriculograms obtained before and after treatment. Premature ventricular contractions were reduced by imipramine but were not consistently changed by doxepin or placebo. Treatment with imipramine and doxepin, but not placebo, was associated with significant improvement ($P < 0.001$) in standard ratings of depression. These findings underscore the need for a reappraisal of the cardiovascular risks of tricyclic antidepressants and suggest that in the absence of severe impairment of myocardial performance, depressed patients with preexisting heart disease can be effectively treated with these agents without an adverse effect on ventricular rhythm or hemodynamic function.[37]

Risch et al[38] discussed two tetracyclic antidepressants (TCAs) and three other drugs relative to their degree of freedom from undesirable side-effects or potential cardiotoxicity:

1. Maprotiline showed less anticholinergic effects than other TCAs and much less of an effect on the noradrenergic system and a lower incidence of cardiovascular side-effects.

Table 9-4
Some Common Side-Effects of Antidepressant Medications

Side-Effect	Intervention
Anticholinergic	
Urinary retention and delayed micturition	Monitor intake and output. Check for abdominal distention. Withhold medication and advise physician if patient is unable to void; catheterization and/or Urecholine may be required.
Blurred vision	Suggest consultation if this persists beyond medication adjustment period. Urecholine or contact lenses may be helpful.
Diaphoresis	Encourage adequate fluid intake (preferably noncaloric) to replace lost fluid. Observe for symptoms of electrolyte imbalance.
Atropine psychosis	Withhold medication.
Dry mouth	Suggest an oral lubricant or diabetic or nonsucrose candy.
Constipation	Maintain adequate fluid intake. Encourage intake of bran, fresh fruits and vegetables, and prunes. When needed, suggest stool softeners or laxatives. Withhold medication; Urecholine may be needed to prevent paralytic ileus when constipation is severe.
Psychiatric	
Mental confusion, psychotic behavior	Discontinue drug; physostigmine (antidote for severe anticholinergic side effects).
Anxiety, restlessness, irritability	Medication may need to be changed to one that produces more sedation such as amitriptyline; sedatives and/or antipsychotics may be required.
Hypomania	Withhold medication; antidepressant may be unmasking a bipolar disorder.
Cardiovascular	
Orthostatic hypotension	Withhold medication if systolic blood pressure drops more than 20 or 30 mmHg or if the patient reports dizziness or falls upon standing.
Tachycardia	Monitor pulse for rate and arrhythmias. Withhold medication if resting pulse is more than 120 bpm.
Arrhythmias and T-wave abnormalities	Monitor pulse for irregularities. Provide for routine ECG and serial ECGs if patient has history of conduction defects.

Reproduced with permission from Dellefield and Miller.[32]

2. Mianserin has no anticholinergic effects, does not block the uptake of norepinephrine according to Kopera,[39] and there are no reports of its causing hypotension, a negative effect on myocardial contractility, or cardiovascular toxicity, even in an overdose. None of these patients developed a significant change in PR interval, heart rate, width of QRS interval, or T wave.

3. Trazodone is at least as effective as imipramine, appears devoid of noradrenergic activity and anticholinergic effects, and does not inhibit monoamine oxidase, antagonize reserpine, or potentiate levodopa as indicated by Stefanini et al.[40] It exhibits alpha-adrenergic antagonism, inhibiting norepinephrine uptake only at high doses. Administration of trazodone to patients with hypertension, coronary artery disease, and hyperthyroidism resulted in minimal ECG changes.[40] This drug may have a special place in the treatment of patients with cardiovascular disease if subsequent results confirm the initial findings.

4. Nomifensine is an effective blocker of both dopamine and norepinephrine, but exerts little effect on serotonin uptake. It is associated with fewer cardiotoxic effects or anticholinergic symptoms than most tricyclic depressants. It was not found to cause significant changes in heart rate, cardiac conduction, or systolic time interval measurements according to Brodgen et al.[41]

EFFECTS OF MONOAMINE OXIDASE INHIBITORS, LITHIUM, AND NEUROLEPTICS

Monoamine oxidase inhibitors have numerous cardiotoxic drug-drug interactions and are probably not appropriate for use in the general management of depression in elderly patients with cardiovascular disease.

Georgotas et al[42] treated 15 patients who manifested a major depressive illness with phenelzine sulfate for 2 to 7 weeks. A 60% success rate was noted utilizing an initial 15-mg dose in the morning which was gradually increased to 75 mg daily in various weekly increments. Six of the 15 patients experienced untoward side-effects, ie, orthostatic hypotension and dizziness, but these subsided upon reducing the dosage by 15 mg to the immediately preceding level. No significant ECG alterations were noted during the study. The authors concluded that:

> The minimal occurrence of anticholinergic side effects or serious myocardial toxic effects provides further support for studying this drug in the depressed elderly in view of cases of possible myocardial toxicity and the frequently associated anticholinergic effects with tricyclic antidepressant treatment. Orthostatic hypotension has also been associated with TCA treatment.[42]

Appropriate levels of lithium (0.8 to 1.5 mEq/L) appear to have minimal and reversible effects on the cardiovascular system if the patient had no pathologic cardiovascular signs prior to lithium administration. T-wave flattening and occasional U-waves on ECG are reversible upon cessation of lithium therapy. A number of case reports of a reversible interference with sinus node and atrioventricular conduction were reported by Hagman et al;[43] it has also been noted that lithium may decrease the frequency of preexisting PACs and paroxysmal supraventricular tachyarrhythmias and may induce or aggravate PVCs and ventricular arrhythmias. Most of these changes take place at therapeutic levels of lithium and all disappear when the lithium is stopped. Stancer and Kivi[44] observed that lithium may cause edema and precipitate or aggravate congestive heart failure. Interactions of lithium with cardiotropic medications indicate that thiazide diuretics, hydroxyzine, and methyldopa should not be given concomitantly.

Major tranquilizers or neuroleptics such as phenothiazines, thioxanthines, and butyrophenones can act directly or indirectly on the cardiovascular system in an additive, synergistic, or antagonistic way. Such effects vary, of course, with the type and dosage given. Cardiomegaly, congestive heart failure, and arrhythmias refractory to treatment have been associated with chronic use of the neuroleptics. Orthostatic hypotension is common with neuroleptic therapy, particularly with chlorpromazine and thioridazine, according to a National Institute of Mental Health Study.[45]

Although several investigators reported favorable use of neuroleptics in the management of acute myocardial infarction, cardiogenic shock, hypertensive crisis, and atrial and ventricular arrhythmias,[46,47] the cardiotoxicity mentioned earlier necessitates further controlled studies before neuroleptics can be recommended as therapeutic agents in the management of cardiovascular disturbances.[38]

The benzodiazepines have been found to be much more suitable than barbiturates from the standpoint of cardiotoxicity.[48] Ikram[49] noted that diazepam causes coronary artery vasodilation and a subsequent increase in coronary blood flow. Although benzodiazepines continue to be used in the management of essential hypertension, their effectiveness in reducing hypertension have been compared to placebo.[50] Salzman et al[51] compared the long and short half-life of benzodiazepines, specifically oxazepam and diazepam, in the elderly. Although the absorption of diazepam and its clinical effects were quicker and more significant, accumulation was excessive, washout was slow, and residual active substances were present two weeks after the last dose. The accumulation of oxazepam was much less and elimination took place significantly faster compared to diazepam. It was of note that the sedative effects of diazepam lasted two weeks after treatment was stopped. Such was not the case with oxazepam. Other long half-life benzodiazepines are nordazepam (desmethyl-diazepam), desalkylflurazepam (formed from its precursor flurazepam), and chlordiazepoxide. Benzodiazepines similar to the actions of oxazepam are lorazepam and temazepam. As Salzman[51] indicated, the above observations would lead one to conclude that the shorter half-life benzodiazepines would be preferable in elderly individuals, but no extensive clinical studies have validated this as yet.

SUMMARY

The elderly population is steadily increasing and yet depression remains a disturbing element in this group just as cardiovascular disease does. Problems of a psychiatric nature, including anxiety, panic, and depression, cardiovascular conditions such as angina, myocardial infarction, arrhythmias, and hypertension are interacting and interfacing constantly in geriatric patients.

Attention is being given to the multiple ways in which psychiatric and cardiovascular medications function and interact with one another and the degree to which each may improve or complicate the illnesses of the other. Although current research is furthering our understanding, it is vital that psychiatrists and cardiologists, internists and family medicine physicians work together in the management of elderly patients.

When anti-anxiety and antidepressant or neuroleptic medications are called for in the treatment of an elderly person, with or without cardiovascular disease, the degree of cardiotoxicity as measured by anticholinergic effects, the blocking of uptake of norepinephrine, the percentage of noradrenergic activity, the severity of orthostatic hypotension, the effect on heart rate and rhythm, the amount of catecholamine potentiation and monoamine oxidase inhibition and other criteria should be known by the treating physician prior to decision-making.

But what is also vital is the doctor-patient relationship and the importance of establishing a positive, meaningful rapport that may lessen psychiatric or cardiovascular problems in the elderly patient before any medications are given.

REFERENCES

1. Wise TN: Pain: The most common psychosomatic problem. *Med Clin North Am* 1977;61:771–780.
2. Kimball CP: Techniques of interviewing. *Ann Intern Med* 1969;71:147–153.
3. Jarvik L: Aging and psychiatry. *Psychiatr Clin North Am* 1982;5:5–9.
4. Garner HH, Falk MA: Recognizing the patient with pseudoangina. *Geriatrics* 1970;25:87–92.
5. Flinn DE: Functional chest pain. *Clin Aviation Aerospace Med* 1967;38:1167–1170.
6. Weiss G: Electrocardiographic indices of emotional stress. *Am J Psychiatr* 1956;113:348.
7. Stevenson IP, Duncan CH, Ripley HS: Variations in electrocardiographic changes in emotional state. *Geriatrics* 1951;6:164.
8. Rakel RE: Differential diagnosis of anxiety. *Psychiatr Ann* 1981;11:11–14.
9. Braunwald E: Coronary artery spasm. *Med World News* 1979;20:43–44.
10. Eliot RS, Todd GL: Stress induced myocardial necrosis. *J SC Med Assoc* 1976;72:27–32.
11. Myers A, Dewar HA: Circumstances attending 100 sudden deaths from coronary artery disease with coroner's necropsies. *Br Heart J* 1975;37:1133–1143.
12. Wolf S, Biorck G, Brunner D, et al: Sudden cardiac death. *Adv Exp Med Biol* 1972;16B:213–276.
13. Bruhn JG, Thurman AE, Chandler BC, et al: Patients' reactions to death in a coronary care unit. *J Psychosom Res* 1970;14:65–70.
14. Jenkins SD, Stanton B, Klein MD, et al: Correlates of angina pectoris among men awaiting coronary bypass surgery. *Psychosom Med* 1983;45:141–153.
15. Cassem NH, Hackett TP: Psychological aspects of myocardial infarction. *Med Clin North Am* 1977; 61:711–721.
16. Shine KI: Early explanation of myocardial infarction curbs anxiety in coronary care unit. *Clin Psychiatry News* 1979;7:3,38.
17. Lutz EG: Tranquilizers and decline in cardiovascular mortality, letter. *JAMA* 1982;248:306.
18. Rahe RH: Stress and strain in coronary heart disease. *J SC Med Assoc* 1976;72(suppl):7–14.
19. Mayou R: Psychological reactions to myocardial infarction. *J R Coll Physicians Lond* 1979;13:103–105.
20. Salzman C, van der Kolk BA: Management of the geriatric patient in a general hospital. *J Geriatr Psychiatry* 1979;12(2):167–176.
21. Hammond JJ, Kirkendall WM: Antihypertensive drugs for the aging. *Geriatrics* 1979;34:27–36.
22. Glassman AH, Bigger JT: Cardiovascular effects of therapeutic doses of tricyclic antidepressants. *Arch Gen Psychiatry* 1981;38:815–820.
23. Gerner R, Estabrook W, Steuer J, et al: A placebo

controlled double blind study of imipramine and trazodone in geriatric depression, in Cole JO, Barret JE (eds): *Psychology in the Aged*. New York, Raven Press, 1980, pp 167–179.
24. Snyder SH, Yamamura HI: Antidepressants and the muscarinic acetylcholine receptor. *Arch Gen Psychiatry* 1977;34:236–239.
25. Davis JM: Antipsychotic drugs, in Cook T, Cohen G (eds): *Physicians Handbook on Psychotherapeutic Drug Use in the Aged*. New Haven, Mark Powley Associates Inc, 1981, pp 23–28.
26. Damovic P, Burrows GD, Chamberlain K, et al: Effect of therapeutic dosage of lithium on the heart. *Br J Clin Pharmacol* 1980;9:599–604.
27. Tilkian AG, Schroeder JS, Kao J, et al: Effect of lithium on cardiovascular performance—A report on extended ambulatory monitoring and exercise testing before and during lithium. *Am J Cardiol* 1976;38:701–708.
28. Jefferson JW, Kalin NH: Serum lithium levels and long term diuretic use. *JAMA* 1979;241:1134–1136.
29. Macfie AL: Lithium poisoning precipitated by diuretics. *Br Med J* 1975;1:516–517.
30. Greenblatt DJ: The psychiatric effects of cardiac drugs. A Medical Insight Reprint. Insight Publishing Co, 1973.
31. Goodman LS, Gilman A: *The Pharmacologic Basis of Therapeutics*. New York, Macmillan Publishing Co, 1975, p 673.
32. Dellefield K, Miller J: Psychotropic drugs and the elderly patient. *Nurs Clin North Am* 1982;17:303–318.
33. Blumenthal MD: Depressive illness in old age: Getting behind the mask. *Geriatrics* 1980;35(4):33–43.
34. Kantor S, Glassman A: The use of tricyclic antidepressant drugs in geriatric patients, in Eisdorfer C, Fann WE (eds): *Psychopharmacology of Aging*. New York, SP Medical and Scientific Books, 1980.
35. Sutherland J: *Depression Today, Part 2, Managing the Acute Episode and Follow up Phase*. New York, CME Communications Inc, 1978.
36. Davidson J, Wenger T: Using antidepressants in patients with cardiovascular disease. *Drug Ther* 1982;12:55–63.
37. Vieth RC, Rasking MA, Caldwell JH, et al: Cardiovascular effects of tricyclic antidepressants in depressed patients with chronic heart disease. *N Engl J Med* 1982;306:954–959.
38. Risch SC, Groom GP, Janowsky DS: The effects of psychotropic drugs on the cardiovascular system. *J Clin Psychiatry* 1982;43(section 2):16–31.
39. Kopera H: Anticholinergic and blood pressure effects of mianserin, amitriptyline, and placebo. *Br J Clin Pharmacol* 1978;5:29S–34S.
40. Stefanini E, Faoca F, Medda L, et al: Selective inhibition of serotonin uptake by trazodone, a new antidepressant agent. *Life Sci* 1976;18:1459–1466.
41. Brogden RN, Heel RC, Speight IM, et al: Nomitensine: A review of its pharmacological properties and therapeutic efficacy in depressive illness. *Drugs* 1979;18:1–24.
42. Georgotas A, Reisberg B, Gershop S, et al: Clinical efficacy and safety of monoamine oxidase inhibitors in the depressed elderly. *Psychiatr Hosp* 1983; 14:93–95.
43. Hagman A, Arnman K, Ryden L: Syncope caused by lithium treatment. Report on two cases and a prospective investigation of the prevalence of lithium-induced sinus node dysfunction. *Acta Med Scand* 1979;205:467–471.
44. Stancer HC, Kivi R: Lithium carbonate and edema. *Lancet* 1970;2:985–989.
45. National Institute of Mental Health, Psychopharmacology Service Center for Collaborative Study Group: Phenothiazine treatment in acute schizophrenia. *Arch Gen Psychiatry* 1964;10:246–261.
46. Lal HB, Bahl AL: Treatment of myocardial infarction with phenothiazine derivatives. *J Assoc Physio India* 1967;15:69–72.
47. Singh KP, Sharma VN: 10-N substituted phenothiazine derivatives in auricular arrhythmias. *Arch Intern Pharmacodynam Ther* 1969;177:168–178.
48. Greenblatt DJ, Shader RI: *Benzodiazepines in Clinical Practice*. New York, Raven Press, 1974.
49. Ikram H, Rubin AP, Jewkes RF: Effect of diazepam on myocardial blood flow of patients with and without coronary artery disease. *Br Heart J* 1973;35:626–630.
50. Diazepam (Valium) in hypertension, letter. *Med Lett Drugs Ther* 1974;16:96–97.
51. Salzman C, Shader RI, Greenblatt DJ, et al: Long v short half-life benzodiazepines in the elderly. Kinetics and clinical effects of diazepam and oxazepam. *Arch Gen Psychiatry* 1983;40:293–297.

CHAPTER 10

Pharmacologic Basis for the Response to Cardiac Drugs in the Elderly

Jay Roberts
Paula Bursztyn Goldberg
Asher Woldow

The pharmacology of an agent is considered to consist of several aspects, namely, its chemistry, pharmacokinetics, pharmacodynamics, side-effects, toxicity, clinical use and indications, and interactions with other drugs. Although there may be general agreement regarding the properties that constitute the pharmacology of an agent, the definition and use of these terms differ widely. For the discussion in the present chapter, chemistry describes the relationship of chemical structure to biological activity; pharmacokinetics is used to indicate those processes involved in determining the concentration of a drug at its site of action, while pharmacodynamics describes those processes influencing the effects of a drug on the end-organ. The more difficult terms to differentiate are side-effects and toxicity. In the present context, side-effects indicate those effects of the drug which are considered undesirable but stem from the primary action of the drug. For instance, certain antiarrhythmic agents may not only depress rhythm disturbances but may also produce atrioventricular (AV) block. Toxicity refers to those effects of the drug which are not directly related to its principal pharmacologic action. An example of drug toxicity is the lupus-like syndrome produced by procainamide on prolonged administration. Clinical use and indications are self-explanatory. Drug interactions refer to alteration in any one of the effects of an agent due to concomitant use of another agent. For example, either verapamil or quinidine administered with digoxin will increase plasma concentration of digoxin, which may result in an increase in the toxicity of digoxin.

The relationship among the different processes that determine pharmacokinetic properties (absorption, distribution, biotransformation, elimination), pharmacodynamic actions (status of the effector organ or receptor site), side-effects, and toxic manifestations are shown in Figure 10-1.[1] All of the factors indicated in the figure are subject to change with age. Absorption of drug from the gastrointestinal (GI) tract can change because of the increasing prevalence of achlorhydria; both basal and stimulated gastric acid secretion are known to decrease with age.[2] Therefore, it can be expected that the degree of ionization, as well as the solubility and absorption characteristics of various substances, might change with age. Furthermore, the blood flow to the GI tract decreases with age, as does gastric motility; this may cause a delay in the absorption of substances from the intestinal tract. These and other factors would have the overall effect of making the absorption of drugs from the GI tract a less efficient and more unpredictable process as aging occurs.

Distribution of drugs may differ in older patients since there is a reduction in the actual lean body mass and an increase in fatty mass.[3] This will directly affect the volume of distribution (V_d) of a drug, ie, the apparent space in the body available to contain the drug. Digoxin, which mainly distributes in the lean body mass, has a reduced V_d in the elderly. Thiopental, a highly lipid solu-

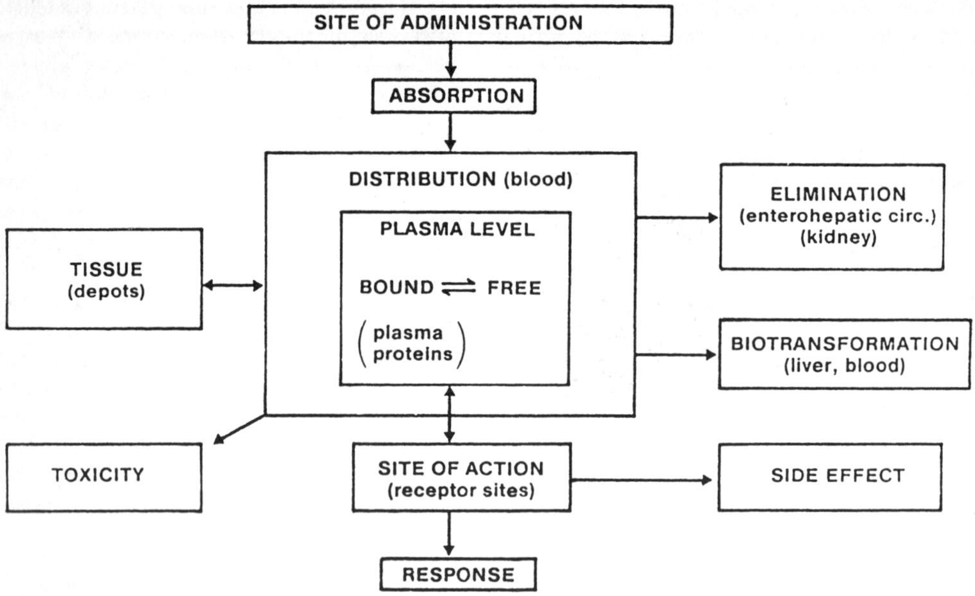

Figure 10-1 The relationship between pharmacokinetics, pharmacodynamics, side-effects, and toxicity of drugs. (Reproduced with permission from Goldberg and Roberts.[1])

ble substance shows a markedly increased V_d in older patients.

Some drugs bind to serum albumin in varying degrees. With respect to distribution and pharmacologic action, it is only the proportion of free drug that is important. It appears that serum albumin concentration decreases in the elderly.[4] Indeed, reductions in binding to albumin with increasing age has been shown for furosemide[5] and warfarin.[6]

The effect of age on drug metabolism by liver microsomal enzyme systems has been studied intensively, especially in relation to drugs that produce central nervous system (CNS) effects. Data indicate that the hepatic metabolism of prazosin,[7] digitoxin,[8] quinidine,[9] and propranolol is altered with age. In general, the plasma half-lives (t½) of these agents are prolonged. Impaired hepatic metabolism seems to play a role in the prolonged half-life of the active metabolite of lidocaine in the aged. The influence of impaired liver function on the dose regimen of commonly administered cardiovascular agents is shown in Table 10-1.

With increasing age there is an observed decrease in renal function. Reduced renal function is the consequence of less efficient renal hemodynamics as well as of poorer nephron function. The overall result of an age-related decline in renal function is less efficient clearance of water-soluble drugs, and therefore for a given dose, higher circulating drug levels in older patients. It follows that dosage schedule must be adjusted accordingly. Drugs excreted by the kidney for which significant age-related changes have been documented include such agents as digoxin, hydralazine, and phenobarbital.

RESPONSIVENESS TO CARDIAC DRUGS IN THE ELDERLY

The incidence of cardiovascular disease among the elderly is high. Among those 65 to 74 years of age, 52% of deaths are caused by cardiovascular disease; the incidence goes up to 75% in those 85 years or older.[10] It is not surprising that drugs which act on the cardiovascular system are frequently used in the elderly population. The discussion of this chapter will be concerned with the effects of drugs that are widely used in elderly patients and affect cardiac contractility or rhythm. The discussion will consider, in particular, the changes that occur with age in the pharmacodynamics and pharmacokinetics of the agents, as well as modification in the clinical indications and use of drugs in the elderly.

ANTIARRHYTHMIC AGENTS

A detailed description of clinically useful antiarrhythmic agents is beyond the scope of this chapter. Only those properties of these agents which have shown to change with age will be treated in this presentation. Their clinical pharmacologic properties are tabulated in Table 10-2.[11]

Pharmacodynamics

Changes in excitable membrane properties of cardiac tissue as a function of age have been reported only in a few cases. Roberts and Goldberg[12] studied the effects of several antiarrhythmic agents on the transmembrane action potential (TAP) and pacemaker tissue of rats. These results are summarized in Table 10-3. The effects of lidocaine (5 mg/L) to abolish the overshoot and prolong the duration of the action potential and plateau phase increased with increasing age. Quinidine (5 mg/L) depressed the rate of rise of the action potential and prolonged the duration of the action potential. Only the effects on membrane responsiveness appeared to be age-related, the depression being greatest in atria from young animals. Propranolol (1 mg/L) prolonged the duration of the action potential and decreased the maximum rate of rise of the action potential; however, these effects did not appear to be age-related. In this concentration propranolol had no effect on any other parameter of transmembrane action potential.

The effects of phenytoin (DPH) and verapamil were also examined. The depressant effect on the overshoot by DPH (10 mg/L) was most evident at the older ages, and in this respect the relationship between its effects on TAP and age resembles the effect of lidocaine on the overshoot. The prolongation by DPH of the action potential duration was significantly greater at the younger ages; de-

Table 10-1
Implications of Impaired Liver and Renal Function on the Use of Certain Drugs

Drug	Impaired Liver Function	Impaired Kidney Function
Clonidine	No change in dose	Use with caution
Digitoxin	Decrease dose	No change in dose
Digoxin	No change in dose	Decrease dose
Guanethidine	Unknown	Decrease dose
Hydralazine	95% metabolized in the liver; monitor for signs of liver damage or toxicity	Administer twice daily at most
Methyldopa	Do not use in patients with end-stage disease	Reduce dose
Reserpine/rauwolfia	No change in dose	No change in dose
Thiazide diuretics	Use with caution	Use with caution
Quinidine	Reduce dosage	Reduce dosage
Disopyramide	Reduce dosage	Reduce dosage

Adapted from Lamy PR: *Prescribing for the Elderly*. Littleton, MA, PSG Publishing Co, 1980.

Table 10-2
Clinical Pharmacologic Properties of Antiarrhythmic Drugs

Drug	Effect on SA Nodal Rate	Effect on AV Nodal Refractory Period	Usefulness in Arrhythmias		Half-Life (hours)
			Supraventricular	*Ventricular*	
Quinidine	↑↓*	↑↓*	+ +	+ + +	6
Procainamide	↑↓*	↑↓*	+ +	+ + +	4
Disopyramide	↑↓*	↑↓*	+ +	+ + +	5
Aprindine (investigational)	↓	↑	+ +	+ + +	12
Amiodarone (investigational)	↓↓	↑↑	+ + +	+ + +	(weeks)
Lidocaine	None	None	None†	+ + +	1
Tocainide (investigational)	None	None	None†	+ + +	12
Mexiletine (investigational)	None	None	None†	+ + +	12
Phenytoin	None	None	None†	+	24
Verapamil	↑↓	↑↑	+ + +	+	6
Propranolol	↓↓	↑↑	+ +	+ +	8
Bretylium	↑↓‡	↑↓‡	0	+ +	4

*Direct depressant action partly counteracted by anticholinergic effect.
†May be effective in atrial arrhythmias caused by digitalis.
‡Initial stimulation by release of endogenous norepinephrine followed by depression.
Reproduced with permission from Hondeghem and Mason.[11]

Table 10-3
Effect of Age on Responsiveness of Heart to Antiarrhythmic Drugs

	Decrease of Pacemaker Rate		Electrical Activity						
Drug	*Atrial*	*Ventricular*	*Level of Resting Potential*	*Amplitude of Action Potential*	*Amplitude of Overshoot*	*Maximum Rate of Rise of Action Potential*	*Action Potential Duration*	*Plateau Duration*	*Membrane Responsiveness*
Quinidine	↓	↓	0	0	0	(−)→	(+)→	0	(−)↓
Lidocaine	↑	↓	0	(−)→	(−)↑	(−)→	(+)↑	(+)↑	—
Propranolol	—	—	0	0	0	(−)→	(+)→	0	—
Phenytoin	—	—	0	(−)→	(−)↑	(−)↑	(+)↓	(+)↓	—
Verapamil	—	—	0	(−)→	(−)↑	(−)↑	(+)↓	(−)↑	—

Reproduced with permission from Roberts and Goldberg.[12]
(+) = increase in TAP parameter; (−) = decrease in TAP parameter; 0 = no effect on TAP parameter; → = effect on TAP parameter not age-related; ↑ = effect on TAP parameter increased with age; ↓ = effect on TAP parameter decreased with age; — = not studied.

pression of maximum rate of rise of the action potential was greatest in 28-month-old animals.

Verapamil (5 mg/L) decreased the maximum rate of rise of the action potential; this increased with age. The most striking difference between the action of verapamil, a calcium antagonist, and other agents (eg, lidocaine and phenytoin) was that verapamil decreased the plateau duration, while the others increased the duration. Only in the case of phenytoin did the effect on plateau duration decrease with age.

Moekler[13] reported on the action of disopyramide in young and old rabbits. As was reported for quinidine, another class I antiarrhythmic agent,[12] disopyramide induced changes in excitability that were for the most part similar in the young and old rabbits.

There have been studies performed in dogs in relation to age; these studies were performed in dogs whose ages were in the ranges equivalent to the young and adult age groups of this species.[14,15] In one of these studies it was observed that the TAP of Purkinje fibers from adult dogs was more sensitive to the depressant actions of lidocaine.[14] In the study by Rosen et al[15] it was noted that the action of a fast sodium channel blocker (tetrodotoxin) on the TAP did not change with age while the action of a slow channel blocker (AHR-2666) on the TAP increased in the older preparations.

Roberts and Goldberg[12] concluded that since the electrophysiologic effects of the cardiac depressants used in their study (see above) related to modification of K^+, Na^+, and CA^{++} currents across membranes,[16,17] the changes in effects of these agents on TAP suggests that the channels involved in ionic currents are altered with age. Thus, further experimentation in this area should be directed towards elucidating the mechanisms underlying age-related changes in ionic channels.

Pharmacokinetics

While there have been relatively few studies performed in animals and humans regarding changes in the cardiac action of antiarrhythmic agents with age, there are reports in humans which indicate that there are important changes in the pharmacokinetic properties of antiarrhythmic agents with age. These changes occur as a result of age-related alterations in physiologic and biochemical function as well as a result of disease.

Some of the pharmacokinetic changes that occur as a result of age are depicted in Table 10-4.[18] In addition, since antiarrhythmic agents are used in patients who may have a multiplicity of diseases which might influence drug distribution and elimination, it is important to take into account this factor as well. The influence of disease states on the pharmacokinetic properties of antiarrhythmic agents are summarized in Table 10-5.[19] It is clear that any disease that modifies cardiac output, renal and liver function, plasma protein content, and hepatic and renal blood flow will require that adjustments be made in the dosage regimen.

Several antiarrhythmic agents for which pharmacokinetic data in relation to increasing age are available will be discussed in detail.

Quinidine Hepatic metabolism accounts for 60% to 85% of total quinidine clearance, while renal elimination is responsible for about 20% of total clearance. The plasma t½ of quinidine has been reported to be about six hours. The t½ of quinidine is prolonged and total clearance is reduced in healthy elderly persons as compared with young control subjects.[9] This is probably due to the reduction in both renal and liver function with age. Plasma quinidine levels following intravenous (IV) drug infusion are consistently higher in patients with congestive heart failure than in patients without congestive heart failure (see Table 10-5).

It is well known that in the elderly AV conduction may be compromised. Quinidine can depress pacemaker automaticity irrespective of underlying abnormalities. Therefore, it should be avoided in elderly patients with the potential for developing AV block. The hazard of pacemaker automaticity depression is of particular concern in older age groups, since the elimination t½ of quinidine is prolonged and total clearance is significantly reduced. To forestall such hazards, one precaution might be to reduce the dosage up to 50%.[20]

Procainamide About 75% of orally administered procainamide is absorbed. Peak blood levels occur approximately one hour thereafter. The amount of orally administered drug excreted in the urine in the unchanged form is approximately 50%. The drug is metabolized in the liver to N-acetylprocainamide, which also has biologic activity. The rate of hepatic metabolism depends on whether the patient exhibits fast or slow drug acetylation. Both the parent compound and the n-acetylated metabolites are eliminated through the kidney. The dose should be decreased in patients with reduced renal function. Furthermore, in patients with renal failure and congestive heart failure the V_d is reduced and the t½ of N-acetylprocainamide and procainamide is prolonged (see Table 10-5). The V_d is 3 to

Table 10-4
Physiologic Changes and Pharmacokinetics

Physiologic Changes	Pharmacokinetic Consequence	Common Cardiovascular Drugs Affected*
Decreased cardiac output; increased circulation time	Delayed onset of action of the drug. Prolonged drug effect.	All cardiac drugs
Changes in body weight and composition; reduced total body weight; reduced lean body mass; per kg body weight; increased body fat	Change in drug distribution and action. With some drugs, the peak concentration is greater and the half-lives are prolonged, increasing the drug effect. However, effects are highly variable, depending on type of drug, solubility, and kidney function. (See pharmacology texts for specific drug effects.)	
Decrease in serum albumin	Decrease availability of protein for binding. Increase serum concentration of free drug increasing pharmacologic effect in some drugs. (For a few drugs, such as phenytoin, increased free state leads to faster clearance and less intense effect.)	Propranolol Quinidine Hydralazine Prazosin Digitoxin Warfarin Chlorthalidone Furosemide Spirinolactone
Altered circulation to liver; other organic liver changes (vitamins C, A, B_{12}, folic acid deficiencies, environmental pollutants can also decrease liver function)	Altered drug metabolism and detoxification in liver. Toxicity can occur more readily.	Oral anticoagulants Propranolol Chlordiazepoxide Quinidine Lidocaine
Decreased renal function. BUN and serum creatinine levels are poor indicators of kidney function in the elderly. Creatinine clearance should be used as a more accurate measurement of kidney function.	Impaired drug excretion. Drug dosage and client response should be monitored closely to prevent toxicity.	Digoxin Procainamide N-acetyl procainamide Furosemide Metolazone Thiazides Diazoxide Guanethidine Methyldopa Chlorthalidone

*These lists are not exhaustive. Only common drugs have been identified. For complete lists, see a pharmacology text.

Table 10-5
Influence of Disease States on the Effects of Antiarrhythmic Drugs

	Condition	Effect of Pharmacokinetics	Therapeutic Action*
Quinidine	Heart failure, low cardiac output	↑ Plasma concentration	↓ Loading dose ↓ Maintenance dose Monitor plasma concentration
	Renal impairment	↑ Plasma concentration	Modify dosage Monitor plasma concentrations
	Hypoalbuminemia, cirrhosis	↓ Protein binding	↓ Maintenance dosage Monitor unbound drug concentration
Procainamide	Heart failure, low cardiac output	↑ Plasma concentration	↓ Bolus or loading dose ↓ Maintenance dose
	Acute myocardial infarction	↓ Oral absorption	Administer IV at least for first dose
	Renal impairment	↑ Plasma concentration	Modify dosage and monitor plasma concentrations
Lidocaine	Heart failure, low cardiac output	↑ Plasma concentration	↓ Bolus or loading dose ↓ Rate of administration Monitor plasma concentrations
	Cardiogenic shock, hepatic failure	↑↑Plasma concentration (virtually no metabolism)	↓ Loading doses and maintenance infusion Monitor plasma concentrations
	Cirrhosis	↑Plasma concentration ↓ Hepatic clearance	↓ Rate of maintenance infusion (50% usual) Monitor plasma concentrations
Verapamil	Liver disease	↓ Protein binding ↑ Plasma concentration	Adjust dosage

Reproduced with permission from Moser.[19]
*Arrows indicate effect increased (↑) or decreased (↓) with age.

4 L/kg of body weight.[21] The t½ is approximately 3 to 4 hours, although the antiarrhythmic action may be longer because of the longer t½ of N-acetylprocainamide.

Lidocaine Lidocaine is ineffective when given orally since only 36% of the orally administered drug appears in the plasma. This is because of a high first-pass clearance by the liver. Hepatic clearance is greatly influenced by the rate of hepatic blood flow. Since the latter is reduced in patients with congestive heart failure or following an acute myocardial infarction[22] (see Table 10-5), and since in persons with heart failure there is a reduction in the V_d and an increase in t½, an increase in associated toxicity will occur unless doses are appropriately reduced. However, since both V_d and total body clearance may be decreased in most patients, these factors may counterbalance each other and the t½ may not decrease as much as would be anticipated from body clearance changes alone.

Liver disease is associated with an increase in the t½, as the liver is responsible for metabolism of the drug. The metabolites retain some antiarrhythmic activity and they contribute to the CNS toxicity of lidocaine. The metabolites and a small amount of unchanged drug are eliminated in the urine when given intravenously. Elimination half-life is approximately 0.5 to 2 hours, but it may be considerably longer with prolonged infusions of 12 to 24 hours. There has been a study[23] of lidocaine kinetics in elderly persons. No difference in lidocaine clearance was found between a group of six elderly men and a group of younger controls.

Hypotension, heart block, and sinus arrest following lidocaine administration have been reported.[24] The principal toxicity is to the CNS, reflecting local anesthetic properties of the drug. As with other local anesthetics, the symptoms reflect mixed stimulation and CNS depression. There may be excitement, confusion, paresthesias, nausea, vomiting, and seizures. Respiratory arrest may occur at very high blood levels. Since changes in the blood-brain barrier may be expected in the elderly, CNS toxicity may be even greater in this group.

Propranolol Propranolol is 70% absorbed from the GI tract and reaches maximum plasma concentration within one to three hours.[25] Propranolol is rapidly inactivated by the liver during its first pass through that organ. Metabolism occurs in the liver via oxidative deamination, dealkylation, and hydroxylation. Only approximately 30% of orally administered propranolol enters the systemic circulation. In the elderly this increases to 55%.[26] After oral administration, plasma $t\frac{1}{2}$ is approximately three hours. Propranolol metabolism (as measured by total body clearance) is reduced in the elderly, which helps to explain the higher plasma concentrations achieved in this group as compared with those in younger persons.[26] Less than 1% of propranolol is excreted unchanged in the urine.

Clinical Uses and Indications

Arrhythmias in the aged are most frequent, and may occur even though myocardial function as measured by the clinical syndrome, ejection fractions, and echocardiography show no significant damage. The conduction system itself may be affected, leading to serious complications. This is in contrast to younger individuals where arrhythmias are often benign and their significance is only a function of underlying myocardial damage.

The heart rate in the elderly patients is slower than in young patients, with rates of 50 to 60 beats per minute (bpm) in many individuals.[27] Isolated premature atrial and ventricular beats, from 6 to 10 bpm, and occurring in the same patient, are usual. Such abnormalities are usually not treated, as they frequently do not respond to drug therapy. They may disappear, stay the same, or increase, the changes being unpredictable. When the rate is slower than 40 bpm or over 140 bpm, dizziness, palpitations, exaggeration of underlying angina pectoris, and congestive heart failure become a risk and even without evidence of myocardial disease should be treated.

Atrial fibrillation is one of the most common chronic arrhythmias. The therapy is to slow the ventricular rate. Digitalis is used in these patients with reasonable results when the ventricular response is rapid. When the ventricular rate is slow, digitalis is frequently of little benefit. Occasionally a spontaneous conversion to sinus rhythm for variable periods of time even without treatment is seen. Since it is felt that the elderly are at increased risk for emboli with atrial fibrillation,[28] long-term anticoagulant treatment should be considered even with the possible risk of bleeding.

Frequent runs of premature atrial contractions, atrial flutter, and paroxysmal junctional tachycardia do occur, often all in the same patient. These are manifestations of the sick sinus syndrome and the only treatment of value is not pharmacologic but placement of a permanent pacemaker.

Premature ventricular contractions, when isolated, probably do not need any medication. But bigeminy, trigeminy, multifocal premature beats, and runs of two or more premature ventricular contractions do occur and should be treated.[19] Quinidine and procainamide are considered the primary drugs even though they may cause syncope and patients must be watched carefully for fever, rashes, and blood dyscrasias. Calcium blockers are becoming more popular in controlling atrial tachyarrhythmias and may be of value in the elderly.[29]

DIGITALIS

Congestive heart failure and atrial tachyarrhythmias, especially atrial fibrillation accompanied by a rapid ventricular rate, are the most common indications for digitalis therapy. The incidence of these cardiovascular conditions increases greatly with increasing age. Thus, it is not surprising that the elderly constitute a large group of those taking digitalis compounds, of which digoxin is the most commonly prescribed. In the United States, digoxin ranks as the seventh most frequently prescribed drug;[30] it ranks as the fourth most frequently used drug in skilled nursing homes. Because the therapeutic index for digoxin is quite narrow and because of its wide use, toxic reactions to digoxin occur with great frequency as high as 15% among hospitalized patients and as high as 20% among geriatric patients.[31] Toxic manifestations with digoxin have quite serious consequences, especially for those who are elderly and frail. An understanding of the pharmacology of digoxin, together with an appreciation of the factors that alter its pharmacology in the elderly is, therefore, of utmost importance. The discussion on digoxin will address the following topics: (1) pharmacodynamics, with respect to the cardiac actions of the drug and the known effects of age on cardiac sensitivity; (2) pharmacokinetics, with emphasis on changing pharmacokinetics in the elderly; and (3) clinical considerations for the use of digitalis in the elderly.

Pharmacodynamics

The most prominent effects of digitalis compounds on the heart are an increase in myocardial contractility and alteration of electrical properties. The positive inotropic effect is believed to be related to an action of digitalis on the plasma membrane Na^+-K^+-adenosine triphosphatase (ATPase).

Changes in responsiveness to digitalis compounds with respect to increasing age have been observed in humans as well as in laboratory animals. Some of the differences can be attributed to altered pharmacokinetics, a topic that will be discussed below. However, some observations indicate that pharmacodynamic properties of these drugs also undergo age-related changes. It has been noted, for example, that children exhibit digitalis toxicity at blood concentrations considerably higher than those at which adults manifest toxicity.[32] Furthermore, older patients can exhibit signs of toxicity often beginning several hours subsequent to peak circulating levels of drug.[33] Although these observations suggest changes at the end-organ such as altered functional status, altered responsiveness, and altered drug binding capacity, among others, no systematic studies have come to our attention which attempted to determine age-related changes of myocardial responsiveness to cardiac glycosides in humans.

That age-related changes in responsiveness occur at the effector organ has been implied primarily from animal studies. As early as 1944, it was reported that in rabbit hearts, smaller amounts of ouabain were required per unit weight of tissue to cause standstill as the rabbits increased in age from very young to 5 years.[34] Later, it was found that the concentration of ouabain lethal to guinea pig hearts perfused in vitro decreased with increasing age between 20 days and 6.5 years.[35] In heart slices from guinea pigs, smaller amounts of ouabain produced progressively greater inhibition of oxygen uptake with increasing age of the animals between 1 day and 6.5 years.[35] Similarly, a study of rat myocardial Na^+-K^+-ATPase showed that ouabain inhibition of this enzyme was greater in tissue from old rats (28 months) than in tissue from younger rats.[36] A histologic study of cat hearts showed that chronic administration of "toxic" doses of digitalis compounds produced more frequent and severe lesions (degeneration of myocardial fibers, scar tissue formation), particularly in ventricular muscle, in old animals than in young animals.[37] With regard to this particular finding, it has been suggested that because the heart of an elderly patient is likely to have foci of degeneration or scar tissue, these may serve as centers for development of ectopic beats, thus explaining in part the increased toxicity of digitalis in this age group. Overall, it appears that the heart's sensitivity to the toxic effects of the glycosides increases with age. On the other hand, some of the beneficial effects of digitalis appear to change in the opposite direction. Thus, a single concentration of ouabain produced a greater decrease in action potential amplitude and greater acceleration of repolarization in Purkinje fibers obtained from young and adult dogs than in Purkinje fibers from neonatal dogs.[38] Old dogs were not included in this study so that further aging effects were not observed. It is not known whether similar changes in responsiveness to digitalis glycosides occur with increasing age in humans, since the problem has not been studied clinically. Further, it is not certain whether such age-related changes as are seen in animals could account for the age-associated changes in responsiveness and in toxicity that are seen in humans.

Pharmacokinetics

Digoxin is the most frequently used digitalis glycoside, with digitoxin second. Both drugs are almost completely absorbed from the GI tract, although digitoxin is the more lipid-soluble of the two and, therefore, more reliably absorbed from its dosage forms. Digoxin absorption is enhanced from a hydroalcoholic vehicle, but problems with bioavailability have been known to occur. Absorption of either drug can be delayed by malabsorption problems, by food in the GI tract and delayed gastric emptying, by the coadministration of certain antibiotics (eg, neomycin, tetracyclines), by antacids, and by steroid-binding resins. Some of the drugs' pharmacokinetic properties, as observed in adults, are summarized in Table 10-6.

Briefly, the glycosides are slowly distributed throughout all body compartments and are bound to plasma proteins, but digoxin is less avidly bound to plasma proteins than is digitoxin. Quinidine can interfere with digitalis binding to tissues, thus increasing levels of circulating drugs. Verapamil can displace digoxin from plasma-protein binding sites, thus also increasing circulating levels of digoxin. The main difference between the two digitalis agents is that digoxin is eliminated primarily through renal clearance, whereas digitoxin is eliminated primarily through biotransformation by the hepatic microsomal enzyme system. One of the metabolites of digitoxin is digoxin. Digoxin clearance would be expected to be influenced primarily by renal function; digitoxin clearance would be expected to be influenced by hepatic function and by drugs known to inhibit (eg, cimetidine) or induce (eg, phenobarbital, phenylbutazone) microsomal enzymes. Both drugs undergo some degree of enterohepatic recirculation. With respect to these glycosides, an important drug interaction with antibiotics might occur

Table 10-6
Digoxin and Digitoxin: Dosages, Time of Effect and Fate in Man

	Digoxin	Digitoxin
Average digitalizing dose		
Oral	1.0–2.5 mg	0.8–1.2 mg
IV	0.5–2.0 mg	0.8–1.2 mg
Average daily maintenance dose		
Oral	0.125–0.75 mg	0.05–0.2 mg
IV	0.25 mg	0.10 mg
Onset of action		
Oral	1.5–6 h*	3–6 h
IV	5–30 min	30–120 min
Maximal effect		
Oral	4–6 h	6–12 h
IV	1.5–3 h	4–8 h
Intestinal absorption	<40–90%† (75%)	90–100%
Plasma protein binding	25%	90%
Enterohepatic circulation	Small	Large
"Therapeutic" plasma concentration	0.5–2.0 ng/ml	10–35 ng/ml
Disposition half-time	1.7 d	7 d
Route of elimination	Renal excretion of unchanged drug; limited hepatic metabolism	Hepatic degradation of molecule; renal excretion of metabolites

*Dependent on relationship of dose to meals, gastric time, and type of preparation.
†About 90% of digoxin in an alcoholic elixir is absorbed from a normal enteric tract; about 75% of a tablet with high bioavailability is absorbed by a normal enteric tract. Absorption may be poor with certain tablets or when there is gastrointestinal malabsorption.

because of this mechanism of drug reabsorption and elimination. Recently, it has been shown that intestinal bacteria metabolize glycosides eliminated into the gut. However, when antibiotics are taken orally and intestinal flora are decreased, the glycosides are available for reabsorption.[39]

With advancing age, several changes in body compartments and in organ system function become important in relation to digitalis glycoside pharmacokinetics. Lean body mass, in relation to fat or total body mass, decreases with age. Because the glycosides bind to muscle, a decrease in this compartment would tend to increase circulating levels of drug.[40] This effect might be particularly serious in patients with malnutrition, and those with chronic disease. With increasing age, hepatic circulation as well as hepatic metabolizing function decrease, although the extent of this varies greatly among individuals. If it occurs to an appreciable extent, then metabolism of digitoxin would be decreased, resulting in higher circulating levels. Decreases in renal function with increasing age, to the extent of 35% to 50%, have been observed in healthy humans between the ages of 20 and 90 years.[41] This can be expected to have important consequences on the pharmacokinetics of digoxin, ie, digoxin clearance would be slowed and circulating levels would be increased.

The theoretical changes in glycoside pharmacokinetics discussed above have indeed been observed clinically. In patients on a given maintenance digoxin dose, the steady-state serum digoxin concentration was approximately twice as high as in those aged 70 to 90 years compared to those in their 20s through 40s.[40] When geriatric patients (mean age 84 years, with no patients under 78 years) are put on a digoxin maintenance dose of 0.125 mg/day (about one half the adult maintenance dose) plasma levels were approximately 0.3 to 0.5 ng/ml, with none exceeding 1.0 ng/ml.[42] The plasma t½ is affected with increasing age, ie, it increases from approximately 40 hours seen in average adult patients to approximately 70 hours in old patients.[40] Indeed, in elderly patients, there is great variability in the range of values found for t½, one study reporting a range between 24 and 129 hours.[40] Thus, treating the elderly with digitalis poses serious problems and it is not surprising that toxicities emerge more frequently than would be anticipated.

Clinical Considerations

As discussed in the introduction to this section, digitalis is indicated primarily for congestive heart failure and for various atrial arrhythmias with a rapid ventricular rate. The most important consideration for use of digitalis in the elderly is a correct diagnosis, since in this age group the symptomatology of congestive heart failure is similar to that in conditions other than left ventricular failure. The various factors to be considered, eg, ECG abnormalities, shortness of breath, ankle edema, and roentgenographic findings, in the elderly may or may not originate from a primary defect in cardiac function. The importance of the diagnosis becomes evident from findings that the elderly often can be removed from digitalis without adverse effects.[31,43-45]

Because plasma levels are likely to be higher in the elderly following a given dose of digoxin, loading doses are usually not necessary. However, because the t½ is also prolonged, and because approximately four to five half-lives are needed to reach steady serum concentrations in the absence of a loading dose, it may take as long as two weeks to reach stable levels in the average elderly patient. Dose of digoxin is recommended to be tailored to the individual, based on a rough assessment of body size and estimation of renal function.[46,47] In treating acute congestive failure or acute atrial tachyarrhythmias, a loading dose of 0.5 mg, followed by a maintenance dose of 0.25 mg/day may be used initially. Subsequently, adjustment of dosage to titrate the patient to a desired effect may be necessary. Again, since the t½ is greatly prolonged in the elderly, there appears no need for divided daily doses.

It is noteworthy, that circulating levels of drug are many times neither predictive of therapeutic nor toxic effects at any *age*. Toxic manifestations in the elderly differ frequently from the pattern observed in younger patients. Thus, elderly patients on digitalis often exhibit CNS effects before other symptoms. These take the form of confusion, depression, delirium, hallucinations, and psychosis. Arrhythmias may also occur before other adverse effects. Visual disturbances occur frequently, differing sometimes in quality from those seen in younger patients, ie, diminished visual acuity and hazy vision occurs rather than colored vision. With respect to GI symptoms, nausea and vomiting are less common, but anorexia is observed more frequently than in younger patients.

Factors that contribute to digitalis toxicity in the elderly include small body size, impaired renal or hepatic function, electrolyte abnormalities, and presence of other drugs. The effects of altered body size and physiology, as well as the interactions with several drugs have already been discussed (see above). Several additional points are worthy of mention here. Diuretics which do not spare potassium (eg, thiazide diuretics), by lowering potassium may increase the likelihood of digitalis toxicity. Drugs that decrease renal clearance or are hepatotoxic will increase circulating digoxin levels and cause toxic reactions in a previously stable patient. Anticholinergics, by delaying gastric motility, may increase the total amount of digoxin absorbed and cause problems. In this respect, interactions with tricyclic antidepressants (TCAs) may occur. Sympathomimetics can interact with digoxin at the effector organ resulting in adverse effects. The important point to keep in mind is that when considering an addition to or removal of a drug from the regimen of a patient on digitalis, or conversely, when considering the addition of digitalis to the regimen of a patient on other drugs, the possibility of interactions must be considered and dosage modified accordingly.

TRICYCLIC ANTIDEPRESSANTS

Depression as an illness of itself, as a symptom of another physical illness, or as a side-effect of medication, is quite common in the elderly. It is estimated that 13% of the general elderly population in the United States has forms of depression warranting health care intervention. For those 65 years and older in acute and long-term health care facilities, estimates for the prevalence of depression range from 5% to 47%. As mentioned before, the incidence of cardiovascular disease among the elderly is also high. Cardiovascular conditions such as myocardial infarction, congestive heart failure, arrhythmia, and pulmonary embolism, as well as the cardiovascular drugs used to treat these conditions, are often accompanied by psychiatric manifestations, including depression.[10]

The tricyclic antidepressants (TCAs) are the most widely used drugs to treat depression. However, this group of drugs is not devoid of actions on the cardiovascular system. The cardiovascular effects of TCAs may have particularly serious consequences for an elderly patient since there may coexist an already diagnosed or a latent cardiovascular abnormality. A thorough familiarity with the pharmacology of TCAs and with the differences in responsiveness of elderly patients to these drugs is necessary to provide for their rational uses in geriatric practice.

Chemistry and Pharmacokinetics

The structures of the most commonly used tricyclic antidepressants are shown in Figure 10-2. As can be seen, these compounds differ only slightly in the chemistry of the middle ring and in the number of methyl groups substituted on the terminal nitrogen of the side chain. They are well absorbed from the GI tract. Because they are strongly lipophilic, they become widely distributed in the body. Thus, the apparent V_d for the TCAs are large, ranging between 10 and 50 L/kg. As a group, these agents are highly bound to plasma proteins, in the range of 85% to 97%. They undergo hepatic biotransformation through oxidation by microsomal enzymes followed by conjugation. The tertiary amines, imipramine, amitriptyline, and doxepin, undergo demethylation to their corresponding secondary amines, desipramine, nortriptyline, and nordoxepin, each having biological activity and pharmacokinetic properties similar to the parent compounds. In addition, the 10-hydroxy metabolites of amitriptyline and nortriptyline possess biological activity. Very little of the parent compound is eliminated through renal excretion. Renal clearance of the metabolites is slow, with the t½ ranging between 10 to 20 hours for imipramine and up to 90 hours for protriptyline.

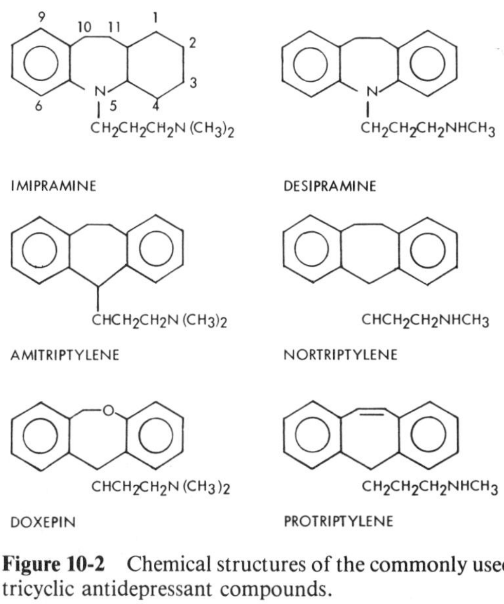

Figure 10-2 Chemical structures of the commonly used tricyclic antidepressant compounds.

As previously described, with increasing age the proportion of fat body mass relative to lean body mass increases, the plasma protein fraction decreases, and hepatic and renal function may be compromised. Thus, for the TCAs, one may expect possibly higher levels of circulating free drug as well as longer clearance times. Indeed, the elimination t½ for imipramine has been found to increase from 19 hours in young adults to 24 hours in the elderly; for desipramine, t½ has been found to double from 34 hours to 75 hours over the same age range.[48] Thus, for an elderly patient, it may be appropriate to initiate therapy with doses of a TCA in the low range and to increase the dosing interval. Moreover, since therapeutic and toxic effects for the TCAs correlate well with circulating levels of drug and since there is great interindividual variability in blood levels relative to dose administered, this is one situation wherein titrating a patient to a desired blood level and periodic monitoring of blood levels is highly recommended. Table 10-7 summarizes currently available information on TCA dosage and plasma levels for obtaining antidepressant therapeutic effects with a minimum of adverse or undesirable effects. Also included is information on plasma t½. Although no rigorous guidelines have as yet been established for dose regimens for elderly patients, the lower range of the "extreme daily dose" is recommended for this group. Dawling et al[49] believe they have developed a means of predicting nortriptyline daily dosage based on the plasma concentration 24 hours after oral administration of a single 50-mg dose.

Pharmacodynamics

The TCAs have several known actions at the cellular level. With regard to actions that bear on cardiovascular effects, four are of importance.[48,50] First, TCAs have prominent anticholinergic actions. Amitriptyline and doxepin are the most potent anticholinergics of the group; imipramine, nortriptyline, and protriptyline are intermediate in anticholinergic potency; and desipramine is the least potent anticholinergic. Second, TCAs block the amine uptake pumps for serotonin and for norepinephrine. There is a differential specificity for this action as well, with amitriptyline being the most potent serotonin uptake blocker and nortriptyline being the most potent norepinephrine uptake blocker. Third, there is evidence that TCAs block alpha-adrenergic receptors.[51] Finally, TCAs have a direct action on cardiac tissue similar to that of quinidine and other type I antiarrhythmic agents. It is not certain whether or not the TCAs

Table 10-7
Dose, Plasma Concentration, and Plasma Half-Life Range for Therapeutic Effects of Tricyclic Antidepressants (TCAs)

Drug (as Hydrochloride)	Usual Daily Dose (mg)[48]	Extreme Daily Dose (mg)[48]	Plasma Concentration (ng/ml)[50]	Plasma Half-Life (hours)[58]
Imipramine	100–200	30–300	150–300	6–20
Desipramine	100–200	25–300	150–300	12–54
Amitriptyline	75–200	50–300	125–250	32–40
Nortriptyline	75–150	20–150	50–150	15–90
Doxepin	75–150	25–300	75–200	8–25
Protriptyline	15–40	10–60	50–150	78 ± 11[48]

Different sources vary on values given for plasma concentration and half-life of the TCAs.

differ in their potency for producing quinidine-like effects. Based on these actions of antidepressants, it is not surprising that significant effects on the cardiovascular system are seen following their administration.

Effects of TCAs on the Cardiovascular System

The cardiovascular effects of TCAs have been reviewed recently.[50,52] Based on epidemiologic and clinical observation, it is seen that TCAs have effects on cardiac rate and rhythm, on cardiac contractility, and on orthostatic blood pressure. Many of the observed effects are dose- or plasma level–related (eg, effects on the heart) whereas others are seen at all doses (eg, orthostatic hypotension), and some effects become important only in the presence of cardiac abnormalities (eg, effect on contractility in the presence of myocardial infarction). The cardiovascular effects will be summarized separately: those associated with therapeutic plasma levels and those associated with toxic plasma levels.

Effects of therapeutic plasma levels of TCA TCAs, in therapeutic doses, increase heart rate, prolong the PR, QRS, and QTc intervals, have both an antiarrhythmic and arrhythmogenic action, produce ST-T wave changes, decrease cardiac contractility, and produce postural hypotension. Some of these effects have relatively greater clinical importance than others, and are influenced by patient factors.

Analyses of ECG records indicate that TCAs have an effect on several phases. Imipramine increases the duration of the PR interval, QRS complex, and the QTc interval at therapeutic concentrations. Nortriptyline produces ECG changes as described for imipramine, but doxepin does not. Doxepin may be a safer antidepressant than nortriptyline. However, those patients who exhibited ECG abnormalities have plasma levels of drug at or above the upper limit for therapeutic effectiveness, whereas those patients on doxepin who are free of ECG changes have plasma levels of drug at or below the lower limit for therapeutic effectiveness. In another study, ECG effects of several TCAs were examined in patients free of overt heart failure and atrial fibrillation and in patients not receiving antiarrhythmic therapy. Heart rate and PR interval were found to increase and T wave flattening was observed, but prolongation of the QRS complex and the QTc interval failed to reach statistical significance.[50,53] After several months of therapy, the ECG changes returned to normal and only heart rate continued to be somewhat increased. Prolongation of the PR interval, when present, is attributed to prolongation of intraventricular conduction.[52]

The effects of TCA on cardiac contractility have not been studied extensively nor systemically. One report indicated that in patients undergoing therapy with TCA, the pre-ejection period (PEP) was increased, as well as the ratio of the PEP to left ventricular ejection time, suggesting decreased contractility.[54] Animal studies also indicate an apparent decrease in contractility following various protocols of TCA administration.

The effects on the ECG and on the intraventricular conduction seen with TCAs resemble the effects of type I antiarrhythmics (quinidine and procainamide). Indeed, in a study of depressed patients, one with premature atrial depolarizations and another with premature ventricular depolarizations, treatment with imipramine improved the arrhythmias independent of improvement of depression.[55] On the other hand, this same action on conduction through the ventricular conducting system might be troublesome to patients with preexisting conduction disturbances (eg, bundle-branch block). Although heart block has been observed during treatment of elderly depressed patients who had preexisting conduction defects,[56] this is not always seen in other similar situations.

The most consistent effect of therapeutic concentrations of TCA is an orthostatic hypotension.[57] Although sometimes recumbent blood pressure is also decreased in humans on TCA therapy, this usually improves with time. However, the orthostatic hypotension, which is seen especially in patients with cardiovascular disease and in older patients with or without cardiovascular disease, does not improve during chronic use of TCAs. The mechanism for the hemodynamic effects of the TCAs has not been firmly established, but it is hypothesized to be related to an alpha-adrenergic blocking action and possibly a blunting of cardiac reflexes.

On the whole, it is felt that TCAs at or just above therapeutic plasma concentrations do produce ECG changes, some of which reflect an action on the ventricular conduction system and on muscle itself. However, the ECG effects are believed to be of minimal clinical significance in depressed young patients free of cardiovascular disease. The quinidine-like effects of this group of drugs may be taken advantage of as antiarrhythmics in some types of rhythm disturbances. Increased age and cardiovascular disease are seen as risk factors in bringing out the arrhythmogenic potential of the TCAs, even at therapeutic plasma levels. The hemodynamic effect, ie, the postural hypotension, is regarded as a troublesome side-effect, and a particular risk factor in elderly patients and in patients with a history of myocardial infarction or symptoms of angina. In the elderly, the orthostatic hypotension is feared as a contributor to accidental falls resulting in fractures. Thus, in the elderly it is particularly important to pay attention to diagnosis of cardiovascular disease and to blood levels of TCA.

Effects of toxic plasma levels of TCA Toxic levels of TCA produce cardiovascular effects as described above, only more exaggerated. Thus, sinus tachycardia, ECG changes, conduction blocks, postural as well as supine hypotension, decreased cardiac contractility, congestive heart failure, and even cardiac arrest and sudden death can result. The ECG changes are accompanied by significant clinical symptoms, including bundle-branch block, second- and third-degree AV block, and various atrial and ventricular arrhythmias. Widening of the QRS complex is especially the one component of the ECG that correlates with toxic plasma levels and is a consistently good indicator of overdose.

The mechanisms for the cardiovascular toxic effects of the TCA stem from the actions of these drugs as mentioned above, ie, the anticholinergic, amine uptake block, quinidine-like action, and alpha receptor blockade. The anticholinergic action of TCAs contribute to serious extracardiovascular side-effects as well. Stemming from a central anticholinergic action are such manifestations as confusion, delirium, psychosis, convulsions, and coma. GI atony and delayed emptying, as well as urinary tract atony, xerostomia, and dry hot skin result from a peripheral action. These effects may occur in elderly patients even at therapeutic levels and are particularly bothersome. Patients with dentures may be especially sensitive to the xerostomia. In the elderly, toxicity on use of TCAs may result from interactions with other drugs that are commonly used. Thus, adverse interactions may occur in elderly hypertensive patients on antihypertensive therapy (eg, interaction with guanethidine results in blockade of guanethidine uptake; interaction with other antihypertensives may result from blockade of uptake of endogenous catecholamines). TCAs are likely to potentiate the effects of quinidine, turning an antiarrhythmic action into a cardiac depressant action. As anticholinergics, TCAs may precipitate or aggravate glaucoma and may delay absorption of drugs by delaying gastric emptying. Other interactions can be deduced from the known pharmacokinetic properties of the drugs, eg, displacement of other drugs from plasma-protein binding sites, which again may have serious consequences in the elderly because of decreased plasma protein fractions.

Clinical Indications and Uses

Properly used, TCAs can be of significant benefit in elderly patients. However, because TCAs can have serious clinical consequences through toxic effects on the cardiovascular system, one should approach their use with caution and respect. Risk factors in the elderly include altered pharmacokinetics, multiple pathologies (in this case cardiovascular abnormalities are of particular concern), and use of other drugs. Risk factors inherent in the drugs are their multiplicity of actions. It is not certain at this time whether any of the TCAs are more efficacious or safer than others. Possibly doxepin may qualify as a relatively safer drug in this group. Above all, careful diagnosis and frequent monitoring of plasma levels of drug are strongly recommended.

Various studies with TCAs suggest that these drugs could increase heart block, cause postural hypotension and sudden death. There are reports of these medications increasing ectopic arrhythmias and also others suggesting improvement in at least ventricular arrhythmias. Increase in heart rate does occur, and more so in patients with an initial bradycardia. The effects of TCAs on myocardial function are still not clear and evidence suggests that in therapeutic dosage myocardial contractility is not significantly effected.

These compounds could be used when needed, even in patients with cardiac conditions, providing side-effects are carefully monitored for. The most frequent problem seen is postural hypotension and this may not be related to dosage schedules. The use of TCAs for patients with high degree AV blocks, and significantly widened QRS complexes is not generally recommended. These drugs should not be used in combination with type I antiarrhythmic drugs like quinidine as the effects are additive unless careful monitoring for side-effects and adjustment of dosages can be readily achieved.

REFERENCES

1. Goldberg PB, Roberts J: Pharmacologic basis for developing rational drug regimens for elderly patients. *Med Clin North Am* 1983;67:315–331.
2. Prescott LF: Gastrointestinal absorption of drugs. *Med Clin North Am* 1974;58:907–916.
3. Novak LP: Aging, total body potassium, fat-free mass and cell mass in males and females between the ages of 18 and 85 years. *J Gerontol* 1972;27: 438–443.
4. Cammarata RJ, Rodnan GP, Fennell RM: Serum anti-gamma-globulin and anti-nuclear factors in the aged. *JAMA* 1967;199:115–118.
5. Adreasen F, Husted S: The binding of furosemide to serum proteins in elderly patients: Displacing effects of phenprocoumon. *Acta Pharmacol Toxicol* 1980;47:202–206.
6. Hayes MJ, Langman MJS, Short AH: Changes in drug metabolism with increasing age: 1. Warfarin binding and plasma proteins. *Br J Clin Pharmacol* 1975a;2:69–72.
7. Rubin PC, Scott PJW, Reid JL: Prazosin disposition in young and elderly subjects. *Br J Clin Pharmacol* 1981;12:401–404.
8. Donovan MD, Castleden CM, Pohl JEF, et al: The effect of age on digitoxin pharmacokinetics. *Br J Clin Pharmacol* 1981;11:401–402.
9. Ochs HR, Greenblatt DJ, Wood E, et al: Reduced quinidine clearance in elderly persons. *Am J Cardiol* 1978;42:481–485.
10. Ouslander JG: Illness and psychopathology in the elderly, in Jarik LF, Small GW (eds): *Psychiatric Clinics of North America*. Philadelphia, WB Saunders Co, 1982, vol 5, p 1.
11. Hondeghem LM, Mason JW: Agents used in cardiac arrhythmias, in Katzung BG (ed): *Basic and Clinical Pharmacology*. Los Altos, Lange Medical Publications, 1982, pp 146–147.
12. Roberts J, Goldberg PB: Changes in responsiveness of the heart to drugs during aging. *Fed Proc* 1979; 38:1927–1932.
13. Moekler CM: Lack of aging effect on responses to disopyramide in rabbit ventricle—A brief note. *Mech Aging Dev* 1982;18:111–114.
14. Rabin ML, Rosen MR: Lidocaine effect on action potentials of purkinje fibers from neonatal and adult dogs. *J Pharmacol Exp Ther* 1978;205:204–211.
15. Rosen MR, Reder R, Hordof AJ, et al: Age-related changes in purkinje fiber action potentials of adult dogs. *Circ Res* 1978;43:931–938.
16. Hoffman BF, Rosen MR, Wit AL: Electrophysiology and pharmacology of cardiac arrhythmias. VII. Cardiac effects of quinidine and procainamide. *Am Heart J* 1975;90:117–122.
17. Rosen M, Hoffman BF, Wit A: Electrophysiology and pharmacology of cardiac arrhythmias. V. Cardiac effects of lidocaine. *Am Heart J* 1975;89:526–536.
18. Potempa K, Roberts KV: Cardiovascular drugs and the older adult. *Nurs Clin North Am* 1982;17:263–274.
19. Moser M: The management of cardiovascular disease in the elderly. *J Am Geriatr Soc (Suppl)* 1982;30:s20–29.
20. Palmer JD: Therapy for cardiovascular disorders, in Conrad KA, Bressler R (eds): *Drug Therapy for the Elderly*. St Louis, CV Mosby Co, 1982.
21. Koch-Weser J, Klein SW: Procainamide dosage schedules, plasma concentration and clinical effects. *JAMA* 1971;215:1454–1460.
22. Stenson RE, Constantino RT, Harrison DC: Interrelationships of hepatic blood flow, cardiac output and blood levels of lidocaine in man. *Circulation* 1971;43:205–211.
23. LeLorier J, Grenon D, Latour Y, et al: Pharmacokinetics of lidocaine after prolonged intravenous infusions in uncomplicated myocardial infarction. *Ann Intern Med* 1977;87:700–702.
24. Benowitz NL: Clinical applications of the pharmacokinetics of lidocaine. *Cardiovasc Clin* 1974;6: 77–101.
25. Shand DG, Rangno RE: The disposition of propranolol. I. Elimination during oral absorption in man. *Pharmacology* 1972;7:159–165.
26. Castleden CM, George CF: The effects of ageing on the hepatic clearance of propranolol. *Br J Clin Pharmacol* 1979a;7:49–53.
27. Kohn RR: Heart and cardiovascular system, in Finch C, Hayflick L (eds): *Handbook of the Biology of Aging*. New York, Van Nostrand Reinhold, 1977, chap 12.
28. Harris R: Disorders of the heart rhythm, in *The Management of Geriatric Disease*. Philadelphia, JB Lippincott Co, 1970, chap 14.
29. Henry PD: Comparative pharmacology of calcium antagonists: Nifedipine, verapamil, and diltiazem. *Am J Cardiol* 1980;46:1047–1058.

30. Tallarida R: *Top 200.* New York, Springer-Verlag, 1981, p 25.
31. Stults BM: Digoxin use in the elderly. *J Am Geriatr Soc* 1982;30:158–164.
32. Giardina ACV, Ehlers KH, Morrison JB, et al: Serum digitoxin concentrations in infants and children. *Circulation* 1975;51:713–717.
33. Taylor BB, Kennedy RD, Caird FI: Digoxin studies in the elderly. *Age Ageing* 1974;3:79–84.
34. Chen KK, Robbins EB: Influence of age of rabbits on the toxicity of ouabain. *J Am Pharmacol Assoc* 1944;33:61–62.
35. Wollenberger A, Jehl J, Kaish ML: The influence of age on the sensitivity of the guinea pig and its myocardium to ouabain. *J Pharmacol Exp Ther* 1953;108:52–60.
36. Kendrick ZV, Goldfarb AH, Roberts J, et al: The effects of age on the activity and ouabain inhibition of Na^+, K^+-ATPase purified from tissues of the Fischer 344 rat, in Adelman RC, Roberts J, Baker GT, III, et al (eds): *Neural Regulatory Mechanism During Aging.* New York, Alan R Liss, Inc, 1980.
37. Dearing WH, Barnes AR, Essex HE: Experiments with calculated therapeutic and toxic doses of digitalis: Effects on the myocardial cellular structure. *Am Heart J* 1943;25:648–664.
38. Rosen MR, Hordof AJ, Hodess AB, et al: Ouabain-induced changes in electrophysiologic properties of neonatal, young, and adult canine cardiac purkinje fibers. *J Pharmacol Exp Ther* 1975;194:255–263.
39. Saha JR, Butler VP, Jr, Neu HC: Digoxin-inactivating bacteria: Identification in human gut flora. *Science* 1983;220(4594):325–327.
40. Cusacks B, Kelly J, O'Malley K, et al: Digoxin in the elderly: Pharmacokinetic consequences of old age. *Clin Pharmacol Ther* 1979;25:772–776.
41. Rowe JW, Andreas R, Tobin JD, et al: The effect of age on creatinine clearance in men. *J Gerontol* 1976;31:155–163.
42. Waldo A: Digoxin levels as indicators of therapeutics and toxicity in the elderly population. *Annual Meeting of the Gerontology Society,* November 1981, Toronto.
43. Dall JLC: Maintenance digoxin in elderly patients. *Br Med J* 1970;2:705–706.
44. Taggart AJ, McDevitt DG: Digitalis: Its place in modern therapy. *Drugs* 1980;20:398–404.
45. Johnson DG, McDevitt DG: Is maintenance digoxin necessary in patients with sinus rhythm? *Lancet* 1979;1:567–570.
46. Moser M: The management of cardiovascular disease in the elderly. *J Am Geriatr Soc* 1983;30:520–529.
47. O'Malley K, Judge TG, Crooks J: Geriatric clinical pharmacology and therapeutics, in Avery GS (ed): *Drug Treatment: Principles and Practice of Clinical Pharmacology and Therapeutics*, ed 2. New York, ADIS Press, 1980 chap 5.
48. Baldessarini RJ: Drugs and the treatment of psychiatric disorders, in Gilman AG, Goodman LS, Gilman A (eds): *Goodman and Gilman's Pharmacological Basis of Therapeutics*, ed 6. New York, Macmillan Publishing Co Inc, 1980, chap 19.
49. Dawling S, Chrome P, Heyer EJ, et al: Nortriptyline therapy in elderly patients: Dosage prediction from plasma concentration at 24 hours after a single 50 mg dose. *Br J Psychiatry* 1981;139:413–416.
50. Marshall JB, Forker AD: Cardiovascular effects of tricyclic antidepressant drugs: Therapeutic usage, overdose, and management of complications. *Am Heart J* 1982;103:401–414.
51. U'Pritchard DC, Greenberg DA, Sheehan PP, et al: Tricyclic antidepressants: Therapeutic properties and affinity for alpha-noradrenergic receptor binding sites in the brain. *Science* 1978;199:197–198.
52. Glassman AH, Bigger JT Jr: Cardiovascular effects of therapeutic doses of tricyclic antidepressants. *Arch Gen Psychiatry* 1981;38:815–820.
53. Burckhardt D, Raeder E, Muller V, et al: Cardiovascular effects of tricyclic and tetracyclic antidepressants. *JAMA* 1978;239:213–216.
54. Muller V, Burckhardt D: Die wirkung tri und tetrazyklischer antidepressiva aus herz und kreislauf. *Schweiz Med Wochenscher* 1974;104: 1911–1933.
55. Bigger JT Jr, Giardina EGV, Perel JM, et al: Cardiac antiarrhythmic effects of imipramine hydrochloride. *N Engl J Med* 1977;296:206–208.
56. Smith RR, Rusbatch BJ: Amitriptylene and heart block, letter. *Br Med J* 1967;3:311.
57. Muller OF, Goodman N, Bellet S: The hypotensive effect of imipramine hydrochloride in patients with cardiovascular disease. *Clin Pharmacol Ther* 1961; 2:300–307.
58. Hollister LE: Psychiatric disorders, in Avery GS (ed): *Drug Treatment: Principles and Practice of Clinical Pharmacology and Therapeutics,* ed 2. New York, ADIS Press, 1980, chap 26.

CHAPTER 11
Epidemiology of Coronary Heart Disease in the Elderly Patient

Erik Agner

During the last century the incidence of coronary heart disease (CHD) has been steadily increasing in industrialized Western countries at the same time as the importance of infectious diseases and malnutrition in these countries has been decreasing. Together with malignant diseases CHD today is responsible for a major part of the mortality in younger as well as in older age groups. This has stimulated a rapidly growing interest in the study of all aspects of CHD.

CHD epidemiology today is descriptive as well as causality-seeking and includes the following items:

1. *Description of the prevalence and incidence of defined CHD manifestations*, ie, the percentage of a defined population showing the manifestations of CHD at a given time, and the percentage of a defined population developing the manifestations of CHD over a defined period. In the many surveys on this subject it is important to note the entry criteria for selection of participants (geography, place of employment, age, sex, referred patients, hospitalized patients).

2. *Definitions of risk factors* or markers of excess risk of existing or developing CHD (retrospectively). Since the finding of such risk factors in the late 1940s and early 1950s in a larger population in the Framingham study[1] an enormous amount of literature has emerged on this subject, which may crudely be subdivided into four groups of risk factors[2]: (*a*) Factors involving fundamental biology, ie, age, sex, and heredity. (*b*) Factors involving endogenous biochemical-physiologic mechanisms, but which may be influenced by exogenous factors, ie, arterial blood pressure, resting heart rate, serum cholesterol, various cholesterol fractions, serum triglycerides, fasting plasma glucose, glucose tolerance, and plasma uric acid. (*c*) Factors involving social environment and life style, ie, smoking, diet, and physical activity. (*d*) Factors involving existing pathologic conditions, ie, history of myocardial infarction, chronic cardiovascular symptoms, and pathologic ECG changes.

3. *Evaluation of such risk factors in new populations* (prospectively) before definite establishment.

4. *Evaluation of the effect when modifying these risk factors* in order to establish possible causality.

This chapter will deal mainly with the first three items, only briefly touching upon the fourth. Emphasis will be placed upon studies of unselected populations. The results presented are mainly based on sections of the Glostrup population studies in Denmark.

DESIGN OF THE GLOSTRUP STUDY

Population at Entry

In 1967 all men and women born in 1897 and living in nine municipalities around the Glostrup University Hospital were invited to participate in a health survey at the hospital. A total of 230 men and 210 women participated, the participation rate being 69%, with no significant differences between participants and nonparticipants and no significant differences between the present population and the total 1897 population in Denmark according to housing conditions or to death and hospitalization in the following decade.[3,4]

Procedure at Age 70

The design of the 70-year survey has previously been described.[5] World Health Organization standardized questionnaires on angina pectoris, possible previous myocardial infarction, intermittent claudication, and smoking habits were filled in and questions on exercise habits were asked. Angina pectoris or intermittent claudication were considered present if pain arose while walking or hurrying, and stopped after nitroglycerine or resting.

A clinical examination was carried out including calculation of body mass index (kg/stature [m] squared) and palpation of the femoral, posterior tibial, and dorsalis pedis arteries on both sides. Distal pulse abnormality was defined as one or more missing pulses. An AP film of the thorax was taken for calculation of the cardiothoracic ratio. Arterial blood pressure was measured after 15 minutes rest in the supine position, using a standardized mercury sphygmomanometer with a fixed bladder dimension of 12.5×25 cm. For the diastolic reading the Korotkoff phase 5 was used. Blood flow in the anterior tibial muscle was measured in both legs by the xenon 133 method after maximal muscular exercise in ischemia.[6,7] Maximal muscular flow (ml/100 g $\times$ min) and delay time until this was achieved after discontinuation of ischemia were registered, and the lowest value of the maximal muscular flow and the highest value of the delay time obtained in both legs were used. A 12-lead ECG was coded according to the Minnesota code.

CHD at ages 70 and 80 was defined by the presence of one or more of the following symptoms: angina pectoris, possible previous myocardial infarction, definite ECG signs of myocardial infarction (Minnesota code 1.1–2).

The following blood tests were obtained in the morning after a 13-hour fast: serum cholesterol, triglycerides, insulin and creatinine, plasma uric acid, and venous whole blood glucose. This was followed by a 2½-hour oral glucose tolerance test (1 g/kg, max 70 g), the results of which were grouped according to WHO into normal glucose tolerance, impaired glucose tolerance, and diabetes mellitus. Cholesterol was measured by the method described by Grafnetter[8] and triglycerides by the method of Laurell.[9]

No intervention was attempted during this survey, but the results were forwarded to the participants' own physicians upon request.

Ten-Year Course

During the following 10 years all hospital admittances and deaths in the population were recorded. Medical records and death certificates were obtained; in 68% of the deaths an autopsy had been carried out. Diseases were coded according to WHO's diagnosis group for CHD (WHO code: 410–429[10]). CHD manifestations in the eighth decade were defined as death or hospitalization because of CHD.

Population and Procedure at Age 80

Of the 361 surviving 80-year-old men and women, 68% participated in a re-examination around the time of their 80th birthdays.[5] No differences were found between participants and nonparticipants at 80 according to hospitalization in the eighth decade. The examination at age 80 was identical to the entry examination except that the high-density lipoprotein cholesterol (HDL cholesterol) fraction was now also being measured by the magnesium-dextran precipitating method,[11] and the xenon 133 leg muscle perfusion was replaced by ultrasonic measurement of blood pressure in the brachial, posterior tibial, and dorsalis pedis arteries on both sides. The decreased distal blood pressure ratio was defined as a difference between the systolic pressure in the brachial and dorsalis pedis arteries of more than 18 mmHg together with an ankle blood pressure of less than 120 mmHg. Care was taken that no drifts of measuring methods had taken place over the 10-year course.

Statistical Evaluation

The statistical evaluation was carried out in the Data Processing Department of the Copenhagen County Hospitals. The χ^2-test with Yates' correction was used when comparing classed variables, Wilcoxon Mann-Whitney's or Kruskal Wallis' test when comparing two or three classed variables with integer variables, Spearmann's rank sum test when testing for correlation, and Wilcoxon's signed rank test when testing for differences between two integer variables. In the multivariate evaluation, Cox's regression analysis was used. The variables included in the latter analysis all fulfilled the criterion of proportional intensities of the end-points, when these intensities were plotted graphically. Statistical level $P < 0.05$.

CHD IN THE EIGHTH DECADE

Prevalence of CHD at Ages 70 and 80

The prevalence of angina pectoris, possible previous myocardial infarction, definite myocardial infarction in ECG and CHD, defined as one or more of these, is shown in Table 11-1. At age 70 a significantly higher prevalence of CHD was found in men than in women, whereas in the surviving 80-year-old population this sex difference had disappeared, the women having reached the level of the men, whose level had not moved significantly over the decade. Interestingly, at age 70 only 23% of the men compared to 30% of the women had an increased cardiac/thoracic ratio (>50%), while in both age groups significantly higher percentages of women than of men (14% and 36% compared to 7% and 28%, respectively) were receiving diuretics.

The Age 70 to 80 Years' Course

During the following 10 years 53% of the men and 34% of the women died, 35% and 34% of the deaths, respectively, being caused by CHD (Table 11-2); 26% of the men and 19% of the women were hospitalized because of CHD during the decade (Table 11-3). The number of hospital days due to CHD, however, was small, the mean being only 7 and 4 days, respectively, compared to a total number of hospital days with means of 33 and 34 days.

The prevalence of CHD manifestations at age 70 were at the same level as other populations above middle age.[12,13] However, the narrowing of the gap between prevalence in men and women noted in some of these surveys could not be found in the present 70-year-olds. Only at age 80 had the gap closed.

The real course and incidence of CHD are difficult to evaluate from a longitudinal study of the present design, where no intermediate questions were asked. On the other hand, the risk of inducing symptoms by repeated questioning has been avoided. The 10-year incidence of 15% to 22% is a little higher than found in the older age groups in the Framingham study[1,14] and the Israeli heart study.[15] It is of special interest that few participants confirming angina pectoris or possible previous myocardial infarction at age 70 denied it at age 80.[5] This gives a repeatability of positive answers equaling that found in studies of younger populations.[16]

Table 11-1
Prevalence of CHD Manifestations at Ages 70 and 80

	Age 70		Age 80	
	Men	*Women*	*Men*	*Women*
Angina pectoris	10	5*	10	9
Possible previous myocardial infarction	5	3*	7	10
Definite myocardial infarction in ECG	6	2*	11	6
One or more of these = CHD	15	9*	20	20

*Significant sex difference, $P < 0.05$.

Table 11-2
Main Causes of Death in the Eighth Decade

	WHO Code	Men (%)*	Women (%)*
Neoplasms	140–239	32	29
Myocardial infarction	410	23	23
Other manifestations of ischemic disease	411–429	12	11
Cerebrovascular disease	430–438	9	10
Other vascular diseases	439–459	4	6
Diseases of respiratory system	460–519	15	7
Others		5	14

*Percent of all deaths.

Table 11-3
Cumulated Morbidity (%) and Mean Duration of Hospitalization (Days) in Eighth Decade

		Men		Women	
	WHO Code	%	*Days*	%	*Days*
Hypertensive disease	400–404	1	0.1	2	0.3
Myocardial infarction	410	9	2.4	8	1.7
Other manifestations of ischemic heart disease	411–429	17	4.8	11	2.7
Cerebrovascular disease	430–438	10	2.6	8	2.3
Other vascular diseases	439–459	8	2.0	10	2.1

CORONARY HEART DISEASE RISK FACTORS AT AGE 70

Ten-Year Prediction

CHD at age 70 in men, but not in women, was significantly connected to excess total mortality in the following decade. Table 11-4 shows the CHD mortality and total CHD manifestations in the eighth decade according to the presence or absence of CHD at age 70. In men alone definite myocardial infarction in ECG and CHD at age 70 were connected to excess CHD mortality and excess total CHD manifestations. Furthermore, angina pectoris in men and women, and CHD in women were connected to excess total CHD manifestations.

The present findings correspond to findings in younger populations.[14] The few connections between CHD and traditional CHD risk factors in both age groups might be taken as evidence for a decreasing importance of these factors in old age.

In the present 70-year-old men, mean systolic blood pressure was 153 mmHg (SD ± 23) and in the present 70-year-old women 157 mmHg (SD ± 28) with no significant sex difference. Diastolic blood pressure on the other hand showed a significant sex difference, the mean in men being 86 mmHg (SD ± 13) and in women 82 mmHg (SD ± 13). Systolic and diastolic blood pressures were closely correlated in both sexes. If WHO's definition of arterial hypertension (⩾160/95 mmHg) is applied, 46% of the men and 45% of the women had arterial hypertension.

At age 80 systolic blood pressure showed a statistical sex difference, the mean in men being 137 mmHg (SD ± 22) and in women 148 mmHg (SD ± 26). Diastolic blood pressure had a mean value in both sexes of 71 mmHg (SD ± 13). Also at this age, systolic and diastolic blood pressures were closely correlated in both sexes. Using WHO's definition of arterial hypertension, 19% of the men and 30% of the women had arterial hypertension.

Table 11-5 shows the relations between blood pressure and CHD and other CHD risk factors at ages 70 and 80. It may be seen that blood pressure was connected to a major part of other CHD risk factors but not to CHD.

A number of external factors might have influenced the blood pressure distribution: (1) At age 70, 8% of the men and 16% of the women were receiving antihypertensive medication (6% and 12%, respectively, were receiving diuretics alone, the others alpha-methyldopa or combinations of these two drugs). At age 80 these percentages had increased to 28% of the men and 39% of the women (67% receiving diuretics alone, 6% receiving alpha-methyldopa or beta-blockers as single therapy, 27% receiving a combination of diuretic and one of the latter two drugs). Mean systolic blood pressure, however, was still significantly higher at both ages and in both sexes in the treated group than in the untreated group. (2) Male smokers who inhaled, on the other hand, had lower systolic and lower diastolic blood pressures

Table 11-4
CHD Mortality in the Eighth Decade According to Presence or Absence of CHD at Age 70 (%)

	Men		Women	
	+	−	+	−
Angina pectoris	32	18	30	8
Possible previous myocardial infarction	45	18	16	8
Definite myocardial infarction on ECG	54	18‡	25	8
One or more of these = CHD	37	16†	22	7

Significant difference between + and −.
*$P < 0.05$, †$P < 0.01$, ‡$P < 0.001$.

Table 11-5
Connections Between Arterial Blood Pressure and CHD and Possible CHD Risk Factors at Ages 70 and 80

	Age 70				Age 80			
	Men		*Women*		*Men*		*Women*	
	Systolic	Diastolic	Systolic	Diastolic	Systolic	Diastolic	Systolic	Diastolic
Cholesterol		*						
Triglycerides	*		†	*				*
Glucose tolerance (three classes)	†	*	†					
Body mass index	‡	‡	‡	†		‡		
Smoking (three classes)	*						*	
Antihypertensive/diuretic treatment	*		*		*		*	
CHD								
Cardiac/thoracic ratio (at age 70)	‡	‡	†	*				
Intermittent claudication		I*				I†		
Distal pulse abnormality								
Maximal distal muscle flow (at age 70)								
Delay time (at age 70)	I‡	I‡	I*					
Distal blood pressure ratio (at age 80)								

Significant connection: *$P < 0.05$, † $P < 0.01$, ‡$P < 0.001$.
I = Inverse connection.
For definitions, see study design.

at both ages compared to nonsmokers, blood pressure values from male smokers who did not inhale being intermediate. (3) Dietary habits also had importance, as high values of body mass index correlated positively with systolic and diastolic blood pressures in both sexes at age 70 and with diastolic blood pressure in men at age 80.

Table 11-6 shows the mean systolic and diastolic blood pressures at age 70 in relation to CHD mortality and CHD manifestations in the eighth decade. In both sexes high systolic blood pressure was connected to excess CHD mortality and excess CHD manifestations, whereas only in women was high diastolic blood pressure connected to excess CHD mortality.

Similarly, hospitalization and number of hospital days in the eighth decade due to CHD were connected to high systolic blood pressure in both sexes, and to high diastolic blood pressure in women. Furthermore, systolic blood pressure in both sexes and diastolic blood pressure in women correlated inversely with time elapsed till development of CHD. Systolic and diastolic blood pressures at age 70 correlated with systolic and diastolic blood pressures at age 80. High systolic blood pressure at age 70 was associated with decreased glucose tolerance in both sexes at age 80, and high systolic and high diastolic blood pressures at age 70 were associated with high plasma creatinine in both sexes at age 80.

In the present study the level of blood pressure at age 70 was considerably higher than that found in population surveys of younger age groups.[17-20] A lower blood pressure in smokers than in nonsmokers has previously been reported from younger populations.[21] This finding has not been explained except by the correlation between nonsmoking and high body weight, as found in the present study in both age groups and sexes. High body weight might falsely contribute to a higher blood pressure.

As in younger and middle-aged populations, where a high blood pressure has been found to be an important predictor of CHD,[22-24] a high systolic blood pressure in old age in the present study was associated with excess 10-year CHD mortality and CHD manifestations. Only in women and only in reference to the former end-point did high diastolic blood pressure show a similar statistical connection.

Hypercholesterolemia[25-29] and—less unanimously—hypertriglyceridemia[27] have been established as significant risk factors for development of CHD in younger and middle-aged persons. Beyond the mid-50s, however, the predictive value of these two measurements seems to diminish.[30,31] Furthermore, several recently published studies and re-evaluations of studies have shown a J-shaped relation between cholesterol values and total mortality,[32-34] high cholesterol being associated with excess CHD mortality and low cholesterol with excess cancer mortality.

At age 70 the mean value of serum cholesterol was in the present men 7.2 mmol/L (SD ± 1.2) and in the present women 7.9 mmol/L (SD ± 1.4), with a significant sex difference. The mean value of serum triglycerides was in men 1.16 mmol/L (SD ± 0.6) and in women 1.12 mmol/L (SD ± 0.5), with no significant sex difference. The mean value of body mass index in the present population was in men 25.6 kg/m^2 and in women 26.6 kg/m^2 with no significant sex difference.

At age 80 mean cholesterol values were in men 6.1 mmol/L (SD ± 1.0) and in women 7.0 mmol/L (SD ± 1.2); mean triglyceride values were in men 1.07 mmol/L (SD ± 0.6) and in women 1.17 mmol/L (SD ± 0.6), both lipids showing significant sex differences.

Mean HDL cholesterol, which was not measured at age 70, was in 80-year-old men 1.37 mmol/L (SD ± 0.3), and in 80-year-old women 1.50 mmol/L (SD ± 0.3), with a significant sex difference.

A highly significant, positive correlation was found between the values of serum cholesterol and serum triglycerides in each sex at age 70 but

Table 11-6
Mean Systolic and Diastolic Blood Pressure (mmHg) at Age 70 Related to CHD Death and all CHD Manifestations in Eighth Decade

		Men		Women	
		Systolic	*Diastolic*	*Systolic*	*Diastolic*
CHD death	+	160*	88	169*	89*
	–	156	85	154	81
CHD manifestations	+	160*	87	169*	85
	–	152	86	156	81

Statistical difference: *$P < 0.05$.

not at age 80. The relations between serum cholesterol and triglycerides and CHD and other possible CHD risk factors at ages 70 and 80 are shown in Table 11-7. Furthermore, at age 80 low HDL cholesterol values were connected to high values of triglycerides in both sexes, and in women alone to high values of body mass index, decreased glucose tolerance, a decreased blood pressure ratio, and antihypertensive treatment. Neither of the lipid fractions measured at age 70 or at age 80 showed any connection to exercise habits.

During the following decade, serum cholesterol at age 70 was not connected to total mortality in either sex. However, in both sexes mean 70-year cholesterol values were significantly higher in those dying from CHD than in survivors and in those dying from noncardiovascular diseases (in men 7.4, 7.2, and 6.8 mmol/L respectively; in women 8.2, 8.0, and 7.4 mmol/L). Figure 11-1 shows total mortality, mortality from CHD, and mortality from malignant neoplasms (WHO code: 140–207 [14]) according to values of serum cholesterol in men. The U- or J-shaped curve of the total mortality seems to be explained by the mortality curves for CHD and for malignant neoplasms. Mortality from CHD tended to be higher (25%) in the upper quartile of the cholesterol distribution than in the lower quartile (15%). On the other hand, mortality from malignant neoplasms was significantly higher (30%) in the lower quartile than in the upper quartile (8%). Similarly, the mean value of serum cholesterol at age 70 was lower in men hospitalized for malignant neoplasms in the eighth decade than in other men (6.7 and 7.3 mmol/L, respectively) and higher in men hospitalized for CHD than in other men (7.9 and 7.1 mmol/L, respectively).

A tendency toward increasing mortality corresponding to increasing values of serum triglycerides was seen in both sexes, but like serum cholesterol the level of serum triglycerides was not significantly connected to total mortality in men or in women ($P = 0.06$ and $P = 0.21$). In men dying from CHD, however, the mean value of serum triglycerides (1.47 mmol/L) was significantly higher than in men surviving the decade or dying from noncardiovascular diseases (1.06 and 1.05 mmol/L, respectively). No difference in CHD mortality (17%) was seen between the lower three quartiles of the triglyceride values in men; in the upper quartile, however, CHD mortality was significantly higher (39%). As for cholesterol a similar, but not significant, trend was seen in women. Furthermore, high values of serum triglycerides were connected to excess hospitalization from CHD and also from acute myocardial infarction

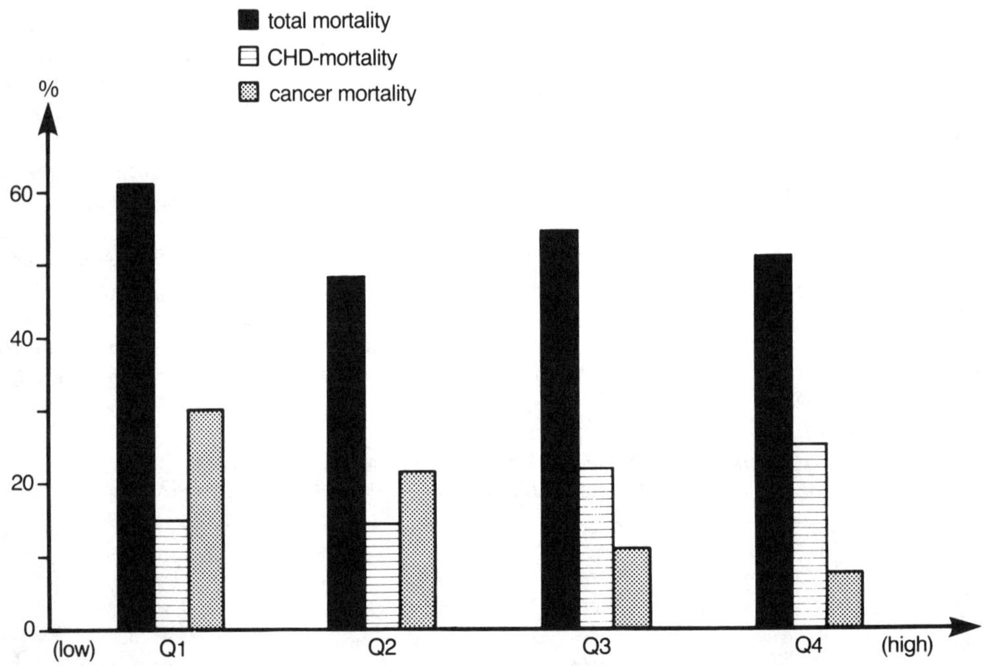

Figure 11-1 Male mortality in the eighth decade according to serum cholesterol quartiles at age 70.

Table 11-7
Connections Between Cholesterol and Triglycerides and CHD and Possible CHD Risk Factors at Ages 70 and 80

	Age 70				Age 80			
	Men		*Women*		*Men*		*Women*	
	Cholesterol	Triglycerides	Cholesterol	Triglycerides	Cholesterol	Triglycerides	Cholesterol	Triglycerides
Systolic blood pressure		*		†				
Diastolic blood pressure				*				*
Glucose tolerance (three classes)		†		†				*
Body mass index	*	‡		*		*		‡
Smoking (three classes)								
Antihypertensive/diuretic treatment		‡		*		†		
CHD					*			
Cardiac/thoracic ratio (at age 70)				*				
Intermittent claudication								
Distal pulse abnormality								*
Maximal distal muscle flow (at age 70)								
Delay time (at age 70)								
Distal blood pressure ratio (at age 80)								I*

Significant connection: * $P < 0.05$, †$P < 0.01$, ‡$P < 0.001$.
I = Inverse connection.
For definitions, see study design.

alone in the eighth decade in men. Low values of serum triglycerides were not connected to increased mortality or hospitalization from malignant neoplasms.

During the 10-year period, the cholesterol and triglyceride measurements were continuously tested against measurements at the Lipid Reference Center in Prague.[31] High precision and accuracy was found in the cholesterol measurements, but it should be noted that using a one-step cholesterol measuring method like the present one,[8] the values obtained will be about 10% higher than when using a two-step technic such as the Abell-Kendall method. The precision of the triglyceride method was high, but it continuously underestimated the triglyceride value by 10% compared with measurements performed at the Lipid Reference Center. Correcting for these factors the presented values are very similar to those found in the Gothenborg population aged 70.

The decreasing cholesterol level and the insignificantly increasing triglyceride level over the decade reflect a concomitant trend in the total population.[31] Thus, these changes can hardly be ascribed to increasing age.

In the present study the high triglyceride level at age 70 was a significant CHD risk factor in men. This might have been mediated through a negative correlation with HDL cholesterol; such a negative correlation was found in both sexes in the present 80-year-olds, as it was in the older age groups in the Framingham study.

The decrease in glucose tolerance with increasing age starts in the second decade and continues through the adult life.[35,36] Decreased glucose tolerance is accompanied by excess mortality.[37-39] Moreover, subjects with minor abnormalities in the oral glucose tolerance test (lately designated impaired glucose tolerance[39,40]) are at a higher risk for development of diabetes mellitus than subjects with a normal glucose tolerance.[35,38-40] However, no longitudinal studies registering variations in glucose tolerance and their influence on longevity have previously been made in old populations.

No agreement exists concerning the interpretation of the results of the oral glucose tolerance test in the elderly.[35,36] Recently three sets of recommendations for classification of the different categories of glucose tolerance have been proposed.[39,40] Although these recommendations were mainly based on long-term studies in younger age groups, no adjustment for age was felt necessary, nor was an upper age limit set for their usefulness.

At age 70 the mean value of fasting blood glucose in men was 4.7 mmol/L (SD ± 1.7)* and in women 4.9 mmol/L (SD ± 1.9); the mean value of 2-hour blood glucose in men was 6.5 mmol/L (SD ± 3.9) and in women 6.9 mmol/L (SD ± 3.3), with no significant sex differences.

At age 80, the mean value of fasting blood glucose in men was 4.9 mmol/L (SD ± 0.9) and in women 5.2 mmol/L (SD ± 1.6); the mean value of 2-hour blood glucose in men was 7.1 mmol/L (SD ± 2.5) and in women 7.7 mmol/L (SD ± 3.9) with no significant sex differences. The connections between glucose tolerance and other possible CHD risk factors at ages 70 and 80 are shown in Table 11-8. At age 70 high levels of systolic blood pressure, triglycerides, body mass index, and in women of cardiac/thoracic ratio, and low levels of maximal distal muscle flow in both sexes were connected to decreased glucose tolerance.

Excess total mortality was seen in men with impaired glucose tolerance and diabetes mellitus, and in women with diabetes mellitus. Moreover, excess mortality was seen in women with diabetes mellitus compared to women with impaired glucose tolerance.

Although total mortality in the present study was high and probably influenced by a multiplicity of factors, the effects of diabetes mellitus on mortality, known from studies of younger populations, were seen in both sexes.[37] Data concerning excess mortality in subjects with impaired glucose tolerance have been conflicting. The excess mortality in the present study could, in men solely, and in women partly, be ascribed to excess mortality from CHD as in the Bedford study,[39] indicating that impaired glucose tolerance in men, as well as diabetes mellitus in both sexes, are risk factors for the development of CHD, and that female diabetes mellitus has an additional connection with excess mortality from noncardiovascular diseases.

In younger populations in the Western industrialized countries smoking has been isolated as a major risk factor for total mortality and cardiovascular and pulmonary diseases, as found in several prospective, epidemiologic surveys.[41] The implications for health in old age, however, have not been specifically evaluated. In our 70-year-old population, 76% of the men and 39% of the women (58% of the population) were smokers. Of these smokers, 32% of the men and 20% of the

*For conversion to mg/dL these values should be multiplied by 18.

women were inhalers, and 14% of the men and 3% of the women were heavy smokers (defined as >15 g tobacco/day plus inhalation [one cigarette = 1 g; one cheroot = 3 g; and one cigar = 5 g]). When evaluated in grams tobacco per day, the mean consumption in men was lower in the cigarette group than in the other smoking groups, while the percentage of inhalers was largest in the cigarette groups in both sexes. At age 70 the male smokers had been smoking for a median of 55 years, the female smokers for a significantly shorter median of 38 years. Table 11-9 shows the relations between smoking and CHD and other possible CHD risk factors at ages 70 and 80. The

Table 11-8
Connections Between Glucose Tolerance (Three Classes) and CHD and Possible CHD Risk Factors at Ages 70 and 80

	Age 70		Age 80	
	Men	*Women*	*Men*	*Women*
Systolic blood pressure	†	†		
Diastolic blood pressure				
Cholesterol				
Triglycerides	†	†		*
Body mass index	‡	‡		†
Smoking (three classes)			*	*
Antihypertensive/diuretic treatment	*	†		*
CHD				
Cardiac/thoracic ratio (at age 70)		‡		
Intermittent claudication				
Distal pulse abnormality				
Maximal distal muscle flow (at age 70)	I*	I†		
Delay time (at age 70)				
Distal blood pressure ratio (at age 80)				

Significant connection: * $P < 0.05$, †$P < 0.01$, ‡$P < 0.001$.
I = Inverse connection.
For definitions, see study design.

Table 11-9
Connections Between Smoking (Three Classes) and CHD and Possible CHD Risk Factors at Ages 70 and 80

	Age 70		Age 80	
	Men	*Women*	*Men*	*Women*
Systolic blood pressure	I*			*
Diastolic blood pressure				
Cholesterol		*		
Triglycerides				
Glucose tolerance (three classes)			*	*
Body mass index	I‡	I†	I*	
Antihypertensive/diuretic treatment				
CHD				
Cardiac/thoracic ratio (at age 70)				
Intermittent claudication	‡		*	
Distal pulse abnormality				
Maximal distal muscle flow (at age 70)				
Delay time (at age 70)	†			
Distal blood pressure ratio (at age 80)				

Significant connection: *$P < 0.05$, †$P < 0.01$, ‡$P < 0.001$.
I = Inverse connection.
For definitions, see study design.

connections to decreased distal perfusion and the inverse relation to body mass index in men are striking.

In the following decade excess total mortality was seen in male cigarette, cheroot, and heavy smokers compared to the other men. In women, but not in men, excess mortality was connected to inhalation. In bivariate, statistical analyses neither heavy smoking nor inhalation at age 70 were connected to excess CHD mortality or hospitalization in the eighth decade, the excess mortality being caused by malignant neoplasms (WHO diagnosis groups 140–239) as well as by nonmalignant pulmonary diseases (WHO diagnosis groups 460–519).

The lower percentage of those who never smoked in the surviving 80-year-olds compared to the 70-year-olds is explained by the excess mortality in the total male group compared to the total female group. Two thirds of the participants remained in their smoking group (in the table marked by dashes); one fourth reported a decreased consumption at the end of the decade; and less than one tenth reported increased consumption. In the re-examined population at age 80, the presence of CHD was not connected to smoking at age 70.

In this cohort nine tenths of the men and a little more than half of the women at age 70 had been smokers. Most of the male smokers had started smoking as young men before World War I, whereas most of the female smokers had started considerably later, between the two world wars. The proportion of cigar/pipe/cheroot smokers in the present population was larger than that found in most countries, and is consistent with the national habit.

Excess mortality in middle-aged smokers is known from several prospective studies.[41–43] The present findings show that even at age 70 smoking is of importance for excess total mortality within the next 10-year period, and with regard to excess CHD mortality and total CHD manifestations. However, no correlations were found in the bivariate analyses.

High values of resting heart rate and plasma uric acid have been included as possible risk factors for CHD.[2] In the present study the values of uric acid were significantly correlated to triglyceride values in both sexes at ages 70 and 80. Neither uric acid nor heart rate, however, were connected to CHD or other CHD risk factors at ages 70 or 80, nor were higher values of these two parameters at age 70 connected to excess CHD mortality or excess total CHD manifestations in the eighth decade.

A MULTIVARIATE MODEL ANALYZING THE DIRECT/INDIRECT PREDICTIVE VALUE OF 70-YEAR CHARACTERISTICS

In order to evaluate which characteristics at age 70 had individual or direct predictive value with regard to total mortality, CHD mortality, and CHD manifestations in the eighth decade, and which characteristics were of indirect predictive value because of their connection to other characteristics, Cox's regression model for competing risks[44] was applied with the three variables mentioned as dependent variables and the following 70-year characteristics as independent variables: cholesterol, cholesterol squared, triglycerides, glucose tolerance, CHD, systolic blood pressure, diastolic blood pressure, body mass index, and heavy smoking (Table 11-10).

It is seen that in men diabetes mellitus, impaired glucose tolerance, heavy smoking, and the presence of CHD were of individual predictive value for *excess total mortality*, whereas in women only diabetes mellitus had such individual predictive value. In men high levels of triglycerides, diabetes mellitus, impaired glucose tolerance, heavy smoking, and the presence of CHD had predictive value for *excess CHD mortality*, whereas in women high levels of systolic blood pressure and presence of CHD were of individual predictive value. Concerning *excess total CHD manifestations*, high levels of triglycerides, diabetes mellitus, and the presence of CHD in men, and high levels of systolic blood pressure, diabetes mellitus, and the presence of CHD in women were of individual predictive value.

These results are not far from those obtained in the Framingham longitudinal study of 50- to 82-year-old men and women when the age groups were pooled (written communication from W.R. Hazzard, MD).

From the present study it is seen that four of the CHD risk factors established in younger and middle-aged populations (high levels of systolic blood pressure, diabetes mellitus, and in men high levels of triglycerides and heavy smoking) still apply at age 70, and a well-defined area for possible CHD intervention thus exists.

ACKNOWLEDGMENTS

This study was supported by grants from the Danish Health Insurance Foundation, the Danish Medical Research Foundation and the Danish Heart Foundation.

Table 11-10
Cox Regression Model for Competing Risks at Age 70 for Total Mortality and CHD Events in the Eighth Decade

	Dependent Variables					
	Men			*Women*		
	Total Mortality	CHD Mortality	CHD Manifestations	Total Mortality	CHD Mortality	CHD Manifestations
Independent variables						
Systolic blood pressure (mmHg)	–	–	–	–	1.02*	1.02*
Diastolic blood pressure (mmHg)	–	–	–	–	–	–
Cholesterol (mmol/L)	–	–	–	–	–	–
Triglycerides (mmol/L)	1.23	1.92†	1.69†	–	–	–
Diabetes/normal glucose tolerance	2.44†	3.86‡	3.86‡	3.25‡	–	2.98*
Impaired/normal glucose tolerance	1.70*	2.80	1.80	1.09	–	1.82
Body mass index kg/m²	1.76	–	–	–	–	–
Heavy smoking +/–	2.95‡	2.82*	–	–	–	–
CHD +/–	2.06	2.66‡	2.94‡	–	4.05*	3.03*

With intensity ratios between classes of units of measurement.
Statistically significant individual predictive value: $*P < 0.05$, $\dagger P < 0.01$, $\ddagger P < 0.001$.
– = Not meeting criterion of inclusion in the model (ie, $P > 0.020$).

REFERENCES

1. Dawber TR, Kannel WB, Lyell LP: An approach to longitudinal studies in a community: The Framingham study. *Ann NY Acad Sci* 1963;107:539–556.
2. Stamler J: *Lectures on Preventive Cardiology*. New York, Grune & Stratton Inc, 1967.
3. Agner E, Damm P, Hansen PF, et al: Causes of hospitalization in different age intervals. *Dan Med Bull* 1982;29:140–144.
4. Agner E, Agner T, Damm P, et al: Hospitalization and medical diagnoses in an aged population. *Dan Med Bull* 1982;29:145–147.
5. Agner E: Natural history of angina pectoris, possible previous myocardial infarction and intermittent claudication during the eighth decade. *Acta Med Scand* 1981;210:271–276.
6. Lassen NA, Lindbjerg I, Munck O: Measurement of bloodflow through skeletal muscle by intramuscular injection of Xenon-133. *Lancet* 1964;1:686–689.
7. Lindbjerg IF: Xenon-133 in the study of peripheral circulation in obliterative arterial disease, thesis. Munksgaard, Copenhagen, 1969, pp 1–18.
8. Grafnetter D, Fodor J, Tepley V, et al: The effect of storage on levels of cholesterol in serum measured by a simple, direct method. *Clin Chim Acta* 1967;16:33–37.
9. Laurell S: A method for routine determination of plasma triglycerides. *Scand J Clin Lab Invest* 1966; 18:668–672.
10. WHO: Manual of the international statistical classification of diseases, injuries and causes of death. Geneva 1967.
11. Kostner GM: Enzymatic determination of cholesterol in high density lipoprotein fractions prepared by polyanion. *Clin Chem* 1976;22:695.
12. Reid DD: Studies of disease among migrants and native populations in Great Britain, Norway and the United States III. Prevalence of cardiorespiratory symptoms among migrants and native-born in the United States. *Natl Cancer Inst Monogr* 1969;19: 321–346.
13. Reid DD, Holland WW, Humerfeldt S, et al: A cardiovascular survey of British postal workers. *Lancet* 1966;1:614–618.
14. Kannel WB, Feinleib M: Natural history of angina pectoris in the Framingham study. *Am J Cardiol* 1972;29:154–163.
15. Medalie JH, Snyder M, Groen JJ, et al: Angina pectoris among 10,000 men. *Am Heart J* 1973;55: 583–594.
16. Werkö L: Risk factors and coronary heart disease—Facts or fancy? *Am Heart J* 1976;91:87–98.
17. Miall WE, Lowell HG: Relation between change of blood pressure and age. *Br Med J* 1967;2:660–664.
18. Berglund G, Andersson O, Wilhelmsen L: Prevalence of primary and secondary hypertension: Studies in a random population sample. *Br Med J* 1976;2:554–556.
19. National Health Survey. Blood pressure of persons 18–74 years. United States 1971–1972. National Center for Health Statistical Series 11, no 150. US Dept of Health, Education and Welfare, 1975.
20. Hypertension Detection and Follow-up Program Cooperative Group. Blood pressures from 14 communities. A two-stage screen for hypertension. *JAMA* 1977;237:2385–2391.
21. Smoking and Health: A report of the Surgeon General. US Department of Health, Education and Welfare 1979;4/57.
22. Rose G, Hamilton PJS, Keen H, et al: Myocardial ischemia, risk factors and death from coronary heart disease. *Lancet* 1977;1:105–109.

23. Wilhelmsen L, Wedel H, Tibblin G: Multivariate analysis of risk factors for coronary heart disease. *Circulation* 1973;48:950–958.
24. Menotti A, Capocaccia R, Conti S, et al: Identifying subsets of major risk factors in multivariate estimation of coronary risk. *J Chronic Dis* 1977;30: 557–565.
25. Chapman JM, Coulson AH, Clark VA, et al: The differential effect of serum cholesterol, blood pressure and weight on the incidence of myocardial infarction and angina pectoris. *J Chronic Dis* 1971;23:631–645.
26. Kannel WB, Castelli WP, Gordon T, et al: Serum cholesterol, lipoproteins and risk of coronary heart disease. The Framingham Study. *Ann Intern Med* 1971;74:1–12.
27. Carlson LA, Böttiger LE: Ischemic heart disease in relation to fasting values of plasma triglycerides and cholesterol. Stockholm Prospective Study. *Lancet* 1972;1:865–868.
28. Wilhelmsen L, Wedel H, Tibblin G: Multivariate analysis of risk factors for coronary heart disease. *Circulation* 1973;48:950–958.
29. Kagan A, McGee DL, Yano K, et al: Serum cholesterol and mortality in a Japanese-American population. *Am J Epidemiol* 1981;114:11–20.
30. Lannerstad O, Isacsson S, Lindell S: Risk factors for premature death in men 56–60 years old. *Scand J Soc Med* 1979;7:41–47.
31. Schroll M, Grunnet K, Hansen PF: Fasting serum cholesterol and triglyceride values in a ten-year prospective study of the 1914-population in Glostrup, 1964–1974. *Dan Med Bull* 1981;28:251–259.
32. Kark JD, Smith AH, Hames CG: The relationship of serum cholesterol to the incidence of cancer in Evans County, Georgia. *J Chronic Dis* 1980;33: 311–322.
33. Oliver MJ: Serum cholesterol – The knave of hearts and the joker. *Lancet* 1981;2:1090–1095.
34. International Collaborative Group. Circulating cholesterol level and risk of death from cancer in men aged 40 to 69 years. *JAMA* 1982;248:2853–2859.
35. Davidson MB: The effect of aging on carbohydrate metabolism. A review of the English literature and a practical approach to the diagnosis of diabetes mellitus in the elderly. *Metabolism* 1979;28:688–705.
36. Editorial: Impaired glucose tolerance and diabetes – WHO criteria. *Br Med J* 1980;281:1512–1513.
37. Kannel WB, McGee DL: Diabetes and cardiovascular disease. *JAMA* 1979;241:2035–2038.
38. Birmingham Diabetes Survey Working Party. Ten-year follow-up report on Birmingham diabetes survey of 1961. *Br Med J* 1976;2:35–37.
39. Keen H, Jarrett RJ, Alberti KGMM: Diabetes mellitus: A new look at diagnostic criteria. *Diabetologia* 1979;16:283–285.
40. National Diabetes Data Group. Classification and diagnosis of diabetes mellitus and other categories of glucose intolerance. *Diabetes* 1979;28:1039–1057.
41. Report of the Royal College of Physicians: *Smoking and Health Now*. Pitman Medical & Scientific Publishing Co, London 1971.
42. Friedmann GD, Dales LD, Ury HK: Mortality in middleaged smokers and nonsmokers. *N Engl J Med* 1979;300:213–215.
43. Goldbourt U, Medalie JH: Characteristics of smokers, nonsmokers and exsmokers among 10,000 adult males in Israel. *Am J Epidemiol* 1977;105:75–82.
44. Cox DR: Regression models and life tables. *J R Statist Soc* 1972;334:187–220.

CHAPTER 12
Measurement of the Ejection Fraction in the Elderly

F. I. Caird

The ejection fraction is defined as:

(end-diastolic volume − end-systolic volume)/end-diastolic volume × 100, or, in the absence of valvular regurgitation; stroke volume/end-diastolic volume × 100.

It will be noted that all four cardiac chambers have an ejection fraction, although those of the atria are rarely considered. The ejection fraction is recognized as a valuable estimate of ventricular performance,[1,2] and change in it is a reliable, early, and direct indicator of myocardial damage or malfunction.

It may be measured in man by one of four technics. Angiocardiographic[3] and thermodilution[4] methods both require cardiac catheterization and are thus invasive, and so not appropriate to the elderly. The geometrical problems in particular that beset the measurement of the ejection fraction by echocardiography[5] result in so many inaccuracies that the measurements made are of doubtful value.[6]

The fourth technic is by radionuclide injection and external counting. This method has been considerably exploited.[7] It is appropriate to the elderly, although technically invasive. A more serious objection is the cost and cumbersome nature of the equipment used. There are two main variants, the first-pass method in which external counting is carried out during the first passage of the isotope through the heart and lungs, and the equilibrium method in which counts from numerous cardiac cycles, aligned by their constant relationship to the R wave of the ECG, are averaged to give an ejection fraction from the difference between systolic and diastolic volumes. Both of these methods have been used in the elderly, and this chapter will discuss the difficulties and inaccuracies of each and outline the results which have been obtained.

First-pass methods may be either of a simple type using a single scintillation counter, eclipse collimation, and two injections,[8,9] or one of the more complex methods using a gamma camera. In both methods in the elderly the injection of radioisotope, commonly technetium pyrophosphate or technetium-labeled human serum albumin, is given rapidly into a peripheral vein.[10] In younger patients more proximal injection can be given by catheter, but there is evidence that the site of injection does not greatly affect the absolute results of the method.[11]

The eclipse-collimated single scintillation counter method is easy to use, and can be applied to comparatively ill patients. It may be combined with estimation of the cardiac output and pulmonary blood volume if two separate venipunctures are carried out, the first for injection and the second for blood sampling. The method is probably not accurate enough to estimate the ejection fraction in single beats, where this varies from beat to beat. The principal disadvantages of the method are that it can only measure the left ventricular ejection fraction, that it is impracticable if the ejection fraction is less than perhaps 20%,[8,9] and that it is uninterpretable in perhaps one patient in five. A study of the inaccuracies in the method[10] shows that approximately half are due to incorrect positioning of the counter in patients whose hearts are not greatly enlarged and whose apex beat is impalpable, to breath-holding by the patient during the injection (this can be avoided by instructing the patient to take deep breaths during the injection), by slow injection, as mentioned above by a low cardiac output, and also by dispersal of the injection bolus by tricuspid incompetence. The value of this method has been demonstrated in the elderly, and the various inaccuracies are easy to recognize and can be correctly assigned.[10]

First-pass methods using the gamma camera are of greater value. Since on anatomical grounds the image of the right ventricle will be very variable and cannot be totally distinguished from that of the left,[11] resolution of the right ventricular ejection fraction is only possible in respect of time. This can only be achieved by first-pass gamma camera methods, from which the right ventricular ejection fraction can be estimated.[11,12] Both the right and the left ventricular ejection fractions of single beats can be determined if an ECG and some method of time marking are employed, and the cardiac output, etc is also calculable if a second venipuncture is carried out. Left ventricular ejection fractions can be calculated down to values of 5% or so. The inaccuracies mentioned above, which result from breath-holding, slow injection, and tricuspid incompetence, remain, together with others resulting from drawing by hand of the outlines of the ventricular cavities. In particular it is difficult to be sure in some cases that the right ventricle has been distinguished clearly from the right atrium, and similarly the left ventricle from the left atrium. Nevertheless the accuracy of the method is adequate, even for the assessment of single beats[12] (Figure 12-1). The method is usable after the patient has exercised, but not during exercise.

Equilibrium methods may be considerably less troublesome to the patient than first-pass methods. He requires only to lie still for some five minutes or so; the radionuclide injection can be given up to several hours previously. Because of the anatomical superimposition of the right over the left ventricle in ap projections and the left atrium over the left ventricle on left lateral and oblique projections, there are difficulties in measuring the right ventricular ejection fraction, although this has been attempted. By definition the ejection fraction cannot be measured during single beats. Only one injection is necessary, but the cardiac output is not calculable. It can be used to measure the response to exercise or rapidly acting drugs.

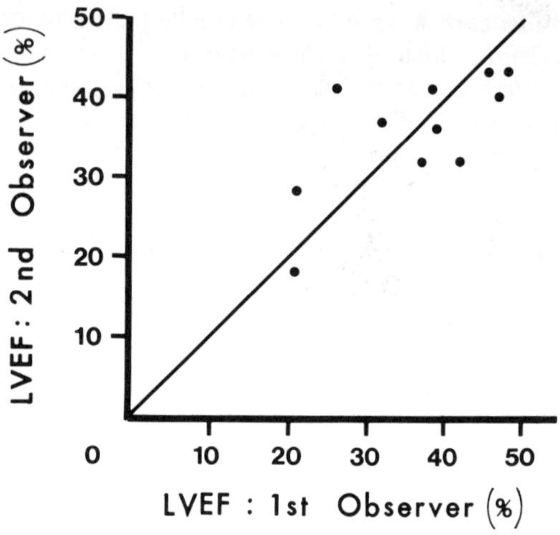

Figure 12-1 Observer variation in left ventricular ejection fraction in 11 single beats in an elderly patient with atrial fibrillation (first-pass gamma camera method). (From Williams and Caird, unpublished.)

RESULTS

Relatively few investigations of the ejection fraction in elderly patients have been reported. It appears that there is no reduction in resting left ventricular ejection fraction in old age despite the reduction in stroke volume. Its normal value by eclipse-collimation methods is around 70%.[10] However, it has been reported[13] that the left ventricular ejection fraction remains unchanged at rest as age advances, but falls with the tachycardia of exercise; it normally rises.[14,15] There is, however, some doubt about the normality of some of the elderly subjects studied. Substantial reductions in ejection fraction in the elderly occur in left ventricular hypertrophy and diseases of the left ventricle,[10] and in relation to heart rate in atrial fibrillation. Rapid heart rates are associated with a decline in ejection fraction rather than a rise, and it may also fall with very slow rates.[16] Changes in anemia are variable.[17]

Even fewer measurements of the right ventricular ejection fraction have been reported, but it generally has a lower mean value of 50% to 60%.[11] Reduction in the right ventricular ejection fraction in inferior myocardial infarction can be inferred from the finding of normal left ventricular ejection fractions in some patients with inferior myocardial infarction and congestive heart failure, and has been directly and convincingly demonstrated.[18] It is probably also reduced in some cases at least of right bundle-branch block (Caird, unpublished observation).

Perhaps one of the most important uses of measurement of the ejection fraction in the elderly is in the validation of truly noninvasive and simple methods such as systolic time intervals[10,19,20] and impedance cardiography.[21,22] Work in the elderly along these lines is actively proceeding (Figures 12-2 through 12-5) and may be expected to show the value and limitations of these noninvasive methods, which are in principle particularly suitable for application in the elderly. Guidelines for their future use in clinical and research situations will thus be given.

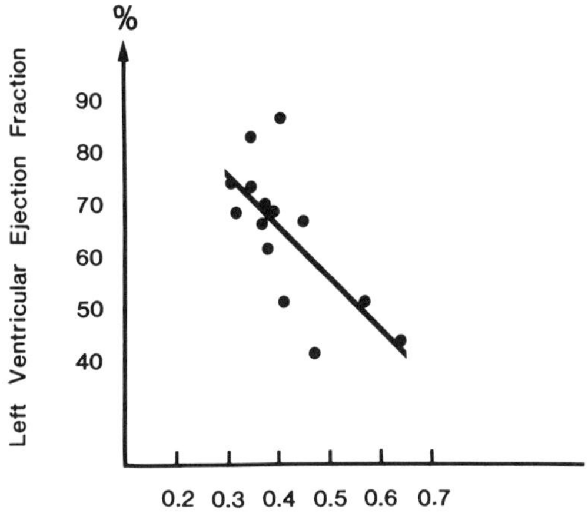

Figure 12-2 Relationship of PEP/LVET (pre-ejection period/left ventricular ejection time) to left ventricular ejection fraction in 14 elderly patients with sinus rhythm (first-pass single scintillation counter method). (From Williams, unpublished.)

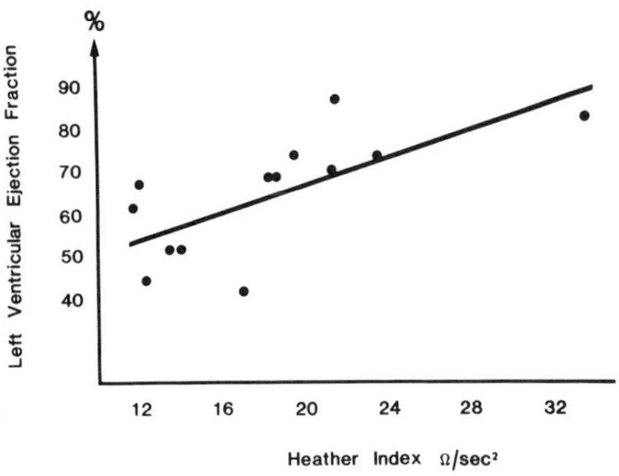

Figure 12-3 Relationship of Heather index[22] of the impedance cardiograph to left ventricular fraction in 14 elderly patients with sinus rhythm (first-pass single scintillation method). (From Williams, unpublished.)

ACKNOWLEDGMENTS

It is a pleasure to acknowledge the close collaboration of Dr. B.O. Williams in much of the work of the department, and for many fruitful discussions.

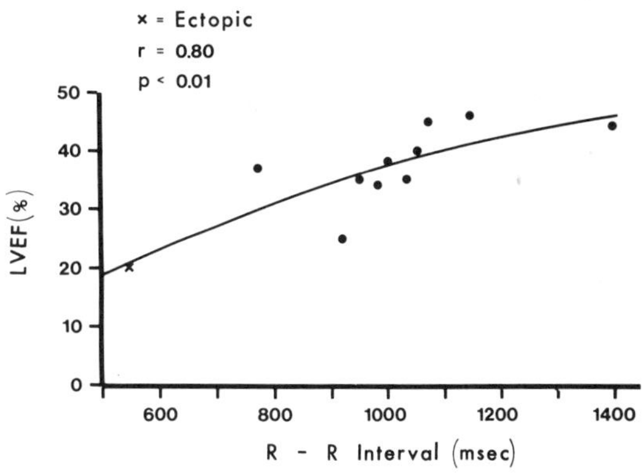

Figure 12-4 Relationship between preceding R-R interval and left ventricular ejection fraction in single beats from an elderly patient with atrial fibrillation (first-pass gamma camera method). (From Williams and Caird, unpublished.)

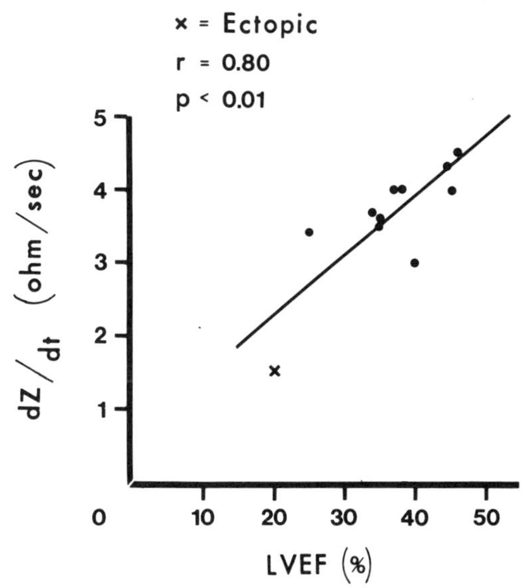

Figure 12-5 Relationship between dZ/dt on impedance cardiogram and left ventricular ejection fraction in single beats from an elderly patient with atrial fibrillation (first-pass gamma camera method). (From Williams and Caird, unpublished.)

REFERENCES

1. Dodge HT, Sandler H, Baxley WA, et al: Usefulness and limitations of radiographic methods for determining left ventricular volume. *Am J Cardiol* 1966; 18:10–24.
2. Dodge HT, Baxley WA: Hemodynamic aspects of heart failure. *Am J Cardiol* 1968;22:24–34.
3. Kennedy JW, Baxley WA, Figley MM, et al: Quantitative angiocardiography: I. The normal left ventricle in man. *Circulation* 1966;34:272–278.
4. Bartle SH, Sanmarco ME: Comparison of angiocardiographic and thermal washout techniques for left ventricle volume measurements. *Am J Cardiol* 1966;18:235–252.
5. Pombo JF, Troyl BL, Russell RO: Left ventricular volumes and ejection fraction by echocardiography. *Circulation* 1971;43:480–490.
6. Folland ED: Assessment of left ventricular function, in Parisi AF, Tow DE (eds): *Noninvasive Approaches to Cardiovascular Diagnosis.* New York, Appleton-Century-Crofts, 1979, p 51.
7. Strauss HW, Pitt B: Evaluation of cardiac function and structure with radioactive tracer techniques. *Circulation* 1978;57:645–654.
8. Steele PP, Van Dyke D, Trow RS, et al: Simple and safe bedside method for serial measurement of left ventricular ejection fraction, cardiac output, and pulmonary blood volume. *Br Heart J* 1974;36:122–131.
9. Berndt T, Alderman EL, Wasnich R, et al: Evaluation of radionuclide method for measurement of left ventricular ejection fraction and cardiac output. *J Nucl Med* 1975;16:289–292.
10. Latour J, De La Fuente R, Caird FI: Measurement of ejection fraction in the elderly. *Age Ageing* 1980;9:157–164.
11. Steele P, Kirch D, LeFree M, et al: Measurement of right and left ventricular ejection fractions by radionuclide angiography in coronary artery disease. *Chest* 1976;70:51–56.
12. Berger HJ, Matthay RA, Loke J, et al: Assessment of cardiac performance by quantitative radionuclide angiocardiography: Right and left ventricular ejection fraction with reference to findings in chronic obstructive pulmonary disease. *Am J Cardiol* 1976;41:897–905.
13. Port S, Cobb FR, Coleman LE, et al: Effect of age on the response of the left ventricular ejection fraction to exercise. *N Engl J Med* 1980;303:1133–1137.
14. Slutsky R, Karliner J, Ricci D, et al: Response of left ventricular volume to exercise in man assessed by radionuclide equilibrium angiocardiography. *Circulation* 1979;60:565–571.
15. Dewhurst NG, Hannan WJ, Muir AL: Prognostic value of radionuclide ventriculography after myocardial infarction. *Q J Med* 1980;49:479–490.
16. Caird FI, Williams BO: Left ventricular performance in atrial fibrillation in the elderly. *Age Ageing* 1981;10:231–236.
17. Caird FI: The effect of age upon the cardiovascular response to anaemia: II. Radionuclide studies in the elderly. *J Clin Exper Gerontol* 1982;4:193–203.
18. Tobinick E, Schelbert HR, Henning H, et al: Right ventricular ejection fraction in patients with acute anterior and inferior myocardial infarction assessed by radionuclide angiography. *Circulation* 1978;57: 1078–1084.
19. Garrard CL, Weissler AM, Dodge HT: The relationship of alterations in systolic time intervals to ejection fraction in patients with cardiac disease. *Circulation* 1970;42:455–462.
20. Sutton R, Hood WP, Koch GG: Noninvasive assessment of left ventricular function in chronic heart disease. *Am Heart J* 1977;93:289–297.
21. Williams BO, Caird FI: Impedance cardiography and cardiac output in the elderly. *Age Ageing* 1980; 9:47–52.
22. Heather LW: A comparison of cardiac output values by the impedance cardiograph and dye dilution techniques in cardiac patients, in Kubicek WG, et al, (eds): *Development and Evaluation of an Impedance Cardiographic System.* NASA Report 1969 NAS-9-4500, p 247.

CHAPTER 13
Exercise Physiology, Testing, and Training in the Geriatric Population

Emmanuel C. Vasilomanolakis
James R. Licht
Myrvin H. Ellestad

With advancing age there is gradual reduction in physical strength and the ability to sustain strenuous physical exercise.[1,2] The factors responsible include the aging effects on the heart and vascular system, and diminishing ability of peripheral tissues to extract circulating oxygen.[1] The net outcome is usually a reduction in hemodynamic capacity by the cardiovascular system resulting in less efficiency and a more sedentary life style.

Expansion of medical knowledge and improvement in socioeconomic conditions have contributed to increasing survival and life expectancy in the United States.[3] The number of persons reaching age 65 and the length of survival past this age are increasing progressively. People are also maintaining a better state of well-being into advanced years and are desiring means to maintain improved fitness. Advanced years also results in an increasing prevalence of cardiovascular diseases. The need for maintaining physical fitness and for diagnosing cardiovascular disease in this unique age group has added urgency to a better understanding of exercise testing. In this communication, current knowledge of changes in exercise physiology with aging will be reviewed.

EXERCISE PHYSIOLOGY

The physiologic requirements for the performance of work involve a coupling of accelerated cardiovascular and respiratory activity to achieve gas (O_2 and CO_2) transport between muscle cells, blood, and the surrounding atmosphere.[4] The capacity to provide oxygen to the body tissues serves as the major limiting factor determining the level of physical activity an individual can perform. Indices employed to quantitate this ability to perform work are many and most notably include: $\dot{V}O_2$ (oxygen uptake), HR (heart rate), SBP (systolic blood pressure), HR × BP (pressure-pulse product), efficiency index, anaerobic threshold, and METs (metabolic equivalents). Each of these variables has a role in assessing fitness, degree of exertion, and status of the cardiovascular system. Each will be reviewed with special attention on its relation with aging.

Oxygen Uptake

$\dot{V}O_2$ is considered to be a critical measure of functional capacity. It correlates well with degree of physical conditioning, being an accepted index of total body fitness. It is readily measured by breath analyzer technics and is a reproducible value when corrected for body weight. $\dot{V}O_{2max}$ (maximal $\dot{V}O_2$) physiologically represents the highest rate of oxygen transport and utilization attainable in an individual. It can best be understood by a rearrangement of the Fick equation:

$$\dot{V}O_2 = HR \times SV \times \text{A-V } O_2 \text{ difference}$$

where $\dot{V}O_2$ = oxygen uptake (L/min); HR = heart rate (bpm); SV = stroke volume (ml/beat); and A-V O_2 difference = arteriovenous oxygen difference (ml/dl blood). $\dot{V}O_{2max}$ would thus represent the maximal oxygen uptake which could be achieved.

The major determinants affecting the $\dot{V}O_{2max}$, ie, the capacity of the organism to take up oxygen, are the pumping capacity of the heart, the adequacy of the vascular system, and the strength and endurance of the muscle groups exercised. Of note, the oxygen demand of the working muscles is directly related to their mass and metabolic efficiency. Therefore, exercise involving a larger mass of muscle is likely to be associated with a higher oxygen uptake.

As exercise progresses the $\dot{V}O_2$ will increase many-fold in the healthy person with a lesser increase in the person with coronary artery disease. This reduction in oxygen transport capacity in the cardiac patient is due to the decreased ability to increase cardiac output (HR × SV) and is also proportional to the degree of deconditioning in these people. The diminished cardiac output results from a decreased contractile force of the left ventricle secondary to local myocardial ischemia or scarring, limiting the ability of stroke volume to increase with exercise. In addition, there is decreased coronary perfusion associated with a shorter diastolic interval with exercise-induced tachycardia.

As age progresses, the reduction in $\dot{V}O_{2max}$, serves as an index of the functional limits of the cardiovascular system. Thus, it provides a frame of reference for estimation of the functional aerobic age of individuals. Persons with higher than average $\dot{V}O_{2max}$ for their chronologic age are functionally equivalent to younger individuals, those with below average $\dot{V}O_{2max}$ are functionally older.[5]

In healthy persons, the following variations in $\dot{V}O_{2max}$ are seen:

1. $\dot{V}O_{2max}$ is highest in adolescence and declines with age in adults[5] (Figure 13-1).
2. $\dot{V}O_{2max}$ is proportional to the amount of skeletal muscle, which helps explain the difference noted between sexes.[5]
3. $\dot{V}O_{2max}$ varies directly with habitual physical activity states[5] (Figure 13-2).

In a cross-sectional sample of men of different ages, the age-predicted $\dot{V}O_{2max} = 56.59 - 0.398 \times$ (years of age) ml/kg/min. For men of 40 to 69 years of age, $\dot{V}O_{2max} = 52.74 - 0.362 \times$ (years of age) ml/kg/min.[5] Furthermore, a longitudinal study following the same men revealed a difference in $\dot{V}O_{2max}$ in relation to activity status (−0.65 for active versus −1.32 ml/kg/min/year for sedentary men).[5,6]

That $\dot{V}O_{2max}$ usually decreases with age raises the question as to whether this is solely an age-related phenomenon or is due to other factors associated with older age. DeVries and Wessel and

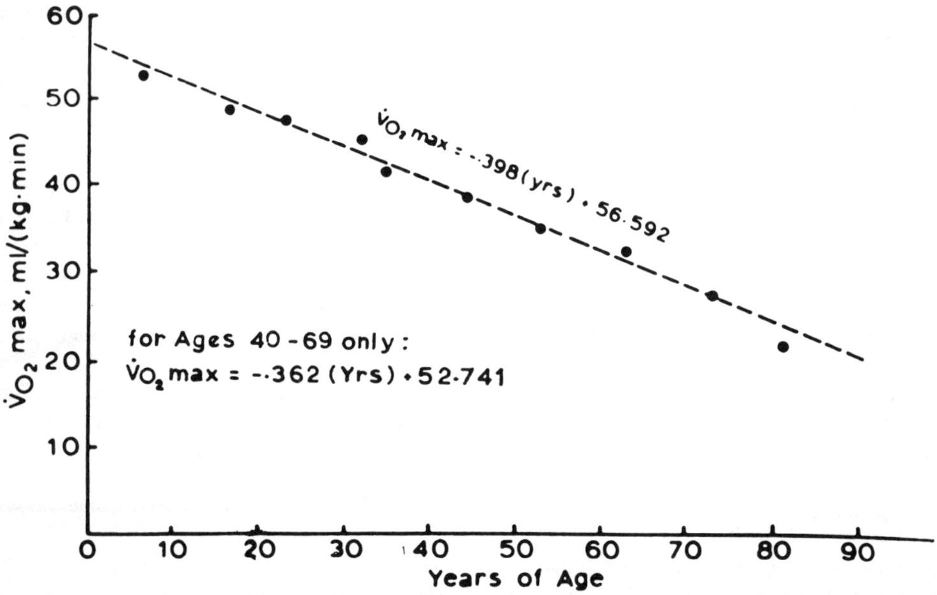

Figure 13-1 Regression of mean VO_{2max} per decade of age for 700 observations in healthy boys and men, recalculated from 17 studies in the literature. (Reproduced with permission from Dehn and Bruce.[5])

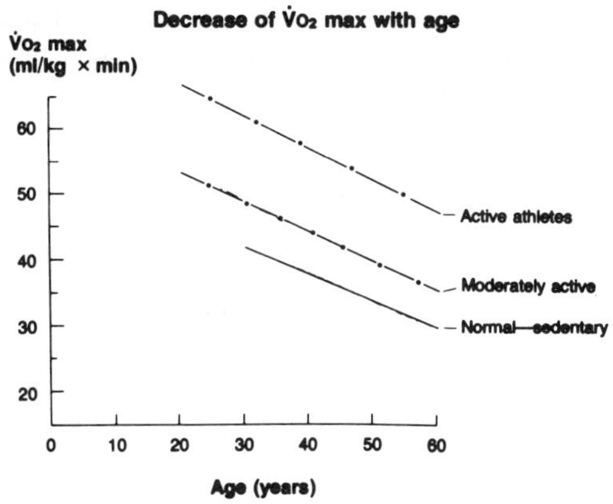

Figure 13-2 The relations of VO_{2max} with activity level and age. (Reproduced with permission from Furlow B, Oberman A, Eggert D: A step-by-step guide to exercise for the CAD patient. *Geriatrics* 1980;35(9):41–47.)

Van Huss[7,8] showed that age-related losses in physiologic variables were more highly related to the decreased habitual activity level than to age itself. For example, many aging-like changes in cardiovascular physiology can be brought about in young well-conditioned men in as little as three weeks by simply enforcing bed rest. In three weeks of bed rest maximal cardiac output diminished by 26%, oxygen consumption by 30%, and even the amount of active tissue declined by 1.5%.[9] It is not even necessary to remain at bed rest for that long in order to feel debilitated. Lamb demonstrated that healthy, active young men subjected to 10 days of chair rest exhibited substantially diminished work capacity and symptoms of dizziness, fainting, and circulatory collapse.[10] Thus, inactivity can produce losses in function similar to those brought about more slowly in the average individual as he or she grows more sedentary as they get older.

In summary, $\dot{V}O_{2max}$ serves as an index of physical fitness and is age-related. However, the age relation is not only that of an effect on cardiovascular tissue but is also due to the tendency for decreased activity and physical conditioning level of the aging person. With the help of periodic exercise, fitness and a higher $\dot{V}O_{2max}$ can be maintained into advanced years.

Heart Rate

Heart rate is the result of a number of physical and emotional influences which are mediated through the autonomic nervous system. Both the vagal and sympathetic nerves are constantly stimulating the sino-atrial node with alternating influences producing the increases and decreases seen in heart rate. Resting heart rate changes little with age with some suggestion of a decrease in older age groups.[11] However, maximum heart rate has an apparent age-related ceiling, decreasing with advancing age in a linear fashion (Figure 13-3). This can roughly be determined by the formula:

$$HR_{max} = 220 - age$$

where HR_{max} refers to the maximum heart rate (bpm) attainable at a certain age. For each age there is a wide variability in resting heart rate; however, the maximum heart rate is fairly predictable.

Resting heart rate is influenced by many factors, including training state. In the well-conditioned subject, the pumping capacity of the heart may be 25% more efficient resulting in a slower heart rate for any given level of exercise. This decrease in heart rate is due to increases in stroke volume and vagal tone and decrease in circulating catecholamines.[1,12]

With exercise, the sinus rate increases progressively with each increase in workload, providing the principal mechanism utilized in the augmentation of cardiac output. As maximal aerobic capacity is approached, heart rate reaches a plateau just as oxygen consumption does.

There may be two kinds of abnormal heart-rate responses to exercise. First, the heart rate incremental rise for any given level of work is lower than normal and heart rate plateau is below the average. This may be the result of a reduction in catecholamines or the presence of excessive vagal tone. Second, the heart rate may be very high at low levels of work. Physical deconditioning, marginal circulatory compensation, or low stroke volume are usually the causes here. Both of these

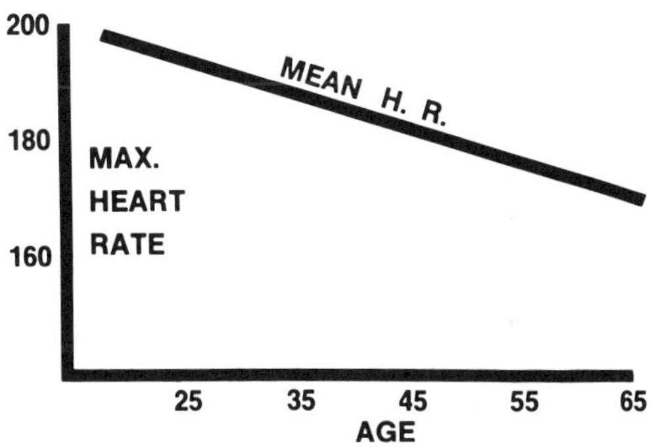

Figure 13-3 The maximum predicted heart rate is linearly related to age. (Reproduced with permission from Ellestad.[24])

abnormal heart rate responses are more common in the elderly person as are the underlying causes mentioned above.

Blood Pressure

Blood pressure is the force developed by the heart against peripheral vascular resistance. It is mediated by many factors and tends to increase with age[13] (Figure 13-4).

The normal blood pressure response to exercise is a progressive rise in systolic pressure with little change in diastolic pressure (±10 mmHg in normals). The total systemic vascular resistance falls with exercise in order to provide an increased flow associated with the increased metabolic demand of the working muscles. However, this fall is usually insufficient to prevent a rise in the blood pressure. Using most exercise testing protocols, systolic blood pressure rises about 8 to 10 mmHg per stage. A pathologic fall in blood pressure, though occasionally encountered early in exercise, is felt to be highly specific for severe left ventricular dysfunction, often due to advanced coronary artery disease.

Older persons demonstrate a greater rise in blood pressure during exercise than do the young.[14,15] This is largely due to increased peripheral resistance and rigidity of arterial vessels.[13,16] The systolic pressure load on the left ventricle during exercise is consequently greater in older persons,[14,15] which may explain some of the inconsistencies seen with exercise responses in the elderly.

Pressure-Pulse Product

The pressure-pulse product is the systolic blood pressure multiplied by the heart rate. This is also known as the double product. The pressure-pulse product rises progressively with exercise and its peak value serves to characterize the normal cardiovascular performance and maximum myocardial oxygen consumption. Normal values (expressed in mmHg × bpm) are in the range of 20,000 to 30,000 and those with coronary disease usually have values less than 25,000. Considerable overlap between people with and without coronary disease is the rule, however. Diagnostically the pressure pulse product is more useful for the comparison of different conditions in the same patient than in comparing one person to another. It may be used in multivariate interpretation, enhancing the test accuracy.

In the older population, blood pressure and heart rate are usually higher at any given workload than in younger subjects. Thus, the product (HR × BP) is often substantially higher, resulting in the older person expending greater energy for a given workload and thus attaining maximum myocardial oxygen capacity earlier.

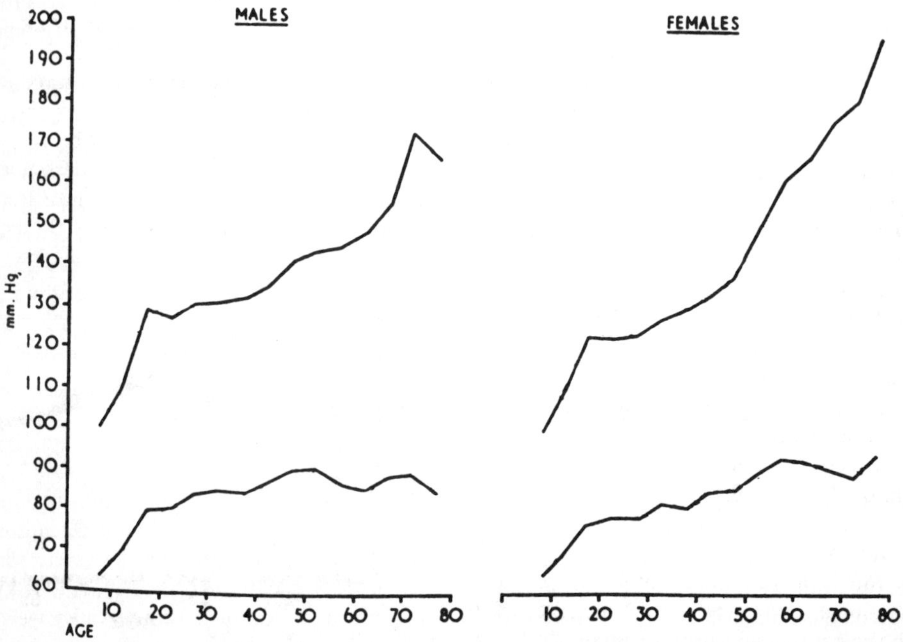

Figure 13-4 Mean resting systolic and diastolic pressures at different ages. (Reproduced with permission from Miall WE and Lovell HG: Relation between change of blood pressure and age. *Br Med J* 1967;2:660–664.)

Efficiency Index

The relationship between a given amount of cardiac work and the quantity of oxygen consumed by the myocardium in order to accomplish this work is an indication of the efficiency of the heart.[17] This can be expressed as:

$$\text{efficiency index} = \frac{\text{external body work}}{\text{myocardial oxygen consumption}} = \frac{\dot{V}O_2}{HR \times SBP}$$

where $\dot{V}O_2$ represents external body work (ie, total body oxygen consumption), and $HR \times SBP$ (pressure-pulse product) serves as an index of myocardial oxygen consumption.

Myocardial efficiency serves as an index of cardiac status and physical fitness. The ratio is lower with deconditioning and with age.[17] Furthermore, the presence of and degree of coronary artery disease also correlates with a lower ratio. Exercise training is associated with an improvement in this index.[17]

Anaerobic Threshold

A noninvasive method of assessing anaerobic threshold involves determining the respiratory gas exchange ratio.[18] In the basal state there is a fairly constant relation of CO_2 produced to O_2 consumed, termed the respiratory quotient (R). With increasing exercise, as the anaerobic threshold is reached CO_2 production increases above that of O_2 consumed. This results from additional CO_2 released when bicarbonate buffers the acids formed from anaerobic metabolism. This is manifested as a rise in the respiratory quotient. The workload at which this rise occurs serves as an index of the conditioning level of the individual.

A second method of determining when anaerobic metabolism has begun is from blood lactate analysis. This requires venipuncture technic. Again by correlating the rise in lactate level with the workload at which this occurs helps determine the fitness state of an individual.

Both with respiratory quotient and blood lactate testing, the fit subject will begin to show rises in these indices (ie, anaerobic threshold) at higher work levels than the deconditioned subject.[19] With age, as with deconditioning, the subject begins anaerobic metabolism at a lower workload level than the younger subject. Similarly, at equivalent work levels the degree of anaerobic metabolism (eg, R, lactic acid production) is greater in the older subject.[19] These effects again are related to the relative inactivity level of the older person but are also influenced by diminished cardiovascular and respiratory reserve associated with age.

Of note, failure of lactic acid or respiratory quotient to rise suggests that the patient has not been stressed beyond his aerobic capacity and this may be due to orthopedic, cardiac, or psychologic problems.

METs

Effective work, or metabolic rate, has been arbitrarily expressed in METs or metabolic equivalents. One MET unit represents the energy requirement at complete rest. It is defined as 3.5 ml O_2 consumed/kg body weight/min.[20] Any steady-state activity may be described in terms of an equivalent number of METs.

Energy expenditure (kcal/hr) is approximated by multiplying METs by kilograms of body weight. Some examples of MET equivalents for various activities[21] are summarized in Table 13-1.

Cardiac Output

Cardiac output, or blood flow per unit time, decreases steadily with age. During exercise the rate of increase in cardiac output with increasing workload is essentially the same in old as in young.[22] However, the mean cardiac output at any workload remains less in elderly groups than in young ones, with an average difference of 1.3 L/min.[13]

In summary, the results of exercise physiologic and hemodynamic testing suggest that the reduced capacity of the elderly to undertake strenuous physical exercise is only partly due to cardiac or pulmonary changes and loss of muscle strength.[1] A second, and preventable cause of these effects is deconditioning, which is more prevalent in older ages. Deconditioning may be produced in healthy young persons by inactivity, as conditioning can be induced in older persons by exercise.

EXERCISE TESTING

Exercise testing remains the principal noninvasive examination of cardiovascular status and disease. There is controversy, however, whether such a stress in older persons is unduly risky and should be avoided. Such a conservative viewpoint fails to recognize that as in all medical testing, patients must be evaluated as individuals and not as members of arbitrary age groups. There is no evidence that age alone increases risk of stress

Table 13-1
Average Work Requirements of Common Activities

MET Range	Prescribed Activity	Recreational Activity	kcal/hr (75 kg)
2–4	Walking at 2–3 mph Cycling (ergometer) at 150–300 kpm Swimming, using float board*	Strolling Light stretching exercise Bicycling at 6 mph*	225
5–6	Walking-jogging at 4 mph Cycling (ergometer) at 450–600 kpm Swimming, treading water	Light calisthenics Golf Bicycling at 8 mph	412
7–8	Walking-jogging at 5 mph Cycling (ergometer) at 750–900 kpm Swimming, doing crawl at 40 yd/min	Noncompetitive tennis, badminton Hiking Bicycling at 11–12 mph	562
9–10	Jogging-running at 5.5–6 mph Cycling (ergometer) at 1050 kpm Swimming, doing crawl at 40 yd/min	Vigorous calisthenics Rope skipping Cross-country skiing Bicycling at 13 mph	712
11–12	Jogging-running at 7 mph Cycling (ergometer) at 1200–1350 kpm Swimming, doing crawl at 50 yd/min	Team sports, eg, basketball, soccer handball	862
13–14	Running at 8 mph Cycling (ergometer) at 1500–1650 kpm	Vigorous team sports Cross-country skiing Vigorous rope skipping	1012
15–16	Running at 10 mph Cycling (ergometer) at 1800 kpm	Sustained performance at level of highly trained athlete	1162

Adapted from Bruce et al.[43]
kpm = kilopond-meter.
*The metabolic cost of swimming and cycling may vary considerably owing to technic, body weight and resistance.

testing. However, special attention is often indicated in older patients undergoing exercise evaluation.

Mode of Exercise

The exercise test may consist of various forms of exercise. Isotonic or rhythmic-type exercises include the use of Master's "2-step" exercise test, the bicycle ergometer, and the treatmill. Isometric exercise such as handgrip is not usually employed for noninvasive stress evaluation although it is sometimes helpful in hemodynamic evaluation in the catheterization laboratory. Bicycle ergometry and treadmill exercise have replaced the 2-step test in most laboratories. By requiring use of a larger muscle mass the treadmill necessitates a larger energy expenditure and thus stresses the cardiovascular system somewhat more than bicycle ergometry. Ergometry on the other hand has the benefit of allowing either leg or arm exercise, the latter one especially, when situations preclude use of the lower extremities.

Exercise testing serves a number of purposes. These include chest pain evaluation, functional capacity evaluation, arrhythmia production and detection, and assessment of therapy. Before beginning the exercise the physician should formulate the questions being asked from the test and should likewise consider what adverse effects may occur from the exercise. A list of indications and contraindications to exercise testing[11] are found in Tables 13-2 and 13-3.

Awareness of the problems peculiar to the elderly during exercise testing is critical. These include early appearance of fatigue and lightheadedness due to muscle weakness and deconditioning. Vasoregulatory insufficiency and a tendency to unsteadiness of gait may occur and require physical or emotional support. Pulmonary insufficiency may also limit performance. These factors will limit the degree of exercise a person can perform. In Table 13-4 are listed reasons for terminating exercise testing.

Protocols

Geriatric patients commonly have difficulty with balance, joint stiffness, and other orthopedic problems which limit their adaptability to perform in standard treadmill protocols. Performance may also be limited by fear and anxiety. Occasionally physical capacity may actually be less than the stress imposed by the first stage or two of many standard testing protocols, although this has been rare even in 70- and 80-year-olds. If this is suspected a protocol may be used that begins at a lower workload and increases more gradually, such as those used for postinfarction testing. Protocols requiring longer exercise at each level may exhaust the patient before his/her maximum cardiovascular capacity is reached. Therefore, attenuation of the time at each workload is often advisable.

The specific protocol employed is not important. If the older patient is without orthopedic handicap and is capable of walking briskly, then maximal exercise protocols such as the Bruce[23] or the Ellestad[24] may be used. If there is some question as to the ability to walk at a brisk pace, then other protocols can be substituted. Such protocols require less initial energy expenditure and increase the workload more gradually. Representative protocols include the Chung protocol,[25] which begins at a level grade (0%), and the Patterson protocol[26] (Table 13-5), which in addition to level grade

Table 13-2
Indications for Stress Testing

1. Evaluation of patient with symptoms suggestive of coronary artery disease
2. Determination of patient's physical work capacity and aerobic capacity
3. Evaluation of functional limitations in patients with valvular or peripheral vascular disease
4. Determination of patient's physical limitations postinfarction and as an aid in the design of a rehabilitation exercise program
5. Evaluation of the post-bypass patient to aid in the rehabilitation exercise program and to detect residual ischemia
6. Evaluation of the asymptomatic patient over age 40 with risk factors for coronary disease
7. Evaluation of arrhythmias
8. Evaluation of therapeutic drug regimens for arrhythmias, angina, or ischemia
9. To stimulate patients to conform to risk-factor modification

Table 13-3
Contraindications to Stress Testing

1. Symptomatology suggestive of unstable angina
2. Rapid atrial arrhythmias
3. Advanced atrioventricular block (second or third degree)
4. Uncompensated congestive heart failure
5. Acute noncardiac illnesses (eg, hyperthyroidism, infection, pulmonary disease)
6. Acute myocardial infarction (However, many centers are routinely subjecting patients to a submaximal 70% symptom-limited test prior to discharge.)
7. Acute myocarditis or pericarditis
8. Aortic stenosis (relative contraindication)
9. Known left main coronary artery disease (relative contraindication)

Table 13-4
Termination of Stress Testing

1. Development of ventricular premature contractions (PVCs) in pairs or with increasing frequency, or of ventricular tachycardia (runs of three or more PVCs)
2. Occurrence of atrial tachycardia or atrial fibrillation
3. Onset of heart block, either second or third degree
4. Progressive anginal pain (grade three pain, if grade four is the most severe in patient's experience)
5. Severe ST segment depression, ie, 6 to 7 mm or more in vigorous asymptomatic subjects
6. ST depression in patient with documented severe coronary disease or angina at low workloads
7. Inability of patient to continue because of dyspnea, fatigue, or feelings of faintness
8. Severe musculoskeletal pain, as might occur with arthritis or claudication
9. Vasoconstricted, ie, pale and clammy, appearance of patient
10. Extreme elevations in systolic and diastolic blood pressure associated with headache or blurred vision
11. Predicted maximum pulse rate reached or exceeded
12. Progressive fall of heart rate or systolic blood pressure with continuing exercise

Table 13-5
Patterson Protocol

Stage	Time (min)	Speed (mph)	Grade (%)	METs
1	0–2	1.0	0	2
2	2–4	1.5	0	3
3	4–6	2.0	0	3
4	6–8	2.0	3.5	3–4
5	8–10	2.0	7	4–5
6	10–12	3.0	5	5
7	12–14	3.0	7.5	6–7
8	14–16	3.0	10	7–8
9	16–18	3.0	12.5	8–9
10	18–20	3.0	15	9–10

Data from Patterson et al.[26]

begins at only 1.0 mph. The latter protocol is one which most ambulatory patients can accomplish without difficulty. A protocol allowing flexibility of speed and slope is that of Naughton.[27] Specifically for the older age groups Schwimmer[28] has modified other standard treadmill protocols. Thus, by carefully selecting the treadmill protocol to match the patient's estimated capability, many apparently disabled patients can undergo meaningful exercise testing. It is important to appreciate that deviation from standard protocols is permissible when the primary goal is to detect an ischemic ECG response. When work capacity is being measured, a structured protocol is preferred.

For patients with fear of or unsteadiness on walking, and for those with musculoskeletal problems precluding sustained unsupported walking, a bicycle ergometer may provide an effective alternative. Allowing the patient to sit down for weight support, to hold onto handlebars for balance, and to be able to terminate the test at will makes bicycle ergometry well tolerated. For unusual circumstances such as severe orthopedic, neurologic, peripheral vascular disease, or leg amputation, the bicycle ergometer can be adapted to cranking with the arms. This may only be possible when patients have retained considerable strength in their arms. Nonetheless, even in handicapped patients exercise can be employed for detection of an ischemic ECG response and as a measurement of cardiorespiratory fitness. A representative protocol for bicycle ergometry is that developed by Fox et al[29] (Table 13-6).

Exercise Parameters

The exercise test is a multivariate test where symptomatic, ECG, and physiologic variables can be monitored. The monitoring of these multiple parameters enhance the accuracy of the exercise test in addition to providing more information about the subject. However, economic, spatial, and time restraints do not make it practical to monitor all parameters in the clinical setting (eg, oxygen uptake, lactate analysis). Instead, certain basic information is sought and decisions are made in combination with the pretest clinical data.

The basic parameters an exercise test should examine include symptoms, duration and degree of exercise, heart rate and blood pressure response, arrhythmias, and ST segment changes. Other ECG features such as R wave[30] and Q wave,[31,32] size and QT interval[33–35] can also be examined readily.

Symptoms Anginal chest pain during exercise testing has been shown to be predictive of the presence and severity of coronary artery disease, as well as risk for subsequent coronary events. Anginal chest pain without ischemic ECG changes is nearly as predictive of multivessel coronary disease as the ischemic ECG is alone. Furthermore, the presence of angina pectoris enhances the predictive significance of the ST segment. When both chest pain and ischemic ECG changes are noted, the incidence of coronary disease has been shown to be between 85% to 93%.[36,37] Together, they carry twice the incidence of coronary events than does ST segment depression alone.[36] When dealing with a young patient (41 to 50 years old) the presence of chest pain alone may carry a threefold increased risk of coronary events compared to older patients.[36] This leads us to the conclusion that exercise-induced chest pain may be a less ominous sign in older people. Whether this is due to better coronary collateral formation or a slower progression of arteriosclerosis remains to be determined.

Table 13-6
Fox Bicycle Ergometer Protocol

Stage	Time (min)	Workload* *kg-m/min*	Workload* *watts*	METs (for 70 kg person†)
1	0–3	150	25	2–3
2	3–6	300	50	4
3	6–9	450	75	5
4	9–12	600	100	6
5	12–15	750	125	7
6	15–18	900	150	8–9
7	18–21	1050	175	10
8	21–24	1200	200	11

Data from Fox et al.[29]
*Pedaling at approximately 50 rpm.
†For a person of greater weight, the METs achieved are proportionately lower; for a person of lesser weight, the METs achieved are proportionately greater.

Exercise capacity As discussed previously, exercise is dependent on age, fitness, and cardiovascular status. The amount of exercise is dependent on both the duration and degree of stress imposed. It is felt that a short duration of exercise tolerance (less than three minutes) suggests either advanced coronary disease or high risk for a cardiac event. Exercise duration is inversely related to the likelihood of coronary artery disease. In the presence of coronary artery disease, longer duration implies a better prognosis. Elderly patients are less able to undergo sustained physical stress due to physiologic constraints of maximal oxygen consumption, as noted. Similarly, coronary disease patients may display angina pectoris or ECG signs of ischemia before they reach their threshold maximum. Although both age and coronary disease impair exercise performance at maximal exercise, the coronary disease patient will often demonstrate impairment at submaximal levels.

In the elderly patient exercise duration is often dependent on the protocol used. Even the first stage of standard protocols in the sedentary elderly patient may produce maximal stress and consequently the patient will exercise little. This should not necessarily imply a poor cardiac prognosis, especially if the patient is able to attain a near maximal predicted heart rate. Thus in the elderly, maximal stress can be obtained at low workloads, and the associated poor prognosis of short exercise duration is not necessarily applicable to these persons.

Heart rate The physiologic changes of heart rate with age have been discussed previously. There appears to be a correlation between achieved heart rate during stress testing and presence or absence of coronary disease. A high risk of sudden cardiac death, coronary events, impaired left ventricular function, and presence of coronary disease have been shown by different investigators to be associated with a failure of heart rate to rise appropriately with exercise (chronotropic incompetence).[38,39] This has been quantitated as either a heart rate below 95% limits for any given workload for age and sex or the failure of heart rate to rise above 120 bpm.[39,40] The ability to increase heart rate above 160 bpm is associated with a low risk for future coronary events.[39]

Older persons have an age-related decrease in maximal heart rate. They increase their heart rate faster and at lower workload levels than do younger persons. However, maximum heart rate recorded in many tests of the elderly may approach only 75% to 85% of the maximum predicted heart rate.[28,41] This is partly because older patients—for psychologic and physical reasons—will not push themselves as much as younger people. In addition, many physicians are reluctant to overexert an older person. For these reasons, achieved heart rate as a variable in evaluating the presence and severity of coronary artery disease loses its specificity in the older population.

Blood pressure To reiterate what was discussed previously, systolic blood pressure increases with age and its rate of rise is also greater with exercise in older persons. The development of abnormally high systolic blood pressure during exercise (ie, >200 mmHg) indicates well-preserved left ventricular function.[42] When such patients are followed for the development of angina, myocardial infarction, or death, their prognosis is more favorable when there is development of a hypertensive response to exercise.[42,43]

It is felt that exertional hypotension manifested at low workloads portends a grave prognosis and is usually associated with severe left ventricular dysfunction.[11,44] This dysfunction is usually ischemic in origin but in geriatric patients a higher incidence of cardiomyopathies, stenotic valvular lesions, and exercise-induced arrhythmias may account for the hypotension.[42] Failure of systolic blood pressure to rise appropriately is also prognostically significant with regards to cardiac events.[43] This applies when systolic blood pressure fails to rise above 140 mmHg, when it fails to increase on the average of 8 to 10 mmHg per stage of standard maximal exercise protocol, or when the rise in systolic pressure is less than 10% above resting levels.[42,43] This finding applies to patients of all ages.

Arrhythmias Exercise-induced ventricular arrhythmias occur in from 35% to 50% of normal middle-aged men.[44,45] This incidence increases with age and with increased stress on exercise testing.[44] Exercise-induced ventricular arrhythmias occur in from 38% to 65% of coronary disease patients with complex forms in 30%.[46] In general, coronary patients manifest arrhythmias at a lower heart rate and are somewhat more reproducible than those seen in clinically normal subjects. By itself, exercise-induced ventricular arrhythmias are not predictive of future cardiac events, even in patients with chronic coronary artery disease.[47] In the presence of ischemic ST-segment depression they are predictive of significant multivessel disease, impaired left ventricular function, and carry a two- to threefold risk of death over a 5-year period.[48,49]

With age, the incidence of ventricular arrhythmias is increased both at rest and with exercise.[45,50]

No study has addressed their predictive value with exercise in the geriatric group. It is presumed to carry the same risks as it does in the younger populations examined.

ST segment Electrocardiographic evidence of ischemia is classically represented by ST segment depression. ST segments are influenced by many factors and may be characterized as upsloping, flat, and downsloping. These carry somewhat different predictive values for evidence of coronary artery disease. There is general agreement that an increased magnitude of ST segment depression denotes more severe ischemia and extent of coronary disease.[38,51,52] In addition, greater ST segment depression also suggests a correlation with location of disease, in particular left main and proximal left anterior descending disease.[38,48,53] Finally, the magnitude of ST segment depression affects the predictive value of the stress test. Thus, a 2-mm ST segment depression versus 1-mm ST segment depression is less sensitive (more false negatives) but more specific (fewer false positives) for coronary disease.

Time of onset of ST segment depression is important. When occurring within 3 minutes of exercise, ST segment depression is associated with more severe coronary artery disease.[11] This includes left main, left anterior descending, and triple vessel coronary artery disease.[54] In addition, from a prognostic standpoint there is an increased incidence of future cardiac events.[41] This incidence has been shown to be 15% per year compared to 8% and 4% in those whose ST segment depression did not develop until 5 and 7 minutes, respectively.[41]

Persistence of ST segment depression also correlates with severity of coronary artery disease. In one study, ST segment depression lasting more than 8 minutes into the recovery period was associated with two- or three-vessel disease in 90% of patients.[54]

ST segment configuration during exercise is important in predicting both presence and severity of coronary disease. One study found that downsloping ST segments were highly specific for the presence of significant coronary disease (1% false positives) compared to a 15% false-positive rate with horizontal ST segments and 32% with slowly upsloping patterns.[54] Likewise, downsloping was associated with higher mortality and more severe coronary artery disease, and persons with a left main lesion were most likely to exhibit this response.[54]

Controversy exists over upsloping ST segments. It is generally agreed that J-point depression with a rapidly upsloping ST segment is a normal phenomenon. Given slowly upsloping ST segments the magnitude of ST depression becomes critical. Presence of ST segment depression of at least 1 mm at 80 ms after the J point suggests a higher incidence of coronary disease.[55] When ST depression is 2 mm or more it is similar in predictive value for coronary disease and mortality to horizontal ST segment depression. However, this remains controversial and probably should be considered abnormal awaiting further interpretation of clinical data.

What is the significance of ST segment depression in the older population? The limited number of studies concerning geriatric exercise testing reveal a greater incidence of ST segment depression at rest and with exercise in normal older persons than in younger persons.[56-60]

Estimates of the incidence of ST segment depression with exercise in normal elderly volunteers has been reported to be as high as 67%,[52] although most studies place this between 10% and 37%.[57-62] These studies have employed use of normal volunteers. In a review of coronary angiography[63] at Memorial Hospital Medical Center of Long Beach, Calif, we found 22 patients over age 65 with normal coronary arteries, who had treadmill stress tests performed prior to angiography. Sixteen of the 22 developed at least 1-mm ST segment depression with exercise, giving a false-positive response of 74%. This may partly reflect a hospital-based population with its increased incidence of diseases affecting ventricular compliance and electrocardiographic repolarization. This suggests that ST segment depression in older populations may have less specificity than in younger populations.

Attempts to explain these findings have been made. Riley et al[57] point out that anxiety, or vasoregulatory asthenia causing ST segment depression may be more prevalent in older people. Alternatively, this may reflect a high workload per unit mass of myocardium in the elderly.[60]

On the other hand, Lester et al[61] argue that the observed ST segment depression in normal older persons is a transient and not a "true" ST segment depression. In their group of normal male volunteers (aged 40 to 75 years) they noted that ST segment depression occurred either during maximal exercise or terminated within 30 seconds after the end of exercise. ST segment depression lasting greater than 30 seconds was seen in less than 1% of their population.

Abnormal ECGs at rest are more common in the elderly, particularly with presence of base-line

ST segment depression. Factors accounting for this include left ventricular hypertrophy, intraventricular conduction defects, and the effect of digitalis,[64] all of which are more prevalent in the geriatric age group. The ability to accurately evaluate exercise-induced ischemic ST response in those with resting ST segment depression is possible when persons with the above abnormalities are excluded. An exception to this, in the geriatric group, appears to be the effect of digitalis. It has been shown that exercise-induced ST segment changes during digitalis therapy maintained predictive accuracy in an elderly population whereas it was unreliable in detecting coronary disease in all other age groups.[65] Causes of false ischemic responses to exercise are listed in Table 13-7.

The predictive ability of exercise-induced ST segment depression in the elderly has been examined. Astrand[66] noted that the risk of developing coronary disease in 10 years was three times greater in these subjects as compared to elderly patients without ST segment depression.

In summary, ST segment depression, although still a sensitive (low false negative) test in detecting coronary artery disease, appears to lose its specificity in older persons. It becomes necessary to evaluate other parameters on the exercise ECG to compensate for the decreased specificity. We have found that checking for other abnormal responses, such as elevation of R wave height or diminution of Q wave depth at peak exercise, add to the true positivity of the test. A multivariate approach such as is used at Long Beach Memorial Hospital where variables such as ECG at rest, minutes exercised, achieved heart rate, presence of anginal pain, R wave changes, sex, age, and ST depression are weighted, improves predictive value. Thus, exercise testing in the elderly still remains a useful method for detecting coronary disease, although the number of false-positive responses based on ST-segment depression is increased.

Functional Evaluation

We have concentrated the discussion on exercise testing to identification of ischemia in the elderly. The geriatric population also affords unique experiences in evaluating other disease states, such as syncope, peripheral vascular disease, and valvular heart disease.

Cardiovascular etiologies of syncope in older persons include myocardial ischemia, valvular lesions (particularly aortic stenosis) and arrhythmias, which are relatively common etiologies of syncope in this age group. These entities can be evaluated by exercise testing.

The prevalence of sinus node disease (sick sinus syndrome) increases with advancing age. An important means of identifying this entity is exercise testing. If the sinus rate does not increase appropriately with increasing exertion, the diagnosis of sinus node disease should be entertained.

Evaluation of functional capacity is also an important part of the assessment of valvular heart disease, particularly regarding timing of surgery. A standardized multistage protocol is employed and measurement of workload or oxygen consumption is made. The diagnosis of subclinical aortic stenosis should be entertained in older persons when fatigue or failure of appropriate blood pressure rise with increasing effort occurs.[67]

EXERCISE PRESCRIPTION

Reduced physical activity and the accompanying reduction in mobility can become a serious problem for the older individual. A systematic physical activity program contributes to increased mobility, improved self-image and self-care capabilities, as well as better general health in persons of all ages.

Static stretching exercises and calisthenics can be used safely if done with slow cadences. Running-jogging exercises produce higher cardiovascular demands and, if undertaken, must be

Table 13-7
Causes of False ST-Segment Responses to Exercise

Causes of False Negatives	Causes of False Positives
1. Single-lead monitoring	1. Digitalis therapy
2. Single-vessel disease	2. Left ventricular hypertrophy
3. Postmyocardial infarction	3. Left intraventricular conduction defects
	4. Wolff-Parkinson-White conduction
	5. Mitral valve prolapse
	6. Hyperventilation
	7. ST abnormalities at rest

monitored carefully. The optimum frequency, intensity, and duration of exercise for older adults depends to a large degree on the individual.[68]

Exercise to 60% of the heart rate range (HRR), the difference between resting and maximal predicted HR, improves conditioning in older patients.[69] For a person at the age of 70 this probably represents a heart rate of 115 to 120 bpm. When dealing with chronically institutionalized geriatric patients an even less vigorous 50% of HRR has proved to be effective.[69]

As to the frequency and duration of exercise, it is known that in younger subjects the amount of improvement in maximal $\dot{V}O_2$ is minimal when exercise frequency is increased above three times per week.[42] For older persons, because of the tendency to exercise at lower intensity and for shorter durations, it is suggested that a frequency greater than three times per week be employed. The exercise period should be at least 20 to 30 minutes per session.

CONCLUSION

It appears that geriatric patients can undergo similar types of exercise evaluations as younger persons. Much of the difference in their response is due to diminished exercise capacity, which in turn is largely due to sedentary habits. Although ECG changes when present carry similar implications in the elderly, ST-segment depression is less specific in this age group. Finally, training effects of exercise are possible and may be obtained with periodic submaximal exertion.

REFERENCES

1. Julius S, Amery A, Whitlock LS, et al: Influence of age on the hemodynamic response to exercise. *Circulation* 1967;36:222–229.
2. Shock NW: Physiological aspects of aging. *J Am Diet Assoc* 1970;56:491–496.
3. Stamford BA: Effects of chronic institutionalization on the physical working capacity and trainability of geriatric men. *J Gerontol* 1973;28:441–446.
4. Wasserman K, Whipp BJ: Exercise physiology in health and disease. *Am Rev Respir Dis* 1975;112: 219–249.
5. Dehn M, Bruce RA: Longitudinal variations in maximal oxygen intake with age and activity. *J Appl Physiol* 1972;33:805–807.
6. McDonough JR, Kusumi F, Bruce RA: Variations in maximal oxygen intake with physical activity in middle-aged men. *Circulation* 1970;41:743–751.
7. DeVries HA: Physiology of exercise and aging, in Woodruff DS, Birren JE (eds): *Aging in Broad Perspective.* New York, Van Nostrand Reinhold Co, 1975, pp 253–276.
8. Wessel JA, Van Huss WD: The influence of physical activity and age on exercise adaptation of women aged 20–69 years. *J Sport Med* 1969;9:173–180.
9. Saltin B, Blomquist G, Mitchell JH, et al: Response to exercise after bed rest and after training: American Heart Association Monograph #23. New York, The American Heart Association, 1968.
10. Lamb LE, Johnson RL, Stevens PM: Cardiovascular conditioning during chair rest. *Aerosp Med* 1964;35:646–649.
11. Ellestad MH, Cooke BM, Greenberg PS: Stress testing: Clinical application and predictive capacity. *Prog Cardiovasc Dis* 1979;21(6):431–460.
12. Schroeder G: Circulatory adaptations at rest and during exercise in normal adults. *Acta Med Scand* 1968;495(suppl):1–120.
13. Kennedy RD, Caird FI: Physiology of aging of the heart, in Noble RJ and Rothbaum D (eds): *Geriatric Cardiology.* Philadelphia, FA Davis, 1981, pp 1–8.
14. Granath A, Jonsson B, Strandell T: Circulation in healthy old men, studied by right heart catheterization at rest and during exercise in supine and sitting position. *Acta Med Scand* 1964;176:425–446.
15. Granath A, Jonsson B, Strandell T: Studies on the central circulation at rest and during exercise in the supine and sitting body position in old men. *Acta Med Scand* 1961;169:125–126.
16. Master AM, Dublin LI, Marks HH: Normal blood pressure range and its clinical implications. *JAMA* 1950;143:1464–1470.
17. Aptecar M, Vazquez A, Aptecar FRM: The assessment of myocardial efficiency by an exercise-testing index. *J Cardiac Rehab* 1982;2:271–279.
18. Wasserman K, McIlroy MB: Detecting the threshold of anaerobic metabolism in cardiac patients during exercise. *Am J Cardiol* 1964;14:844–852.
19. Montoye HJ: Age and oxygen utilization during submaximal treadmill exercise in males. *J Gerontol* 1982;37:396–402.
20. Hanson PG, Giese MD, Corliss RJ: Clinical guidelines for exercise training. *Postgrad Med* 1980; 67(1):120–138.
21. Bruce RA: Maximal exercise testing. *Postgrad Med* 1981;70(6):161–168.
22. Strandell T: Cardiac output in old age, in Caird FI, Dall JLC, Kennedy RE (eds): *Cardiology in Old Age.* New York, Plenum Press, 1976.
23. Bruce RA: Methods of exercise testing: Step test, bicycle, treadmill, isometrics, in Amsterdam EA, Wilmore JH, and DeMaria AN (eds): *Exercise in Cardiovascular Health and Disease.* New York, Yorke, 1977, pp 149–160.
24. Ellestad MH: *Stress Testing.* Philadelphia, FA Davis, 1980.
25. Chung EK: *Exercise Electrocardiography: Practical Approach.* Baltimore, Williams and Wilkins, 1979.
26. Patterson JA, Naughton J, Pietras RJ, et al: Treadmill exercise in assessment of the functional capacity of patients with cardiac disease. *Am J Cardiol* 1972;30:757–762.
27. Naughton J: Stress electrocardiography, in Rios JC (ed): *Clinical Electrocardiographic Correlations.* Philadelphia, FA Davis, 1977, p 127.
28. Schwimmer J: A new geriatric application of electrocardiographic treadmill testing in an office testing. *J Am Geriatr Soc* 1979;27(8):337–344.
29. Fox SM, Naughton JP, Haskell WL: Physical activity and the prevention of coronary heart disease. *Ann Clin Res* 1971;3:404–432.

30. Bonoris PE, Greenberg PS, Christison GW, et al: Evaluation of R wave changes vs ST segment depression in stress testing. *Circulation* 1978;57:904-910.
31. Morales-Ballejos M, Greenberg P, Ellestad MH, et al: The septal Q wave in exercise testing: Angiographic correlation. *Am J Cardiol* 1981;48:247-251.
32. Famularo MA, Paliwal Y, Redd R, et al: Identification of septal ischemia during exercise by Q wave analysis. *Am J Cardiol* 1983;51:440-443.
33. Yu PNG, Soffer A: Studies of electrocardiographic changes during exercise. *Circulation* 1952;6:183-192.
34. Greenberg PS, Frischa DA, Ellestad MH: Comparison of the predictive accuracy of ST depression, R wave amplitude, QX/QT and QT_c during stress testing. *Am J Cardiol* 1979;44:18-23.
35. Yu PNG, Bruce RA, Lovejoy FW, et al: Observation on changes of ventricular systole (QT interval) during exercise. *J Clin Invest* 1950;29:279-289.
36. Cole JP, Ellestad MH: Significance of chest pain during treadmill exercise: Correlation with coronary events. *Am J Cardiol* 1978;41:227-232.
37. Bartel AG, Behar VS, Peter VS, et al: Graded exercise stress test in angiographically-documented coronary artery disease. *Circulation* 1974;49:348-356.
38. Hinkle LE, Carver ST, Plakun A: Slow heart rates and increased risk of cardiac death in middle-aged men. *Arch Intern Med* 1972;129:732-748.
39. McNeer JF, Margol SJR, Lee KL, et al: The role of the exercise test in the evaluation of patients for ischemic heart disease. *Circulation* 1978;57:64-70.
40. Ellestad MH, Wan MKC: Predictive implications of stress testing. *Circulation* 1975;51:363-369.
41. Morse CE, Smith EL: Physical activity programming for the aged, in Smith EL, Serfass RC (eds): *Exercise and Aging*. Hillside, New Jersey, Enslow Publishers, 1981, pp 101-120.
42. Schrager BR, Ellestad MH: The importance of blood pressure measurement during exercise testing. *Cardiovasc Rev Rep* 1983;4(3):381-394.
43. Bruce RA, De Rouen T, Peterson DR, et al: Noninvasive predictors of sudden cardiac death in men with coronary heart disease. *Am J Cardiol* 1977;39:833-840.
44. McHenry PL, Fisch C, Jordan JW, et al: Cardiac arrhythmias observed during maximal treadmill exercise testing in clinically normal men. *Am J Cardiol* 1972;29:331-336.
45. Blackburn H, Taylor H, Hamrell B: Premature ventricular complexes induced by stress testing. Their frequency and response to physical conditioning. *Am J Cardiol* 1973;31:441-469.
46. Crawford M, O'Rourke RA, Ramakrishna N, et al: Comparative effectiveness of exercise testing and continuous monitoring for detecting arrhythmias in patients with previous myocardial infarction. *Circulation* 1974;50:301-305.
47. Vasilomanolakis EC, Kennedy HL: Ambulatory electrocardiography versus exercise testing. *Pract Cardiol* 1983;9(7):205-222.
48. Goldschlager N, Cake D, Cohn K: Exercise-induced ventricular arrhythmias in patients with coronary artery disease. *Am J Cardiol* 1973;31:434-440.
49. McHenry PL, Morris SN, Kavalier M, et al: Comparative study of exercise-induced ventricular arrhythmias in normal subjects and patients with documented coronary artery disease. *Am J Cardiol* 1976;37:609-616.
50. Hinkle LE, Carver ST, Argyros DC: The prognostic significance of ventricular premature contractions in healthy people and in people with coronary heart disease. *Acta Cardiol (Brux)* 1974;18(suppl):5-32.
51. Ellestad MH, Allen WH, Stuart RJ: Diagnostic and prognostic information derived from exercise testing. *Cardiovasc Clin* 1978;9(3):33-55.
52. Martin CM, McConahay DR: Maximal treadmill exercise electrocardiography: Correlations with coronary arteriography and cardiac hemodynamics. *Circulation* 1976;46:956-962.
53. Goldman S, Tselos S, Cohn K: Marked depth of ST-segment depression during treadmill exercise testing. Indicator of severe coronary artery disease. *Chest* 1976;69:729-733.
54. Goldschlager N, Selzer A, Cohn K: Treadmill stress tests as indicators of presence and severity of coronary artery disease. *Ann Intern Med* 1976;85:277-286.
55. Stuart RJ, Ellestad MH: Upsloping ST segments in exercise stress testing. *Am J Cardiol* 1976;37:19-22.
56. Nohara Y, Takeuchi T: Age change in circulatory adjustments to exercise in normal subjects, in Orimo H, Shimada K, Iriki M, et al (eds): *Recent Advances in Gerontology*. Amsterdam, Excerpta Medica, 1979, pp 651-654.
57. Riley CP, Oberman A, Lampton TD, et al: Submaximal exercise testing in a random sample of an elderly population. *Circulation* 1970;42:43-52.
58. Kavanagh T, Shephard RJ: The application of exercise testing to the elderly amputee. *Can Med Assoc J* 1973;108:314-317.
59. Kasser IS, Bruce RA: Comparative effects of aging and coronary heart disease on submaximal and maximal exercise. *Circulation* 1969;39:759-774.
60. Sidney KH, Shephard RJ: Training and electrocardiographic abnormalities in the elderly. *Br Heart J* 1977;39:1114-1120.
61. Lester FM, Sheffield LT, Reeves TJ: Electrocardiographic changes in clinically normal older men following near maximal and maximal exercise. *Circulation* 1967;36:5-14.
62. Doan EA, Peterson DR, Blackman JR, et al: Myocardial ischemia after maximal exercise in healthy men. *Am Heart J* 1965;69:11-21.
63. Vasilomanolakis EC, Damian A, Ellestad MH, et al: Treadmill stress testing in geriatric patients. *J Am Coll Cardiol* 1984;3(2)II:520.
64. Kansal S, Roitman D, Sheffield LT: Stress testing with ST-segment depression at rest. *Circulation* 1976;54:636-639.
65. Sketch MH, Mooss AN, Butler ML, et al: Digoxin-induced positive exercise tests: Their clinical and prognostic significance. *Am J Cardiol* 1981;48:655-659.
66. Astrand I: Prognostic value of exercise electrocardiogram in older men. *Scand J Clin Lab Invest* 1969;23(3):271-276.
67. DeVries HA: Exercise intensity threshold for improvement of cardiovascular-respiratory function in older men. *Geriatrics* 1971;26(4):94-101.
68. DeVries HA: Prescription of exercise for older men from telemetered exercise heart rate data. *Geriatrics* 1971;26(4):102-111.
69. Stamford BA: Physiological effects of training upon institutionalized geriatric men. *J Gerontol* 1972;27(4):451-455.

CHAPTER 14
Echocardiographic Evaluation of the Elderly

Julius M. Gardin

The ability to image cardiac structures and to evaluate left ventricular function noninvasively has made echocardiography extremely useful in the evaluation of individuals known to have or suspected of having heart disease. The noninvasive character of the technic has made it particularly applicable to an older population. The discussions in this chapter will focus on: (1) a basic description of M-mode and two-dimensional echocardiography; (2) changes in cardiac structure and function which have been documented to occur by M-mode echocardiography in normal subjects with aging; and (3) a description of a number of cardiac conditions which are common in an older population and in the evaluation of which echocardiography has been shown to have a role.

BASIC PRINCIPLES OF ECHOCARDIOGRAPHY

Echocardiography involves the application of reflected ultrasound, ie, sound waves of frequency above the normally audible range, to the evaluation of the heart. Pulsed ultrasound waves in the frequency range of 1.6 to 5 MHz are emitted from a transducer that also acts as a receiver for reflected waves. Since ultrasound is reflected at interfaces having different acoustic impedances, internal structures of the heart possessing different densities, such as myocardium, valves or cardiac chambers, can be readily imaged.

The two basic cardiac ultrasound imaging modalities in clinical use are M-mode and two-dimensional echocardiography. The M-mode (time-motion) technic utilizes a single beam of ultrasound which begins at the chest wall and traverses identifiable cardiac structures at various depths. The reflected ultrasound waves ("echoes") can be displayed on an oscilloscope or television monitor (1) in proportion to the depth and density of the tissues from which they are reflected (on the vertical axis), and (2) as a function of time (on the horizontal axis). Structures can then be identified by the intensity and motion of the reflected echoes as well as by the characteristic anatomical relationships of the various structures to each other. The transducer is usually placed in the second to fourth intercostal spaces to the left of the sternum, and a "sweep" is performed from the region of the ventricles to the interface of the left atrium and the aorta[1] (Figures 14-1 and 14-2). Additional views of the heart may be obtained from the apical, subxiphoid, and suprasternal positions.

Two-dimensional echocardiography is an attempt to provide a two-dimensional image rather than the single dimension (over time) afforded by the M-mode technic. Various methods have been developed to produce a continuous (real-time) display of cardiac function in up to a 90° arc (sector). The two most popular two-dimensional methods involve mechanical and electronic ("phased array") sector scanning. In mechanical sector scanning, one or a few ultrasound crystal(s) is (are) mechanically rotated directly on the chest wall or within a housing in contact with the chest wall. A simultaneous display of echoes from each position in a 30° to 90° arc is possible with this approach. In phased-array sector scanning, a small transducer with multiple crystals—eg, 32 individual elements—is held stationary on the chest while the ultrasound beam is steered back and forth electronically by controlling the sequence of firing of the individual elements. Imaging in an arc of up to 90° is also possible with this technic.

With both the mechanical and phased-array approaches, imaging in multiple views—including longitudinal, short-axis, apical, subxiphoid, and suprasternal—usually allows visualization of most areas of the heart and proximal great arteries (Figure 14-3). Both M-mode and two-dimensional echocardiography have the advantages of being painless, relatively rapid to perform—in general, requiring 15 to 45 minutes—and, unlike radiation exposure, without known biologic ill effects as used clinically in humans. Consequently, both technics can be utilized repetitively in a given

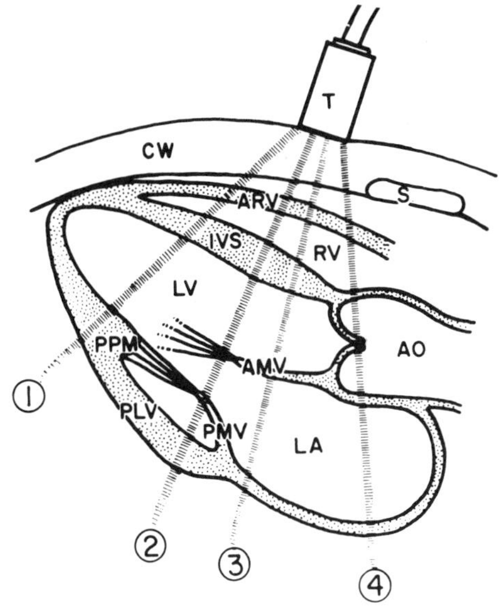

Figure 14-1A Diagrammatic representation of the heart in longitudinal section, depicting structures through which the ultrasound beam passes as it is directed from the apex toward the base of the heart. Numbers (1 through 4) refer to standard positions for recording the M-mode echocardiogram. CW = chest wall, T = transducer, S = sternum, ARV = anterior right ventricle, RV = right ventricular cavity, IVS = interventricular septum, LV = left ventricle, PPM = posterior papillary muscle, PLV = posterior left ventricular wall, AMV = anterior mitral valve leaflet, PMV = posterior mitral valve leaflet, AO = aorta, LA = left atrium.

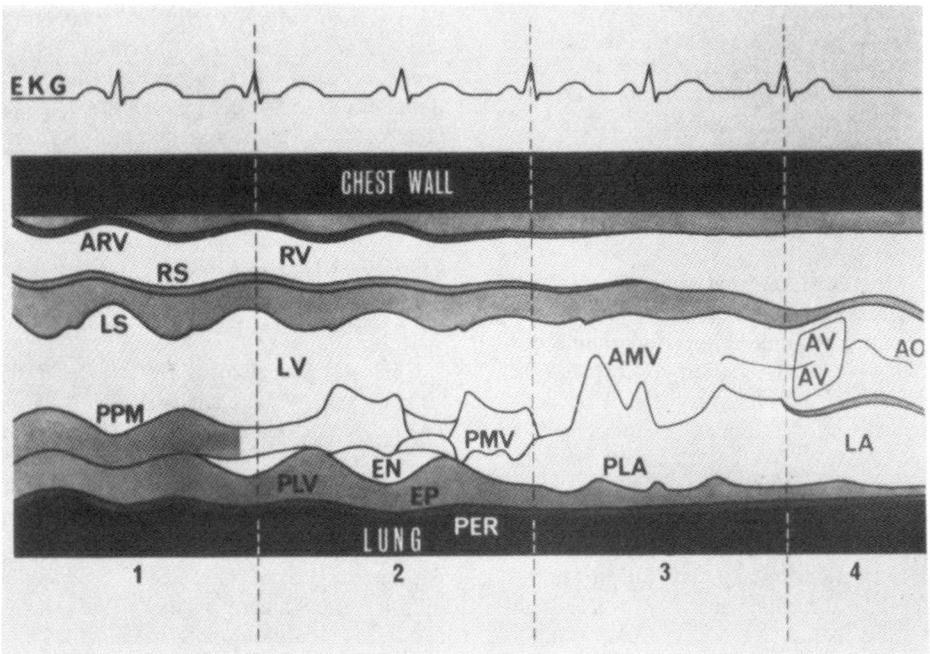

Figure 14-1B Diagrammatic representation of M-mode echocardiogram as transducer is directed from cardiac apex (position 1) to base (position 4). Areas between the dotted lines correspond to the transducer positions as depicted in Figure 1A. AV = aortic valve, EN = endocardium of left ventricle, LS = left septum, PER = pericardium, PLA = posterior left atrial wall, RS = right septum, other abbreviations as in Figure 1A. (Reproduced with permission from Feigenbaum H: Clinical applications of echocardiography. *Prog Cardiovasc Dis* 1972;14:531.)

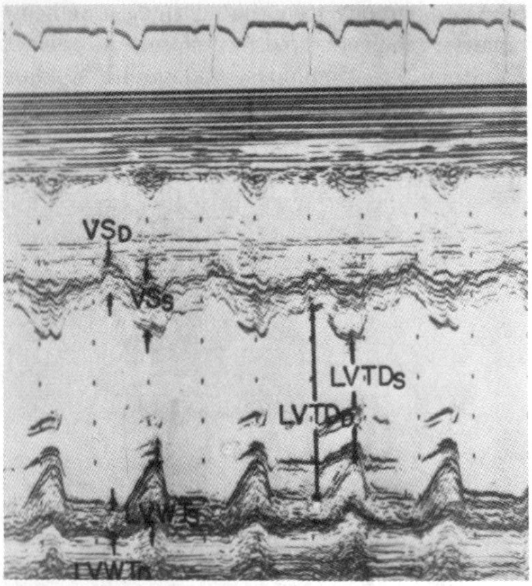

Figure 14-2 Echocardiographic recording of the left ventricle indicating measurements of parameters of left ventricular muscle mass. VS_D = interventricular septal thickness measured during diastole, VS_S = interventricular septal thickness measured during systole, PW_D = left ventricular posterior wall thickness measured during diastole, PW_S = left ventricular posterior wall thickness measured during systole, $LVTD_D$ = left ventricular transverse dimension measured during diastole, $LVTD_S$ = left ventricular transverse dimension measured during systole. (Reproduced with permission from Drayer J, Gardin JM, Weber MA, Aronow WS: Changes in cardiac anatomy and function during therapy with alpha-methyldopa: An echocardiographic study. *Curr Ther Res* 1982;32:856.)

patient for serial evaluation of cardiac anatomy and function.

In the absence of localized disorders of left ventricular function, eg, as may be seen in coronary artery disease, M-mode echocardiographic measurements have been reported to correlate well with left ventricular volume and ejection fraction measurements as determined angiographically.[1] Although ejection fraction does not perfectly characterize the functional state of the left ventricle, this measurement is accepted as providing an overall assessment of pump performance. Furthermore, ejection fraction is thought to be a more sensitive measurement of myocardial contractile state than are either cardiac output or left ventricular end-diastolic pressure. The left ventricular ejection fraction is defined as the ratio of ventricular stroke volume to end-diastolic volume. The approach to echocardiographic determination of left ventricular volumes, and ejection fraction, relies on the assumptions that (1) the left ventricle is a uniformly contracting prolate ellipsoid, and (2) the volume of the left ventricle in systole and diastole approximates the cube of its internal transverse dimension in systole and diastole, respectively. Left ventricular internal dimensions are measured from the left ventricular septal surface to the endocardium of the posterior left ventricular wall (Figure 14-2). Left ventricular ejection fraction, it follows, equals

$$\frac{(LVID_d)^3 - (LVID_s)^3}{(LVID_d)^3} \times 100\%$$

where $LVID_d$ and $LVID_s$ are the left ventricular internal dimensions in diastole and systole, respectively.[2] Left ventricular stroke volume can be obtained by multiplying the left ventricular ejection fraction by $(LVID_d)^3$ (left ventricular diastolic volume). Cardiac (ie, left ventricular) output can be derived by multiplying the stroke volume by the heart rate. In conditions which give rise to segmental abnormalities of left ventricular wall motion—eg, coronary artery disease—the above geometric assumptions regarding calculation of left ventricular volumes cannot be utilized. Consequently, in patients with coronary artery disease, two-dimensional echocardiography has been much more useful in evaluating left ventricular anatomy and function. Various approaches have been developed utilizing two-dimensional echocardiography to evaluate left ventricular volumes and ejection fraction[3] and segmental left ventricular function[4] in patients with coronary artery disease.

ECHOCARDIOGRAPHIC EVALUATION OF NORMAL CHANGES WITH AGING

Clinical and necropsy studies have demonstrated that several changes occur in the human heart with advancing age.[5-11] Nonetheless, the initial published echocardiographic data defining normal adult cardiac dimensions were derived mainly from younger volunteers or from data in older subjects without systematic consideration of age and/or body surface area.[12-14] Gerstenblith et al[15] have documented age-related changes in several echocardiographic measurements. However, they did not use their data to derive age-corrected normal changes, nor did they examine the relationship between the size (weight or body surface area) of the individual and his heart dimensions. Furthermore, their study population did not include women and they did not report measurements for left atrial dimension or left ventricular mass.

We have had the opportunity to study 136 adult subjects (78 men and 58 women) without evidence of heart disease (Table 14-1).[16] These subjects, whose ages ranged from 20 to 97 years, all underwent history-taking and physical examination, chest roentgenography, electrocardiography, and M-mode echocardiography. In no subject did this evaluation reveal the presence of heart disease, hypertension, other serious illness, or obesity. Furthermore, all subjects had a normal ECG, normal chest film, and no evidence of mitral valve prolapse or pericardial effusion on M-mode echocardiogram. M-mode echocardiography was performed in the left lateral decubitus position and the following measurements were made: left ventricular internal dimensions at end-diastole and

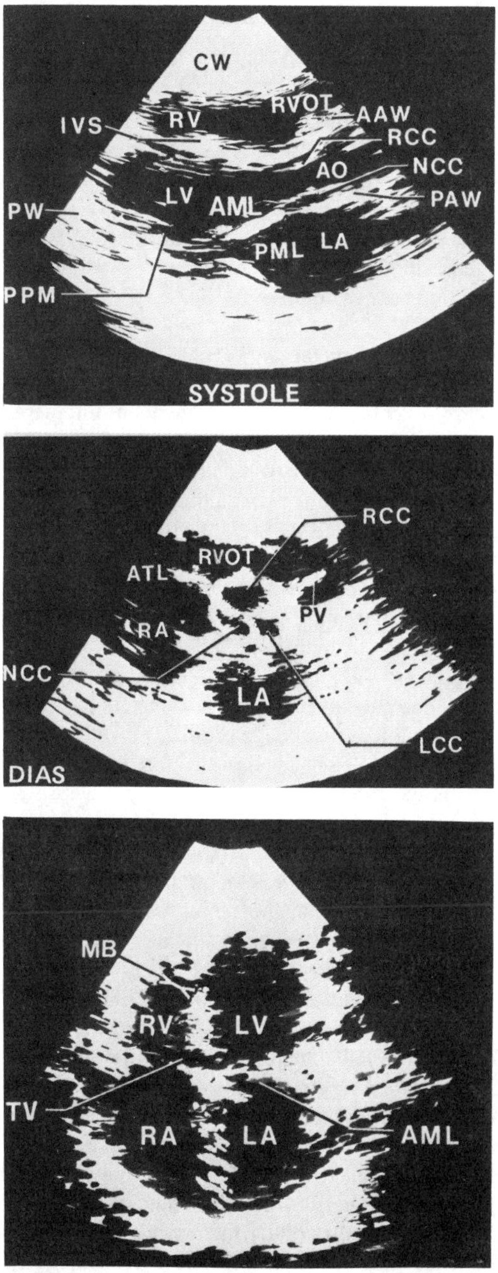

Figure 14-3 Panel A. Labeled drawing of the heart, in systole, in the parasternal long-axis view. P = posterior, I = inferior, S = superior, AAW = anterior aortic wall, AO = aortic root, PAW = posterior aortic wall, LA = left atrium, RCC = right coronary cusp, NCC = noncoronary cusp, AML = anterior mitral leaflet, PML = posterior mitral leaflet, LV = left ventricle, PW = posterior left ventricular wall, PPM = posterior papillary muscle, IVS = interventricular septum, RV = right ventricle, RVOT = right ventricular outflow tract, CW = chest wall.

Panel B. Labeled drawing of the heart at the level of the great arteries in the parasternal short-axis view. ATL = anterior tricuspid leaflet, PV = pulmonic valve, LCC = left coronary cusp, RA = right atrium, DIAS = diastole.

Panel C. Labeled drawing of the heart in systole in the apical four-chamber view. MB = moderator band, TV = tricuspid valve. (Reproduced with permission from Koenigsberg D. and Ganote C: Cardiac anatomy, in Talano JV, Gardin JM (eds): *Textbook on Two-Dimensional Echocardiography.* New York, Grune & Stratton, Inc, 1983.)

Table 14-1
Population Characteristics

Age Group (yr)	Sex Distribution		BSA (m^2)		Blood Pressure (mmHg)			Heart Rate (bpm)
	Men	*Women*	*Range*	*Mean*	*Systolic*	*Diastolic*	*Mean*	
21–30	15	10	1.48–2.25	1.80	120	71	87	74
31–40	9	15	1.47–2.38	1.80	117	76	90	69
41–50	16	13	1.42–2.20	1.83	120	76	91	73
51–60	19	10	1.51–2.17	1.84	120	71	87	73
61–70	9	8	1.52–2.10	1.75	130	72	92	73
71–97	10	2	1.42–2.13	1.73	131	61	84	70
Total (n = 136)	78	58	Mean	1.80	122	72	89	72

Reproduced with permission from Gardin et al.[16]
BSA = body surface area.

end-systole; ventricular septal and posterobasal left ventricular free-wall thicknesses at end-diastole; aortic root and left atrial dimensions; and mitral valve E-F slope, which corresponds to the rate of early diastolic closure of the anterior mitral valve leaflet (see Figures 14-1 and 14-2). In addition, the following parameters were derived from these echocardiographic measurements:

$$\text{LV mass} = (1.05)\{(\text{LVID}_d + \text{septal thickness} + \text{posterior wall thickness})^3 - (\text{LVID}_d)^3\}, \quad (1)$$

$$\text{LV ejection fraction} = \frac{(\text{LVID}_d)^3 - (\text{LVID}_s)^3}{(\text{LVID}_d)^3} \times 100\% \quad (2)$$

and

$$\text{LV \% FS} = \frac{(\text{LVID}_d - \text{LVID}_s)}{\text{LVID}_d} \times 100\% \quad (3)$$

where LV % FS denotes the left ventricular percentage fractional shortening and gives information similar to that obtained from LV ejection fraction.

Echocardiographic measurements were analyzed for the influence of age, sex, and body surface area. When the data for each echocardiographic parameter was analyzed separately for men and women, using the appropriate function of body surface area, statistically significant differences between men and women were found for three parameters: (1) ventricular septal thickness, (2) posterobasal free-wall thickness, and (3) estimated left ventricular mass. However, since the sex differences for these three parameters were relatively small (range 6.2% to 7.2%), we chose for the sake of simplicity to combine data for men and women in our calculation of regression equations and prediction intervals.

In analyzing our data for each echo parameter, we found that data for each parameter could be expressed according to a general regression equation which was dependent on age and body surface area, and which would contain normal 95% confidence intervals for the parameter. This general equation was as follows:

$$\text{Echo parameter} = B\,(\text{BSA}) + A \pm C$$

where A represented the age-dependent intercept, B represented an age-independent slope which was unique for each parameter, and C represented the width of the 95% prediction interval, ie, the interval into which, with 95% confidence, a new normal observation would fall.[17] The width of the 95% prediction interval ($\pm$C) was shown to be nearly constant and not appreciably influenced by age or body surface area.

Table 14-2 gives the values for B, A, and $\pm$C for seven echocardiographic parameters for adult normal subjects in six age groups. For all parameters except left ventricular ejection fraction and percentage fractional shortening, there were statistically significant changes with increasing age. Left ventricular ejection fraction was demonstrated to be 75% ± 9%, and left ventricular percentage fractional shortening was 36% ± 8% independent of age or body surface area.

Figure 14-4 depicts the changes in mean left ventricular internal dimensions in diastole and systole in the six age groups. The mean left ventricular internal dimension in diastole decreased 6% from 48.1 mm in the 30-and-under age-decade to 45.3 mm in the over-70 group. Likewise, the mean left ventricular internal dimension in systole decreased 5% from 30.0 mm in the youngest group to 28.4 mm in the oldest age group.

The mean ventricular septal thickness increased from 9.8 mm in the 30-and-under age-decade to

Table 14-2
Regression Equations Using Linear Function Approach

Equation		Intercepts (Age-Dependent)						Prediction
		21-30	*31-40*	*41-50*	*51-60*	*61-70*	⩾ 70	Interval
$LVID_d$	= 6.94(BSA) +	35.5	36.2	34.4	34.1	34.8	32.7	± 5.60
$LVID_s$	= 4.24(BSA) +	22.4	22.6	21.5	21.1	21.7	20.8	± 5.81
Septum	= 2.53(BSA) +	5.27	5.47	6.27	6.53	6.84	7.20	± 1.75
PWT	= 2.18(BSA) +	6.11	6.02	6.94	6.97	7.34	7.81	± 1.43
Ao	= 8.31(BSA) +	12.3	13.1	14.7	15.6	16.4	18.5	± 5.76
LA	= 9.98(BSA) +	16.3	16.7	17.6	18.0	19.3	21.7	± 7.01
E-F slope	= 20.1(BSA) +	99.9	90.2	78.3	66.6	62.2	43.5	± 62.2

Reproduced with permission from Gardin et al.[16]
BSA = body surface area.

11.8 mm in the over-70 age group, an increment of 20%, whereas the mean left ventricular posterior wall thickness increased 18% from 10.1 mm in the 30-and-under age group to 11.8 mm in the over-70 group. The mean values of septal and posterior wall thicknesses for each age group were within 0.3 mm of each other. Therefore, only the relationship of the mean left ventricular posterior wall thickness to age is illustrated in Figure 14-5. Increases in septal and posterior wall thicknesses occurred despite the absence of significantly higher systolic, diastolic, or mean pressures in our older-age study population (Table 14-1). It is of interest that Roberts and Perloff have noted that hearts of older individuals studied at necropsy appear to have smaller ventricular chambers and thicker walls than those of their younger counterparts.[5]

Figures 14-6 and 14-7 illustrate the age-related changes in aortic root dimension and left atrial dimension. The mean aortic root dimension was 22% larger in the over-70 age group (33.5 mm) when compared with the under-30 age group (27.4 mm). The mean left atrial dimension showed a 16% increase from the youngest (33.4 mm) to the oldest (39.7 mm) age groups. Krovetz[8] has reviewed a number of published reports of measurements of aortic valve annulus size made at necropsy. When aortic annulus size was corrected for body surface area, progressive increases with age were noted in both males and females over 20 years of age. With regard to changes in left atrial dimension with increasing age, Roberts and Perloff have noted an increase in left atrial dimension in older individuals at necropsy.[5] This finding is a particularly important consideration in echocardiographic studies designed to make quantitative statements about the effects of various diseases—eg, hypertension, valvular or coronary artery disease—on left atrial dimension.

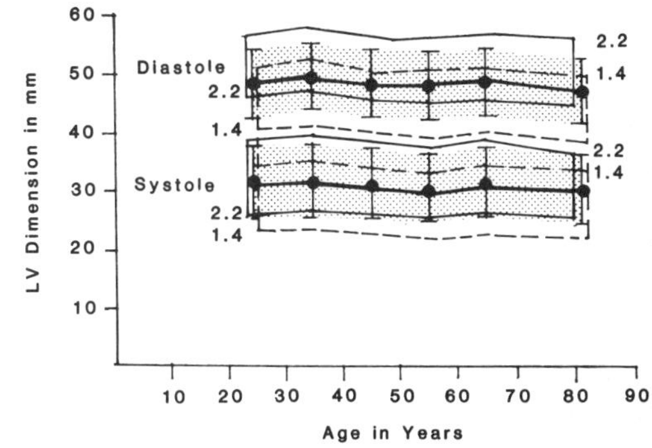

Figure 14-4 Plot of left ventricular end-diastolic and end-systolic dimensions (in millimeters) versus age (in years). In this figure and Figures 14-5 through 14-9, the mean value for each age group is depicted by a solid dot plotted at the mean age in the age group. The bracketed shaded area on either side of the solid dot represents the 95% prediction interval for normal values for a subject with a body surface area of 1.8 m². The 95% prediction intervals are also shown for subjects with body surface area values of 1.4 m² (dotted lines) and 2.2 m² (solid lines). (Reproduced with permission from Gardin et al.[16])

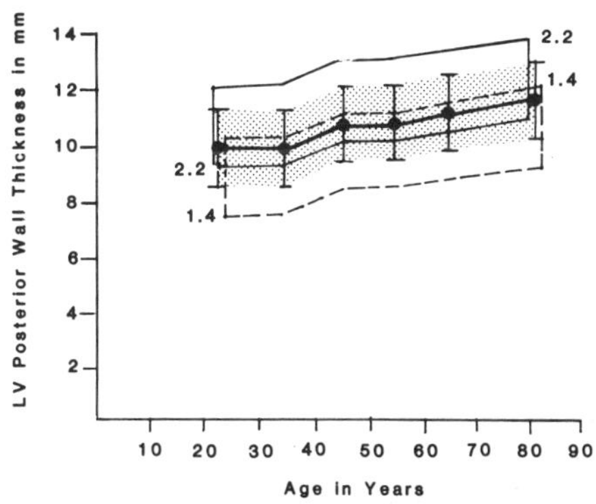

Figure 14-5 Plot of left ventricular posterior wall thickness in late diastole (in millimeters) versus age (in years). For each age group, the mean and 95% prediction interval for normal values are depicted. (Reproduced with permission from Gardin et al.[16])

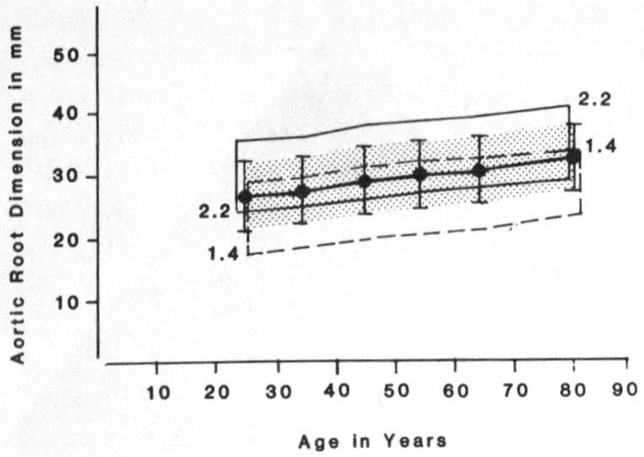

Figure 14-6 Aortic root dimension in late diastole is plotted (in millimeters) versus age (in years). For each age group, the mean and 95% prediction interval for normal values are depicted. (Reproduced with permission from Gardin et al.[16])

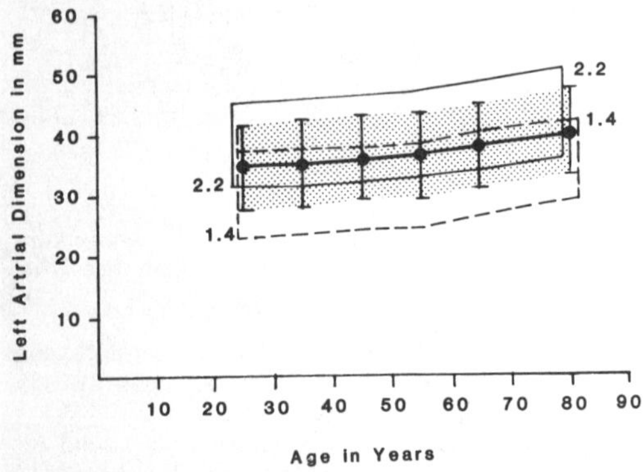

Figure 14-7 Plot of left atrial dimension in late diastole (in millimeters) versus age (in years). For each age group, the mean and 95% prediction interval for normal values are depicted. (Reproduced with permission from Gardin et al.[16])

The mean mitral valve E-F slope, plotted for each age group in Figure 14-8, decreased progressively from 136 mm/sec in the 21 to 30 age group to 77 mm/sec in the over-70 age group, a mean decrease of 43%. Various investigators have reported functional changes with age in the mitral valve echocardiogram consistent with our findings, including prolonged diastolic closure time[9] and decreased E-F slope.[10] Factors postulated to explain this decrease in the rate of early diastolic closure of the anterior mitral valve leaflet have included sclerosis of the mitral leaflets and/or decreased compliance of the left ventricle.[9,10]

With regard to the left ventricular mass (in grams) there was a 15% increase in mean left ventricular mass from 214 g in the youngest to 246 g in the oldest age group. The left ventricular mass showed a small but progressive increase from the 21 to 30 age group to the over-70 age group. This increase reflected an increase in wall thickness that was relatively greater than the decrease in left ventricular diastolic dimension.

Although it is highly likely that the echocardiographic changes reported above in the different age groups are related to the aging process, one cannot be certain that this explanation is correct until these changes are documented during serial studies in the same patient. Nonetheless, the above analysis makes it clear that it is important to use normal echocardiographic values corrected for both age and body surface area when evaluating adult patients suspected of having heart disease.

ECHOCARDIOGRAPHIC EVALUATION OF VARIOUS DISEASE STATES

Although various textbooks have been written outlining the utility of M-mode and two-dimensional echocardiography in the evaluation of patients with congenital and acquired heart disease,[1,18–20] it seems appropriate to briefly outline the use of echocardiography in the evaluation of some of the more common cardiac lesions seen in the elderly.

Mitral Valve Disease

Mitral annular calcification A later chapter in this text discusses the general topic of mitral annular calcification in the elderly. Both M-mode and two-dimensional echocardiography are ex-

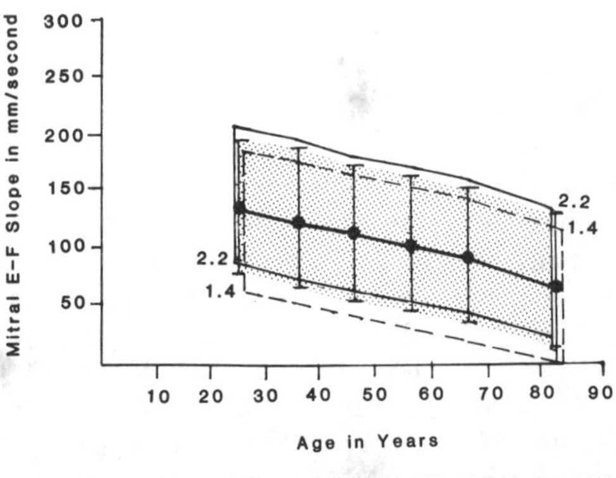

Figure 14-8 Mitral E-F slope (in millimeters per second) is plotted versus age (in years). For each age group, the mean and 95% prediction interval are depicted. (Reproduced with permission from Gardin et al.[16])

tremely useful and more sensitive than the chest roentgenogram in making this diagnosis.[21]

Mitral stenosis Whereas M-mode echocardiography has proved extremely helpful in diagnosing the *presence* of mitral stenosis, two-dimensional echocardiography has proved far superior in estimating the severity of stenosis. Henry et al[22] and others[23,24] have shown that parasternal short-axis two-dimensional echocardiographic measurements of mitral orifice area correlate well with mitral orifice size measured at surgery or estimated invasively by cardiac catheterization. Figure 14-9 shows parasternal short-axis two-dimensional images in patients with a normal mitral valve and with severe mitral stenosis.

Other mitral valve abnormalities Other mitral valve abnormalities, which may be detected by M-mode and/or two-dimensional echocardiography in both younger and older patients, include mitral valve prolapse, flail posterior mitral leaflet due to ruptured chordae tendineae, acute and chronic aortic insufficiency, mitral valve vegetations, and atrial myxoma.

Aortic Valve Disease

Aortic stenosis Aortic stenosis has several etiologies, but the most frequent etiology in the child or adult is congenital.[25] It is extremely important to diagnose the presence of severe aortic stenosis since the first clinical presentation of the severe form may be syncope, myocardial infarction, or sudden death.[26] In patients over the age of 35 years, it is extremely unusual to find significant aortic stenosis in the absence of calcification of the aortic valve.[27]

Both M-mode and two-dimensional echocardiography can be useful in the evaluation of the patient with suspected aortic stenosis. The absence of dense echoes corresponding to calcification of the aortic valve virtually excludes the diagnosis of significant aortic stenosis in an elderly individual. Figure 14-10 illustrates diagrammatically the M-mode echocardiographic findings in severe aortic stenosis. Weyman et al[28,29] utilized two-dimensional echocardiography to estimate the severity of aortic stenosis by noting the maximum aortic leaflet separation in the parasternal long-axis view. In the absence of left ventricular systolic failure, maximum aortic cusp separation should have a direct relationship to the severity of aortic stenosis. In normal subjects, the maximum cusp separation should be nearly equal to the aortic annulus diameter. The presence of a maximum aortic cusp separation of less than

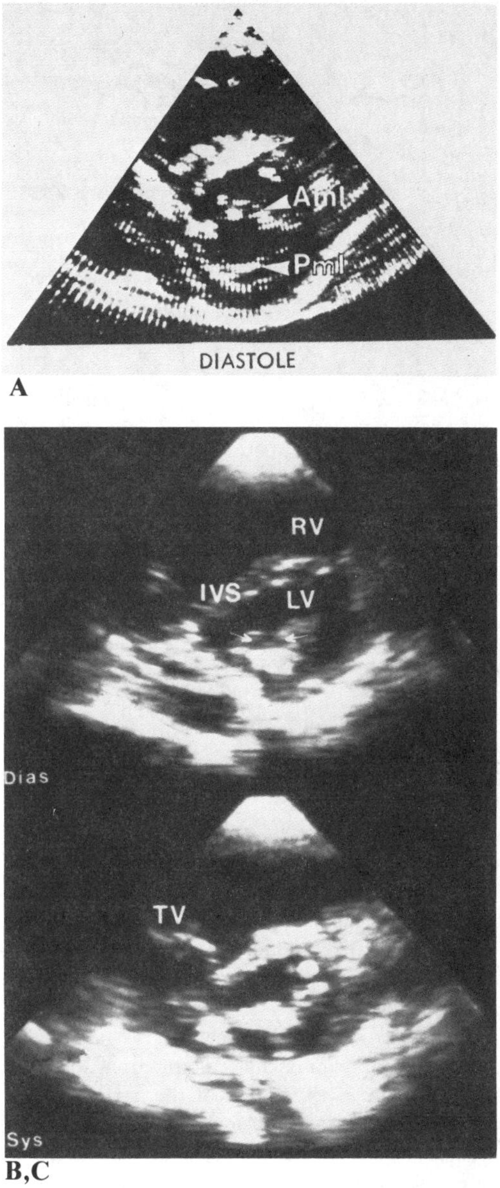

Figure 14-9 Panel A. Parasternal short-axis view in a normal subject. This echocardiographic recording demonstrates the maximal diastolic mitral valve orifice in a normal subject.

Panels B and C. Parasternal short-axis views in a patient with a severe calcific mitral stenosis. In diastole (DIAS), Panel B, the mitral valve orifice (arrows) measured 0.35 cm^2 in area. There is heavy calcification of the mitral leaflets and annulus. Abbreviations: ATL = anterior tricuspid leaflet, PV = pulmonic valve, LCC = left coronary cusp, RA = right atrium, DIAS = diastole. (Reproduced with permission from Gardin JM, Butman S, Talano JV: Mitral valve disease, in Talano JV, Gardin JM (eds): *Textbook on Two-Dimensional Cardiography*. New York, Grune & Stratton, Inc, 1983.)

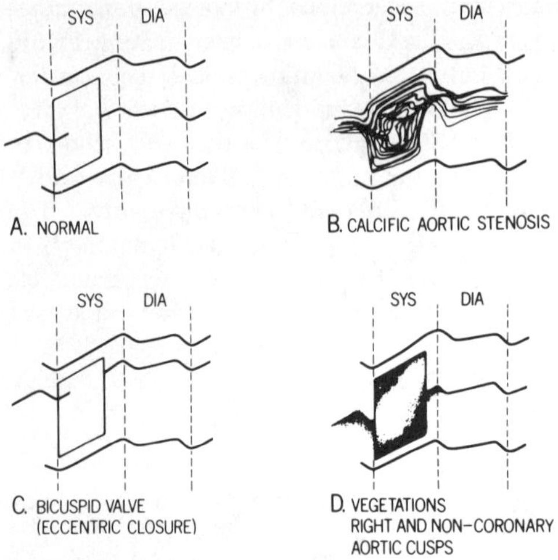

Figure 14-10 Composite of aortic valve echocardiograms seen in various normal and abnormal states. SYS = systole, DIA = diastole. (Reproduced with permission from Gardin JM, Askenazi J, Lesch M: Assessment of cardiovascular function, in Sciarra JJ, Depp R [eds]: *Maternal and Fetal Medicine, Gynecology and Obstetrics,* vol 3. Hagerstown, Md, Harper & Row, 1979, pp 1–19.)

8 mm favors the diagnosis of significant aortic stenosis.

Aortic sclerosis The presence of aortic leaflet or aortic root thickening without a gradient across the aortic valve (aortic sclerosis) can also be inferred from echocardiography. In this condition, the aortic leaflets and/or the aortic root appear increased in thickness relative to normal, but there is normal leaflet opening (separation) noted on the echocardiogram. Echocardiography may be helpful in confirming that calcification noted on the chest film in the region of the aortic valve is associated with aortic sclerosis without a significant aortic valve gradient. It may be difficult, however, to differentiate aortic sclerosis from mild, and occasionally even significant, aortic valve stenosis on the basis of echocardiography.

Bicuspid aortic valve In the elderly, bicuspid aortic valves are usually calcified.[25] Figure 14-10 illustrates diagrammatically the appearance of a bicuspid aortic valve in a younger individual in whom it is still uncalcified. It should be noted that sometimes calcification of the aortic leaflets may be confused with the presence of vegetations on the leaflets (Figure 14-10).

Ischemic Heart Disease

It is well-known that the incidence of atherosclerotic cardiovascular disease increases with advancing age. Echocardiography is particularly useful in detecting the complications of myocardial infarction, such as left ventricular aneurysm with or without associated thrombus, ruptured chordae tendineae with flail mitral leaflet, and ventricular septal rupture.

Left ventricular aneurysm Two-dimensional echocardiography is particularly useful for delineating the presence of left ventricular wall motion abnormalities, ranging from hypokinesis to dyskinesis. Figure 14-11 depicts an area of severe left ventricular dyskinesis, consistent with left ventricular aneurysm. Within the area of the aneurysm is a distinct apical layered area consistent with an intraventricular thrombus.[30] In the setting of acute myocardial infarction, left ventricular thrombi are most common in patients who develop apical left ventricular aneurysms[31] (Figure 14-11).

Flail mitral leaflet Ruptured chordae tendineae may result in a flail mitral leaflet. Note that in Figure 14-12 the posterior mitral leaflet is shown not to coapt normally with the anterior mitral leaflet; rather, the posterior leaflet demonstrates erratic systolic motion into the left atrium.

Ventricular septal rupture Rupture of the ventricular septum can be a severe, and often fatal, complication of acute myocardial infarction. Figure 14-13 demonstrates sequential systolic two-dimensional echocardiographic frames from a patient with an acute ventricular septal defect after myocardial infarction. At the onset of systole, there is no defect; during systole, the septum bulges into the right ventricle.[32] Other investigators have demonstrated that the peripheral venous injection of saline may be used to outline a ventricular septal defect. The saline acts as an echo-contrast material, probably through the production of microcavitations within the blood stream.

Normally, this contrast effect would proceed from the venae cavae through the right atrium into the right ventricle and out the main pulmonary artery. The microbubbles would be then dissipated in the pulmonary circulation. In the presence of a left-to-right shunt at ventricular septal level, a "negative contrast" effect would be seen in which contrast-free blood would outline an area (relatively echo-free) around the defect on the right side of the ventricular septum.[33] The presence of a right-to-left shunt would be accompanied by the appearance of echo contrast in the left ventricle after the echo bubbles had passed through the septal defect.[34]

Cardiomegaly

Echocardiography is extremely useful in differentiating the causes for cardiomegaly noted on the chest film. Conditions that are readily identifiable by both M-mode and two-dimensional echocardiography include pericardial effusion, congestive (dilated) cardiomyopathy, and concentric and asymmetric left ventricular hypertrophy.

Pericardial effusion There are numerous etiologies for pericardial effusion, including idiopathic, viral, tuberculous, neoplastic, postirradiation, uremic, and congestive heart failure. Figure 14-14 illustrates two-dimensional echocardiographic findings in a patient with pericardial effusion. Note the presence of a relatively echo-free space behind the posterior left ventricular wall.[35]

Congestive (dilated) cardiomyopathy The presence of global left ventricular hypokinesis in association with normal ventricular septal and left ventricular free-wall thickness and increased

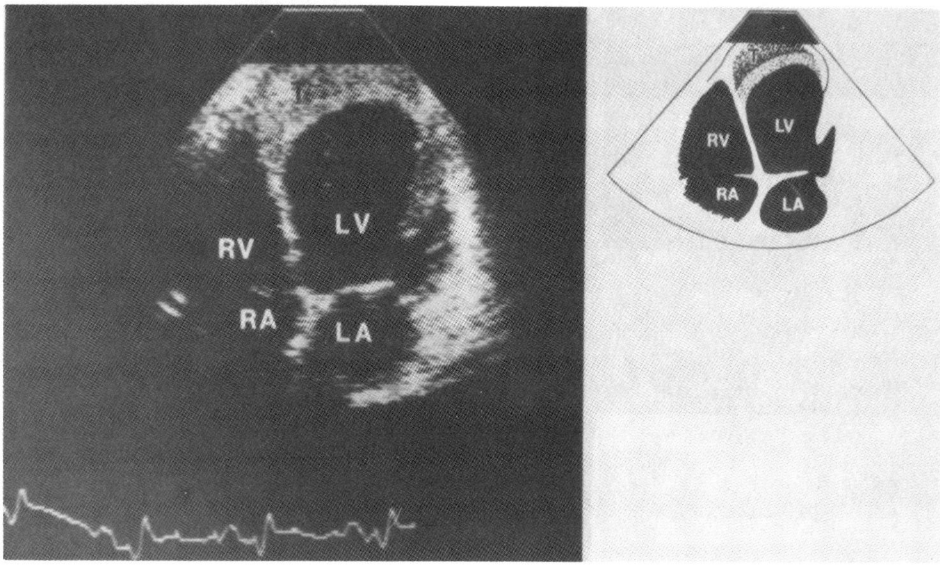

Figure 14-11 Two-dimensional apical four-chamber view demonstrating a large layered apical mural thrombus (T). LA = left atrium, LV = left ventricle, RA = right atrium, RV = right ventricle. (Reproduced with permission et al.[30])

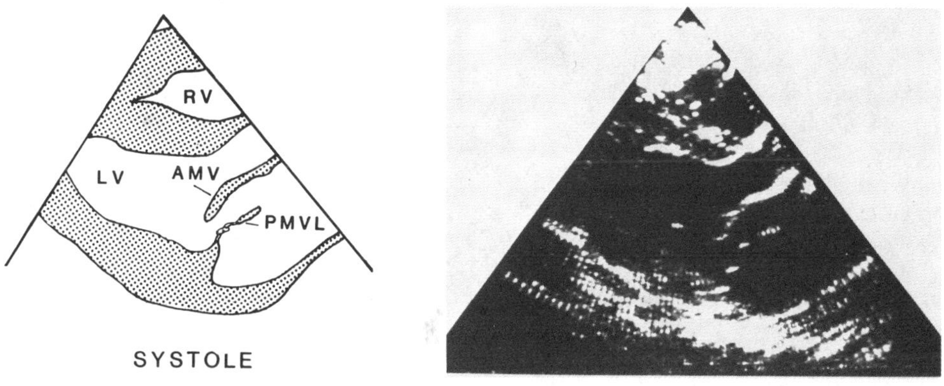

Figure 14-12 Diagram (left panel) and two-dimensional echocardiogram in a parasternal long-axis view in systole (right panel) from a patient with a flail posterior mitral leaflet. Patient developed acute mitral regurgitation secondary to ruptured chordae tendineae. AMV = anterior mitral valve leaflet, PMVL = posterior mitral valve leaflet. (Reproduced with permission from Gardin JM, Butman S, Talano JV: Mitral valve disease, in Talano JV, Gardin JM (eds): *Textbook on Two-Dimensional Echocardiography*. New York, Grune & Stratton, Inc, 1983.)

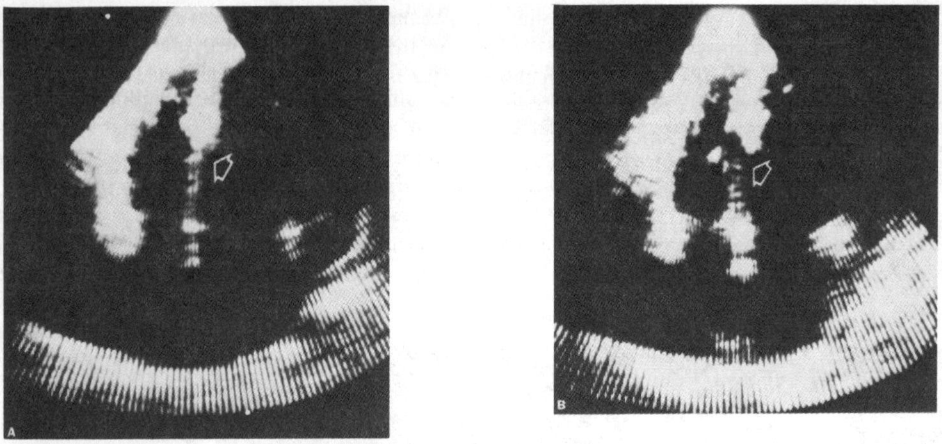

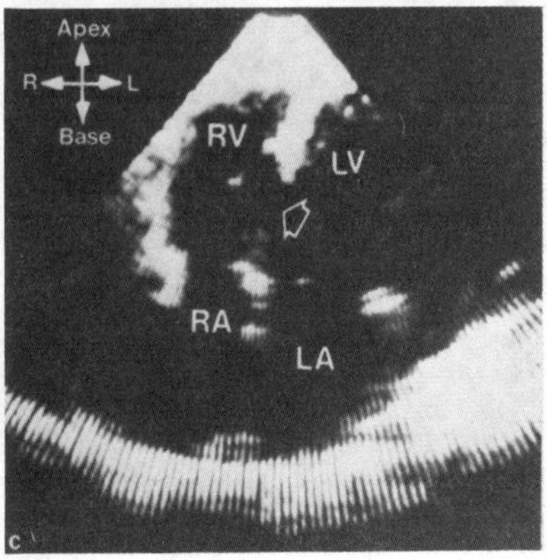

Figure 14-13 Sequential systolic frames from a two-dimensional echocardiographic study in the apical four-chamber view. The patient had an acute ventricular septal defect following a myocardial infarction. At the onset of systole (A), there is no defect. During systole (B and C), the septum bulges into the right ventricle (RV). The open white arrow indicates the defect in the middle of the septal aneurysm. R = right, L = left, other abbreviations as in previous figures. (Reproduced with permission et al.[32])

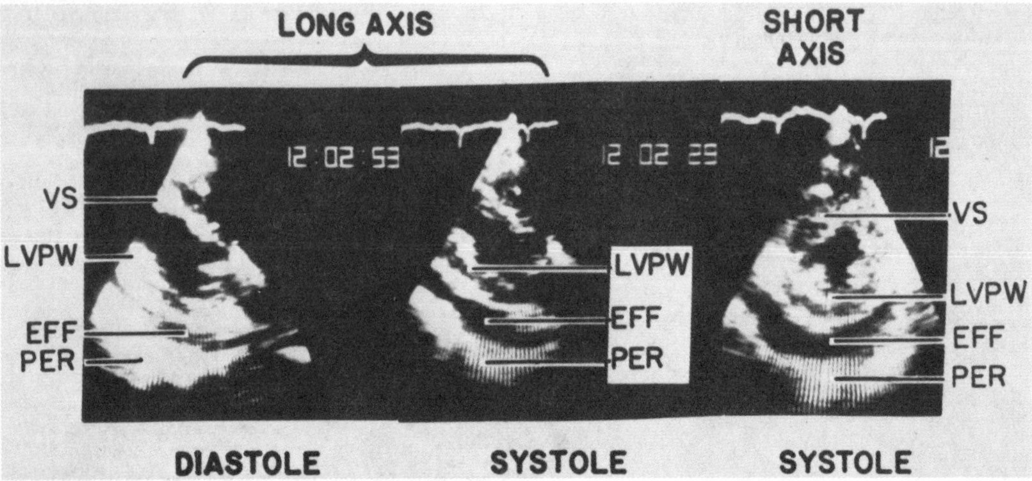

Figure 14-14 Two-dimensional echocardiographic views in a patient with a small- to medium-sized pericardial effusion. The parasternal long-axis frames are from the same cardiac cycle. The posterior pericardial echo-free space is wider in systole (center frame) than in diastole (left frame) and is also demonstrated in the parasternal short-axis view (systole). EFF = pericardial effusion, LVPW = left ventricular posterior wall, PER = pericardium, VS = ventricular septum. (Reproduced with permission from D'Cruz IA: Pericardial disease, in Talano JV, Gardin JM (eds): *Textbook on Two-Dimensional Echocardiography*. New York, Grune & Stratton, Inc, 1983.)

chamber dimensions is consistent with the diagnosis of congestive cardiomyopathy.[1,36]

Concentric and asymmetric left ventricular hypertrophy There are many causes for concentric left ventricular hypertrophy, including hypertension, aortic stenosis, hemochromatosis and amyloidosis. Asymmetric septal (or ventricular free-wall) hypertrophy has been described as one of the hallmarks in patients with hypertrophic cardiomyopathy. Figure 14-15 depicts asymmetric septal hypertrophy in a patient with hypertrophic cardiomyopathy who did not have a left ventricular outflow tract gradient.[36]

SUMMARY

Echocardiography is an extremely useful noninvasive tool for assessing cardiac anatomy and function in normal subjects and in patients with heart disease. In order to take full advantage of this technic in elderly individuals, it is important to be aware of the changes in cardiac anatomy that occur in apparently normal subjects with aging. There are many applications of both M-mode and two-dimensional echocardiography in the evaluation of valvular and ischemic heart disease, pericardial effusion, cardiomyopathy, and other cardiac abnormalities in our older population.

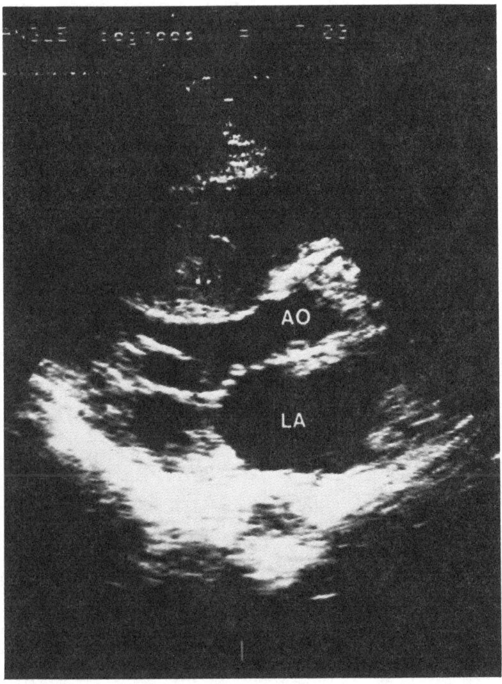

Figure 14-15 Two-dimensional parasternal long-axis view in systole from a patient with hypertrophic cardiomyopathy without left ventricular outflow tract obstruction. Note marked asymmetric septal hypertrophy (septal-to-free-wall thickness ratio = 3.1). Abbreviations as in Figure 14-3.

ACKNOWLEDGMENTS

Wilma Mottin, Nancy Hagerty Futty, and Carol West assisted in the preparation of the manuscript and Jack Newby and the Medical Media Department at the Long Beach (California) Veterans Administration Medical Center provided expert assistance in preparing a number of the figures.

REFERENCES

1. Feigenbaum H: *Echocardiography*, ed 3. Philadelphia, Lea & Febiger, 1982.
2. Pombo JF, Troy BL, Russell RO Jr: Left ventricular volumes and ejection fraction by echocardiography. *Circulation* 1971;43:480.
3. Folland ED, Parisi AF, Moynihan PF, et al: Assessment of left ventricular ejection fraction and volumes by real-time, two-dimensional echocardiography. A comparison of cineangiographic and radionuclide techniques. *Circulation* 1979;60:760.
4. Parisi AF, Moynihan PF, Folland ED, et al: Quantitative detection of regional left ventricular contraction abnormalities by two-dimensional echocardiography. II. Accuracy in coronary artery disease. *Circulation* 1981;63:761.
5. Roberts WC, Perloff JK: Mitral valve disease. A clinicopathologic survey of the conditions causing the mitral valve to function abnormally. *Ann Intern Med* 1972;77:1939.
6. Gerstenblith G, Lakatta EG, Weisfeldt ML: Age changes in myocardial function and exercise response. *Prog Cardiovasc Dis* 1976;19:1.
7. Caird FI, Dall JLC, Kennedy RD: *Cardiology in Old Age.* New York, Plenum Publishing Corp, 1976, p 11.
8. Krovetz J: Age-related changes in size of the aortic valve annulus in man. *Am Heart J* 1975;90:569.
9. Luisada AA, Watanabe K, Bhat PK, et al: Correlates of the echocardiographic waves of the mitral valve in normal subjects of various ages. *J Am Geriatr Soc* 1975;23:216.
10. Derman U: Changes of the mitral echocardiogram with aging and the influence of atherosclerotic risk factors. *Atherosclerosis* 1972;15:349.
11. Brandfonbrener M, Landowne M, Shock NW: Changes in cardiac output with age. *Circulation* 1955;12:557.
12. Feigenbaum H: *Echocardiography*, ed 2. Philadelphia, Lea & Febiger, 1976, p 464.
13. Longo MR, Guzman AW, Triebwasser JH: Normal values in commonly used echocardiographic formulae for adults. *Aviat Environ Med* 1975;46:1062.
14. Francis GS, Hagan AD, Oury J, et al: Accuracy of echocardiography for assessing aortic root diameter. *Br Heart J* 1975;37:376.

15. Gerstenblith G, Frederiksen J, Yin CP, et al: Echocardiographic assessment of a normal adult aging population. *Circulation* 1977;56:273.
16. Gardin JM, Henry WL, Savage DD: Echocardiographic measurements of normal subjects: Evaluation of an adult population without clinically apparent heart disease. *J Clin Ultrasound* 1979; 7:439.
17. Kendall MG, Stuart A: *Advanced Theory of Statistics,* New York, Hafner Publishing, 1961, vol 3.
18. Weyman AE: *Cross-Sectional Echocardiography.* Philadelphia, Lea & Febiger, 1982.
19. Talano JV, Gardin JM (eds): *Textbook of Two-Dimensional Echocardiography.* New York, Grune & Stratton, 1983.
20. Schapira JN, Charuzi Y, Davidson RM (eds): *Two-Dimensional Echocardiography.* Baltimore, Williams and Wilkins, 1982.
21. D'Cruz I, Panetta F, Cohen H, et al: Submitral calcification or sclerosis in elderly patients: M-mode and two-dimensional echocardiography in "mitral annulus calcification." *Am J Cardiol* 1979;44:31.
22. Henry WL, Griffith JM, Michaelis LL, et al: Measurement of mitral orifice area in patients with mitral valve disease by real-time, two-dimensional echocardiography. *Circulation* 1975;51:827.
23. Nichol PM, Gilbert BW, Kisslo JA: Two-dimensional echocardiographic assessment of mitral stenosis. *Circulation* 1977;55:120.
24. Wann LS, Weyman AE, Feigenbaum H, et al: Determination of mitral valve area by cross-sectional echocardiography. *Ann Intern Med* 1978;88:337.
25. Roberts WC: The congenitally bicuspid aortic valve. A study of 85 autopsy cases. *Am J Cardiol* 1970; 26:72.
26. Wood P: Aortic stenosis. *Am J Cardiol* 1958;1:553.
27. Glancy DL, Freed TA, O'Brien KP, et al: Calcium in the aortic valve: Roentgenologic and hemodynamic correlations in 148 patients. *Ann Intern Med* 1969;71:245.
28. Weyman AE, Feigenbaum H, Dillon JC, et al: Cross-sectional echocardiography in assessing the severity of valvular aortic stenosis. *Circulation* 1975;52:828.
29. Weyman AE, Feigenbaum H, Hurwitz RA, et al: Cross-sectional echocardiographic assessment of the severity of aortic stenosis in children. *Circulation* 1977;55:773.
30. Asinger RW, Mikell FL, Sharma B, et al: Observations on detecting left ventricular thrombus with two-dimensional echocardiography: Emphasis on avoidance of false positive diagnoses. *Am J Cardiol* 1981;47:15.
31. Asinger RW, Mikell FL, Elsperger J, et al: Incidence of left ventricular thrombosis after acute myocardial infarction. Serial evaluation by two-dimensional echocardiography. *N Engl J Med* 1981;305:297.
32. Mintz GS, Victor MF, Kotler MN, et al: Two-dimensional echocardiographic identification of surgically correctable complications of acute myocardial infarction. *Circulation* 1981;64:91.
33. Weyman AE, Wann LS, Caldwell RL, et al: Negative contrast echocardiography: A new method for detecting left-to-right shunts. *Circulation* 1979;59: 498.
34. Drobac M, Gilbert B, Howard R, et al: Ventricular septal defect after myocardial infarction: Diagnosis by two-dimensional contrast echocardiography. *Circulation* 1983;67:335.
35. D'Cruz I: Pericardial diseases, in Talano JV, Gardin JM (eds): *Textbook of Two-Dimensional Echocardiography.* New York, Grune & Stratton, 1983.
36. Gardin JM, Henry WL: Echocardiographic evaluation of dilated, hypertrophic, and infiltrative cardiomyopathy, in Linhart JW, Joyner CR (eds): *Diagnostic Echocardiography.* St Louis, The CV Mosby Co, 1982.

CHAPTER 15
Left Ventricular Thrombus Detection by Two-Dimensional Echocardiography

John R. Stratton

Left ventricular thrombi occur frequently in patients with either transmural anterior myocardial infarction or congestive cardiomyopathy and may lead to systemic embolization. The detection of a ventricular thrombus is of potential clinical importance in influencing decisions regarding anticoagulation. However, until recently, the premortem diagnosis of intracardiac thrombi was limited and usually unsuspected until the time of an embolic event. Several noninvasive methods are now available which are capable of diagnosing left ventricular thrombi. Most of these technics, including two-dimensional echocardiography, radionuclide angiography, and computed tomographic (CT) scanning detect the anatomic defect a thrombus creates. Additionally, thrombi can be detected by the external imaging of radiolabeled blood components which are incorporated into thrombi, as with indium 111 platelet imaging. For reasons which will be discussed, two-dimensional echocardiography has clear advantages over the other noninvasive diagnostic methods for the diagnosis of left ventricular thrombi.

Left ventricular thrombi, which are usually due to prior myocardial infarction, occur primarily in the elderly. It is very uncommon for the younger cardiac patient, who typically has congenital or valvular heart disease, to have associated left ventricular thrombus. Although there is no firm data regarding the presentation of ventricular thrombi in the two age groups, the older patient is probably less likely to have idiopathic cardiomyopathy as a cause of ventricular thrombus than the younger patient. Because the risks of anticoagulation may be increased in the older patient, diagnostic certainty as to the presence or absence of thrombus is even more imperative in the older than in the younger patient.

This chapter will review the clinical features of patients who develop left ventricular thrombi, describe echocardiographic examination technics in patients with suspected left ventricular thrombi, review the echocardiographic characteristics of thrombi, define the accuracy and limitations of the echocardiographic diagnosis of thrombi, compare the accuracy of echocardiography to other noninvasive diagnostic methods, and discuss the clinical implications of the echocardiographic detection of thrombi.

CLINICAL FEATURES ASSOCIATED WITH LEFT VENTRICULAR THROMBI (Table 15-1)

Most patients with left ventricular thrombi are elderly. Slightly more than half of patients with definite left ventricular thrombi are aged 60 or above, and the mean age for all patients with thrombi has been approximately 60 years in most series. Left ventricular mural thrombi occur predominantly in two patient groups. One group consists of patients with advanced congestive cardiomyopathy and the other of patients with coronary artery disease and transmural myocardial infarction. Rarely, patients with other cardiac or systemic disorders such as endomyocardial fibrosis,[1] thrombocytosis secondary to myeloproliferative disorders,[2] or polycythemia vera[3] develop mural thrombi, but such patients are infrequently encountered and will not be discussed further. Patients with advanced congestive cardiomyopathy

Table 15-1
Clinical Features Associated with Left Ventricular Thrombi

Advanced congestive cardiomyopathy
Transmural anterior myocardial infarction by ECG
Combined transmural anterior and inferior infarctions by ECG
Left ventricular aneurysm
Low ejection fraction, congestive heart failure, cardiomegaly
Systemic embolization

frequently have associated left ventricular thrombi. In autopsy series, approximately one third of patients dying with congestive cardiomyopathy have left ventricular mural thrombi.[4] A similar prevalence of mural thrombi (36%) has been noted in an echocardiographic study of living patients with congestive cardiomyopathy.[5]

The other group of patients who develop left ventricular thrombi consists of patients with coronary artery disease. On the basis of autopsy and clinical studies, several overlapping clinical findings can be used to define subsets of this large population of patients with coronary artery disease who are at low or high risk for the presence of a thrombus. Patients with coronary artery disease but without prior myocardial infarction virtually never have ventricular thrombi. In contrast, one quarter to two thirds of patients with fatal myocardial infarction have left ventricular thrombi detected at autopsy.[6-8] By electrocardiography, most patients (approximately 80%) with ventricular thrombi have transmural anterior infarctions.[9-12] Patients with both transmural anterior and inferior infarctions appear to be at particular risk for thrombus formation, probably due to the large extent of myocardial scarring.[9] However, patients with only isolated inferior myocardial infarctions rarely have thrombi unless there is an associated aneurysm or pseudoaneurysm.[9-12] The natural history of left ventricular thrombi following myocardial infarction will be discussed below. It should be noted that many patients who have thrombi detected by echocardiography are months to even years following their acute infarction.[10]

Another feature associated with thrombus formation is the presence of a left ventricular aneurysm. In patients with aneurysms, the prevalence of left ventricular thrombi is very high (44% to 78%) as documented at autopsy[8,13,14] or cardiac surgery.[15-17] Patients with congestive heart failure or a decreased ejection fraction are also more likely to have ventricular thrombi than patients without these features.[18] In one study, 11 of 13 patients (85%) with proved left ventricular thrombi had a left ventricular ejection fraction of less than 0.45.[19] Additionally, approximately 65% of patients with left ventricular thrombi have cardiomegaly by chest film.[20] Left ventricular regional wall motion, as assessed by either radionuclide angiography, two-dimensional echocardiography, or contrast angiography, is abnormal in virtually all patients with ventricular thrombi. Most commonly there are localized areas of akinesis or dyskinesis. Occasionally diffuse hypokinesis is present, as in patients with multiple infarctions or idiopathic cardiomyopathy. Regional stasis of blood due to decreased wall motion appears to be a prerequisite for left ventricular thrombus formation.

As would be predicted, systemic embolization is also associated with the presence of a left ventricular thrombus. In autopsy series, the presence of pathologically proven emboli in patients with left ventricular thrombus has been approximately 30% to 40%; however, many of these embolic events were clinically silent, particularly when the embolus lodged in the kidney or spleen.[13,18,21] Clinically documented systemic embolism is a significant problem since the in-hospital mortality rate is high (15% to 40%).[22-24] In a recently reported clinical study of 2789 men followed for five years after a myocardial infarction, 6% had a definite or suspect peripheral arterial occlusion and 10% had a definite or suspect stroke or transient ischemic attack.[25] Although the presence or absence of ventricular thrombus was not determined in these patients, it is possible that many of these events were secondary to left ventricular thrombi which formed at the time of infarction. Once a thombus is diagnosed in a patient, the risk of subsequent embolization has not been well defined. The available data will be reviewed below.

In one study of 22 patients with proven left ventricular thrombus and 56 patients without thrombus, the relative prevalences of several of the above mentioned clinical features were noted. Compared with patients who had no thrombus, patients with proven thrombus had a higher prevalence of ECG transmural anterior infarction (86% vs 13%, $P < 0.001$), left ventricular aneurysm (73% vs 5%, $P < 0.001$), and clinically apparent systemic emboli (36% vs 7%, $P < 0.01$).[10]

Careful patient selection is important if echocardiography is to be used in a cost-effective manner in the detection of ventricular thrombi. Awareness of the frequently overlapping clinical features mentioned above should increase the clinical suspicion of thrombus and lead to early identification of patients at risk for systemic embolization. Equally important, the absence of these clinical features defines a group of patients who are at very low risk for left ventricular thrombus. This low-risk group is comprised of patients who do not have transmural anterior infarction, low ejection fraction, left ventricular aneurysm, or systemic emboli. Such low-risk patients are unlikely to benefit from a study performed to determine the presence or absence of thrombus.

ECHOCARDIOGRAPHIC EXAMINATION OF PATIENTS WITH SUSPECTED LEFT VENTRICULAR THROMBI

While conventional M-mode echocardiography has occasionally been able to detect left ventricular thrombi,[26–28] this technic is usually unsuccessful, in large part because the apex, where most ventricular thrombi occur, is not well imaged by the M-mode examination. Thus, the remainder of this discussion will concern only the two-dimensional echocardiographic detection of thrombi.[10,20,29–32] A standard systematic examination should be performed using the parasternal, apical, and subcostal windows. Apical views, including those obtained with the transducer placed near, but not necessarily on, the point of maximal impulse while the patient is supine or in the left lateral decubitus position, are the most useful for thrombus evaluation; standard parasternal long- and short-axis projections generally do not visualize the apex. In addition to the standard apical two- and four-chamber views, multiple nonstandard periapical views are frequently helpful and should be attempted before concluding that a thrombus is not present. Nonstandard views which may be useful include views intermediate between the apical two-chamber and four-chamber views, short-axis views obtained from the apex (ie, apical short-axis views) and views obtained by inferior and medial transducer angulation from the standard apical two-chamber view. Commonly, such views more convincingly demonstrate a thrombus than the standard orientations, as shown in Figure 15-1. Thus, a thorough echocardiographic exploration of the apex is necessary. The use of multiple gain and reject settings is helpful when evaluating an area for possible thrombus. Multiple settings aid in distinguishing artifacts, which are often present at the apex, from thrombus, as well as helping to optimally define the endocardium, epicardium, and pericardium. In addition, shallow depth-of-field settings or the use of higher frequency transducers are occasionally useful in defining apical thrombi. Careful attention should be taken to record wall motion in the area of a suspected thrombus, since thrombi rarely occur in regions of normal wall motion. Typically, thrombi are located in akinetic

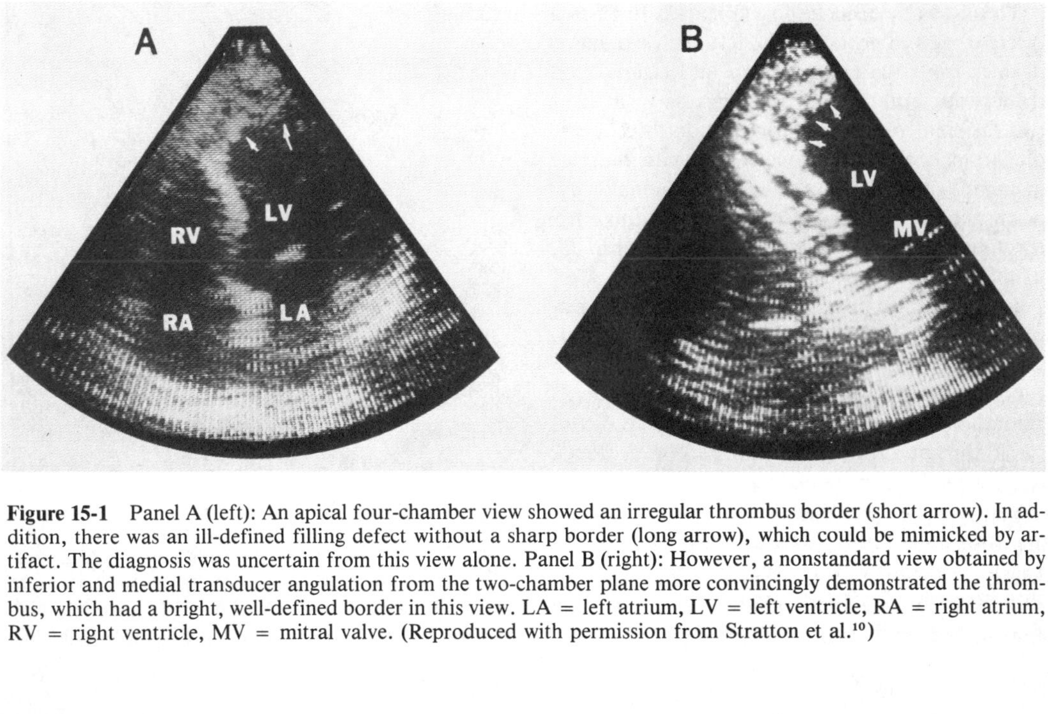

Figure 15-1 Panel A (left): An apical four-chamber view showed an irregular thrombus border (short arrow). In addition, there was an ill-defined filling defect without a sharp border (long arrow), which could be mimicked by artifact. The diagnosis was uncertain from this view alone. Panel B (right): However, a nonstandard view obtained by inferior and medial transducer angulation from the two-chamber plane more convincingly demonstrated the thrombus, which had a bright, well-defined border in this view. LA = left atrium, LV = left ventricle, RA = right atrium, RV = right ventricle, MV = mitral valve. (Reproduced with permission from Stratton et al.[10])

or dyskinetic areas. Frequently the underlying myocardium appears thinned or scarred. In this context, the finding of apparently normal or increased wall thickness in an aneurysmal segment should raise the suspicion of a mural left ventricular thrombus.[33]

Despite close attention to echocardiographic imaging details, technically adequate examinations are not always obtainable. Approximately 10% to 20% of patients have technically inadequate examinations for thrombus assessment. In our experience we have not found a clear superiority for thrombus imaging between phased array and mechanical sector scanners. Both types of instruments are adequate for thrombus assessment.

ECHOCARDIOGRAPHIC FEATURES

The differentiation of a thombus from other apparent intraventricular masses which may be artifactual is often difficult. From studies in which there has been independent confirmation of the presence or absence of ventricular thrombus, several echocardiographic features have been noted that help to distinguish true positive echocardiographic studies (ie, thrombus independently proved) from false-positive studies. The characteristics of true-positive and false-positive studies will be reviewed.

Features of True-Positive Echocardiograms

Thrombus by echocardiography is defined as a discrete mass of echoes in the left ventricle that is distinct from the endocardium and clearly seen throughout both systole and diastole in at least two different (not necessarily standard) echocardiographic views. Additionally, the mass must be in an area of asynergy (akinesia, dyskinesia or hypokinesia). Equivocal echocardiograms for thrombus are those which meet some, but not all, of these criteria.

In evaluating a possible mass by echocardiography, it is useful to consider its location, border, reflectance, approximate size, and motion. In echocardiographic studies of patients with proven thrombus, several features have helped to distinguish thrombi from other masses or artifacts. Most thrombi (approximately 90%) are located at the apex and all are attached to the endocardium (Figures 15-2–15-4). Nearly all thrombi have bright, well-delineated free margins (ie, the thrombus-blood interface), in at least some views. A clear delineation of thrombus from ventricular blood is essential for the diagnosis of thrombus. The thrombus-blood interface is frequently smooth, although some thrombi have shaggy, irregular borders. Approximately one half to two thirds of thrombi are mural and relatively flat while the remainder protrude into the ventricular cavity. Some thrombi are multilobulated. The echo reflectance or density of thrombi varies from patient to patient, possibly related to thrombus age or activity. Most thrombi have a homogeneous, grainy appearance similar to or slightly denser than that of normal myocardium. In some patients, the thrombus is clearly more echo-dense than normal myocardium. Rarely, central areas of lucency can be seen within the thrombus[20,33]; the significance or histologic correlate of these echolucent areas is unknown. In addition, a few thrombi exhibit a layered appearance in which the most echo-dense layer is usually adjacent to the left ventricular cavity. We found an estimation of the thrombus size as small (< 1 cm in greatest dimension), medium (1–2 cm), or large (> 2 cm) helpful, since all but one of our true-positive studies appeared greater than 1.0 cm in size, in contrast to most studies which we interpreted falsely as positive.[10] Similarly, Asinger et al also noted that the smallest thickness of a definite thrombus on echocardiography was 1.0 cm.[33] Very large thrombi (> 2 cm in diameter) may be more common in patients with idiopathic dilated cardiomyopathy and left ventricular thrombi (11 of 17 patients, 65%) than in patients with prior myocardial infarction and thrombi (7 of 42 patients, 17%).[20]

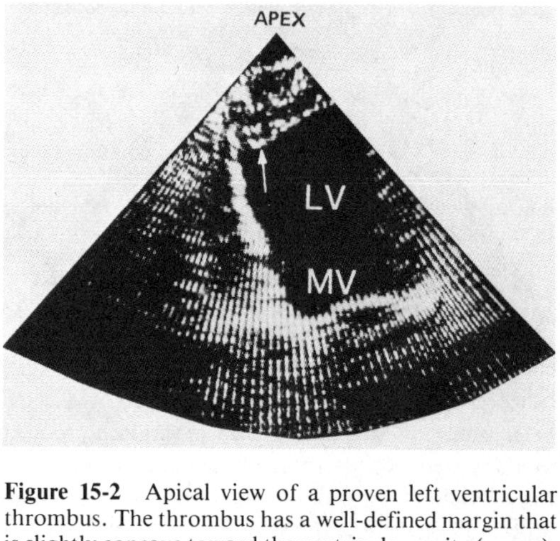

Figure 15-2 Apical view of a proven left ventricular thrombus. The thrombus has a well-defined margin that is slightly concave toward the ventricular cavity (arrow). The thrombus measures greater than 2 cm in its largest dimension. LV = left ventricle, MV = mitral valve. (Reproduced with permission from Stratton et al.[9])

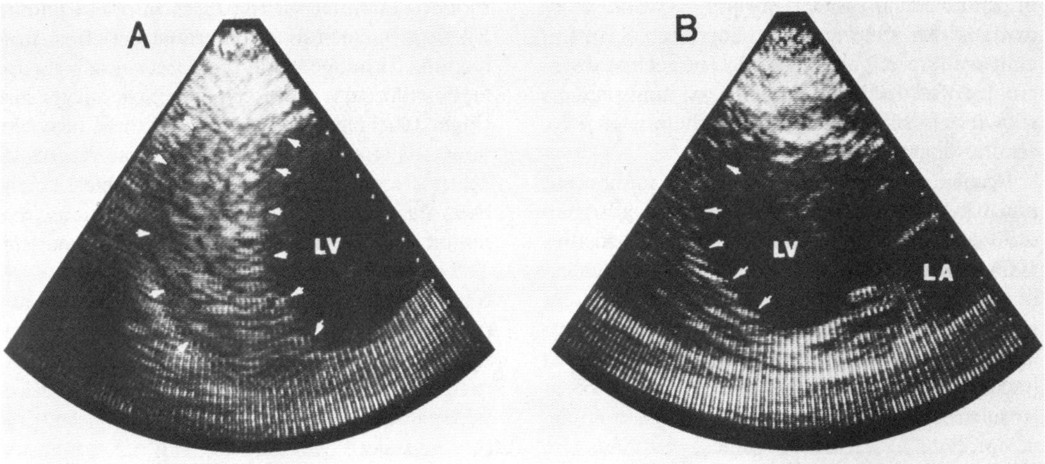

Figure 15-3 A very large thrombus is seen in the parasternal long axis views of the cardiac apex (panel A) and base (panel B). The thrombus has a homogeneous, grainy consistency similar to normal myocardium. The thrombus border is smooth, well-defined (arrows), and concave toward the ventricular cavity in contrast to most false-positive studies, which have convex borders that bulge into the ventricle. Most thrombi have at least some areas where the border is concave. LA = left atrium, LV = left ventricle. (Reproduced with permission from Stratton et al.[10])

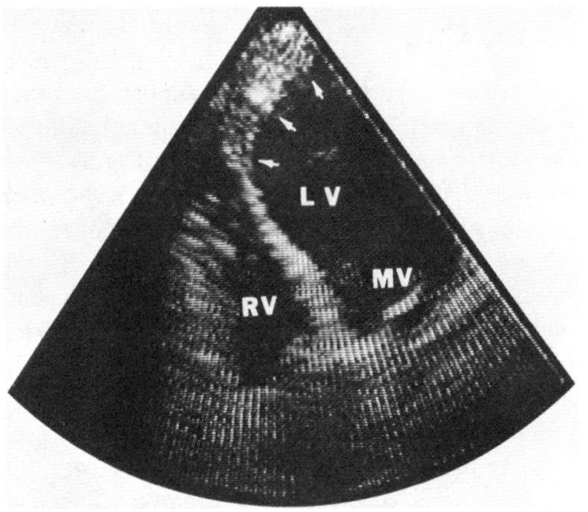

Figure 15-4 This apical thrombus has a discrete, bright border and was approximately 3 cm in its greatest dimension. LV = left ventricle, MV = mitral valve, RV = right ventricle. (Reproduced with permission from Stratton et al.[10])

Most thrombi do not exhibit motion different from that of the adjacent myocardial wall; however, some thrombi (approximately 15%) do have areas of free intracavitary random motion that are asynchronous with the ventricular wall.[10,33] In a preliminary report, such motion has been noted to correlate with systemic embolization.[34] In addition to motion of the thrombus itself, Mikell et al[35] have noted a pattern of slowly, circularly moving intracavitary echoes of varying amplitude and density at the apex, typically in patients who also had thrombi. These echoes lacked a well-defined border and were distinct from left ventricular thrombi.[35] In dogs with experimentally induced myocardial infarctions, Mikell et al demonstrated that these dynamic echoes were probably due to regional stasis of blood, not frank thrombosis. The significance of these echoes is unclear, except that they were typically associated with ventricular thrombi (in seven of nine patients) and were uniformly associated with severe underlying wall-motion abnormalities.

Features of False-Positive Echocardiograms

One or more of the features suggestive of possible ventricular thrombus noted above are relatively common in patients with diffuse or regional wall motion abnormalities but without thrombus. Thus, it is frequently difficult to distinguish true-positive echocardiograms, in which the apparent mass is in fact a thrombus, from false-positive echocardiograms, in which the apparent mass is caused by some other intracardiac structure or artifact. There are several echocardiographic and anatomic causes of intracavitary masses of echoes. These causes include echocardiographic artifact, aneurysmal shelves, chordal structures, and prominent papillary muscles and muscular trabeculae, particularly in hypertrophied ventricles. Another potential cause of a false-positive study is anatomical alterations resulting from prior ventricular surgery. Awareness of these potential pitfalls may improve diagnostic accuracy. Unfortunately, no clinical (nonechocardiographic) feature is reliable in separating patients with true-positive from those with false-positive echocardiographic studies.

Detailed review of false-positive studies has identified several characteristics that may help to distinguish true thrombi from falsely positive masses. In false-positive studies, the border between the apparent thrombus and the ventricular cavity often does not appear as bright or discrete as in true-positive studies. In addition, estimated thrombus size in false-positive studies is often smaller than in true-positive studies. For example, in our eight false-positive studies, thrombus size was rated as small (< 1.0 cm in largest dimension) in half of the misdiagnosed studies and medium (1–2 cm) in the remainder. In our experience, most of the echocardiograms (four of five) interpreted as showing small thrombi were falsely positive. Visser et al have also noted that false positive studies appeared as small, poorly defined masses.[39] Echocardiographic artifacts probably account for most false-positive studies. These artifacts apparently represent reverberations from the transducer itself, from the chest wall, or from dense, highly reflectant apical myocardial scar. Such artifacts can appear as convincing apical intraventricular masses. However, the borders of many artifacts are often convex or bulging into the ventricular cavity in contrast to true-positive studies, which usually have at least a portion of thrombus that is concave toward the blood pool. Also, a few artifacts have multiple bright radial lines, which in part simulate the bright borders of most proven thrombi. When artifactual lines or masses of echoes project beyond the myocardium they are easily distinguishable from thrombus, but when they appear completely within the ventricle, as in patients with enlarged hearts, distinguishing artifact from thrombus can be difficult or impossible. Another feature of some artifacts is their inconsistent size or shape from one echocardiographic view to another. In some false-positive studies, the mass of artifacts appear large in one view but markedly smaller in another view. Such inconsistency in thrombus size or appearance when the same area of the ventricle is imaged from different orientations is not observed in true-positive studies, and may be an important clue that intracavitary echoes are artifactual.

Misinterpretation of the echocardiogram may also be due to alterations in ventricular anatomy caused by cardiac surgery or by normal anatomical variants such as heavy trabeculation or false tendons. Prominent trabeculation (usually associated with ventricular hypertrophy) may cause bright echo masses in the apex as may false tendons. False tendons, which are also known as heart strings, are thin structures which course from the apex to the septum, papillary muscle to septum, or papillary muscle to papillary muscle. These tendons typically have a sharply delineated echo-bright border. When false tendons or heavy trabeculation occur in areas of hypokinesis or akinesis, they may simulate the margin of a ventricular thrombus as shown in Figure 15-5. Most false tendons and heavy trabeculae have echo-free spaces on both sides of the structure, and thus do not closely mimic the appearance of a thrombus. However, artifactual filling-in of the space between the tendon or trabeculation and the endocardium can at times resemble a thrombus (Figure 15-5).

DIAGNOSTIC ACCURACY OF ECHOCARDIOGRAPHY

As shown in Table 15-2, the diagnostic accuracy of the two-dimensional echocardiographic detection of thrombus is high. In reported series[10,31,32] the sensitivity has ranged from 77% to 92%; when the cases from the three studies are pooled, the sensitivity is 87% (53 of 61). The specificity has been similarly high, ranging from 88% to 96% with a pooled value from all three studies of 93% (115 of 123). Thus, echocardiography can be reliably utilized to detect thrombi. In considering an individual patient, it is more useful to examine the positive (or negative) predictive value of a test, ie, the percentage of positive (or negative) diagnoses that are correct. For the echocardiographic detection of left ventricular thrombi, the predictive value of a positive test is 85% (ranging from 83% to 86% in three studies) and the predictive value of a negative test is 93% (range 90% to 95%). The agreement between experienced observers for the diagnosis of the presence or absence of thrombus in these three studies was high. The observer agreement was 93% (40 cases, two observers),[32] 93% (67 cases, two observers)[31] and 88% (78 cases, three observers).[10]

These figures for the diagnostic accuracy of echocardiography were obtained in patient groups with a high prevalence (approximately 33%) of ventricular thrombi. When echocardiography is applied to a patient population with a lower prev-

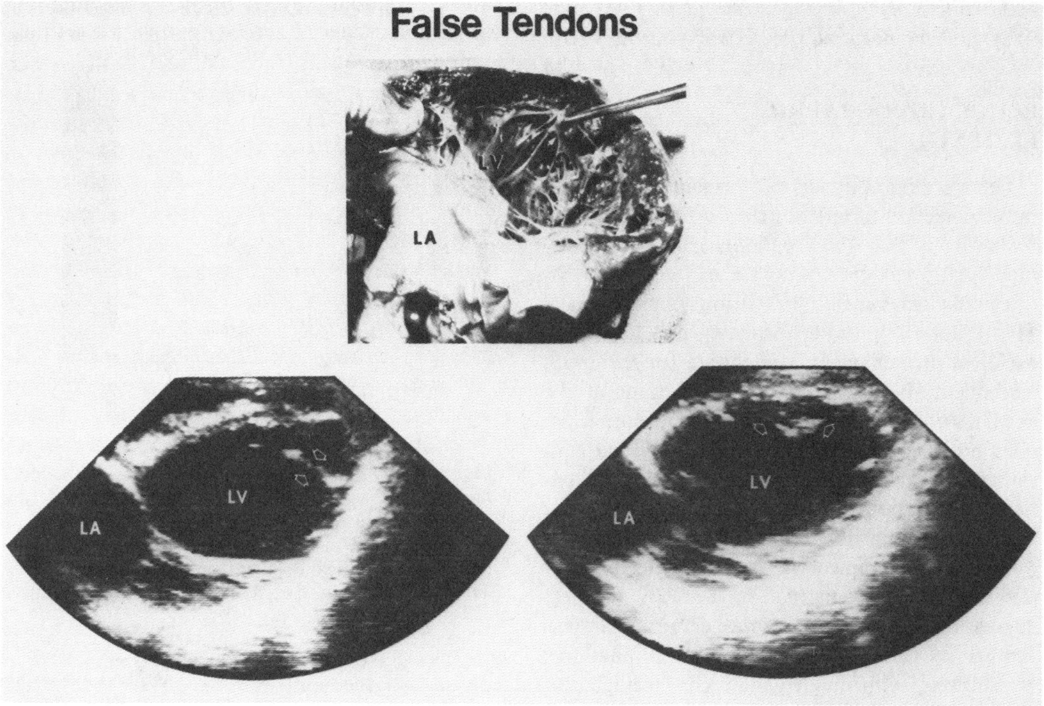

Figure 15-5 False tendons. In the top panel a lengthy false tendon is present (arrow) as well as several shorter ones. In addition, many prominent trabeculae are present. In an echocardiogram obtained shortly before death there was artifactual filling-in of the space between the tendon and endocardium (lower right), which resembled a thrombus. At autopsy, only prominent trabeculae and false tendons, but no thrombus, were present. Echocardiograms courtesy of Mr. Eric J. Sisk.

alence of thrombi, it would be anticipated that the results would be less favorable, particularly for the positive predictive value. Similarly accurate results have been obtained with both mechanical sector scanners[10,31] and with phased array scanners,[10,32] indicating that both types of instruments appear highly suitable for the diagnosis of thrombus.

Although the diagnostic accuracy of echocardiography for left ventricular thrombi is high, the accuracy for left atrial thrombus detection is less satisfactory, largely because approximately 20% of left atrial thrombi are isolated to the atrial appendage, which frequently cannot be imaged. The sensitivity of echocardiography for left atrial thrombus detection is only 59%, while the

Table 15-2
Sensitivity, Specificity, and Predictive Value of Two-Dimensional Echocardiographic Detection of Left Ventricular Thrombi†

	Patients with Thrombi	Patients without Thrombi	Sensitivity	Specificity	Predictive Value of a Positive Test	Predictive Value of a Negative Test
Visser et al[31]	26	41	92% (24/26)	88% (36/41)	83% (24/29)	95% (36/38)
Ezekowitz et al[32]*	13	27	77% (10/13)	96% (26/27)	91% (10/11)	90% (26/29)
Stratton et al[10]*	22	56	86% (19/22)	95% (53/56)	86% (19/22)	95% (53/56)
Overall[10,31,32]	61	124	87% (53/61)	93% (115/124)	85% (53/62)	93% (115/123)

*For the results of Ezekowitz et al and Stratton et al, equivocal or possible studies were considered as negative. Visser et al did not classify any studies as equivocal.
†Sensitivity = true positives/(true positives + false negatives); specificity = true negatives/(true negatives + false positives).
Predictive value of a positive test = true positives/[all positives (true + false)].
Predictive value of a negative test = true negatives/[all negatives (true + false)].

specificity is 99%, the positive predictive value 91%, and the negative predictive value 92%.

ECHOCARDIOGRAPHIC LIMITATIONS

Echocardiography has two principal limitations in the detection of left ventricular thrombus. One limitation is that some patients have technically inadequate echocardiographic examinations for thrombus assessment. In various series, 6%,[33] 11%,[10] and 25%[32] of echocardiograms have been excluded as technically inadequate for thrombus assessment. Because most thrombi occur at the apex, a study that fails to demonstrate the apex well does not exclude thrombus and should be considered inadequate. However, in a study of 200 patients undergoing echocardiography for a wide variety of indications, Bansal et al[36] were able to obtain adequate apical views in a higher proportion (99%) of patients than in the above studies, suggesting that persistence may decrease the percentage of technically inadequate examinations. In subjects with inadequate echocardiographic studies, one of the alternative noninvasive diagnostic technics discussed below may be useful.

The second principal limitation of the echocardiographic diagnosis of thrombus is the relatively high percentage (9% to 33%) of falsely positive echocardiograms.[10,20,31,32] The percentage of falsely positive echocardiograms is highly dependent on whether equivocal or possible studies (ie, studies in which there is diagnostic uncertainty) are considered as negative or positive for thrombus. If equivocal or possible studies are considered as negative for thrombus, the percentage of falsely positive studies is relatively low (9% to 14%).[10,32] In contrast, if equivocal or possible studies are considered as positive for thrombus, the percentage of falsely positive studies increases greatly (28% to 33%), since nearly all (9 of 11) such studies have been in patients without documented thrombus. The difference between the predictive value of an equivocal study (29%), a positive study (86%, $P < 0.001$ vs equivocal studies), and a negative study (95%)[10] is shown graphically in Figure 15-6. Thus, to minimize diagnostic errors, equivocal or possible studies should be considered as negative.

As noted above, the agreement between trained observers is high. However, in the few cases in which experienced observers disagreed, diagnostic accuracy was poor. Studies in which observers disagreed were much more likely to be falsely positive (6 of 8, 75%) than studies in which there was

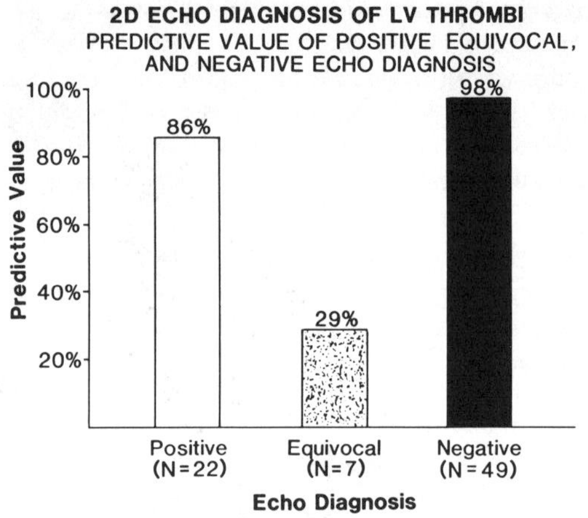

Figure 15-6 The predictive value of a positive echocardiographic diagnosis (86%) or a negative echocardiographic diagnosis (98%) is high. In contrast, an equivocal diagnosis, if considered as indicating thrombus, has a significantly lower predictive value (29%).[10] Thus, equivocal studies should be considered negative.

observer agreement (2 of 20, 10%) ($P < 0.01$).[10] Thus, in difficult cases, if multiple experienced observers disagree, the study should probably be interpreted as negative.

Close attention to several echocardiographic details, including the size, shape, and margin of the mass may also help minimize false-positive diagnoses. As previously noted, false-positive masses tend to be small (< 1.0 cm in the largest dimension) and have less clearly demarcated borders which are frequently convex with respect to the ventricular cavity. In addition, false-positive masses frequently are inconsistent in size and appearance from view to view. True echocardiographic targets are generally constant and reproducible when the same region of the ventricle is imaged. Although attention to these guidelines may be useful in decreasing false-positive studies, no criteria are foolproof. Visser et al[31] also noted that false-positive studies decreased as the experience of the echocardiographer increased. In the future, further development of echocardiographic tissue characterization may help to distinguish thrombus from artifact or nonthrombotic masses. False-negative studies are uncommon. The principal means of minimizing false-negative studies is by obtaining complete echocardiographic examinations at multiple gain and reject settings in patients with suspected thrombi.

A last potential source of diagnostic error is that a ventricular mass may be due to a cardiac tumor, not a thrombus. Since standard echocardiography cannot readily distinguish tissues of different histologies, tumors and thrombi can be confused. However, cardiac tumors are very rare and frequently do not have associated significant wall-motion abnormalities, as opposed to virtually all thrombi.

COMPARISON OF ECHOCARDIOGRAPHY WITH OTHER DIAGNOSTIC METHODS

Other diagnostic modalities which are capable of detecting left ventricular thrombi include x-ray CT scanning,[37,38] equilibrium radionuclide angiography,[19,40] and contrast left ventriculography,[4,17,31] all of which can define the anatomic defect created by a thrombus. In addition, thrombus can be diagnosed by the external imaging of radiolabeled blood components which are incorporated into thrombi, as with indium 111 platelet imaging.[9,32,39] Although CT scanning can detect thrombi, the sensitivity and specificity are not currently defined. The diagnostic accuracies of two-dimensional echocardiography, indium 111 platelet imaging, radionuclide ventriculography, and contrast ventriculography are compared in Table 15-3. Contrast left ventriculography and equilibrium radionuclide ventriculography are clearly inferior to the other methods. In several reported series, the sensitivity of contrast ventriculography for the detection of ventricular thrombi has been low, ranging from 20% to 50%.[4,17,31] In the largest series of 100 patients, the sensitivity was 31%, specificity 75%, the positive predictive value 54%, and the negative predictive value 54%.[17] Equilibrium radionuclide angiography also has a relatively low diagnostic accuracy, in part because of its intrinsically poorer resolution compared to echocardiography. Although radionuclide angiography can detect thrombi, diagnostic certainty is greater with two-dimensional echocardiography. In one small study in which the two technics were directly compared in eight patients with proven thrombus and five patients without, echocardiography was correct in all cases while radionuclide angiography failed to detect two patients with thrombi.[19] In a study of 70 patients, 22 of whom had thrombi, the sensitivity of the radionuclide angiographic diagnosis of thrombus was only 55%, the specificity 94%, the positive predictive value 80%, and the negative predictive value 82%.[40]

Indium 111 platelet imaging detects left ventricular thrombi by imaging labeled platelet deposition on the thrombus surface with conventional gamma cameras.[9,32] Platelet imaging is positive only if ongoing thrombosis is occurring. It has the potential advantage over echocardiography and the other technics of being able to define thrombus activity, ie, the extent of platelet incorporation into the thrombus. Presumably, fresh and hematologically active thrombi are more likely to embolize. The sensitivity (71%) of platelet imaging is lower than that of echocardiography, presumably because some chronic thrombi are hematologically inactive or endothelialized or because platelet uptake on some thrombi is present but of inadequate magnitude for external detection. However, the specificity appears to be excellent at 100% (ie, there appear to be no false-positive diagnoses).[9,32] Platelet imaging may be particularly useful in the

Table 15-3
Comparative Diagnostic Accuracies of Echocardiography, Indium 111 Platelet Imaging, Equilibrium Radionuclide Ventriculography, and Contrast Ventriculography for Detection of Left Ventricular Thrombi

	Patients with Thrombi	Patients without Thrombi	Sensitivity	Specificity	Predictive Value of a Positive Test	Predictive Value of a Negative Test
Two-dimensional echocardiography[10,31,32]*	61	124	87%	93%	85%	93%
Indium 111 platelet imaging[32]	14	38	71%	100%	100%	90%
Radionuclide ventriculography[19,40]	22	48	55%	94%	80%	82%
Contrast ventriculography[17]	48	52	31%	75%	54%	54%

*Results of three studies pooled.

patient who has a technically inadequate or equivocal echocardiogram. In one study, four patients with falsely positive echocardiograms also had platelet imaging, which was correctly negative in all cases.[10] Additionally, platelet imaging may prove superior to echocardiography for the detection of left atrial thrombi, 40% of which are missed by echocardiography. However, as currently performed, platelet labeling and imaging is costly, time-consuming and is not widely available.

Two-dimensional echocardiography has clear advantages over these other modalities for left ventricular thrombus detection since it involves no radiation exposure, is relatively rapid, can be used at the bedside, has acceptable diagnostic accuracy, is widely available, and often gives valuable additional information. Thus, two-dimensional echocardiography is the initial procedure of choice for determining the presence or absence of left ventricular thrombus.

NATURAL HISTORY, DRUG EFFECTS, AND EMBOLIC POTENTIAL

There are many unanswered clinical questions regarding the natural history and optimal therapy of patients with left ventricular thrombi. The recent development of echocardiography and other noninvasive diagnostic technics facilitates studies designed to answer these questions. This section will briefly review available data regarding the natural history, embolic potential, and therapy of patients with documented left ventricular thrombi.

The natural history of left ventricular thrombi, ie, the frequency with which they resolve or progress, has not been precisely determined, since there are no reports of the long-term follow-up of a large number of patients with either acute or chronic thrombi. Studies to date have largely been preliminary and have involved small numbers of patients with thrombi. Most thrombi due to myocardial infarction form during the first one to two weeks following infarction. In 12 patients with acute myocardial infarction who developed thrombi in one study, the mean time of thrombus detection was five days after admission (range one to 11 days); only one of the 12 patients had thrombus at the initial study performed within 72 hours of hospital admission.[11] In another study of 18 patients who developed thrombi, 83% (15 of 18) occurred within the first three days after hospital admission; however, an additional three patients developed thrombi at some point in the interval between three days following infarction and the time of their next examination at four months.[41] McEntee et al[42] serially studied 94 patients with acute infarction, initially at less than 48 hours following admission and again at 10 days. Seventeen patients developed thrombi; in seven patients thrombi were present at both the initial and late study, while the remaining 10 patients had thrombi only at the late study. Thus, in the setting of acute myocardial infarction some thrombi are not present within the first 48 to 72 hours after hospital admission, but nearly all are present by 10 days. The data are inconclusive as to whether thrombi ever develop following hospital discharge in such patients. It has been postulated that some newly formed thrombi may not be detectable because their tissue acoustic properties are not sufficiently different from flowing blood. However, animal data do not support this hypothesis. Echocardiography appears capable of detecting thrombi that form early in the course of acute infarction in humans.

When thrombi are detected in a patient with acute myocardial infarction, we consider them as acute thrombi; likewise, thrombi that are demonstrated in patients months to years following infarction are considered as chronic thrombi. Although definitive studies are lacking, the fate of thrombi appears to vary with their age. Some acute thrombi resolve spontaneously without anticoagulant therapy and without clinical evidence of embolization.[11,42] However, the frequency with which spontaneous resolution of acute thrombi occurs has not been determined accurately.

In contrast, complete resolution of chronic thrombi does not appear to occur spontaneously. We have serially studied 19 patients with definite chronic left ventricular thrombi. Patients had a mean of 3.4 ± 3.0 echocardiograms over 12 ± 7 months ($\pm$ SD). In these patients, resolution was seen only in two patients who received full-dose warfarin therapy and in one patient who had aneurysmectomy. In another series, no thrombus resolution occurred during follow-up in four nonanticoagulated patients with thrombi due to chronic cardiomyopathy.[40]

The frequency with which acute or chronic left ventricular thrombi cause clinically significant embolic events has not been determined prospectively in a large number of patients with myocardial infarction. In largely retrospective studies in which thrombus was diagnosed by contrast angiography, echocardiography, cardiac operation, or autopsy, the prevalence of clinically diagnosed emboli in patients with thrombi has been extremely variable, from 0% to 47%.[10-12,17,41-43] This variability is difficult to explain but may relate to differences in patient populations or diagnostic criteria for either thrombus or embolus, which were not defined in most studies. In autopsy series, the prevalence of pathologically proven emboli in patients with left ventricular thrombi has been consistently higher (approximately 30% to 40%) than in most clinical series, since many emboli are clinically silent.[13,15,18,21] As determined from autopsy studies, the most common sites of systemic embolization are the brain (15% to 30% of emboli), the kidneys (30% to 40%), the spleen (16% to 28%), and the limbs (10% to 15%).[6,18] In the setting of acute myocardial infarction, most emboli probably occur within the first two weeks. Thus, the embolic potential is probably greatest for recently formed thrombi. The risk of embolization in patients with chronic thrombi due to remote myocardial infarction is probably lower than in patients with acute thrombi. However, prospective studies are needed to determine the true incidence of clinically significant embolization in patients with documented left ventricular thrombi. Whether or not echocardiographic features can be used to define those patients at greatest risk of embolization from left ventricular thrombi is uncertain. Haugland et al[34] in a preliminary report suggested that thrombi with independent chaotic motion were more likely to embolize than thrombi without such motion.

Data regarding the proper therapy of patients with left ventricular thrombi due to acute myocardial infarction or those with thrombi due to remote infarction are scant. Serial echocardiographic studies have demonstrated the resolution of thrombi in small numbers of patients on full-dose warfarin or heparin.[11,41,43] Low-dose heparin did not prevent thrombus formation in four patients with acute myocardial infarction.[44] In the two randomized trials of full-dose anticoagulation in acute myocardial infarction in which autopsy data was reported, left ventricular mural thrombi occurred in 49% of the 53 control patients but in only 19% of the 59 treated patients, suggesting that inhibition of fibrinogen deposition by warfarin reduced thrombus formation or led to thrombus resolution.[45,46] No prospective trials assessing full-dose warfarin or heparin using the presence or absence of left ventricular thrombus as the endpoint have been reported in living patients. The randomized trials of full-dose anticoagulation in acute myocardial infarction also found a significant reduction in both stroke and all systemic embolic events in the anticoagulated groups, suggesting that a reduction in ventricular thrombus formation was beneficial (Table 15-4). Due to the risks of anticoagulation, we reserve full-dose heparin or warfarin therapy for the patients most likely to develop ventricular thrombus, ie, those with acute transmural anterior infarction. Since the elderly patient with this type of infarction may be at increased risk for the bleeding complications of anticoagulation, it may be reasonable to document the presence of a thrombus by echocardiography prior to the institution of anticoagulation. The optimal duration of therapy is unknown, but it may be reasonable to discontinue therapy after three months, since the thrombus may resolve or organize by that time. However, some thrombi will recur once anticoagulation is discontinued.[11] Further studies using two-dimensional echocardiography may help define the influence of anticoagulation on ventricular thrombus formation, resolution and embolization in the setting of acute infarction. In patients with chronic ventricular thrombi, the correct therapy is even less clear. The rare patient with an embolic event thought to be due to a chronic thrombus should be anticoagulated with heparin or warfarin. However, when the embolic event is cerebral, some authorities

Table 15-4
Clinically Diagnosed Systemic Emboli in Acute Myocardial Infarction: Randomized Anticoagulant Trials

Study	No. of Patients	Stroke (%)		All Systemic Emboli (%)	
		Control	*Anticoagulant*	*Control*	*Anticoagulant*
Wright et al[53]	800	3.4	1.4	6.4	2.4
V.A.[46]	999	3.8	0.8	5.6	0.8
Medical Research Council[52]	1427	2.5	1.1	3.4	1.3
Drapkin and Merskey[45]	1136	2.3	1.7	—	—

recommend delaying anticoagulation for about three days, because of the potential of causing intracranial bleeding.[47] In other patients with chronic thrombi due to past infarction, we do not use full-dose warfarin anticoagulation since the risks of anticoagulation may outweigh the embolic risk. Although platelet inhibitory agents may interrupt platelet deposition in some chronic left ventricular thrombi, it has not been determined if such agents can lead to thrombus resolution or a reduction in embolic events.[48]

Patients with left ventricular thrombi due to idiopathic dilated cardiomyopathy may be at a greater risk of embolization than patients with thrombi due to prior myocardial infarction,[49] and, such patients should probably be chronically anticoagulated. In addition, Fuster et al in a retrospective review of patients with idiopathic dilated cardiomyopathy (in whom the presence or absence of ventricular or atrial thrombi was unknown) found the incidence of systemic embolization to be 3.5% per year in 103 nonanticoagulated patients but 0% per year in 32 anticoagulated patients,[50] further strengthening the argument for chronic anticoagulation in patients with idiopathic dilated cardiomyopathy, regardless of the presence or absence of a left ventricular thrombus.

With the proven ability of echocardiography to detect left ventricular thrombi and other potential sources of systemic embolization, elderly patients with stroke syndromes are increasingly referred for echocardiographic examination to rule out an intracardiac source of embolus. In addition to left ventricular thrombus, other embolic sources detectable by echocardiography include left atrial thrombi, valvular vegetations, cardiac tumors, and possibly mitral valve prolapse. However, several series have now documented that the diagnostic yield in unselected patients is very low for finding any cardiac abnormality responsible for the cerebral event.[51] In particular, only nine of 408 unselected patients in three series had left ventricular thrombi as a potential cause of their cerebral ischemia. In addition, five patients had left atrial thrombi, six had vegetations, one had a tumor and eight had mitral valve prolapse. Thus, the routine use of echocardiography to look for an embolic source in unselected elderly patients with stroke syndromes is of extremely low yield, costly, and not justified. The group of patients in whom echocardiography may be beneficial are those with a reasonable clinical suspicion of vegetations, myxoma, mitral valve prolapse, prosthetic valve thrombus, or left atrial or left ventricular thrombus.[52]

SUMMARY AND CONCLUSIONS

Several clinical features define a group of patients who are at increased risk for having left ventricular thrombi. In particular, patients with transmural anterior myocardial infarction or advanced congestive cardiomyopathy are prone to left ventricular thrombus formation. Two-dimensional echocardiography can detect thrombi in such patients reliably; sensitivity and specificity both approximate 90%. Hence, echocardiography, which is widely available, radiation-free, and relatively rapid is the initial procedure of choice for the diagnosis of ventricular thrombus. Echocardiography has two main limitations in the detection of ventricular thrombi. One is that 10% to 20% of studies are technically inadequate for thrombus assessment. One of the alternative noninvasive diagnostic approaches, in particular indium 111 platelet imaging or CT scanning, may be helpful in such patients. The second main limitation is the relatively high percentage of false-positive studies (approximately 10% to 15%). Attention to several echocardiographic features may help minimize false-positive diagnoses. Echocardiograms appearing to have defects which are small (<1.0 cm in the largest dimension), have a variable appearance from one view to another, or which have indistinct or hazy borders should not be accepted as diagnostic for thrombus.

The natural history of ventricular thrombi has not been well defined. Currently, it is not known how frequently thrombi cause clinically significant embolic events. Patients with thrombi due to myocardial infarction are probably at greatest embolic risk in the acute period. The embolic risk in patients with chronically formed thrombi or in patients with thrombi due to congestive cardiomyopathy has not been determined. The optimal therapy for patients with ventricular thrombi in any of these groups is also not known. Tentative recommendations regarding anticoagulation are discussed above, but definitive data is lacking. Further studies using echocardiography and other noninvasive technics should answer the important remaining questions about the course and optimal treatment of patients with ventricular thrombi.

ACKNOWLEDGMENTS

This work was supported by the Research Service of the Veterans Administration. The author thanks Mrs. Maxine Cormier and Mrs. Patricia Jenkins for typing the manuscript and Dr. Alan S. Pearlman for his critical review.

REFERENCES

1. Oakley CM, Olsen EGJ: Eosinophilia and heart disease. *Br Heart J* 1977;39:233–237.
2. Baker KM, Hess CE, Ayers CR, et al: Left ventricular mural thrombus in a patient with thrombocytosis and agnogenic myeloid metaplasia. *Arch Intern Med* 1981;141:1527–1529.
3. Ali M, Fayemi AO, Malcolm D, et al: Intraventricular thrombosis in polycythemia vera: A cause of intractable cardiac failure. *Am Heart J* 1980;100: 520–522.
4. Segal JP, Stapleton JF, McClellan JR, et al: Idiopathic cardiomyopathy: Clinical features, prognosis and therapy. *Cur Probl Cardiol* 1978; 3(September):14–18.
5. Gottdiener J, Gay J, Van Voorhees L, et al: Frequency and embolic potential of left ventricular thrombus in dilated cardiomyopathy: Assessment by 2-dimensional echocardiography, abstracted. *Am J Cardiol* 1983;52:1281–1285.
6. Bean WB: Infarction of the heart: Clinical course and morphological findings. *Ann Intern Med* 1938;12:71–94.
7. Garvin CF: Mural thrombi in the heart. *Am Heart J* 1941;21:713–720.
8. Wartman WB, Hellerstein HK: The incidence of heart disease in 2,000 consecutive autopsies. *Ann Intern Med* 1948;28:41–64.
9. Stratton JR, Ritchie JL, Hamilton GW, et al: Left ventricular thrombi: In vivo detection by indium-111 platelet imaging and two dimensional echocardiography. *Am J Cardiol* 1981;47:874–881.
10. Stratton JR, Lighty GW, Pearlman AS, et al: Detection of left ventricular thrombus by two-dimensional echocardiography: Sensitivity, specificity and causes of uncertainty. *Circulation* 1982;66: 156–166.
11. Asinger RW, Mikell FL, Elsperger J, et al: Incidence of left-ventricular thrombosis after acute myocardial infarction. *N Engl J Med* 1981;305: 297–302.
12. Hamby RI, Wisoff BG, Davidson ET, et al: Coronary artery disease and left ventricular mural thrombi: Clinical, hemodynamic, and angiocardiographic aspects. *Chest* 1974;66:488–494.
13. Berman B, McGuire J: Cardiac aneurysm. *Am J Med* 1950;8:480–489.
14. Gorlin R, Klein MD, Sullivan JM: Prospective correlative study of ventricular aneurysm. *Am J Med* 1967;42:512–531.
15. Raphael MJ, Steiner RE, Goodwin JF, et al: Cine angiography of left ventricular aneurysms. *Clin Radiol* 1972;23:129–139.
16. Swan HJC, Magnuson PT, Buchbinder NA, et al: Aneurysm of the cardiac ventricle. *West J Med* 1978;129:26–40.
17. Reeder GS, Lengyel M, Tajik AJ, et al: Mural thrombus in left ventricular aneurysm: Incidence, role of angiography, and relation between anticoagulation and embolization. *Mayo Clin Proc* 1981; 56:77–81.
18. Miller RD, Jordan RA, Parker RI, et al: Thromboembolism in acute and in healed myocardial infarction. II. Systemic and pulmonary arterial occlusion. *Circulation* 1952;6:7–15.
19. Stratton JR, Ritchie JL, Hammermeister KE, et al: Detection of left ventricular thrombi with radionuclide angiography. *Am J Cardiol* 1981;48:565–571.
20. Reeder GS, Tajik AJ, Seward JB: Left ventricular mural thrombus: Two dimensional echocardiographic diagnosis. *Mayo Clin Proc* 1981;56:82–86.
21. Abrams DL, Edelist A, Luria MH, et al: Ventricular aneurysm: A reappraisal based on a study of sixty-five consecutive autopsied cases. *Circulation* 1963;27:164–169.
22. Thompson JE, Weston AS, Sigler L, et al: Arterial embolectomy after acute myocardial infarction. *Ann Surg* 1971;171:979–986.
23. Lary BG, de Takats G: Peripheral arterial embolism after myocardial infarction. *JAMA* 1954;155: 10–13.
24. Thompson JE, Sigler L, Raut PS, et al: Arterial embolectomy: A 20 year experience with 163 cases. *Surgery* 1970;67:212–220.
25. Schlant RC, Forman S, Stamler J, et al: The natural history of coronary heart disease: Prognostic factors after recovering from myocardial infarction in 2789 men. The 5-year findings of the Coronary Drug Project. *Circulation* 1982;66:401–414.
26. Horgan JH, Shiel FO'M, Goodman AC: Demonstration of left ventricular thrombus by conventional echocardiography. *J Clin Ultrasound* 1976;4: 287–288.
27. Kramer NE, Rathod R, Chawla KK, et al: Echocardiographic diagnosis of left ventricular mural thrombi occurring in cardiomyopathy. *Am Heart J* 1978;96:381–383.
28. Come PC, Markis JE, Vine HS, et al: Echocardiographic diagnosis of left ventricular thrombi. *Am Heart J* 1980;100:523–530.
29. Ports TA, Cogan J, Schiller NB, et al: Echocardiography of left ventricular masses. *Circulation* 1978;58:528–536.
30. DeMaria AN, Bommer W, Neumann A, et al: Left ventricular thrombi indentified by cross-sectional echocardiography. *Ann Intern Med* 1979;90:14–18.
31. Visser CA, Kan G, David GK, et al: Two-dimensional echocardiography in the diagnosis of left ventricular thrombus: A prospective study of 67 patients with anatomic validation. *Chest* 1983;83: 228–232.
32. Ezekowitz MD, Wilson DA, Smith EO, et al: Comparison of indium-111 platelet scintigraphy and two-dimensional echocardiography in the diagnosis of left ventricular thrombi. *N Engl J Med* 1982; 306:1509–1513.
33. Asinger RW, Mikell FL, Sharma B, et al: Observations on detecting left ventricular thrombus with two dimensional echocardiography: Emphasis on avoidance of false positive diagnosis. *Am J Cardiol* 1981;47:145–156.
34. Haugland JM, Asinger RW, Mikell FL, et al: Embolic potential of left ventricular thrombus (LVT) detected by two-dimensional echocardiography (2DE), abstracted. *Am J Cardiol* 1981;47:471.
35. Mikell FL, Asinger RW, Elsperger J, et al: Regional stasis of blood in the dysfunctional left ventricle: Echocardiographic detection and differentiation from early thrombosis. *Circulation* 1982;66:755–763.
36. Bansal RC, Tajik AJ, Seward JB, et al: Feasibility of detailed two-dimensional echocardiographic ex-

aminations in adults: Prospective study of 200 patients. *Mayo Clin Proc* 1980;55:291–308.
37. Nair CK, Sketch MH, Mahoney PD, et al: Detection of left ventricular thrombi by computerized tomography: A preliminary report. *Br Heart J* 1981;45:535–541.
38. Lackner K, Thurn P: Computed tomography of the heart: ECG-gated and continuous scans. *Radiology* 1981;140:413–420.
39. Ezekowitz MD, Leonard JC, Smith EO, et al: Identification of left ventricular thrombi in man using indium-111-labeled autologous platelets: A preliminary report. *Circulation* 1981;63:803–810.
40. Stratton JR: Identification of left ventricular thrombi by radionuclide angiography. *Primary Cardiology* 1984;10:133–147.
41. Visser CA, Kan G, Durrer D: Incidence and natural history of left ventricular thrombus during the first three days and four months after acute myocardial infarction, abstracted. *Circulation* 1981;64:IV- 94.
42. McEntee CW, Van Reet RE, Winters WL, et al: Incidence and natural history of mural thrombi in acute myocardial infarction by two-dimensional echocardiography, abstracted. *Circulation* 1981;64: IV–92.
43. Mikell FL, Asinger RW, Sharma B, et al: Serial evaluation of left ventricular thrombi (LVT) by two-dimensional echocardiography (2DE): Effect of anticoagulant therapy, abstracted. *Circulation* 1979;60:II–19.
44. Ezekowitz MD, Smith EO, Fahmy A, et al: The effect of subcutaneous heparin on the incorporation of indium-111 labeled platelets into mural left ventricular thrombi developed during the acute phase of myocardial infarction, abstracted. *J Nucl Med* 1982;23:P47.
45. Drapkin A, Merskey C: Anticoagulant therapy after myocardial infarction: Relation of therapeutic benefit to patient's age, sex, and severity of infarction. *JAMA* 1972;222:541–548.
46. VA Cooperative Clinical Study Group: Anticoagulants in acute myocardial infarction. *JAMA* 1973;225:724–730.
47. Genton E: Intracardiac thrombosis, in Colman RW, Hirsh J, Marder VJ, et al (eds): *Hemostasis and Thrombosis: Basic Principles and Clinical Practice*. Philadelphia, JB Lippincott Company, 1982, p 926.
48. Stratton JR, Ritchie JL: The effects of antithrombotic drugs in patients with left ventricular thrombi: Assessment with indium-111 platelet imaging and two-dimensional echocardiography. *Circulation* 1984;69:561–568.
49. Cabin HS, Roberts WC: Left ventricular aneurysm, intraaneurysmal thrombus and systemic embolus in coronary heart disease. *Chest* 1980;77:586–590.
50. Fuster V, Gersh BJ, Giuliani ER, et al: The natural history of idiopathic dilated cardiomyopathy. *Am J Cardiol* 1981;47:525–531.
51. Greenland P, Knopman DS, Mikell FL, et al: Is routine echocardiography useful in the evaluation of patients with stroke? *Ann Intern Med* 1981;95: 51–53.
52. Larson EB, Stratton JR, Pearlman AS: Selective use of two-dimensional echocardiography in stroke syndromes. *Ann Intern Med* 1981;95:112–114.
53. Report of the Working Party on Anticoagulant Therapy in Coronary Thrombosis to the Medical Research Council: Assessment of short-term anticoagulant administration after cardiac infarction. *Br Med J* 1969;1:335–342.
54. Wright IS, Marple CD, Beck DF: Report of the committee for the evaluation of anticoagulants in the treatment of coronary thrombosis with myocardial infarction. *Am Heart J* 1948;36:801–815.

CHAPTER 16
The Role of Computed Tomography of the Heart in the Elderly Patient

Bruce H. Brundage

During the past decade many exciting developments have occurred in the field of cardiovascular imaging. Echocardiography and nuclear medicine in particular have established themselves as useful noninvasive diagnostic technics. However, both suffer from less than ideal image resolution and the search for better methods has continued.

The development of x-ray transmission computed tomography (CT) created a revolution in the diagnostic approach to central nervous system disorders by reducing the number of invasive imaging studies by 40%. Continued progress in CT technology has now resulted in scan times of 1 to 5 seconds. These "fast" body scanners are capable of producing images of the heart and great vessels with sufficient resolution to be clinically applicable for the diagnosis of cardiovascular disease. Furthermore, most of the current uses for this technic involve diseases common to the elderly patient. Cardiac CT scanning is minimally invasive, thereby adding further to its utility in the older patient.

SCANNING METHODS

Blood and muscle have approximately the same density and therefore a similar CT attenuation number. Consequently, enhancement of the blood pool with iodinated contrast medium is necessary for differentiating most cardiovascular structures (Figure 16-1). The contrast medium is administered intravenously either by bolus injection or drip infusion during CT scanning.

Currently two scanning protocols are utilized for imaging cardiovascular structures. One addresses the rapid temporal changes associated with cardiac function and blood flow, and is known as dynamic scanning. With this protocol scanning is rapidly repeated at the same body level. The scanner used to produce the images in this chapter completes a 360° scan in 2.4 seconds and is able to repeat scans after a 1-second delay. With computer assistance, an overscan of 540° obtained in 3.5 seconds can be divided into two complete images each with overlapping, but also different information. Therefore 12 sequential images can be produced from a series of six overscans in 26 seconds. Coupling this particular scanning protocol with a 25 ml intravenous bolus of contrast medium, a "poor man's angiogram" can be produced (Figure 16-2). We have found this method to be particularly useful for evaluating cardiovascular problems related to blood flow, such as coronary bypass graft patency.

The other scanning protocol employed delineates the three-dimensional nature of cardiovascular anatomy and pathology. The region of interest is evaluated by scanning at 5-mm to 10-mm adjacent levels. Usually only one scan is needed at each level. For cardiac imaging with currently available scanners, 10-mm slices are best and 12 to 16 scanning levels usually will encompass all of the heart and great vessels (Figure 16-3). With this so-called conventional scanning methodology, contrast enhancement is best achieved by an intravenous drip infusion of approximately 1.5 ml/kg body weight of contrast medium administered over 5 to 10 minutes. The images are usually obtained at the end of the infusion period when the blood pool density has reached a fairly constant level. Some

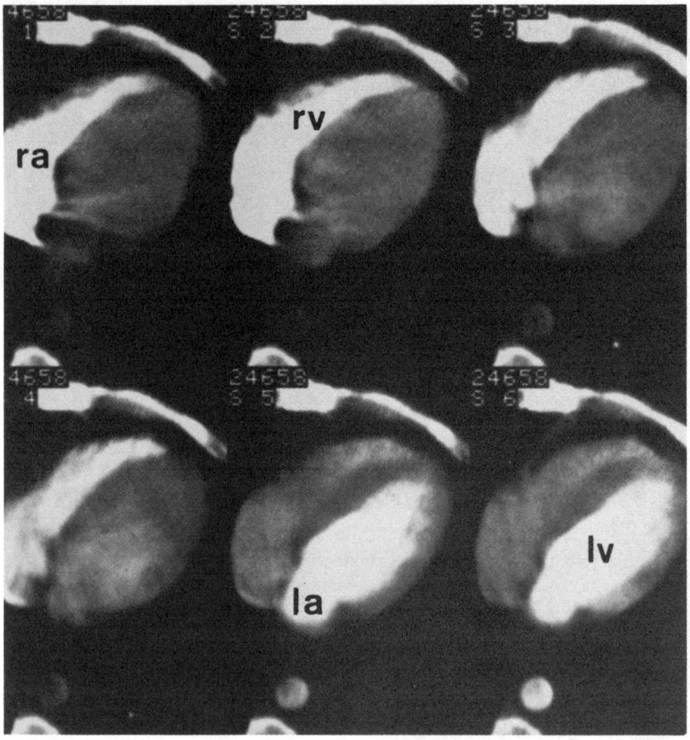

A

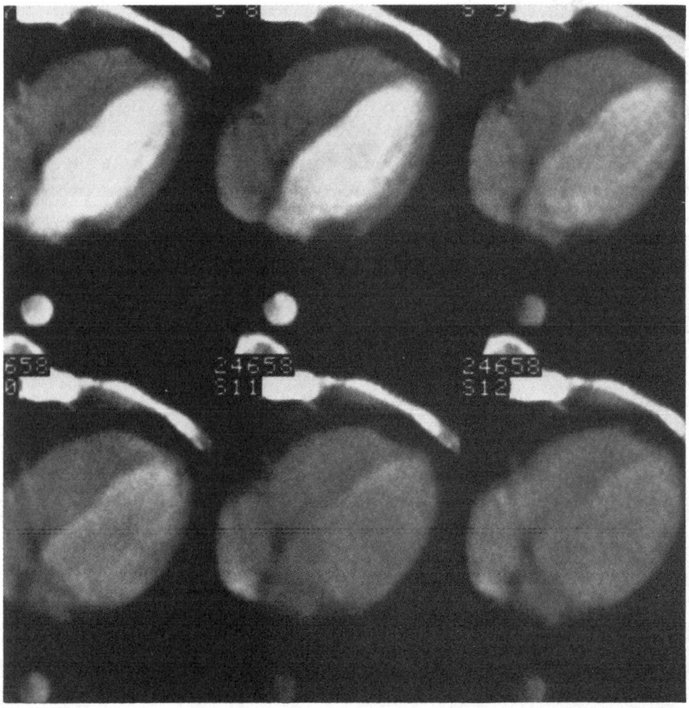

B

Figure 16-1A and B Cardiac anatomy is difficult to differentiate without contrast enhancement of the blood pool. During sequential contrast enhancement, the right atrium (ra), right ventricle (rv), left atrium (la), and left ventricle (lv) are easily distinguished. After contrast washout in the last two scans, cardiac anatomy is poorly recognized.

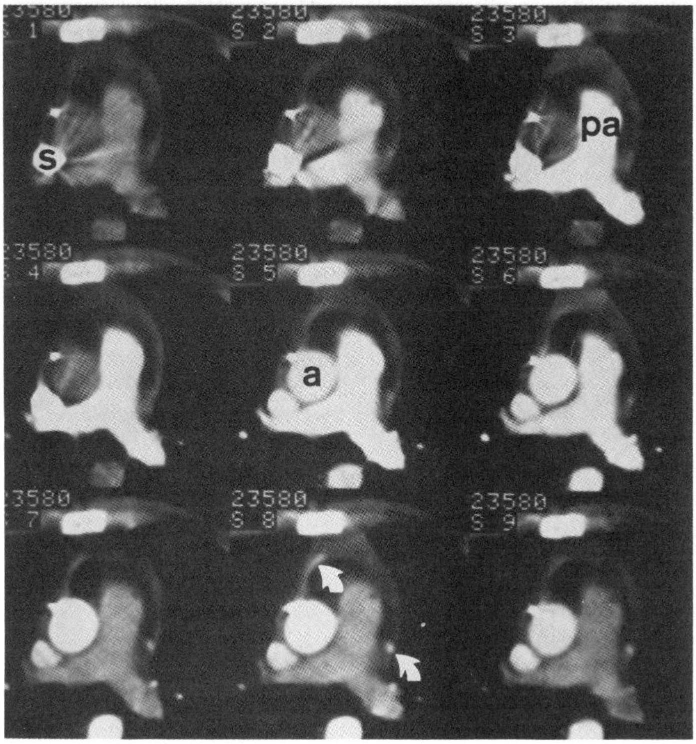

Figure 16-2 A series of nine sequential scans obtained during an intravenous bolus of contrast medium demonstrates patent coronary bypass grafts (arrows). s = superior vena cava, pa = pulmonary artery, a = aorta.

CT scanners have computer software that permits "stacking" of the individual adjacent scans so cardiovascular images can be reformatted along any desired longitudinal plane (Figure 16-4). Reformatting maximizes the ability of CT to define spatial relationships and enhances one's three-dimensional understanding of cardiovascular anatomy and pathology.

CONTRAST MEDIUM AND THE ELDERLY PATIENT

The usual dose of contrast medium needed for CT imaging is between 75 ml and 150 ml. This is significantly less than used in cardiac catheterization, but still can be a source of potential problems in the elderly patient. The dose of contrast should be kept to a minimum in patients with congestive heart failure because all contrast media are hyperosmotic and cause an increase in the circulating blood volume, and may exacerbate heart failure symptoms. Contrast medium produces negative inotropic effects on the myocardium, but when administered in small intravenous doses or by drip infusion this effect is probably not clinically significant.

The most worrisome effect of contrast medium in the elderly patient is impairment of renal function that on occasion can progress to overt renal failure. This complication is most likely to occur in patients with diabetes mellitus or pre-existing renal dysfunction. Fortunately this effect of contrast on renal function is usually self-limited. The state of a patient's renal function should be known prior to performing CT with contrast enhancement.

Allergic reactions to contrast medium are rare and no more frequent in the elderly patient than in other patient groups. Contrast medium should not be administered to patients with a known iodine allergy.

We have obtained contrast-enhanced CT scans on several hundred patients over the age of 65 without any serious complications. We have scanned many patients over the age of 80 without difficulty.

RADIATION DOSE

The radiation exposure obtained during CT scanning varies with the protocol employed. With the cardiovascular imaging sequences described, the x-ray exposure is limited to the region of the heart and great vessels with little scatter to adjacent areas. Typical radiation doses for cardiovascular CT are in the range of 3 to 10 rads,

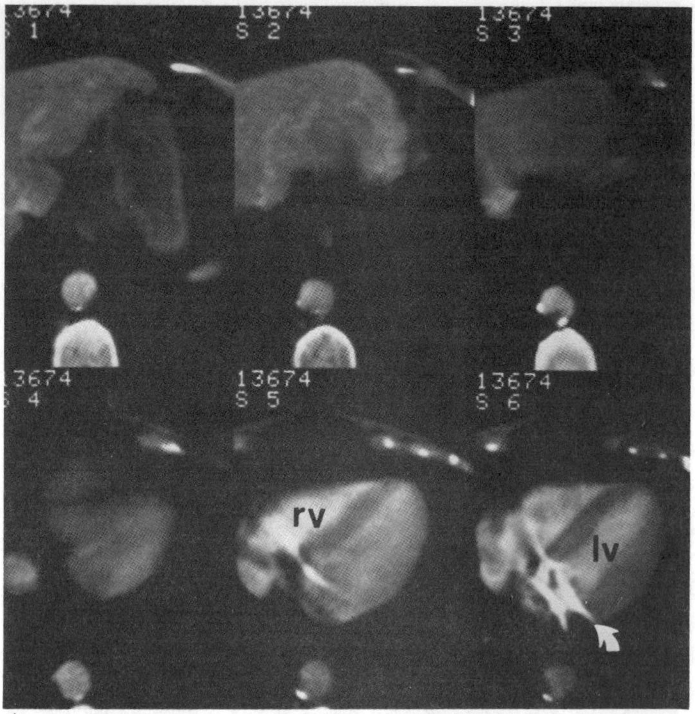

A

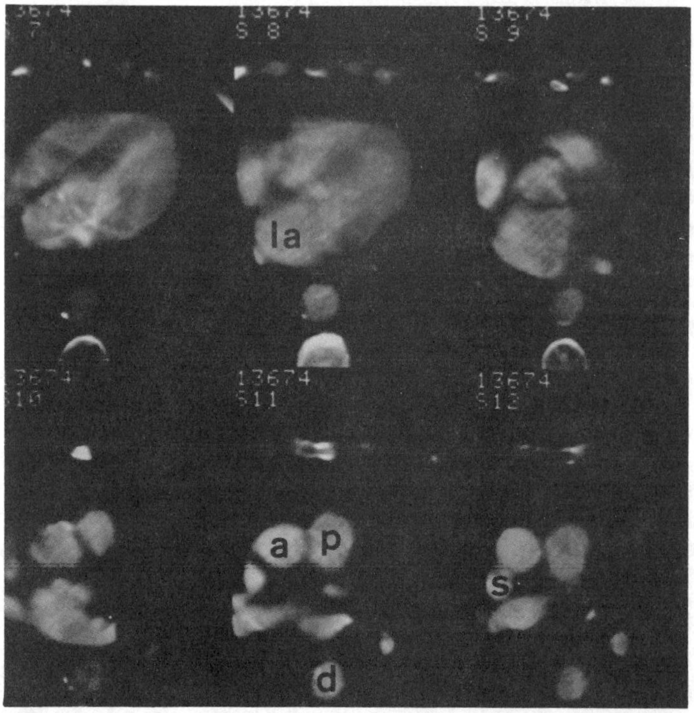

B

Figure 16-3A and B Twelve 1-cm adjacent transverse scans during contrast infusion define cardiac anatomy from the diaphragm to the base of the heart. Note the calcified mitral annulus (arrow). rv = right ventricle, lv = left ventricle, la = left atrium, a = ascending aorta, p = pulmonary artery, d = descending aorta, s = superior vena cava.

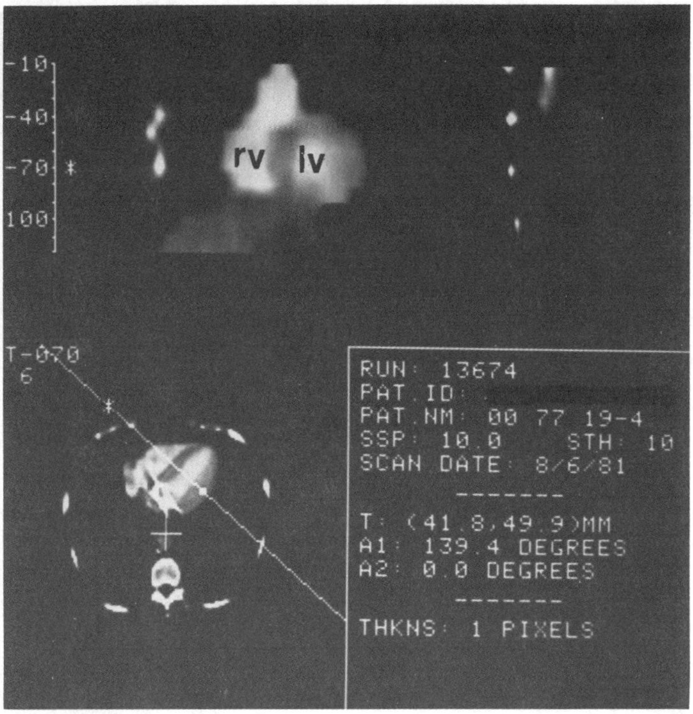

Figure 16-4 An oblique reconstruction of the scans in Figure 16-3 along the plane indicated by the dotted line. The hypertrophied interventricular septum is well visualized.

significantly less than the dose obtained from conventional cineangiographic studies. Furthermore, cinefluoroscopic technics produce a great deal more scatter and x-ray exposure to other parts of the body.

CURRENT CLINICAL APPLICATIONS OF CT

Coronary Bypass Grafts

In 1978, the first clinically useful cardiovascular application of contrast-enhanced CT was reported: the assessment of coronary artery bypass graft (CABG) patency.[1] Dynamic scanning during an intravenous bolus of 25 ml of contrast medium can be used to identify patent CABGs by characteristic contrast enhancement (Figure 16-2). When the aorta is maximally enhanced by the contrast bolus, patent grafts are well visualized but occluded CABGs do not enhance. With dynamic scanning, CT has a predictive accuracy (sensitivity and specificity) that exceeds 90%.[2] CABGs patency can also be evaluated by scanners without dynamic capability.[3,4] The accuracy is somewhat lower than with dynamic scanning, but the technic has proved to be clinically useful. Without dynamic capabilities a single scan is obtained prior to injecting the contrast bolus, followed by a second scan 12 to 15 seconds after the injection, the usual time of peak aortic enhancement. By comparing the two scans, patent grafts can usually be correctly identified.

Occasionally patent bypass grafts will not be identified by CT. The most frequent causes of a false-negative diagnosis include: inability to deliver a compact bolus of intravenous contrast, confusing grafts with native coronary arteries, excessive cardiac motion with resultant poor scan registration, obscuring artifacts produced by metal clips attached to the graft (Figure 16-5), and scanning an area not transversed by the graft. This latter problem can be avoided by obtaining a digital radiograph at the beginning of the study to locate the metal clip that usually identifies the graft's aortic anastomoses (Figure 16-6). By selecting a scanning level 2 to 3 cm below this clip, one ensures the x-ray beam will transect the graft.

Infrequently occluded grafts may be misinterpreted to be patent. Among the causes for false-positive diagnoses are the presence of a residual graft diverticulum, confusion with native coronary arteries, and calcification of an occluded graft. With experience, most false-positive and false-negative diagnoses of graft patency can be avoided.

Internal mammary artery bypass grafts can also be evaluated by CT. However, the multiple distal anastomoses of sequential or "skip" grafts cannot

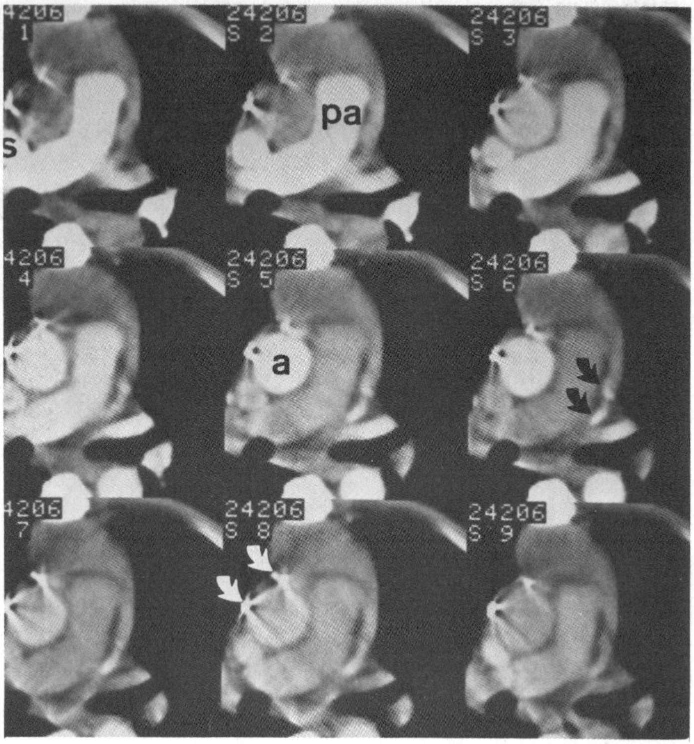

Figure 16-5 Dense artifacts produced by metal clips (white arrows) near a right coronary bypass graft make determination of patency by contrast-enhanced CT difficult. However, two left coronary bypass grafts well removed from the clips are easily seen (black arrows). s = superior vena cava, pa = pulmonary artery, a = aorta.

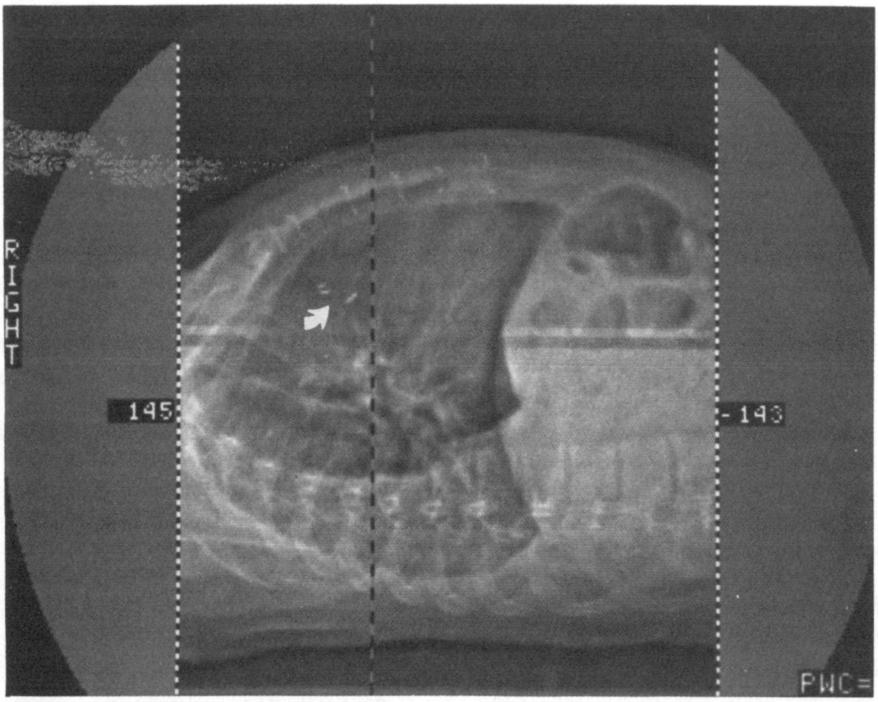

Figure 16-6 This digital radiograph of the chest identifies the position of three metal clips (arrow) marking the proximal anastomoses of three bypass grafts.

be completely assessed because the resolution of current scanners usually cannot define each individual anastomosis.

Experimentally and clinically we have shown that dynamic scanning can detect gross differences in graft flow. By plotting the changing graft density (CT number) against time, a characteristic indicator-dilution curve is produced. Prolongation of this curve when compared to a theoretical curve (gamma variate) indicates reduced graft flow, usually less than 40 to 50 ml/min.[5] Future scanners, able to scan two levels simultaneously, will measure absolute graft flow.

Successful evaluation of graft patency by CT has been performed in patients as early as 24 hours after surgery and as late as 10 years. This noninvasive evaluation of graft patency in the early postoperative period can be helpful in planning the management of patients with perioperative infarction, recurrent chest pain, arrhythmias, or myocardial dysfunction.[6] CT may also be a useful technic for screening postoperative patients for early graft occlusion that could be treated by thrombolysis, angioplasty, or reoperation.

Since 1970, almost 1 million people in the United States have had coronary bypass surgery. Currently nearly 200,000 operations are being performed yearly and an increasing percentage of these patients are over 70 years of age. Based on available studies, at least 30% of these patients will experience the reoccurrence of angina within five years due to graft occlusion or progression of native coronary disease.[7] Contrast-enhanced CT offers a minimally invasive method for the initial evaluation of graft patency in these patients and may save some from the more costly, complicated and dangerous cardiac catheterization.

Aortic Dissection

The management of patients with aortic dissection is very difficult. Many of these patients are elderly, often critically ill, and frequently the diagnosis is uncertain. Contrast-enhanced CT is proving to be a valuable diagnostic method for screening patients suspected of having an aortic dissection.[8] No invasive catheterization is required, only the intravenous drip infusion of approximately 100 ml of contrast medium over 10 minutes while obtaining 10 to 15 scans at adjacent 1-cm intervals. CT appears to be as accurate as invasive aortography in identifying dissection and is probably more safe in these often unstable patients. The cross-sectional image format of CT provides an excellent spatial representation of the intimal flap (Figure 16-7), the finding essential for making the correct diagnosis and one sometimes missed by conventional aortography. By scanning the entire length of the thoracic aorta, ascending and descending aortic dissections can be differentiated. Currently popular surgical technics usually do not attempt to obliterate the dissection's false lumen and focus on repairing only the dissection's entry point. Therefore, in some cases contrast-enhanced CT may be the only diagnostic test required prior to surgery. However, if information regarding the patency of major aortic branches or the degree of aortic regurgitation is necessary, then cineaortography is required.

Computed tomography is also a valuable method for long-term follow-up of aortic dissections whether the patients are treated medically or surgically.

Aortic Aneurysms

Body CT scanners in use today provide excellent images of thoracic and abdominal aortic aneurysms because these structures move very little during scanning compared to the heart. The superb density resolution of CT with contrast enhancement permits easy differentiation of vessel wall, calcification, thrombus, and lumen (Figure 16-8). CT can be used as an adjunct to ultrasound in screening for aortic aneurysms, particularly when the physician has difficulty differentiating between aortic ectasia and true aneurysm formation. This problem is common in the elderly patient and CT offers a new diagnostic approach to this sometimes confusing dilemma.

Cardiovascular Thrombus

As already emphasized, the density resolution of CT makes it an ideal technic for identifying the large thrombi often associated with aortic dissection and aneurysm. CT has also been found to be useful for the detection of thrombus formation in the cardiac chambers. Using contrast enhancement, Tomoda et al were able to accurately diagnose left atrial thrombosis preoperatively in patients having mitral valve replacement.[9] We have demonstrated CT to be equally sensitive to echocardiography, and possibly more specific in diagnosing left ventricular thrombosis.[10] CT has also been useful in following the resolution of thrombus while the patient is receiving anticoagulants (Figure 16-9).

Pedunculated cardiac thrombi that move rapidly during cardiac contraction, however, may be missed by current CT scanners.

Recently we demonstrated that contrast-enhanced CT can be a valuable method for

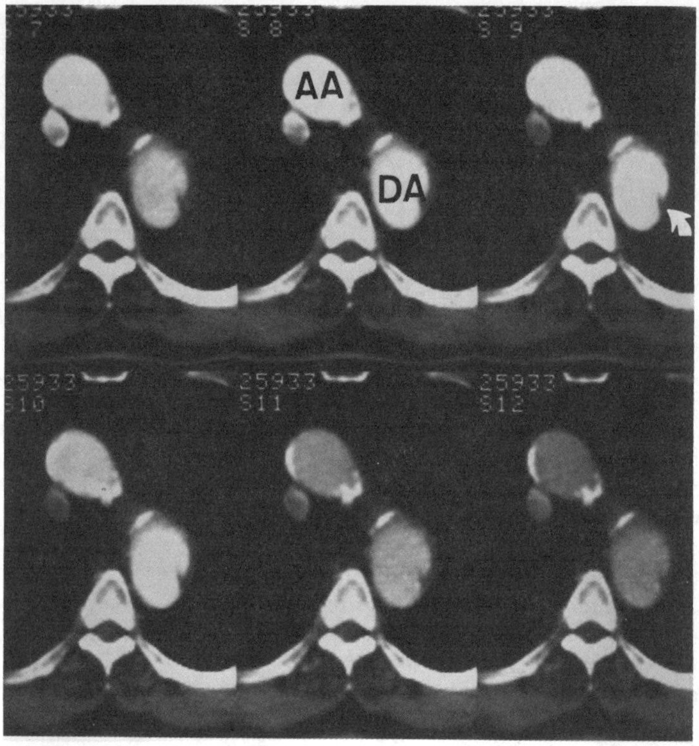

Figure 16-7 The intimal tear (arrow) of a type III aortic dissection is demonstrated by contrast enhancement during dynamic scanning. Note the calcification of the ascending (AA) and descending (DA) aorta.

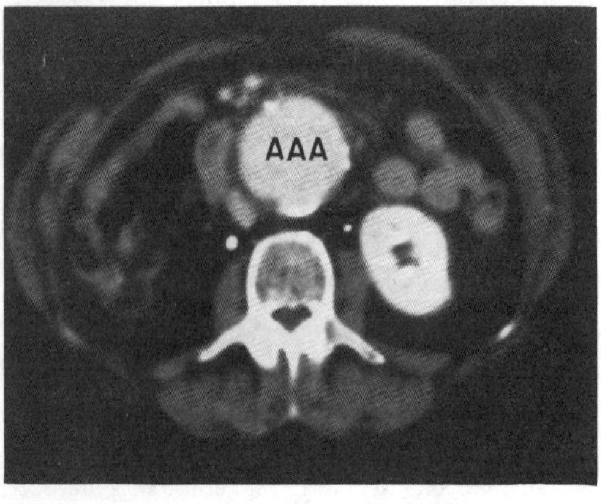

Figure 16-8 An abdominal aortic aneurysm (AAA) is well demonstrated on this abdominal scan by contrast infusion.

screening patients with pulmonary hypertension for the presence of large proximal chronic pulmonary emboli.[11] Sometimes these organized thrombi can be removed surgically to produce a permanent reduction in pulmonary artery pressure. However, successful surgery requires that the emboli reside in the proximal surgically accessible portion of the pulmonary artery. In several patients CT scans have demonstrated the proximal extent of the thrombus better than pulmonary angiography and changed the surgeon's opinion about operability.

As with aortic dissection patients, physicians are reluctant to perform invasive pulmonary arteriography in patients with severe pulmonary hypertension. CT offers a safer method of screening such patients for the presence of proximal emboli that may be amenable to surgical removal.

Neoplasms

Cardiac neoplasms that extend into the cavities of the heart, similar to thrombi, are well visualized by contrast-enhanced CT. The most frequent cardiac tumors are secondary in origin and result from extension or metastasis of the primary tumor that arose in some other thoracic structure. The excellent spatial resolution of CT makes it an ideal technic for assessing the degree of cardiac involvement by invading tumors and can be a useful noninvasive means for determining the effectiveness of tumor therapy (Figure 16-10).

Pericardial Disease

Echocardiography is an extremely useful diagnostic tool for evaluating effusive pericardial disease, but has significant difficulty in diagnosing constructive pericarditis. On occasion, even after complete hemodynamic evaluation by cardiac

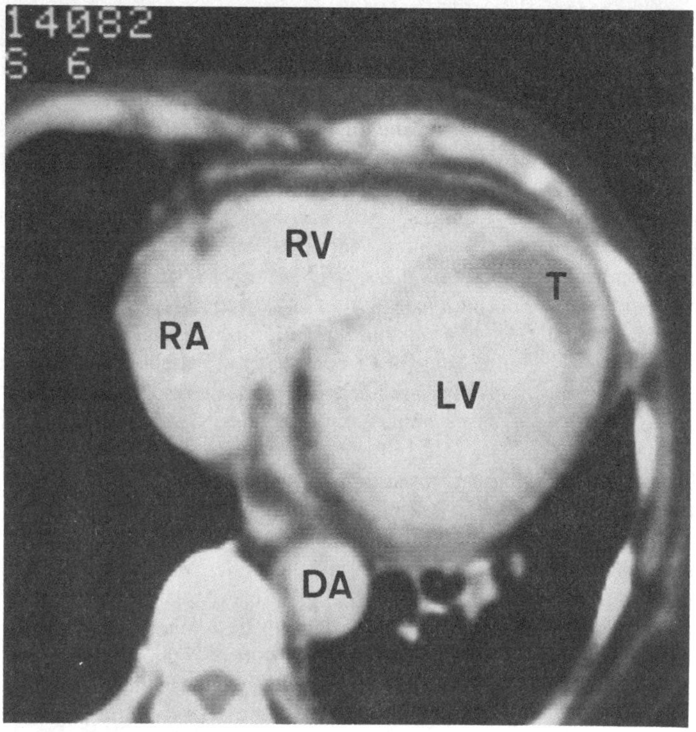

Figure 16-9 A large left ventricular (LV) thrombus (T) is clearly depicted by contrast infusion in this scan. RA = right atrium, RV = right ventricle, DA = descending aorta.

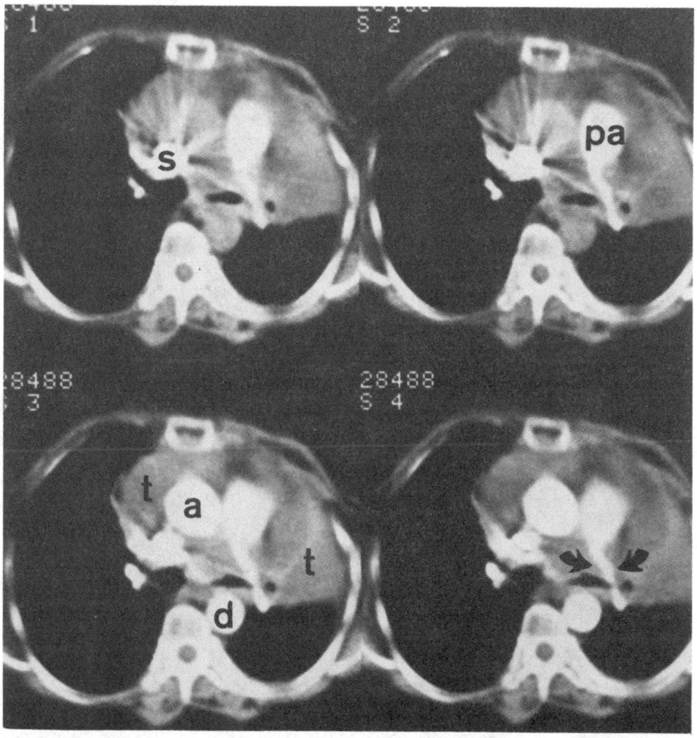

Figure 16-10 Dynamic scanning during an intravenous bolus of contrast medium shows severe constriction of the left pulmonary artery (arrows) by an extensive metastatic tumor (t). S = superior vena cava, pa = pulmonary artery, a = ascending aorta, d = descending aorta.

catheterization, pericardial constriction cannot be separated from myocardial restriction. CT appears to be the first diagnostic method that can reliably make this important differentiation by defining the thickened pericardium that must be associated with pericardial constriction (Figure 16-11). Scanners in current clinical use can show as little as 5 mm of pericardial thickening. Contrast enhancement is often not necessary to detect pericardial disease. Other pericardial abnormalities that have been diagnosed by CT are pericardial effusion, cyst, calcification, and congenital defects.[12]

FUTURE APPLICATIONS OF CT

Current investigation by us indicates that CT may be a useful method for evaluating and sizing myocardial infarction. Measurement of infarct size in animals at autopsy correlates well with CT assessment.[13] At the present time septal, anterior, and lateral infarctions are well visualized (Figure 16-12), but imaging inferior infarctions has been difficult because this wall of the heart is parallel to the scanning plane. With the development of faster scanners or the use of gated scanning, this problem should be resolved.

The increasing enthusiasm for the use of streptokinase thrombolysis to treat acute myocardial infarction in the hopes of salvaging heart muscle has created a real need for a method that can accurately measure infarct size before and after this type of therapy. Certainly CT shows great promise for fulfilling this need.

In the future, cardiac CT will also be employed to evaluate ventricular aneurysm, measure myocardial mass, and accurately determine cardiac chamber volumes and ejection fraction.

The spatial resolution of CT makes it an ideal technic for evaluating cardiovascular anatomy in congenital heart disease. The resolution of ultrafast scanners currently under development is likely to affect the diagnostic approach to congenital heart disease in a way similar to the revolutionary effect of head CT scanners on the diagnostic approach to central nervous system disease.

A new ultrafast scanner which is currently undergoing testing is able to scan multiple levels simultaneously, and this technology will make the noninvasive measurement of regional myocardial blood flow and coronary bypass graft flow possible. This scanner can make accurate measurements of regional ventricular wall motion and thickening.

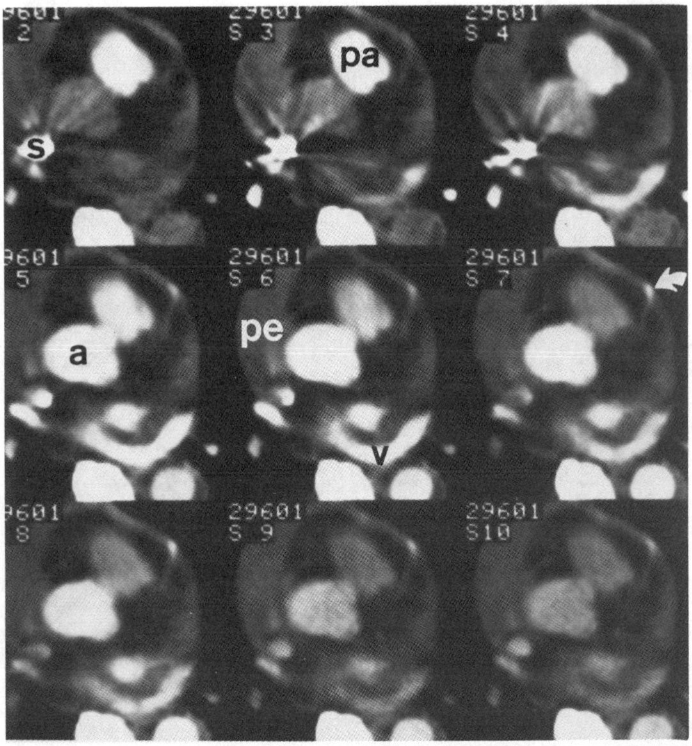

Figure 16-11 Extensive pericardial thickening (pe) is seen on these scans in a post-coronary artery bypass (arrow) patient. s = superior vena cava, pa = pulmonary artery, a = aorta.

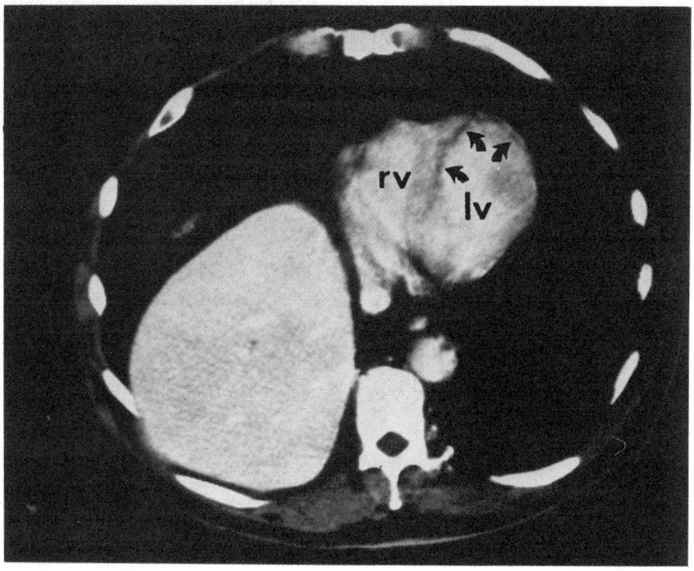

Figure 16-12 An acute anteroseptal myocardial infarct (arrows) is seen as a contrast-deficient area on this contrast-enhanced CT scan. rv = right ventricle, lv = left ventricle.

Cardiac CT has arrived and its future, with the current development of scanners with millisecond scan times, is indeed bright. The minimally invasive nature of this imaging technic and its excellent spatial resolution make it a promising diagnostic tool for the evaluation of degenerative cardiac disorders often encountered in elderly patients.

ACKNOWLEDGMENT

Supported by an NIH Grant from the National Heart, Lung and Blood Institute, HL 29420.

REFERENCES

1. Brundage B, Lipton M, Berninger W, et al: The use of contrast enhanced computerized axial tomography to assess coronary bypass graft patency. *Circulation* 1978;58:2-26.
2. Brundage B, Lipton M, Herfkens R, et al: Detection of patent coronary bypass grafts by computed tomography: A preliminary report. *Circulation* 1980;61:827-832.
3. Moncada R, Salinas M, Churchill R, et al: Patency of saphenous aortocoronary-bypass grafts demonstrated by computed tomography. *N Engl J Med* 1980;303:503-507.
4. Daniel W, Dohring W, Lichtler P, et al: Noninvasive assessment of aortocoronary bypass graft patency by computed tomography. *Lancet* 1980;1: 1023-1025.
5. Goldstein J, Brundage B, Herfkens R, et al: Evaluation of coronary bypass graft flow by contrast enhanced computed tomography. *Circulation* 1981;64:682-684.
6. McKay CR, Brundage BH, Ullyot D, et al: Evaluation of early postoperative coronary artery bypass graft patency by contrast-enhanced computed tomography. *JACC* 1983;2:312-317.
7. Bourassa MG, Campeau L, Lesperance J, et al: Changes in grafts and coronary arteries after saphenous vein aortocoronary bypass surgery: Results at repeat angiography. *Circulation* 1982;65: 2-90-95.
8. Godwin J, Herfkens R, Skioldebrand C, et al: Evaluation of dissections and aneurysms of the thoracic aorta by conventional and dynamic CT scanning. *Radiology* 1980;136:125-129.
9. Tomoda H, Mitsumoto H, Furuya H, et al: Evaluation of left ventricular thrombus with computed tomography. *Am J Cardiol* 1981;48:573-576.
10. Goldstein JA, Lipton MJ, Schiller NB, et al: Evaluation of intracardiac thrombi with contrast enhanced computed tomography and echocardiography. *Am J Cardiol* 1982;49:972.
11. DiCarlo LA, Schiller NB, Herfkens RL, et al: Noninvasive detection of proximal pulmonary artery thrombosis by two-dimensional echocardiography and computed tomography. *Am Heart J* 1982;104:879-881.
12. Moncada R, Baker M, Salinas M, et al: Diagnostic role of computed tomography in pericardial heart disease: Congenital defects, thickening, neoplasma, and effusion. *Am Heart J* 1982;103:263-268.
13. Dougherty PW, Lipton MJ, Berninger WH, et al: The detection and quantification of myocardial infarction in vivo using transmission computed tomography. *Circulation* 1981;63:597-601.

CHAPTER 17
Electrocardiographic Changes Associated with Aging

Eugene L. Coodley
Gregg Coodley

With the rapid development of an aged population, the problem of cardiac diagnosis assumes increasing importance. Since such diagnosis is partially dependent upon electrocardiographic (ECG) changes, a number of studies have attempted to correlate such laboratory changes with the aging process. Inability of many such patients to give an accurate history together with the presence of other systemic disease increases the reliance of the physician on ECG data.

One of the difficulties encountered in prior studies has been the problem of securing data on relatively healthy aged subjects.

This study is designed to review the ECG patterns found in a series of aged subjects in relatively good health and without the existence of associated clinical heart disease.

METHOD OF STUDY

The records of 54 patients from the Veterans Administration Medical Center Nursing Home and 103 subjects from Leisure World (an ambulatory, healthy population) were reviewed for clinical symptoms, laboratory data, and ECG data.

Clinical heart disease was excluded by: (1) the absence of symptoms of angina pectoris and/or myocardial infarction; (2) absence of cardiomegaly; (3) absence of auscultatory signs of heart disease; (4) absence of history of hypertension, diabetes, or hypercholesterolemia. The 12-lead ECGs were reviewed by two separate observers. Subjects were rejected from the study if any disease known to affect the ECG were present or if any history of or signs of heart disease were present.

The age distribution was approximately equal between the two institutions with the mean age at the VA Medical Center being 72.5 and the mean age at Leisure World being 74.2. Sex distribution varied considerably, however, with the males constituting 92% of the population at the VA Medical Center vs 48% of the subjects at Leisure World.

RESULTS OF STUDY

The results of our study are shown in Table 17-1. Of interest are the abnormalities noted in the 103 subjects from Leisure World. The most common kind of abnormalities noted was that of nonspecific ST-T wave changes, while sinus bradycardia and low voltage of the limb leads was the next most common finding. The only other abnormality noted in more than 5% of the subjects was left anterior hemiblock. Only one subject showed evidence of an old myocardial infarction.

Contrast those results with the abnormalities noted in the 54 patients from the VA Medical Center Nursing Home (these patients tended to have more chronic diseases). Again, nonspecific ST-T changes were the most common abnormality noted. However, as cited in the table, certain ECG abnormalities were much more common in this group of patients, eg, first-degree AV block, low voltage, bundle-branch block, atrial abnormalities, atrial premature contractions (PACs), left anterior hemiblock, and old infarction. This

Table 17-1
ECG Abnormalities in 103 Subjects from Leisure World and 54 Patients from VA Medical Center

	No. Abnormal			
Abnormal Finding	*Leisure World*	*VA Medical Center*	Total Series (%)	
Atrial enlargement, left	3	4*	7(4.5)	
Atrial enlargement, right	2	1	3(1.9)	
Old MI, anterolateral	–	2*	2(1.3)	
Old MI, anteroseptal	2	2*	4(2.5)	15(9.6)
Old MI, inferior	3	5*	8(5.1)	
Old MI, nonspecific	1	–	1(0.6)	
Sinus tachycardia	4	2	6(3.8)	
Sinus bradycardia	8	2	10(6.4)	
Bundle branch-block, right	4	8†	12(7.6)	
Bundle branch-block, left	–	2†	2(1.3)	
Low-voltage limb leads	8	7†	15(9.6)	
Left anterior hemiblock	6	7*	13(8.3)	
First-degree AV block	5	7†	12(7.6)	
Poor R progression	–	2*	2(1.3)	
Atrial fibrillation	2	3*	5(3.2)	
Multifocal atrial tachycardia	–	2*	2(1.3)	
Nonspecific ST-T wave changes	12	29†	41(26.1)	
Intraventricular conduction defect	5	3	8(5.1)	
Atrial abnormality, left	–	6†	6(3.8)	
LVH	1	1	2(1.3)	
RVH	–	2†	2(1.3)	
PACs	4	6*	10(6.4)	
PVCs	3	4*	7(4.5)	

MI = myocardial infarction, LVH = left ventricular hypertrophy, RVH = right ventricular hypertrophy, PACs = atrial premature contractions, PVCs = ventricular premature contractions.
*More frequent occurrence than in similar group from Leisure World.
†Two to three times the frequency of the group from Leisure World.

group included nine patients with ECG criteria of myocardial infarction, although none of these patients had any clinical history of such event.

The fourth column in Table 17-1 tabulates the number of ECG abnormalities noted in the total series of 157 elderly persons. Nonspecific ST-T changes are the most common, occurring in 41 of 157 (26.1%); myocardial infarction occurred in 15 of 157 (9.6%); low voltage was noted in 15 of 157 (9.6%); left anterior hemiblock was noted in 13 of 157 (8.3%); and right bundle-branch block occurred in 12 of 157 (7.6%) persons. Ectopic beats were only noted in 17 of 157 (10.9%) persons. The lower incidence of ECG abnormalities noted in the Leisure World population was not related to higher number of female subjects since no statistical difference was noted.

DISCUSSION

A number of studies have attempted to evaluate changes in the ECG associated with aging independent of underlying cardiac disease. Many of these studies have differed somewhat in their conclusions as to which ECG changes are due solely to age. These studies have included both cross-sectional and longitudinal studies and a good correlation has been found between the two.

Among the early studies were those of Gorman et al.[1] They examined the effect of age on the QRS axis of over 600 patients between the ages of 60 and 95. Half of the patients had underlying cardiovascular disease and another half had no apparent disease. In the group without cardiovascular disease the mean of the QRS axis showed no significant trend to the left with age whereas in the group with underlying cardiovascular disease there was a marked leftward trend in the ninth and tenth decades. They concluded that aging alone is not a significant factor in the production of left axis deviation of $-30°$ or greater and that such axis deviation was usually associated with underlying heart disease.

Blackburn et al[2] had previously reported that women in the United States between the ages of 20 and 60 years of age had less steep trends with age than men for certain conventional ECG measurements. They studied the question of whether ECG changes are common to aging men and independent of latent coronary artery disease. Their study concluded that while small ECG changes associated with age might be sensitive as indices of clinically silent coronary artery disease, the same changes might be related to changes in heart muscle mass, heart position in the chest, electrical activation pathways, and also the composition of the population under study. They also demonstrated reduced wave amplitude and leftward upward QRS vector orientation.

In a separate study by DelVecchio,[3] a total of 1094 patients over the age of 65 were studied for ECG changes. Approximately two thirds of these patients were found to have underlying cardiac disease. The ECG was likewise excluded on an additional 211 patients because of inadequate history, conclusion of the ECG prior to recording the history, or related reasons. Therefore, a total of 139 patients with no evidence of cardiac disease were analyzed with regard to ECG changes. The group was divided between 60 men and 79 women. The patients were divided into four groups with group A being males aged 65 to 74 years, group B males aged 75 years or more, group C females aged 65 to 74 years, and group D females aged 75 years or more. The results of this study showed the average heart rate for the entire group to be 83.1/min with only males over the age of 75 showing a significant deviation ie, a rate of almost 90. Sinus rhythm was present in the vast majority of all groups with the principal abnormalities being sinus tachycardia or bradycardia in 5 of 37 patients in group A, and sinus tachycardia in 6 of 23 patients in group B, and in 7 of 49 patients in group C. P-R intervals were within normal ranges. There were seven patients in the four groups combined with QRS intervals greater than .11 second and the majority of these were in groups A and B. The overall QRS axis was +13.7. The final diagnosis in 61 cases was entirely normal and this included 55.1% in group C, 46.0% in group A, 34.8% in group B, and 30% in group D. A total of 13 patients had multiple ventricular premature contractions (PVCs) or PACs, 8 patients showed left ventricular hypertrophy, 7 patients showed first degree AV block, 5 patients showed intraventricular conduction defects, 3 patients showed right bundle-branch block, and 7 patients had miscellaneous abnormalities including left bundle-branch block in two cases, cor pulmonale in two cases and right ventricular hypertrophy in one case. This study concluded that the changes noted did not appear to be correlated with age or sex except for the fact that the women in the younger group had the highest percentage of normal tracings.

A later study by Simonson[4] indicated that there were significant ECG age trends in adult healthy populations from the third to the fifth decade in QRS and T amplitudes (decrease with age) and direction (left axis shift with age) in conventional ECG leads. The decrease of amplitude was found to be more pronounced in men than women. In addition, he found an increased incidence of premature supraventricular and ventricular beats with age. He also described a poor progression of the R wave in the anterior leads as being a normal age trend. The final conclusion of this study was that the frequency of ischemic response to exercise is greater with more pronounced age trends in populations with high prevalence of coronary artery disease and that the ECG age trends in asyptomatic patients are due to a large extent to latent coronary artery disease.

A review of ECG findings in the aged by Mihalick and Fisch[5] cited the literature dealing with ECG changes in the aged and presented data in a study of 671 subjects over the age of 65. This population represented nonhospitalized subjects or elderly patients hospitalized for noncardiac disease. The presence of heart disease was ruled out by detailed history, standard 12-lead ECG, roentgenographic, and other laboratory criteria. Abnormal ECGs were considered to be present when unequivocal and clearly defined axis and pattern changes and arrhythmias were noted. In addition, the ECG was considered abnormal if ST-T changes were present in leads other than leads III and V_1. Sinus arrhythmias, sinus bradycardia and tachycardia, fewer than six premature ventricular systoles and less than six atrial premature systoles per 12-lead ECG were included in the normal group. Conduction defects were felt to be present when the PR interval was greater than .22 seconds and when the QRS interval was equal to or greater than .11 seconds. Of the total population 49% were found to have clinical evidence of heart disease and 46% showed abnormal ECGs. They found that a clearly abnormal ECG was a reliable index of heart disease in that 56% of patients with clinical heart disease had an abnormal ECG as opposed to 37% of normal subjects. The most frequent abnormality encountered was nonspecific ST-T wave changes which were recorded in 106 subjects (65 of whom had clinical heart disease). There was a significant correlation between the ST-T change and heart disease at the 1% level. There was no significant increase in frequency with age. The second most frequent abnormality was left anterior hemiblock occurring in 11% and found twice as often in patients with heart disease. There was a significant increase in frequency with age. First-degree AV block occurred in 67 subjects but was not correlated with heart disease. There was a significant increase with age, however. Right bundle-branch block pattern was seen in 7.1% of subjects and was equally present in normal subjects and those with heart disease. The ECG in 30 subjects exhibited evidence of myocardial infarction and this was equally present between the clinically normal population and abnormal patients. PVCs were present in 11% of patients, PACs in 10.4%, and atrial fibrillation in 5%. There was a relationship between developing age and the occurrence of PVCs. When Mihalick and Fisch reviewed the literature there was a 5% discrepancy between ECG abnormalities noted in the literature and those in their study. Of 2482 patients selected from the literature over the age of 70, 52% had an abnormal ECG. Most studies showed a leftward shift of the frontal QRS axis as well as low voltage of R- and S-waves. The ECG signs of left ventricular hypertrophy (LVH) were found to increase with age and be correlated with the presence of heart disease. Most studies confirmed some increase in frequency of first degree AV block with age. The incidence of both right and left bundle-branch block was shown to increase with age and in the case of the latter was usually correlated with underlying heart disease. A review of the literature indicated that the incidence of ST-T wave changes was increased in subjects over age 70 and appeared to be correlated with underlying heart disease. The overall conclusion of the study was that the incidence of abnormal ECGs increases with age as does the incidence of clinical heart disease. No modification of ECG criteria was felt warranted for the aged patient and it was suggested that the incidence of abnormal ECGs and clinical heart disease with age suggests that the ECG may be a highly reliable indicator of heart disease even up to the ninth or tenth decade.

Another large review of ECGs in aging patients was conducted by Caird et al.[6] In this study 2254 persons aged 65 or over were reviewed. Mortality curves were calculated with patients having no ECG abnormalities as compared to specific ECG abnormalities. The mortality was 1.8 times greater for patients with Q/QS patterns, 3.7 times greater for patients with left ventricular hypertrophy, and 2.7 times greater for patients with left bundle-branch block. This paper concluded that the majority of common ECG abnormalities must be regarded as significant when encountered in the older patient and this was particularly true of changes of QRS patterns and P-wave flattening or inversion.

A later study[7] by Mihalick and Fisch again raised the question of whether ECG criteria should be modified for geriatric patients. The conclusion of this study was that ECG criteria should not be changed for geriatric patients regardless of age. In addition, it was pointed out that with aging both heart disease and abnormal ECGs increased in incidence in a somewhat parallel fashion. Specific abnormalities that increased in frequency in aging included first-degree block, bundle-branch block, ST-T wave changes, premature systoles, left anterior hemiblock, left ventricular hypertrophy, and atrial fibrillation. Those abnormalities that correlated most closely were atrial fibrillation, left bundle-branch block, and intraventricular conduction defect.

The study of Bachman et al[8] has also shown that aging is associated with lowering of amplitude and a leftward frontal plane axis. This study confirmed that previously described cross-sectional age differences clearly parallel longitudinal trends in ECG patterns.

Hamer[9] has indicated that atrial fibrillation is the functional disturbance which represents the most specific cardiac arrhythmia of the elderly patient. It tends to appear in middle age and occurs in the older healthy patient in an incidence of 10%.[10] Atrial fibrillation without underlying heart disease accounted for 31% of the total in a report from the Framingham study.[11] The possibility of thyrotoxicosis must be considered in any patient with atrial fibrillation.[12] The association of senile atrial fibrillation with sinus node disease is often accompanied by evidence of AV block.[13]

Heart block in the elderly may be the result of a diffuse fibrosis of the conduction system[14] or may result from extension of Lev's mitral valve calcification.[15] Shaw and Kelwick have indicated that sinus node disease is being increasingly recognized as a cause of bradycardia and syncope requiring pacing in the elderly.[16]

Cullen et al[17] have reviewed abnormalities in resting ECGs and demonstrated that these have an increased 13-year mortality as compared with the remainder of an age-adjusted population without such abnormality. They included patients with Q waves, left axis deviation. ST depression, atrial fibrillation or flutter, and ventricular extrasystoles.

With regard to the prognosis of abnormalities in resting ECGs of older patients, Rose et al[18] indicated that abnormal Q waves had a 5-year adjusted mortality ratio of 4.1:1 while Caird et al[19] described a mortality risk ratio of 1.8:1. Kannel et al[20] described increased cardiovascular mortality in patients with left ventricular hypertrophy. ST depression in symptom-free patients did not result in an increased risk ratio over a 5-year period according to Medalie et al.[21] Patients with left axis deviation did not show an increase in their risk ratio.[22]

Fleg and Kennedy[23] reported on 24-hour Holter monitoring in 98 healthy subjects ranging in age from 60 to 65. They reported a high prevalence of both supraventricular ectopic beats and ventricular ectopic beats, both isolated and complex. They found a high degree of AV block, severe bradycardia, and sinus pauses to be rare in normal elderly subjects. Hinkle et al[24,25] also reported a high prevalence of supraventricular (76%) and ventricular ectopy (63%) in middle-aged men but their study group included some patients with latent heart disease.

Fisch[26] has reviewed the status of the ECG in the aged and indicated that the conflicting views expressed stem from varying populations, lack of uniform criteria, and inadequate sample sizes. He emphasized that the major problems included: correlation of the tracing with advancing age and criteria of normality of the ECG in the elderly population. His studies considered: (1) AV delay, (2) significant axis shift, (3) right bundle-branch block, (4) left bundle-branch block, (5) intraventricular conduction delay, (6) ST-T changes, (7) infarction pattern, (8) presence of arrhythmias. The results of his study, the present study, and five pooled[27] prior studies are shown in Table 17-2. With regard to left axis deviation (LAD), this is frequently encountered in the ECG of the aging patient but each author uses a different degree of LAD.

In contrast to the distribution described above, Camm et al[28] utilized ambulatory 24-hour monitoring of 106 elderly subjects and found 23% of the records to be normal. Supraventricular arrhythmias and ventricular arrhythmias were found in more than one third of the patients.

Since prior studies of younger patients have shown a very low incidence of the abnormalities described above, Fisch has suggested that such abnormalities in the aged are acquired and that the increasing incidence of such abnormalities in the aged parallel the incidence of clinical heart disease in such patients. Abnormalities which are highly correlated with clinical heart disease include left bundle-branch block, intraventricular conduction delays, ST-T changes, and atrial fibrillation. However, ECG patterns infrequently show a correlation with either severity or prognosis of disease.

Our study illustrates that a number of ECG abnormalities can be expected to occur in older patients without any known underlying cardiac disease. However, 9.6% of the subjects had silent myocardial infarction and others without clear-cut ECG criteria of infarction may indeed have latent coronary heart disease. This would account for the most common abnormalities noted, viz, conduction blocks, and nonspecific ST-T wave changes. It is generally accepted that low voltage and axis shift are commonly found in the older patient. The incidence of arrhythmias in this group was certainly no greater than expected in the general population. First-degree AV block is another common finding in older patients but only noted in 7.6% of our study group. The higher incidence of abnormalities noted in the VA Medical Center Nursing Home population was probably related to the greater incidence of chronic disease in that population. While the incidence of abnormalities in the male subjects of

Table 17-2
ECG Abnormalities in Older Patients

	No. ECGs	RBBB	LBBB	ST-T Changes	PACs	PVCs	Atrial Fibrillation	First Degree AV Block	Left Axis Deviation
Pooled[27]	2482	5%	3%	16%	10%	6%	8%	9%	57%
Fisch[26]	671	7%	5%	15%	10%	11%	8%	10%	11%
Coodley	157	7.6%	1.3%	26.1%	6.4%	4.5%	3.2%	7.6%	Not measured

RBBB = right bundle-branch block, LBBB = left bundle-branch block, PACs = atrial premature contractions, PVCs = ventricular premature contractions.

the Leisure World population was greater than that noted in the female population, this did not reach statistical significance. Our data agrees with other studies in the incidence of first-degree block and low voltage but we found a lower incidence of both right and left bundle-branch block than previously reported. Our incidence of ST-T changes was similar to that reported in combined series. Ventricular hypertrophy did not correlate with aging as has been described in other series.

It would appear that several other series reported a higher incidence of underlying cardiac disease, whereas our population of healthy subjects were screened more successfully to exclude such latent heart disease.

This study indicates that while certain ECG abnormalities eg, low voltage, first-degree block, and probably conduction disease and nonspecific ST-T changes, will be associated with aging, other ECG changes do not occur from aging alone and represent latent cardiac disease. A realization of the incidence of changes associated with aging as opposed to the changes indicating underlying heart disease will help to place in perspective the ECG abnormalities noted in a specific patient.

SUMMARY

One hundred fifty-seven subjects (mean age 72.8) were studied with regard to the relationship between ECG changes and aging. The group was selected so as to exclude those with coronary heart disease or having disease processes known to affect the ECG.

The major abnormalities noted were: silent myocardial infarction in almost 10%, and nonspecific changes in slightly more than 25%.

The study suggests that first-degree heart block, low voltage, and conduction defects are associated with aging while other ECG abnormalities probably represent underlying cardiac disease. The low incidence of PACs and PVCs probably reflects the difference between resting ECGs and Holter monitors, the latter being more useful in demonstrating the extent of these arrhythmias.

REFERENCES

1. Gorman P, Calatayud J, Abraham S, et al: Effects of age and heart disease on the QRS axis during the seventh through the tenth decades. *Am J Med* 1964; 67:39–43.
2. Blackburn H, Vasquez C, Keys A: The aging electrocardiogram, A common aging process or latent coronary artery disease? *Am J Cardiol* 1967;20: 618–627.
3. Del Vecchio P: Electrocardiographic findings in hospitalized noncardiac geriatric patients. *J Am Geriatr Soc* 1967;15:340–345.
4. Simonson E: The effect of age on the electrocardiogram. *Am J Cardiol* 1972;29:64–73.
5. Mihalick M, Fisch C: Electrocardiographic findings in the aged. *Am Heart J* 1974;87:117–128.
6. Caird F, Campbell A, Jackson T: Significance of abnormalities of electrocardiogram in old people. *Br Heart J* 1974;36:1012–1018.
7. Mihalick M, Fisch C: Should ECG criteria be modified for geriatric patients? *Geriatrics* 1977;27:65–72.
8. Bachman S, Sparrow D, Smith K: Effect of aging on the electrocardiogram. *Am J Cardiol* 1981;48: 513–515.
9. Hamer J: The modern treatment of hypertension, in Hamer J, Rowlands D (eds): *Recent Advances in Cardiology*. London, Churchill-Livingston, 1981, pp 1- 28.
10. Camm AJ, Evans KL, Ward DE, et al: The rhythm of the heart in active elderly subjects. *Am Heart J* 1980;99:598–603.
11. Kannel WB, Abbot RD, Savage DD, et al: Epidemiologic features of chronic atrial fibrillation. The Framingham Study. *N Engl J Med* 1982; 306:1018–1022.
12. Forfar JC, Toft AD: Thyrotoxic atrial fibrillation: An underdiagnosed condition? *Br Med J* 1982; 285:909–910.
13. Parsonnett V: The proliferation of cardiac pacing: Medical, technical and socio-economic dilemmas. *Circulation* 1982;65:841–845.
14. Lenegre J, Moreau P: Lebloc auriculo-ventriculaire chronique. Etude anatomique, clinique et histologique. *Arch Mal Coeur* 1963;56:867–888.
15. Lev M: Anatomic basis for atrioventricular block. *Am J Med* 1964;37:742.
16. Shaw DB, Kelwick C: Potential candidates for pacemakers. Survey of heart block and sino-atrial disorder (sick sinus syndrome). *Br Heart J* 1978;60: 98–105.
17. Cullen KJ, Stenhouse NS, Wearne KL, et al: Electrocardiograms and thirteen year cardiovascular mortality in Busselton study. *Br Heart J* 1982;47: 209–212.
18. Rose G, Baxter PJ, Reid DD, et al: Prevalence and prognosis of ECG findings in middle-aged men. *Br Heart J* 1978;40:636–643.
19. Caird FI, Campbell A, Jackson TFM: Significance of abnormalities of electrocardiogram in old people. *Br Heart J* 1974;36:1012–1018.
20. Kannel WB, Gordon T, Offutt D: Left ventricular hypertrophy by electrocardiogram. *Ann Intern Med* 1969;71:89–105.
21. Medalie JH, Snyder M, Groen JJ: Angina pectoris among 10,000 men. Five year incidence and univariate analysis. *Am J Med* 1973;55:583–594.
22. Ostrander LD: Left axis deviation: Prevalence associated conditions and prognosis. An epidemiologic study. *Ann Intern Med* 1971;75:23–28.
23. Fleg JL, Kennedy HL: Cardiac arrhythmias in a healthy elderly population, Detection by 24-hours ambulatory electrocardiography. *Chest* 1982;81: 302–307.
24. Hinkle LE, Carver ST, Stevens M: The frequency of asymptomatic disturbances of cardiac rhythm

and conduction in middle-aged men. *Am J Cardiol* 1969;24:629–650.
25. Hinkle LE, Carver ST, Argyrus DC: The prognostic significance of ventricular premature contractions in healthy people and in people with coronary heart disease. *Acta Cardiol* 1974;18(suppl):5–32.
26. Fisch C: Electrocardiogram in the aged: An independent marker of heart disease? *Am J Med* 1981; 70:4–6.
27. Pipberger HV, Schiederman MA, Klingman JD: The love-at-first-sight effect in research. *Circulation* 1968;38:822–824.
28. Camm AJ, Evans KE, Ward DE, et al: The rhythm of the heart in active elderly subjects. *Am Heart J* 1980;99:598–602.

CHAPTER 18
Postural Hypotension

Michael Lye
Enrique Vargas

A drop in blood pressure on changing from the supine to the standing position is termed postural hypotension. The elderly are particularly vulnerable to the distressing consequences of small reductions in cerebral perfusion manifesting as nervous system dysfunction, eg, dizziness and falls. Postural hypotension in the elderly may lead to direct trauma and fractures or, more commonly, to loss of confidence. If the symptoms are frequent the patient may become immobile and totally dependent. The cost in terms of personal discomfort and the considerable burden placed upon health and social support systems are considerable.

Blood pressure is maintained during postural stress by a number of complex homeostatic reflexes. However, most physiologic studies on the subject are characterized by the limited number of old people studied—the very group most at risk. This chapter is focused upon the more practical aspects of managing patients with the syndrome giving due emphasis to where neurophysiologic or pharmacologic knowledge may now or in the near future be applied with benefit. At the present time the treatment of old people with postural hypotension is difficult and incomplete.

DEFINITION

Surveys of the prevalence of postural hypotension in populations have relied upon measurements of a change in arterial blood pressure following a change in posture. Unfortunately, there is no general agreement as to what change in blood pressure is normal. Equally, the resting control period prior to the stimulus and the timing of measurements after application of the stimulus have varied among studies. These differences exacerbate difficulties in the comparison of different physiologic studies. The postural stimuli used have varied from active standing to passive tilting.

Criteria

There is a wide variation as to what constitutes a significant change in blood pressure on postural change. Thus, Nylin and Lavender[1] defined a normal response as that in which the blood pressure did not fall by more than 20 mmHg systolic and the diastolic either rose or did not fall by more than 4 mmHg. The American Civil Aeronautics Authority stated that the response was normal if the systolic and diastolic blood pressures did not fall below 90 mmHg and 54 mmHg, respectively.[2] This was irrespective of the supine levels. Many workers who have studied the elderly consider that a fall of 20 mmHg or more in systolic blood pressure alone constitutes postural hypotension.[3–6] Others, however, require a decrease in diastolic blood pressure of 10 mmHg[7] or 20 mmHg[8] in addition to a fall in systolic blood pressure.

One review paper[9] suggested that the systolic blood pressure should fall by at least 30 mmHg or, alternatively, that systolic blood pressure should fall to a level of 80 mmHg or lower. These criteria are meant to apply to all age groups but obviously are irrelevant to the elderly. In practice some patients show symptoms with falls in blood pressure defined as being normal. Perhaps of more relevance than changes in systolic or diastolic levels of blood pressure, in terms of cerebral perfusion, are changes in mean arterial blood pressure. Only two studies of old people have specified changes in mean arterial pressure; Myers et al[10] required a fall of 20 mmHg or more in mean pressure, while others required 25 mmHg or more before diagnosing postural hypotension. Clinicians see patients with classical postural symptoms with small falls in blood pressure and asymptomatic patients with gross falls. The reason for this is undoubtedly due to differences in efficiency of autoregulation of cerebral blood flow.[8] Further studies of the relationship between postural change in blood pressure and cerebral blood flow are required.

Control Period

The response of blood pressure to changes in posture depends upon preceding activity. In the elderly, rising from a warm bed after a night's sleep or getting out of a hot bath are common precursors to serious postural symptoms. The observation does emphasize the importance of a standardized protocol. Unfortunately, surveys of the elderly are characterized by the variety of protocols and in particular control periods used.

A number of studies[4,11] have not specified either the position or time spent in the period before applying the postural stress. Others have required a control period of 5 minutes,[3,10] 10 minutes,[11] or 15 minutes. Still others have arbitrarily chosen 20 minutes supine rest[12] and this would accord with our own observations.[13] Thus, we have shown that on average the pulse rate and blood pressure of healthy elderly subjects and also of patients with the syndrome of postural hypotension decrease with supine rest and reach a plateau between 15 and 20 minutes. Application of the postural stress before 20 minutes is likely to blunt changes in the blood pressure and thus lead to underdiagnosis of the syndrome. This period may be difficult to achieve in a busy office practice, but certainly should be adhered to in the experimental or research situation.

Postural Stimulus

The variety of postural stresses used in studies of old people with and without postural hypotension is considerable. These include changes induced by moving from the supine to the sitting position whereas the majority have used the change from supine to supported or unsupported standing. In these latter studies the period of time before recording blood pressure changes on standing have varied between 1[7] and 7 minutes. Others have recorded blood pressures at 30- or 60-second intervals for periods ranging from 3 to 7 minutes.

Physiologic studies of postural stress, whether invasive or not, have mainly used passive, head-up (or feet down) tilt to produce postural stress.[11,12] The angle of head-up tilt has varied between 45°[12] and 90°.[11] Matalon and Farhi[14] demonstrated that the hemodynamic response during passive tilt is linearly related to the sine of the angle of tilt. They showed no significant difference in hemodynamic responses between 60° and 90° head-up tilt, and further that lesser degrees of tilt were insufficient to elicit a full response. Finally "postural" stress may be induced by lower body negative pressure,[15] but has not found favor in studies of the elderly with a single exception.[16] As we[17] and others have argued, the cardiovascular or hemodynamic responses to sitting, active standing, passive tilting, and lower body negative pressure are all different. In order to compare results between different research studies a standardized methodology is required.

PREVALENCE

One of the largest surveys of the change in blood pressure on standing was reported by Currens[18] in 1948. This survey of 1000 subjects who were mainly young has formed the basis of the defined normal response. His conclusion, confirmed by others,[1] was that a change of ± 10 mmHg in systolic and ± 4 mmHg in diastolic blood pressure represents the normal response to standing. Subsequent workers have found wider ranges in healthy elderly subjects and in geriatric patients.

The study of Norris et al[11] involving 140 subjects aged 20 to 92 years showed changes in blood pressure following 45° head-up tilt. While there was a significant age-related increasing fall in systolic pressure on passive tilting, the magnitude of the change was minimal. Diastolic pressure did not change in any age group. Unfortunately the period of supine rest was too short to stabilize blood pressures and the degree of tilt (45°) too small to elicit a maximum hemodynamic response. In the same study Norris et al also used 90° tilt and all groups showed significant falls in systolic blood pressure and small falls in mean diastolic pressures compared with 45° tilt. Increasing age enhanced these responses but the report does not allow the extraction of quantifiable data.

Table 18-1 summarizes the data obtained in three surveys of elderly people. Rodstein and Zeman[3] studied ambulatory residents from a home for the aged and Johnson et al[5] studied consecutive admissions to a hospital geriatric unit. Caird et al[6] surveyed healthy old people living independently at home. The stimulus was the same in all three studies, ie, standing after a variable period of supine rest. The results of all these studies,[3,11] spanning two decades, are remarkably consistent. Thus, in any elderly population, on average, 20% will show a fall in systolic blood pressure of 20 mmHg or more and 5% a fall of 40 mmHg or more. These figures are higher than expected on the basis of Curren's[18] results and imply that aging alone does have a significant detrimental effect on compensatory mechanisms (see below). Some workers have implied that age-related diseases, diabetes and varicose veins and in particular cerebrovascular disease, underlie this aging phenomenon,[3] but this has not been the conclusion of others. Indeed some workers have suggested that aging has little effect on postural reflexes,[10] but these studies, with the exception of one,[10] have been confined to small numbers of subjects. Myers et al[10] unfortunately allowed an insufficient control period of 5 minutes supine rest before standing, which would tend to blunt any postural stress. We have shown in a group of carefully screened healthy individuals quite definite age-related loss of efficiency.

PHYSIOLOGY OF POSTURAL CHANGE

When standing, the force of gravity increases the hydrostatic pressure in body fluid spaces below the level of the heart. The effective intravascular volume is reduced by the pooling of blood in the lower parts of the body and by the filtration of plasma out of capillaries. After standing for about 20 minutes with minimal or no muscle movement, the volume of plasma lost varies between 290 and 590 ml. Variation in these results is explained by differences in the methods used to measure plasma volume and biological variations in the studied populations.

Both pooling of blood and plasma efflux from veins reduce venous return to the heart.[14] Pulmonary and intrathoracic blood volumes are mobilized to compensate for these changes. Nevertheless, a reduction in ventricular filling pressure and hence in stroke volume and cardiac output occurs on standing. In healthy young people stroke volume may decrease by 35% or more on standing. Cardiac output is found to decrease less (25%) than stroke volume, because there is an acceleration of heart rate which reduces the drop in cardiac output relative to the reduction in stroke volume. There are, however, differences in published results for stroke volume and cardiac output change with posture, which can be explained[19,20] by the methods of measurement, protocols followed (eg, active standing or passive tilting), and the criteria for selection of subjects.

Arterial blood pressure falls immediately after standing. The drop in pressure is restored after 30 to 60 seconds by the operation of regulatory mechanisms.[21] Systolic and diastolic pressures may vary but the mean arterial pressure usually remains unchanged.[18]

Autonomic nervous system activity and local vascular control are important mechanisms in the regulation of arterial blood pressure during changes in posture.[22] Other mechanisms[21] are less important since they take longer to respond to changes in hydrostatic pressure, eg, the renin-angiotensin system.[23] On standing, the initial drop in blood pressure elicits a reflex change in autonomic nervous output. Aortic and carotid baroreceptors are stimulated which results in a vagal parasympathetic nervous withdrawal and increased sympathetic nervous activity. Reflex sympathetic nervous discharge, on standing, increases myocardial contractility and total

Table 18-1
Proportion (%) of Individuals Showing Significant Falls in Systolic Blood Pressure on Standing

	Rodstein & Zeman[3]	Johnson et al[5]	Caird et al[6]	
Age (years)	61–95	70+	65–74	75+
Number	250	100	268	226
Decrease in systolic blood pressure mmHg 20+	11	17	16	30
mmHg 40+	4	5	3	8

peripheral resistance, and reduces venous capacitance. Local "intrinsic" control of blood flow[24] also participates in changing peripheral resistance and redistributes blood flow to vital organs, eg, the brain and heart, etc.[22]

In spite of these local protective mechanisms, in a young healthy subject a net decrease in cerebral blood flow of between 15% and 20% occurs on assuming the standing position;[25] the intrathoracic blood pools are depleted, and moderate decreases in renal, hepatic, and gastrointestinal blood flow occur.

Venous capacitance is reduced by sympathetic nervous activity in the standing position. Such reduction would increase venous return although the venomotor response is time-dependent and not as effective as arteriolar resistance changes in compensating for changes in posture.[26] Reflex sympathetic nervous activity also stimulates the release of renin and probably of other vasoactive substances, eg, prostacyclin and vasopressin.[27] The role of such substances is poorly understood in the normal cardiovascular response to changes in posture.

Norepinephrine is the sympathetic postganglionic neurotransmitter.[28] The measurement of plasma norepinephrine concentration under standardized conditions is a reliable index of overall sympathetic nervous activity.[28,29] Evaluation of sympathetic nervous activity in response to posture change requires standardization of the procedure before and during stimulation. Before standing, at least 20 minutes of rest in the supine position are required to reach a relative "basal state" of sympathetic nervous system activity.[28] This time is also appropriate to show a decline in plasma norepinephrine concentration after insertion of an indwelling needle. Plasma norepinephrine concentration increases shortly after assuming the upright position. An increase in plasma norepinephrine of at least 100% has been observed after adoption of the standing position for 2 to 5 minutes.[30] Furthermore, there is no difference in plasma norepinephrine concentration after 5 or 10 minutes of standing. Head-up tilting may result in a smaller increase in plasma norepinephrine concentration than active standing. The differences between tilting and standing on plasma norepinephrine responses have not been investigated in detail.

Other mechanisms that compensate for changes in blood pressure with posture include respiratory movements and skeletal muscle contraction which maintain venous return to the heart, especially during active standing. The contribution of these mechanisms to the overall compensatory response to standing is limited, however.

Aging and age-related changes in the cardiovascular system affect the response to a change from the supine position to the standing position. This effect, however, is not completely understood. Qualitatively the cardiovascular response is the same, ie, plasma volume, stroke volume, and cardiac output, peripheral resistance, plasma norepinephrine, etc, all change on standing in the same direction as in the young. Quantitatively, however, there are differences which have been difficult to explain because of the selection of subjects, and the methods and experimental designs of reported studies,[5,6,12] as already mentioned.

The cardiovascular response to changes in posture in the elderly is characterized by smaller decreases in stroke volume (20%) and cardiac output (10%) on standing.[12] Plasma volume decreases by the same proportion (15%) in old and young healthy subjects after 10 to 20 minutes standing or tilting. Reflex compensatory increases in heart rate and peripheral resistance are also attenuated by increasing age.

The hemodynamic changes in the elderly are difficult to interpret. However, they resemble those observed in patients with mild chronic congestive cardiac failure. The reduced compensatory response to standing can be explained by the diminished baroreceptor sensitivity with increasing age.[31] Equally many efferent mechanisms acting in blood pressure regulation show an age-related change.

The study by Gribbin et al[31] has been criticized,[32] although the reduction in baroreceptor sensitivity explains the problems in the short-term control of blood pressure in the elderly, ie, the higher incidence of postural drop in blood pressure, as shown in Table 18-1. Arteriosclerosis, by increasing the rigidity of the walls of the vessels, increases the resistance to blood flow at rest and reduces the response achieved by normal sympathetic venous stimulation. Hence, arteriosclerosis must always be considered an important factor determining vascular function in old age.

Plasma norepinephrine concentration at rest, an index of overall sympathetic nervous system activity, increases with increasing age.[33] On standing, the concentration of plasma norepinephrine rises by a greater amount in elderly as compared with young subjects. These higher concentrations of norepinephrine in the elderly have been related to reduced metabolic clearance, reduced responsiveness of adrenoreceptors, and structural changes in effector organs, ie, heart and blood vessels.[28] Thus, sympathetic nervous system activity is probably normal in healthy old age. Aging changes in the heart and blood vessels might be the more important factors relating to impairment of the compensatory response to changes in posture.

There is an age-related decrease in the activity of the renin-angiotensin-aldosterone system. Differences between young and old subjects are more pronounced after standing and during ambulation or with the stress of sodium depletion.[34] Further, vasopressin release during changes in blood pressure or blood volume brought about by standing might be impaired in a considerable proportion of elderly people. In summary, the capacity of the cardiovascular system to respond to stress decreases with age. The effects of aging on blood pressure regulation are more apparent during acute stresses such as changes in posture. These changes help to explain why elderly people are prone to develop postural hypotension.

Table 18-2
Conditions Associated with Autonomic Failure and Postural Hypotension

Primary Autonomic Failure
Iodiopathic orthostatic hypotension
Secondary Autonomic Failure
Cerebrovascular disease
Parkinsonism
Diabetes mellitus
Drugs
Neoplasia (eg, carcinoma of bronchus or pancreas)
Alcoholism
Spinal cord lesion
Porphyria
Tabes dorsalis
Transverse myelitis
Syringomyelia
Guillain-Barré syndrome
Hyperbradykininism
Familial dysautonomia (Riley-Day syndrome)
Anorexia nervosa
Long-term hemodialysis
Wernicke's encephalopathy
Multiple sclerosis
Primary aldosteronism
Pheochromocytoma

ETIOLOGY OF POSTURAL HYPOTENSION

In young people autonomic nervous dysfunction is the most common etiologic factor in postural hypotension. In the elderly, however, a number of precipitating factors are as important as autonomic nervous dysfunction. The principal causes of autonomic dysfunction are listed in Table 18-2. In the list are some clinical conditions which are unlikely to be found in old age because they affect young or middle-aged people.

Idiopathic Orthostatic Hypotension

Primary autonomic failure can be acute, subacute, or chronic. The chronic form affects middle-aged to elderly subjects. Acute and subacute autonomic failure may last for a few weeks to months and usually the recovery of the patients is complete.

The term idiopathic orthostatic hypotension (IOH) includes a group of chronic neurologic syndromes. The pure form of autonomic failure with IOH was recognized in 1925 by Bradbury and Eggleston.[35] Later, Shy and Drager[36] described the form with neurologic features of multiple system atrophy and Graham and Oppenheimer[37] reported its association with typical parkinsonism. Lesions found in some patients include degeneration of cells in the dorsal nucleus of the vagus, in the brain stem, and pigmented nuclei containing melanin.[38] The etiology of the selective degeneration of autonomic and nonautonomic structures is unknown.

Patients with IOH can be divided clinically into two groups.[38] In the first group a variety of neurologic disturbances, such as parkinsonism, bulbar palsy, and sometimes cerebellar ataxia develop before or after the onset of autonomic symptoms. This group corresponds to the Shy-Drager syndrome with multiple system atrophy.[36] In the second group, autonomic failure occurs either in isolation or in association with signs of parkinsonism without ataxia or other neurologic manifestations. In the second group the age of onset is later (60+ years), the course is more benign, and the prognosis better when compared with the first group.[36,38] Patients with IOH usually die from cerebral ischemic episodes during hypotension. In a series of 57 cases followed up by Schirger and Thomas[39] death occurred on average 7 to 8 years (range 3 to 33 years) after symptoms appeared and 4 years after neurologic signs were initially noted.

The presenting complaints of patients with IOH are sphincter disturbance in the form of incontinence and/or retention of urine.[36] Postural dizziness or faintness develop together with weakness and giddiness on standing and walking. These episodes may culminate in syncope; thus orthostatic hypotension is perhaps the most incapacitating feature of these patients. Several years after the onset of autonomic failure some patients develop progressive parkinsonian signs, attacks of altered consciousness, etc.[37] Some patients present neurologic signs of widespread involvement of somatic nervous structures.

Tests of autonomic nervous activity[40] in patients with IOH have demonstrated impaired cardiovascular reflexes and altered hemodynamics. The tests have also been used to locate the lesion in the autonomic nervous system, ie, whether the lesion is in the afferent or efferent pathways, and if the latter, to distinguish between preganglionic and postganglionic defects. Many of the tests are invasive, complex, and lack adequate control measurements.[40] Some others are nonspecific and require careful interpretation. The available tests furthermore have limitations when applied to the elderly[17,40] because they are affected by changes induced by aging rather than the disease itself. The common physiologic defects in IOH are a reduced reflex vasoconstriction in resistance vessels and an absent increase in venous distensibility and unchanged heart rate during standing or tilting.

Variations in the supine arterial blood pressure and a lower than normal cardiac output and plasma volume have been found in patients with IOH.[41] In some of them cardiac output can fall on standing more than in normal subjects.[42] There is, nevertheless, a large variation in the results published. Studies in middle-aged and in a few elderly patients with IOH indicate that the pattern of norepinephrine release may be used to distinguish the type of autonomic nervous dysfunction. Thus, patients with IOH who have isolated autonomic dysfunction (and parkinsonism) have plasma norepinephrine levels that are only one third of the normal after 20 minutes rest in the supine position.[43] When the patient stands, the concentration of norepinephrine in plasma remains unchanged; even the combined effects of standing and exercise do not increase the level of norepinephrine. In these patients, infusion of tyramine, which acts by releasing the stores of norepinephrine in nerve endings, has no pressor effect. The autonomic lesion in these patients seems to be a depletion of norepinephrine stores in sympathetic postganglionic nerves, ie, a "peripheral" lesion. Alternatively, patients with IOH and the Shy-Drager syndrome may have normal levels of norepinephrine in plasma at rest in the supine position, but on standing the concentration of norepinephrine fails to increase.[43] These patients have a normal pressor response to the infusion of tyramine which indicates intact peripheral nerves. Hence, the lesion is probably "central" or preganglionic and affects autonomic nuclei, ganglia, and the spinal cord.

Diabetic Orthostatic Hypotension

Autonomic neuropathy is a late but serious complication of diabetes.[44] Ewing et al[45] studied the natural history of diabetic autonomic neuropathy in 73 patients. At entry, there were 40 patients with abnormal tests of autonomic function (Valsalva maneuver and handgrip test); of these 25 had postural hypotension. There were no differences in the age and duration of diabetes between the patients with normal or abnormal tests. The survival of those patients with abnormal tests was on average 18.6 months while the group with normal tests survived 28.6 months. Postural hypotension, gastric symptoms, and hypoglycemic unawareness were more frequent among the patients who died.

Patients with diabetic autonomic neuropathy have been divided into two groups, hypo- and hyperadrenergic responders, according to their pattern of norepinephrine concentration in plasma.[46] Patients with the hypoadrenergic syndrome have lower than normal supine levels of norepinephrine in plasma. There is no increase in plasma norepinephrine on standing. The lesion in this group of patients is in the peripheral or postganglionic nerves[46] (*cf* IOH with isolated autonomic neuropathy). Hyperadrenergic postural hypotension is characterized by abnormally high supine levels of norepinephrine in plasma. On standing, patients demonstrated excessive increase in plasma norepinephrine. In those patients, Tohmek et al[47] could not demonstrate a reduced vascular responsiveness to norepinephrine or sodium depletion. The patients had, however, a lower than normal red cell volume. Plasma renin activity, urinary sodium, and potassium excretion in patients with diabetic orthostatic hypotension are no different from normal subjects or control patients with diabetes mellitus without autonomic neuropathy.

Cerebrovascular Disease and Postural Hypotension

Cerebrovascular disease can produce postural hypotension in the acute and chronic phases of the disease.[48] The mechanism underlying the hypotension is not clear, however. Underlying loss of elasticity of blood vessels is probably an important factor since it increases the risk of cerebrovascular disease and alters hemodynamic reflexes in the elderly.[47] Impaired regulation of cerebral blood flow precipitates the development of symptoms of postural hypotension. Regulation of cerebral blood flow depends in part on sympathetic nervous activity. Thus, elderly patients with cerebrovascular disease would develop postural hypotension when sympathetic dysfunction occurs. Plasma norepinephrine levels in patients with cerebrovascular and postural hypotension might be normal in the supine position, but the concentration of norepinephrine does not increase on standing, particularly in those patients with damaged vasomotor centers.

Orthostatic Hypotension in Parkinson's Disease

Patients with Parkinson's disease may develop postural hypotension, although it is not clear whether Parkinson's disease is an incomplete form of the Shy-Drager syndrome.[36,37] Furthermore, postural hypotension in patients with parkinsonism can be due to drugs, in particular to the use of levodopa.[49] The use of carbidopa has reduced the side-effects of levodopa on the cardiovascular system.[50]

Precipitating Factors in Postural Hypotension

In Table 18-3 are listed the most important precipitating factors of postural hypotension in old age. These factors precipitate postural hypotension by impairing the main determinants of arterial blood pressure; eg, reduction in plasma or red cell volume after hemorrhage, dehydration, or anemia can result in postural hypotension; examples of impairment in cardiac function are myocardial ischemia and cardiac arrhythmias; vascular resistance is affected by environmental and other conditions such as a hot bath, hot weather, etc. Clearly, the operation of several factors increases the risk of postural hypotension. Chapman and Asmussen[51] described a series of patients with dizziness, fainting, and precordial distress when standing. The patients had extensive varicose veins in the legs which presumably would precipitate postural hypotension by accommodating more blood when standing. Bandaging of the legs prevented fainting during 80° head-up tilt in this series of patients.

Iatrogenic Postural Hypotension

A list of drugs commonly used in the elderly and associated with postural hypotension is also included in Table 18-3. A single drug at therapeutic doses may or may not produce postural hypotension; however, since they are usually prescribed in combinations or are associated with precipitating factors, they often will result in postural hypotension. Drugs may account for more than half of the incidence of postural hypotension in the elderly.[52,53]

Table 18-3
Common Precipitating Factors in Postural Hypotension in Old Age

Changes in Blood Volume
Hemorrhage
Anemia
Dehydration
Hyponatraemia
Hypokalemia
Varicose veins
Drugs
Myocardial Insufficiency
Cardiac infarction
Cardiac arrhythmias
Valvular disease
Peripheral Vasodilatation
Hot weather or bath
Exercise
Micturition
Infections
Drugs
Drugs
Hypotensive agents
ganglion blockers
alpha-methyldopa
beta-blockers
reserpine
Diuretics
Phenothiazines
Tricyclic antidepressants
Tranquillizers
Barbiturates
Antihistamines
Monoamine oxidase inhibitors

INVESTIGATION OF ELDERLY PATIENTS WITH POSTURAL HYPOTENSION

Elderly patients in whom postural hypotension is suspected require a complete medical history and detailed physical examination with particular emphasis on drug intake and adequate blood pressure measurements. Blood pressure measurements should be obtained after the patient has been placed in the supine position for 20 minutes, at the end of the physical examination. Then, the patient stands unaided for at least 2 minutes, during which time the blood pressure is recorded at 30- or 60-second intervals with the arm held at the same level of the heart. It is also helpful to record heart rate (or pulse rate), in both the supine and standing positions.

Hematologic and biochemical profiles are useful to uncover patients with anemia, diabetes mellitus, and other metabolic disorders which may underlie postural hypotension in the elderly. Other studies, such as electrocardiography help in the diagnosis of patients with cardiac arrhythmias, coronary heart disease, etc. Twenty-four-hour ECG monitoring would also help in patients with syncope and cardiac arrhythmias.

Tests of autonomic function are difficult to interpret and validate in the elderly. A tilt test or simply having the patient stand while simultaneously measuring blood pressure and heart rate are quite good predictors of autonomic nervous function. A recorded fall of more than 20 mmHg in mean arterial blood pressure suggests significant postural hypotension. The diagnosis is virtually confirmed if this fall is accompanied by symptoms. It may be necessary to repeat the tests over several days because of variability in expression. Patients who fail to accelerate heart rate are likely to have some degree of sympathetic autonomic denervation. If the heart rate is higher than normal supine and again fails to increase on standing, complete autonomic neuropathy is likely. Sophisticated tests, nevertheless, may be required in some patients. Plasma norepinephrine measurement, if available, is the most useful test, as described above.

MANAGEMENT OF POSTURAL HYPOTENSION

The range of drugs and physical maneuvers used in the management of postural hypotension in patients of all ages is great. The wide variety of treatment approaches implies that none are entirely satisfactory for all patients and this underlies the observation that the etiology of postural hypotension is often inadequately investigated in the individual patient. As we have discussed earlier, postural hypotension in old people is not a single syndrome—there are a number of subsets and management should be directed to the presumed underlying mechanisms.

Precipitating Factors

In the individual patient with postural hypotension a search for precipitating factors should be made before resorting to potent and possibly dangerous drug therapy. The simple warning of old people about the dangers of hot baths coupled with the provision of bath support rails can prevent much serious trauma. Avoidance of rapid postural changes during hot weather, especially where subclinical dehydration may be present and unrecognized, are obvious factors to be considered. Constipation, prostatism, or severe coughing may lead to defecation, micturition, and cough syncope, respectively. These mechanisms probably all act by the induction of reflex vasodilatation rather than by a Valsalva maneuver.

Elderly patients with minimally impaired postural reflexes may manifest symptoms of postural hypotension following the introduction of certain drugs. Thus, dehydration and loss of body sodium may be induced by overzealous use of diuretic agents. In many elderly patients with chronic fluid retention the diuretic dosage required to treat the problem in the initial stages is continued unchanged leading to volume and salt depletion and thus aggravating postural hypotension. Dosage reduction monitored by careful weighing can usually be accomplished. In the treatment of hypertension in the elderly the doctor must be prepared to trade off the potential benefits of lowering the supine blood pressure against the aggravation of postural symptoms.

Other drugs inhibit postural reflexes directly. Thus the phenothiazines (chlorpromazine, haloperidol), barbiturates, imipramine, and other tricyclic antidepressants have all been associated with postural hypotension in otherwise physically fit young and old patients.[52,54] Such drugs and also potent hypnotics should be used with care in the elderly, especially if given at night to the patient with nocturia. Levodopa inhibits postural reflexes by central and peripheral actions[55–57] and may aggravate postural symptoms in parkinsonian patients, especially if elderly.[58] The addition of a decarboxylase inhibitor reduces to some extent the extracerebral adverse effects of levodopa[59,60] though minor degrees of postural hypotension may persist.[61] An increased proportion of decarboxylase inhibitor to levodopa may be better tolerated in patients with postural hypotension.[62]

Treatment of Established Postural Hypotension

Developments in biochemistry and pharmacology, particularly in the fields of neurotransmitters and prostaglandins, have led to some exciting therapeutic possibilities in the treatment of the elderly patient with established symptoms from postural hypotension. However, these innovations should not obscure the simple methods discussed previously in relation to precipitating and aggravating factors. Equally, some older methods, both physical and pharmacologic, are still valid. Unfortunately, few comparative studies have been published and many reports have been confined to small numbers of inadequately investigated patients.

Physical methods Simple manipulation of the patient's environment can go far to relieve the symptoms of postural hypotension in the elderly. Thus, a shower may be safer than a bath, the provision of bathroom rails, high chairs, and low overhead cupboards are all useful. Training the patient to change posture with dignity and not speed—to sit on the side of the bed on first rising and to pause before walking after sitting—is useful.

Developments in the aerospace field have led to the introduction of antigravity suits for the treatment of postural hypotension. Their action is to increase venous return and prevent venous pooling on standing. However, our experience is that while such suits are effective, in old people their cumbersome nature precludes their use for the length of time required to treat the condition. Full length, ie, to waist height, firm elastic stockings, while not as effective as antigravity suits, are a satisfactory compromise in the elderly.

There is some evidence that the reflex mechanisms (see above) involved in maintenance of postural hypotension can be "trained" by physical methods. Sleeping in a foot-down position produced by raising the head of the bed may be useful in some elderly patients, but sleeping in the sitting position, a popular treatment a few decades ago, is not a good idea in old people as it may lead to other problems (contractures, stiffening of joints, edema, venous ulceration). Repeated graded postural stress over a number of days is useful in patients who develop symptoms after a period of recumbency. Finally, a recent new physical therapy was reported by Moss et al.[63] The use of fixed atrial pacing at a rate of 100 bpm in a 77-year-old man with severe postural hypotension abolished symptoms and the postural fall in blood pressure was attenuated. He had not responded to other therapies and was asymptomatic 10 months after pacemaker insertion. This innovative approach may be used more often in the future for carefully selected patients.

Drug therapy

Vitamins and minerals Occasionally B_{12} deficiency with peripheral neuropathy may present with symptomatic postural hypotension.[64] In these cases the postural hypotension responds to replacement therapy.

While sodium repletion increases pressor response to exogenous norepinephrine we and others,[65] do not believe sodium deficiency, as evidenced by hyponatremia, is a common etiologic agent in postural hypotension in the elderly. We have been impressed by the lack of efficiency of potassium supplementation unless there is an underlying endocrine disturbance such as hyperaldosteronism.[66]

Dihydroergotamine Dihydroergotamine is a direct vascular alpha-receptor stimulant said to affect capacitance vessels (veins) rather than resistance vessels (arterioles).[67] Its use has been widely advocated in the treatment of postural hypotension and in the prevention of falls in blood pressure during spinal anesthesia. Unfortunately, dihydroergotamine in the doses required to treat postural hypotension does have significant effects on resistance vessels producing supine hypertension.[68,69] Also, as Bobik et al[69] emphasize, this adverse effect is significantly more pronounced in the elderly. Unfortunately, the oral bioavailability of dihydroergotamine is reduced markedly via the hepatic first-pass mechanism which itself is affected by aging. The lack of effectiveness of oral, as opposed to parenteral, dihydroergotamine in postural hypotension is well recognized.

Sympathomimetic amines Sympathomimetic agents can act in postural hypotension in two ways. Firstly, they may act indirectly by enhancing the release of norepinephrine from remaining intact sympathetic nerve endings in patients with partial autonomic denervation. Drugs which have been used in this way include amphetamines, methylphenidate, and tyramine combined with a monoamine oxidase inhibitor.[70] Secondly, a sympathomimetic agent may act directly on the vascular smooth muscle and induce vasoconstriction in the absence of sympathetic innervation. The agents which have been used include norepinephrine, phenylephrine, and midodrine. Ephedrine probably acts both directly and indirectly and has been used in postural hypotension for more than 50 years.

While the theoretical basis for the use of both direct- and indirect-acting sympathomimetic agents is attractive, their adverse effects preclude their extensive use in the elderly. Thus, the responses of postural change in blood pressure vary greatly from individual to individual. Even when the agent has no effect on postural hypotension it often produces intolerable supine hypertension necessitating emergency correction. The adverse effects of sympathomimetic agents on cardiac conduction and the central nervous system should be considered before using these drugs in elderly patients who are likely to be at risk because of underlying cardiac and cerebral disease.

Mineralocorticoids The hypothesis that postural hypotension is related in some way to reduction in circulating blood volume naturally led to attempts to increase plasma volume. If postural hypotension is associated with significant dehydration or volume depletion secondary to endocrine dysfunction, eg, hypopituitarism or Addison's disease, this approach is valid. Treatment should, however, be directed at the underlying condition rather than the volume depletion per se. It should be appreciated that most patients with postural hypotension have a normal or even an increased blood volume; presumably their own remaining homeostatic mechanisms (vasopressin and aldosterone) have been activated in response to the stimulus of the recurrent hypotension. Thus, attempts to increase plasma volume carry the inherent danger of precipitating volume overload and cardiac failure. This is especially likely in the elderly.[71]

In spite of these objections, mineralocorticoids have been used extensively to treat postural hypotension, especially in younger patients. Of the various mineralocorticoids available, the most commonly prescribed agent has been 9-alpha-fluorohydrocortisone, a synthetic analogue of aldosterone. The main problem with all mineralocorticoids is excess fluid retention. Fluid retention tends to decrease with time[71] and if the patient can be followed through the initial introduction of relatively low-dose 9-alpha-fluorohydrocortisone, perhaps by maintaining a semirecumbent posture even at night, then an equilibrium may be achieved.

Prostaglandin synthetase inhibitors Since their discovery and naming in 1934,[72] the prostaglandins have been a group of lipids in search of exploitation. Two varieties of prostaglandins—PGE_1 and PGI_2 (prostacyclin)—have vasodilator properties. In 1978 Kochar and Itskovitz[73] demonstrated that indomethacin, prostaglandin synthetase inhibitor, decreased blood pressure falls in four patients with postural hypotension and the Shy-Drager syndrome. There was no effect in the single patient with cerebral ischemia and mild diabetes. Others have subsequently shown that indomethacin may benefit some, but not all patients with postural hypotension,[74] although headache tends to limit its long-term value.

Flurbiprofen is a more potent prostaglandin synthetase inhibitor and better tolerated than indomethacin. Flurbiprofen has little effect on supine blood pressure and when combined with 9-alpha-fluorohydrocortisone is effective in controlling standing blood pressure at least initially. Others have found flurbiprofen ineffective.[75]

Other drugs Beta-blocking agents, eg, propranolol, have been used to counteract the supine hypertension produced by sympathomimetics, but the results are less than satisfactory. Beta-blockers on their own have been used in the treatment of postural hypotension secondary to the rare syndrome of hyperbradykininemia. The likelihood of precipitating cardiac failure is a particularly limiting factor in elderly patients.

ACKNOWLEDGMENTS

We are grateful for the continued support to our studies of CONACYT (Mexico), the British Foundation for Age Research, and Smith Kline & French Laboratories Ltd.

REFERENCES

1. Nylin R, Lavender S: Studies on circulation with aid of tagged erythrocytes in a case of orthostatic hypotension. *Ann Intern Med* 1948;28:723–746.
2. Foley HT: Clinical observations on value of orthostatic tolerance test in normal man. *J Aviat Med* 1949;20:230–237.
3. Rodstein M, Zeman FD: Postural blood pressure changes in the elderly. *J Chronic Dis* 1957;6: 581–588.
4. Hickler RB, Hoskins RG, Hamlin JT: The clinical evaluation of faulty orthostatic mechanisms. *Med Clin North Am* 1960;44:1237–1250.
5. Johnson RH, Smith AC, Spalding JMK, et al: Effect of posture on blood pressure in elderly patients. *Lancet* 1965;1:731–733.
6. Caird FI, Andrews GR, Kennedy RD: Effect of posture on blood pressure in the elderly. *Br Heart J* 1973;35:527–530.
7. White NJ: Heart rate changes on standing in elderly patients with orthostatic hypotension. *Clin Sci* 1980;58:411–413.
8. Wollner L, McCarthy ST, Soper NDW, et al: Failure of cerebral autoregulation as a cause of brain dysfunction in the elderly. *Br Med J* 1979;1: 1117–1118.
9. Management of orthostatic hypotension, editorial. *Lancet* 1981;1:963–964.
10. Myers MG, Kearns PM, Kennedy DS, et al: Postural hypotension and diuretic therapy in the elderly. *Can Med Assoc J* 1978;119:581–585.
11. Norris AH, Shock NW, Yiengst MJ: Age changes in heart rate and blood pressure responses to tilting and standardized exercise. *Circulation* 1953;8: 521–526.
12. Lee TD Jr, Lindeman RD, Yiengst MJ, et al: Influence of age on the cardiovascular and renal responses to tilting. *J Appl Physiol* 1966;21:55–61.
13. Vargas E: *Cardiovascular Mechanisms in the elderly,* thesis. University of Manchester, Manchester, England, 1983.

14. Matalon SV, Farhi LE: Cardiopulmonary readjustments in passive tilt. *J Appl Physiol* 1979;47: 503–507.
15. Brown E, Grei JS, Greenfield ADM, et al: Circulatory responses to simulated gravitational shifts of blood in man induced by exposure of the body below the iliac crests to subatmospheric pressure. *J Physiol* 1966;183:607–627.
16. Collins KJ, Exton-Smith AN, James MH, et al: Functional changes in autonomic nervous responses with ageing. *Age Ageing* 1980;9:17–24.
17. Vargas E, Lye M: The assessment of autonomic function in the elderly. *Age Ageing* 1980;9: 210–214.
18. Currens JH: A comparison of the blood pressure in the lying and standing position: A study of 500 men and 500 women. *Am Heart J* 1948;35:646–654.
19. Wade OL, Bishop KW: *Cardiac Output and Regional Blood Flow.* Oxford, Blackwell Scientific Publications, 1962.
20. Hamilton WF: Measurement of cardiac output, in Hamilton WF, Dow P (eds): *Handbook of Physiology.* Washington DC, American Physiological Society, 1962, vol 1, sect 2, pp 551–584.
21. Guyton AC: Essential cardiovascular regulation—The control linkage between bodily needs and circulatory function, in Dickinson CJ, Marks J (eds): *Developments in Cardiovascular Medicine.* London, MTP Press, 1978, pp 265–302.
22. Folkow B, Neil E: *Circulation.* London, Oxford, 1971.
23. Cowley AW Jr, Miller JP, Guyton AC: Open-loop analysis of the renin-angiotensin system in the dog. *Cir Res* 1971;28:568–581.
24. Mellander S: Systemic circulation: Local control. *Ann Rev Physiol* 1970;32:313–344.
25. Lassen NA: Cerebral blood flow and oxygen consumption in man. *Physiol Rev* 1959;39:183–238.
26. Gaskell P, Burton AC: Local postural vasomotor reflex arising from the limb veins. *Cir Res* 1953;1: 27–44.
27. Johnston CI, Newman M, Woods R: Role of vasopressin in cardiovascular homeostasis and hypertension. *Clin Sci* 1981;61:129s–139s.
28. Cryer PE: Physiology and physiopathology of the human sympathoadrenal neuroendocrine system. *N Engl J Med* 1980;303:436–444.
29. Ziegler MG: Postural hypotension. *Ann Rev Med* 1980;31:239–245.
30. Cryer PE, Silverberg AB, Santiago JV, et al: Plasma catecholamines in diabetes. The syndromes of hypoandrenergic and hyperadrenergic postural hypotension. *Am J Med* 1978;64:407–416.
31. Gribbin B, Pickering TG, Sleight P, et al: Effect of age and high blood pressure on baroreflex sensitivity in man. *Circ Res* 1971;29:424–431.
32. Kidd C, Linden RJ: Recent advances in the physiology of cardiovascular reflex, with special reference to hypotension. *Br J Anaesth* 1975; 47: 767–776.
33. Rowe JW, Troen BR: Sympathetic nervous system and aging in man. *Endocr Rev* 1980;1:167–178.
34. Weidmann P, Demyttenaere-Bursztein S, Maxwell MH, et al: Effect of aging on plasma renin and aldosterone in normal man. *Kidney Int* 1975;8:325–333.
35. Bradbury S, Eggleston C: Postural hypotension: A report of three cases. *Am Heart J* 1925;1:73–86.
36. Shy GM, Drager GA: A neurological syndrome with orthostatic hypotension. *Arch Neurol* 1960;2: 511–527.
37. Graham JG, Oppenheimer DR: Orthostatic hypotension and nicotine sensitivity in a case of multiple system atrophy. *J Neurol Neurosurg Psychiatry* 1969;32:28–34.
38. Bannister R, Oppenheimer DR: Degenerative disease of the nervous system associated with autonomic failure. *Brain* 1972;95:457–474.
39. Schirger A, Thomas JE: Idiopathic orthostatic hypotension: Clinical spectrum and prognosis. *Cardiology* 1976;61(suppl 1):144–149.
40. Ewing DJ: Cardiovascular reflexes and autonomic neuropathy. *Clin Sci Mol Med* 1978;55:321–327.
41. Magrini F, Ibrahim MM, Tarazi RC: Abnormalities of supine hemodynamics in idiopathic orthostatic hypotension. *Cardiology* 1976;61(suppl 1): 125–135.
42. Hickman JB, Pryor WW: Cardiac output in postural hypotension. *J Clin Invest* 1951;30: 401–405.
43. Bannister R, Sever P, Gross M: Cardiovascular reflexes and biochemical responses in progressive autonomic failure. *Brain* 1977;100:327–344.
44. Henrich WL: Autonomic insufficiency. *Arch Intern Med* 1982;142:339–344.
45. Ewing DJ, Campbell IW, Clarke BF: The natural history of diabetic autonomic neuropathy. *Q J Med NS* 1980;49:95–108.
46. Grover-Johnson N, Kim GE: Ultrastructural evidence of a decrease in autonomic nerves which innervate small blood vessels in diabetes. *J Neuropathol Exp Neurol* 1976;35:336–347.
47. Tohmek JF, Shah SD, Cryer PE: The pathogenesis of hyperadrenergic postural hypotension in diabetic patients. *Am J Med* 1979;67:772–778.
48. Gross M: The effect of posture on subjects with cerebrovascular disease. *Q J Med NS* 1970;39: 485–491.
49. McNay JL: Effect of selected drugs on arterial response to upright posture. *Cardiology* 1976;61 (suppl 1):191–198.
50. Watanabe AM, Parks LC, Kopin IJ: Modification of the cardiovascular effects of L-dopa by decarboxylase inhibitors. *J Clin Invest* 1971;50: 1322–1328.
51. Chapman EM, Asmussen E: On the occurrence of dyspnea, dizziness and precordial stress occasioned by the pooling of blood in varicose veins. *J Clin Invest* 1942;21:393–399.
52. Barraclough MA, Sharpey-Schafer EP: Hypotension from absent circulatory reflexes. *Lancet* 1963; 1:1121–1126.
53. Jackson G, Pierscianowski TA, Mahon W, et al: Inappropriate antihypertensive therapy in the elderly. *Lancet* 1976;2:1317–1318.
54. Blackwell B: Adverse effects of antidepressant drugs. *Drugs* 1981;21:201–219.
55. Henning M, Rubenson A, Trolin G: On the localization of the hypotensive effect of L-dopa. *J Pharm Pharmacol* 1972;24:447–451.
56. Kaplan HR, Barker JW, La Sala SA: Direct evidence for a centrally-mediated hypotensive action of L-dopa in anesthetized dogs. *Eur J Pharmacol* 1972;17:273–278.

57. Reid JL, Calne DB, George CF, et al: The action of L-dopa on baroreflexes in Parkinsonism. *Clin Sci* 1972;43:851–859.
58. Godwin-Austen RB, Tomlinson BE, Frears CC, et al: Effects of L-dopa in Parkinson's disease. *Lancet* 1969;2:165–168.
59. Calne DB, Petrie A, Rao S, et al: Action of L-alpha-methyldopa-hydrazine on the blood pressure of patients receiving levodopa. *Br J Pharmacol* 1972;44:162–164.
60. Marsden CD, Parkes JD, Rees JE: A year's comparison of treatment of patients with Parkinson's disease with Levodopa combined with Carbidopa versus treatment with Levodopa alone. *Lancet* 1973;2:1459–1462.
61. Barbeau A, Mars H, Botez MI, et al: Levodopa combined with peripheral decarboxylase inhibition in Parkinson's disease. *Can Med Assoc J* 1972;106: 1169–1174.
62. Hoehn MH: Increased dosage of carbidopa in patients with Parkinson's disease receiving low doses of levodopa. *Arch Neurol* 1980;37:146–149.
63. Moss AJ, Glaser W, Topol E: Atrial tachypacing in the treatment of a patient with primary orthostatic hypotension. *N Engl J Med* 1980;302:1456–1457.
64. White WB, Reik L, Cutlip DE: Pernicious anaemia seen initially as orthostatic hypotension. *Arch Intern Med* 1981;141:1543–1544.
65. Lye M: The interieur milieu and aging, in Brocklehurst JC (ed): *Textbook of Gerontology and Geriatric Medicine*, ed 3, Edinburgh, Churchill Livingstone Inc, 1983, pp 94–101.
66. Biglierri EG, McIlroy MB: Abnormalities of renal function and circulating reflexes in primary aldosteronism. *Circulation* 1966;33:80–86.
67. Mellander S, Nordenfelt I: Comparative effects of dihydroergotamine and noradrenaline on resistance exchange and capacitance functions in the peripheral circulation. *Clin Sci* 1970;39:183–201.
68. Bevegard S, Castenfors J, Lindblad L-E: Haemodynamic effects of dihydroergotamine in patients with postural hypotension. *Acta Med Scand* 1974; 196:473–477.
69. Bobik A, Jennings G, Skews H, et al: Low oral bioavailability of dihydroergotamine and first-pass extraction in patients with orthostatic hypotension. *Clin Pharmacol Ther* 1981;30:673–679.
70. Davies B, Bannister R, Sever P: Pressor amines and monoamine oxidase inhibitors for treatment of postural hypotension in autonomic failure: Limitations and hazards. *Lancet* 1978;1:172–175.
71. Chobanian AV, Volicer L, Fift P, et al: Mineralocorticoid-induced hypertension in patients with orthostatic hypotension. *N Engl J Med* 1979;301: 68–73.
72. Von Euler US: Zur Kenntnis der pharmakalogischen Wirkungen von Nativsekreten und Extrakten männlicher accessorischer Geschlectsdrüsen. *Arch Pharmakol Exp Pathol* 1934;175:78–84.
73. Kochar MS, Itskovitz HD: Treatment of idiopathic orthostatic hypotension (Shy-Drager Syndrome) by indomethacin. *Lancet* 1978;1:1011–1014.
74. Davies B, Bannister R, Sever P: Indomethacin treatment of postural hypotension in autonomic failure. *Br Med J* 1980;1:181.
75. Sutcliffe RLG: Indomethacin treatment of postural hypotension. *Br Med J* 1980;1:1229.

CHAPTER 19
Hypertension in the Aged: Special Procedures in Diagnosis and Evaluation

Jan I. M. Drayer
Michael A. Weber

The evaluation of the patient with mild to moderate hypertension now focuses on characterizing the nature of the hypertension itself rather than on the search for secondary causes. The main purpose of the initial evaluation of the hypertensive patient is to establish the presence of high blood pressure levels. A secondary goal is the assessment of hypertension-induced end-organ damage and to determine the presence or absence of other risk factors for cardiovascular complications. Finally, the workup of the hypertensive patient includes tests which will help to determine the appropriate therapeutic approach to the patient's hypertension. The basic studies can easily be accomplished in one or two outpatient visits and are fairly inexpensive. Obviously, in patients with severe hypertension the initial workup should focus on defining the best therapeutic approach. Blood pressure should be lowered quickly in these patients so as to prevent serious cardiovascular complications or the development of accelerated or malignant hypertension. Moreover, in these patients with severe hypertension future workup should focus on identifying possible secondary forms of hypertension. The search for secondary hypertension also should be undertaken in patients in whom the physical examination or the laboratory tests provide evidence for renovascular hypertension, renal forms of hypertension, mineralocorticoid excess, or a pheochromocytoma. Such forms of hypertension, however, are rare in elderly patients whose hypertension is mild.

In this chapter, we will focus on the evaluation of the elderly patient with mild to moderate systolic hypertension, diastolic hypertension, or both.

CHARACTERIZING HYPERTENSION IN THE ELDERLY PATIENT

The diagnosis of mild to moderate hypertension can only be made in patients who never have used antihypertensive agents or in patients who have discontinued their medication for at least two weeks. Patients who have been using spironolactone or reserpine should discontinue their medication for at least three weeks prior to the diagnostic workup. It is known that some antihypertensive agents actually may increase blood pressure in certain patients.[1,2] Moreover, in patients whose blood pressure has been controlled during long-term administration of antihypertensive therapy, blood pressure may not return to abnormally high levels after discontinuation of the treatment.[3]

Blood pressure should be measured on at least two occasions, several days apart, in the untreated patient. During the first visit blood pressure should be measured in both the right and the left arm. This can most easily be done with the patient seated. In some patients, especially older individuals, blood pressure may be higher in the right arm. The difference in systolic blood pressure between the right and left arm may be as high as 30 mmHg in some patients. This usually is a consequence of the particular anatomical pattern of the blood vessels in that patient. In some patients, however, the difference is due to a partial stenosis of one of the main arteries such as the subclavian or brachial artery. Arteriosclerotic changes of the arteries are more commonly found in older than in younger patients; in any case, the higher reading should be regarded as representative for the blood pressure in the systemic circulation in that patient. And the arm in which the higher pressure is found should be used as the reference for monitoring antihypertensive therapy in these patients. The next step in the diagnosis of hypertension is the measurement of blood pressure (in the reference arm) in the supine and upright postures. Blood pressure is first measured after 10 minutes of supine rest and then after 2 minutes of passive standing. Heart rate is counted immediately after blood pressure is taken. An abnormal response of blood pressure is often found in the elderly population.[4] Marked decreases in systolic blood pressure (an average 30 mmHg) after assuming the upright posture are found in 23% of the elderly; in another 6% of patients, moderate falls in systolic blood pressure may occur. These decreases in systolic blood pressure may be observed with or without decreases in heart rate. The presence of orthostatic hypotension is at least partly dependent upon blood pressure–related abnormalities of the sino-aortic baroreceptor reflex.[5] The severity of the orthostatic response can further be established by the presence or absence of symptoms such as dizziness and the response of blood pressure after further periods, eg, 5 minutes of passive standing. Prolonged hypotension is more likely to cause symptoms than short-term posture-induced changes in blood pressure and heart rate. The presence of orthostatic hypotension in the elderly patient should be taken into consideration in choosing antihypertensive therapy. Antihypertensive agents with peripheral sympatholytic properties, such as prazosin or high doses of alpha-methyldopa, especially when given in combination with a diuretic, may worsen the orthostatic hypotension in these patients. Increases in blood pressure after standing are observed in approximately 7% of the elderly population.[4] The prognostic importance of orthostatic hypertension has not yet been evaluated.

Special care should be taken in the measurement of blood pressure in patients with arrhythmias; eg, atrial fibrillation or patients with multiple ventricular premature beats. Ventricular premature beats are more common in elderly patients than in young hypertensives. Systolic blood pressure in these patients is defined as the blood pressure level at which the first of a series of Korotkoff sounds (phase I) are heard. Diastolic blood pressure is that pressure at which the last of a series of Korotkoff sounds (phase V) is heard. Thus, infrequent extra sounds are not used in the measurement of blood pressure in these patients.

As mentioned earlier, blood pressure should be taken on at least two occasions several days apart in the elderly patient. The main reason for repeated blood pressure measurements is the increased variability in blood pressure found in older patients. We have shown recently that the variability of systolic blood pressure is significantly greater in older than in younger patients.[6–8] In these studies, variability of blood pressure was defined as the standard deviation of the mean of all blood pressures measured at 7.5-minute intervals during a full day. We found that whereas the variability of systolic blood pressure, pulse pressure, and diastolic blood pressure are greater in older than in younger patients, the variability of heart rate is less in older than in younger patients (Table 19-1). The data also show that the variability of systolic blood pressure is greater than that of diastolic blood pressure, consistent with the finding by others that variability of blood pressure is proportional to its height. It is established that systolic blood pressure is significantly greater in older than in younger patients.[9] However, the correlation between the variability of systolic blood pressure and age is not significant.[7,10] Therefore, systolic blood pressure itself rather than age seems to be the chief determinant of its variability. In only one study has a differing trend been observed.[11]

Variability of blood pressure in most studies has been based on data obtained during long-term monitoring of blood pressure. We have attempted to define variability of blood pressure using short-term (2-h) monitoring of blood pressure. However, the correlation between the variability of blood pressure observed during two hours and that obtained during whole-day monitoring of blood pressure was not significant.[7]

It is evident that the variability of blood pressure directly is related to the predictability of the whole-day average of pressure by a single, casual blood pressure measurement. The variability of blood pressure does not seem to have predictive significance for the presence of cardiovascular complications.[12] Gross[13] reported that although blood pressure was significantly higher in patients with impaired vertebro-carotid circulation than in controls (175/96 vs 144/87 mmHg), the diurnal range in pressures were similar between these groups (33/20 vs 32/19 mmHg). Others have found that patients with cardiac left ventricular hypertrophy have higher pressures and a smaller

Table 19-1
Variability of Blood Pressure and Heart Rate in 24 Younger and 26 Older Hypertensive Patients (mean ± SEM)

	Younger Patients	*P*	Older Patients
Age (yr)	36 ± 2	< 0.001	64 ± 1
Variability of*			
Systolic blood pressure	15 ± 1	< 0.01	18 ± 1
Pulse pressure	13 ± 1	< 0.1	15 ± 1
Diastolic blood pressure	13 ± 1	ns	14 ± 1
Heart rate	13 ± 1	< 0.01	11 ± 1

*Defined as the standard deviation of all measurements obtained during a 24-hour monitoring period. See Drayer et al[7] for full details.

variability of blood pressure than those without left ventricular hypertrophy on the ECG.[14] Both Richardson et al[11] and Soholow et al[15] found that patients without cardiovascular complications tended to have a greater variation in blood pressure during the day than patients with cardiovascular complications.

It should be stressed that elderly patients with mild to moderate hypertension have a circadian pattern of blood pressure similar to that found in younger hypertensive patients.[7] In both subgroups of patients lowest pressures are found most often during the night (between 10 PM and 6 AM) and highest pressures most often during the day (between 6 AM and 10 PM). A clear difference in the circadian pattern of blood pressure between the two subgroups, however, is that systolic blood pressure is consistently higher and diastolic blood pressure consistently lower in the older patients throughout the 24-hour day. The parallelism of the blood pressure–time curves between the two groups reveals that pulse pressure is greater in older than in younger patients at all times of the day.

It has been speculated that a better knowledge of the variability of blood pressure during the day might help predict the time of day at which patients are most vulnerable to cardiovascular complications. Moreover, possible changes in the variability and the circadian pattern could help explain the increased prevalence of these complications in the elderly. Marshall[16] reported that 40% of all ischemic cerebrovascular events occur between midnight and 6 AM. Gyarfas et al[17] and Johanssen[18] reported that the peak incidence of myocardial infarction is between 8 AM and 9 AM, with a smaller peak between 5 PM and 6 PM. It is unlikely that the relatively small changes in variability and circadian patterns observed in younger and older patients can explain the rhythmicity of these complications. The fall in blood pressure during the night is not more pronounced in older patients than in younger patients, and the pre-morning rise in blood pressure is also similar in the two groups.

ASSESSMENT OF BLOOD PRESSURE-INDUCED END ORGAN DAMAGE

The importance of the age-related increase in systolic blood pressure as a risk factor for cardiovascular complications has been clearly demonstrated. Increased systolic or diastolic blood pressures may lead to cardiovascular complications such as cerebrovascular accidents, heart failure, and renal failure. Moreover, abnormal blood pressures also are directly related to preclinical signs of heart disease such as cardiomegaly on the chest film and cardiac left ventricular hypertrophy on the ECG.

However, we have shown that the sensitivity of the chest film and the ECG in the detection of left ventricular hypertrophy is poor, but that M-mode echocardiography can detect abnormalities in cardiac anatomy or function in approximately 50% of patients with mild or moderate hypertension.[19] It is of interest to note that the correlation between voltages on the ECG and age is significantly negative; $r = -.72$, $n = 12$, $P < 0.05$.[20] In contrast, echocardiographic measurements of cardiac muscle mass seem to increase with age, although the relationship between cardiac muscle mass and age is not a strong one. However, one must remember that with age, systolic blood pressure increases rapidly. Many investigators have found significant correlations between age-related increases in systolic blood pressure and echocardiographic signs of left ventricular hypertrophy.[21–23] This correlation is found in hypertensive as well as in normotensive subjects.[24] The known relationship between systolic blood pressure and the development of cardiac hypertrophy helps to explain the process of cardiac hypertrophy and its regression following antihypertensive therapy.[25] The correlations between systolic blood pressure and cardiac muscle mass are stronger than those between diastolic blood pressure and cardiac muscle mass. Similarly, systolic hypertension is much more common in the elderly population than diastolic hypertension. Therefore, it is not surprising that increases in cardiac muscle mass often are seen in the elderly. The thickness of the interventricular septum increases strikingly with age, whereas the thickness of the posterior free wall increases less markedly. In our study, hypertensive patients aged 60 to 70 years had a systolic blood pressure which was 22% higher and a diastolic blood pressure which was only 4% higher than that in hypertensive patients aged between 20 and 30 years. The marked increase in systolic blood pressure was related to the 25% increase in septal thickness and the 12% increase in the thickness of the posterior free wall.[19] It is likely that increased systolic pressures have a more direct effect on the interventricular septum than on the posterior wall of the left ventricle. Thus, it is more appropriate to measure muscle mass separately as septal and posterior wall thicknesses rather than as calculated total left ventricular mass, because of this preferential increase in septal thickness found in many elderly patients with systolic hypertension. The presence of cardiac hypertrophy can help define appropriate antihypertensive therapy in the elderly population.[25]

Cardiac function, measured during rest using M-mode echocardiography, does not change significantly with age in hypertensive patients. However, exercise-induced increases in ejection fraction are less pronounced in older than in younger patients.[26] The only signs of a possible decrease in diastolic cardiac function that we have found is the decrease in mitral valve E-F slope of more than 50% that occurs between the ages of 20 and 70.[19] Interestingly, this change in E-F slope is not related to age-induced changes in systolic blood pressure, and might reflect a specific age-related phenomenon.

The data presented here clearly show that both age and age-related increases in systolic blood pressure are related to echocardiographic signs of a change in cardiac anatomy and function. The M-mode echocardiogram helps to determine the presence of even mild forms of cardiac hypertrophy and moderate decreases in cardiac function in the elderly population with systolic or diastolic hypertension. Often, these changes will not be found on the chest film or the routine ECG.

Blood pressure and age are important factors in the development of left ventricular hypertrophy. Other factors that may attenuate the hypertrophic response are intrinsic biochemical abnormalities within myocardial fibers (eg, collagen deposits), the presence of concurrent arteriosclerosis and myocardial fibrosis, and a relative absence of humoral factors which usually stimulate cardiac growth. These humoral factors include age-related decreases in renin activity and in the activity of beta-adrenergic sympathetic activity. However, other factors actually may enhance the development of hypertrophy in the elderly hypertensive population. These may include age-related increases in blood viscosity. These considerations should be kept in mind in the judgment of the degree of cardiac hypertrophy in the hypertensive patient.

The presence of arrhythmias also should be considered as a possible risk factor for cardiovascular complications. The routine ECG or, in selected cases, Holter monitoring might be helpful in the diagnosis of arrhythmias in the elderly hypertensive patients. One should keep in mind that diuretics, which are one of the first choices for antihypertensive treatment in the elderly, might induce or worsen the incidence of potentially dangerous ventricular premature beats.[27,28] Therefore, the presence of arrhythmias might be used as a consideration in the more careful precription of diuretic agents in the elderly.

THE PREDICTION OF WHOLE-DAY BLOOD PRESSURE LEVELS IN THE ELDERLY

The variability of systolic blood pressure increases with its height. Higher systolic blood pressures are found in older patients. Because of these two observations it is not very likely that a single, casual blood pressure level will accurately reflect the average of blood pressures observed during the 24-hour day. The data in Table 19-2 reveal that the correlations between casual systolic blood pressure and the 24-hour average of systolic blood pressures are fairly weak in younger or older patients with hypertension as well as in patients with very mild hypertension or those with predominant systolic hypertension. However, when the average of multiple blood pressures measured during a 2-hour morning period (between 8 and 10 AM) are correlated with the full 24-hour average of systolic blood pressure, it is evident that predictability increases markedly in all subgroups of hypertensive patients.[7,29,30] Similarly, the 2-hour averages of multiple diastolic blood pressures better predict the full 24-hour diastolic blood pressure than do casual measurements (Table 19-3).

Thus, blood pressure is better defined by the average of multiple blood pressures than by casual (single) blood pressure measurements.[7,9,15,29,30] The importance of the better prediction of the whole-day blood pressure is further confirmed by the significant correlation found between multiple blood pressure averages and the degree of cardiac hypertrophy.[20,23] Thus, the average of blood pressures measured during 2 or 24 hours better predicts the degree of left ventricular hypertrophy than does casual blood pressure. This observation is more pronounced for systolic blood pressures than for diastolic blood pressures (Table 19-4).

Table 19-2
Relationships Between Casual Systolic Blood Pressure and Average of Systolic Blood Pressures*

	Systolic Blood Pressure	
	Casual vs *24-hour Average*	*2-hour Average* vs *24-hour Average*
Younger patients n=24	$r = +.69$ $P < 0.001$	$r = +.88$ $P < 0.001$
Older patients n=26	$r = +.42$ $P < 0.1$	$r = +.84$ $P < 0.001$
Patients with mild hypertension n=19	$r = +.14$ ns	$r = +.84$ $P < 0.001$
Patients with isolated systolic hypertension n=11	$r = +.68$ $P < 0.05$	$r = +.85$ $P < 0.001$

*Obtained during monitoring of blood pressure during 2 hours in the morning and whole-day average systolic blood pressure in different subgroups of hypertensive patients.
See Mancia et al[8] and Drayer et al[29] for full details.

Table 19-3
Relationships Between Casual Diastolic Blood Pressure and Average of Diastolic Blood Pressures*

	Diastolic Blood Pressure	
	Casual vs *24-hour Average*	*2-hour Average* vs *24-hour Average*
Younger patients n=24	$r = +.71$ $P < 0.001$	$r = +.88$ $P < 0.001$
Older patients n=26	$r = +.43$ $P < 0.1$	$r = +.70$ $P < 0.001$
Patients with mild hypertension n=19	$r = +.21$ ns	$r = +.61$ $P < 0.01$
Patients with isolated systolic hypertension n=11	$r = +.33$ ns	$r = +.82$ $P < 0.01$

*Obtained during monitoring of blood pressure during 2 hours in the morning and whole-day average diastolic blood pressure in different subgroups of hypertensive patients.

Table 19-4
Correlations Between Various Measurements of Blood Pressure and Echocardiographically Determined Left Ventricular Mass (n = 12)

Blood Pressure	Left Ventricular Mass	
Casual systolic	$r = +.55$	$P < 0.1$
Casual diastolic	$r = +.10$	ns
2-hour average systolic	$r = +.76$	$P < 0.01$
2-hour average diastolic	$r = +.60$	$P < 0.05$
24-hour average systolic	$r = +.81$	$P < 0.01$
24-hour average diastolic	$r = +.56$	$P < 0.05$

EVALUATION OF ADDITIONAL RISK FACTORS FOR CARDIOVASCULAR DISEASE

The workup of the elderly patient with hypertension may be completed by tests for the presence or absence of other cardiovascular risk factors. Such risk factors include tests for diabetes mellitus, hyperlipidemia, potassium deficiency, and abnormal kidney function. The importance of blood viscosity and its determinants, hematocrit and fibrinogen, for the development of cardiac hypertrophy have been discussed previously.[30,31] It is well accepted that the presence of diabetes mellitus or hyperlipidemia might change the initial approach to antihypertensive therapy in these patients.

The whole workup of the elderly hypertensive patient is fairly simple and is not necessarily different from that in the younger patient. However, certain age-related phenomena need to be recognized. The differences between younger and older hypertensive agents might demand special tests. The tests listed in Table 19-5 will help to assess the risk-status of the elderly hypertensive patient and may be of help in defining the most appropriate antihypertensive therapy.

The use of simple noninvasive technics such as short-term monitoring of blood pressure, Holter monitoring, or the M-mode echocardiogram should be considered in the evaluation of some of the elderly patients. Patients with ischemic heart disease or ventricular premature beats on the routine ECG might benefit from a complete Holter monitoring. Patients with relatively high casual blood pressures but a surprising absence of signs of left ventircular hypertrophy on the chest film or ECG might benefit from the more sensitive M-mode echocardiogram. Similarly, patients with a low casual blood pressure but surprising signs of cardiac hypertrophy on the ECG or chest film might benefit from short-term or long-term monitoring of blood pressure so as to better assess their true level of blood pressure. It has to be emphasized that such recommendations are based on the exciting results from recent studies in this area. Obviously, long-term follow-up studies are needed to fully substantiate the role of these special diagnostic tests in the elderly population with hypertension. However, the initial studies provide promising results that should help to better define those patients in need of antihypertensive medication and those in whom this therapeutic decision can safely be delayed.

Table 19-5
Evaluation of Elderly Patient with Hypertension

Diagnostic Workup
- Blood pressure measurements in right and left arm
- Blood pressure and heart rate measurements in supine and standing position
- Multiple blood pressures taken over a period of several days
- Short-term (2-hour) blood pressure monitoring (optional)
- Long-term (24-hour) blood pressure monitoring (optional)

Evaluation of Cardiovascular Complications
- Chest film
- ECG
- 24-hour Holter monitoring (optional)
- M-mode echocardiogram (optional)

Evaluation of Other Risk Factors
- Renal function
- Serum electrolytes
- Hematocrit, fibrinogen, and blood viscosity (optional)
- Fasting glucose and lipid levels

REFERENCES

1. VA Cooperative Study Group on Antihypertensive Agents: Comparison of propranolol and hydrochlorothiazide for the initial treatment of hypertension. *JAMA* 1982;248:1996–2003.
2. Drayer JIM, Keim HJ, Weber MA, et al: Unexpected pressor responses to propranolol in essential hypertension. *Am J Med* 1976;60:897–903.
3. Garbus SB, Weber MA, Priest RT, et al: The abrupt discontinuation of antihypertensive treatment. *J Clin Pharmacol* 1979;19:476–486.
4. Steen B: Orthostatic tests in 85 geriatric patients in inpatient long-term care. *Scand J Soc Med* 1977;14:146–150.
5. Watson RDS, Stallard TJ, Littler WA: Factors determining the variability of arterial pressure in hypertension. *Clin Sci* 1979;57(suppl):283–285.
6. Watson RDS, Stallard TJ, Flint R, et al: Factors determining direct arterial pressure and its variability

in hypertensive men. *Hypertension* 1980;2:333-341.

7. Drayer JIM, Weber MA, De Young JL, et al: Circadian blood pressure monitoring in younger and older ambulatory hypertensive patients. *Am J Med* 1982;73:493-499.
8. Mancia G, Ferrari A, Gregorini L, et al: Blood pressure variability in man: Its relation to high blood pressure, age and baroreflex sensitivity. *Clin Sci* 1980;59(suppl):401-404.
9. Drayer JIM, Weber MA, Laragh JH, et al: Renin subgroups in essential hypertension. *Clin Exp Hypertens* 1982;A4:1817-1834.
10. Kain HK, Hinman AT, Sokolow M: Arterial blood pressure measurements with a portable recorder in hypertensive patients. *Circulation* 1964;30:882-892.
11. Richardson DW, Honowr AJ, Fenton GW, et al: Variation in arterial pressure throughout the day and night. *Clin Sci* 1964;26:445-460.
12. Kannel WB, Sorlie P, Gordon T: Labile hypertension: A faulty concept? The Framingham Study. *Circulation* 1980;61:1183-1187.
13. Gross M: Diurnal blood pressure variations in cerebrovascular disease. *Ann Intern Med* 1970;72:823-833.
14. Raftery EB, Millar-Graig MW: Information derived from direct 24-hour recordings, in Clement DL (ed): *Blood Pressure Variability*. Baltimore, University Park Press, 1979, pp 67-81.
15. Sokolow M, Perloff D, Cowan R: Contribution of ambulatory blood pressure to the assessment of patients with mild to moderate elevation of office blood pressure. *Cardiovasc Rev Rep* 1980;4:295-303.
16. Marshall J: Diurnal variation in occurrence of strokes. *Stroke* 1977;8:230-231.
17. Gyarfas I, Csukas I, Gandi H: Analysis of the diurnal periodicity of acute myocardial infarction attacks. *Sante Publique Bucur* 1976;19:77-84.
18. Johansson BW: Myocardial infarction in Melius 1960-1968. *Acta Med Scand* 1972;191:505-510.
19. Savage DD, Drayer JIM, Henry WL, et al: Echocardiographic assessment of cardiac anatomy and function in hypertensive subjects. *Circulation* 1979;59:623-632.
20. Drayer JIM, Weber MA, DeYoung JL: Blood pressure as a determinant of cardiac left ventricular muscle mass. *Arch Intern Med* 1983;143:90-92.
21. Cohen A, Hagan AD, Watkins J, et al: Clinical correlates in hypertensive patients with left ventricular hypertrophy diagnosed with echocardiography. *Am J Cardiol* 1981;47:335-341.
22. Ibrahim MM, Madkour MA, Mossallam R: Factors influencing cardiac hypertrophy in hypertensive patients. *Clin Sci* 1981;61(suppl):105-108.
23. Rowlands DB, Ireland MA, Glover DR, et al: The relationship between ambulatory blood pressure and echocardiographically assessed left ventricular hypertrophy. *Clin Sci* 1981;61(suppl):101-103.
24. Sutton MStJ, Reichek N, Lovett J, et al: Effects of age, body size, and blood pressure on the normal human left ventricle, abstracted. *Circulation* 1980;62:3-305.
25. Drayer JIM, Gardin JM, Weber MA: Echocardiographic left ventricular hypertrophy in hypertension. *Chest* 1983;84:217-221.
26. Port S, Cobb RF, Coleman RE, et al: Effect of age on the response of the left ventricular ejection fraction to exercise. *N Engl J Med* 1980;303:1133-1137.
27. Hollifield JW, Slaton PW: Thiazide diuretics, hypokalemia and cardiac arrhythmias. *Acta Med Scand* 1981;647(suppl):67-73.
28. Holland OB, Nixon JV, Kuhnert LV: Diuretic-induced ventricular ectopic activity. *Am J Med* 1981;70:762-768.
29. Drayer JIM, Weber MA, DeYoung JL: The use of short-term ambulatory blood pressure monitoring in differing forms of hypertension. *Clin Exp Hypertens* 1983;A5(10):1597-1610.
30. Weber MA, Drayer JIM, Wyle FA, et al: A representative value for the whole-day blood pressure. *JAMA* 1982;248:1626-1628.
31. Letcher RL, Chien S, Pickering TG, et al: Direct relationship between blood pressure and blood viscosity in normal and hypertensive subjects: Role of fibrinogen concentration. *Am J Med* 1981;70:1195-1202.

CHAPTER 20
Left Ventricular Aneurysm

C. A. Visser
G. Kan
G. K. David
D. Düren
K. I. Lie

As early as 1757, a ventricular aneurysm was described by the English surgeon John Hunter.[1] The association with coronary artery disease, however, was not made until the early twentieth century. The major cause of ventricular aneurysm in Western society is acute transmural myocardial infarction.[2] Occasionally bacterial endocarditis, cardiac trauma, sarcoidosis, syphilitic gumma, and congenital anomaly are responsible.[3,4] The incidence of aneurysm formation in survivors of a transmural infarction has been reported to vary between 10% and 38%, depending on the definition employed.[5,6] The vast majority of aneurysms develop two weeks to two years after acute myocardial infarction,[7] although earlier formation has been documented.[2]

DEFINITION

There is no uniformly accepted definition of a left ventricular aneurysm. An aneurysm may be defined anatomically as a localized protrusion beyond the ventricular surface, involving the free wall or the septum or both[8] (Figure 20-1). A characteristic of such aneurysms is their tendency to collapse at surgery or autopsy. Usually the wall is markedly thinned and consists of fibrous tissue with or without myocardial fibers. This anatomical definition, however, is difficult to use clinically because the surface of the left ventricle is not visualized angiographically. Furthermore, except in extreme cases, it is difficult to define with precision localized abnormalities in the diastolic shape of the left ventricle.

From a functional or clinical point of view a left ventricular aneurysm may be defined as a localized portion of the ventricular wall that exhibits systolic dyskinesia or akinesia by fluoroscopy or contrast ventriculography. Using these criteria, however, a thin-walled resectable aneurysm may be found at surgery in one half to two thirds of patients.[9]

The distinction between anatomical and functional aneurysms is useful because in the latter the wall may consist of ischemic (potentially reversible) myocardium. It is obvious that in clinical practice the incidence of a functionally defined left ventricular aneurysm will exceed the incidence of an anatomically defined aneurysm.

Apart from the aneurysms discussed above, which can be called true aneurysms, there are also so-called false or pseudoaneurysms (Figure 20-2). A true aneurysm is composed of elements of the left ventricular wall. A false or pseudoaneurysm of the left ventricle develops from rupture of recently infarcted myocardium forming a localized hemopericardium confined by adherent parietal pericardium. The wall of a pseudoaneurysm is composed of fibrous tissue, derived from the organization of the pericardial hematoma and contains no endocardial or myocardial elements[10] (Figure 20-2).

TRUE POSTINFARCTION ANEURYSM

The common type of left ventricular aneurysm is a true aneurysm. Gradual widening of the left

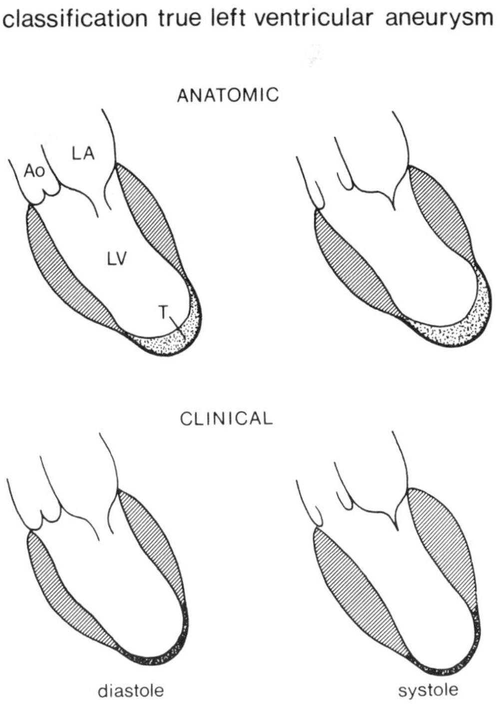

Figure 20-1 Diagrams of hearts in diastole and systole. An anatomically defined aneurysm protrudes beyond the ventricular surface during the whole cardiac cycle. The functional aneurysm protrudes only during the ventricular systole. An anatomic aneurysm has a thin wall and often contains a thrombus (T). Ao = aorta, La = left atrium, LV = left ventricle.

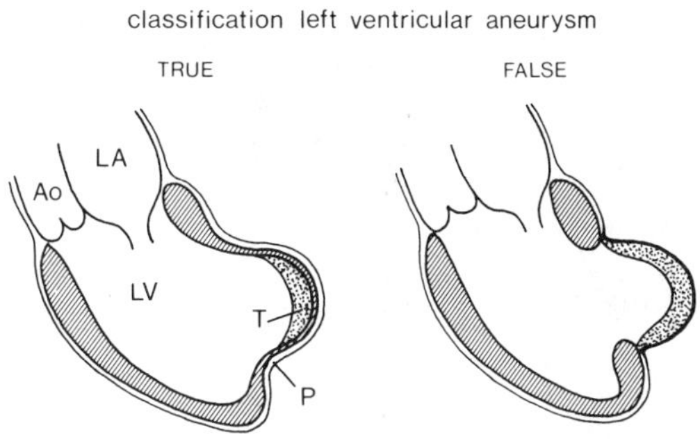

Figure 20-2 Diagrams of a true and false aneurysm. A true aneurysm has a mouth that is as wide or wider than the maximal diameter of the aneurysm. The wall is composed of fibrous tissue with or without residual myocardial elements. The false left ventricular aneurysm protrudes during the whole cardiac cycle and has a mouth that is considerably smaller than the maximal diameter of the aneurysm. The wall is composed of pericardium (P) and often ruptures. For abbreviations, see Figure 20-1.

ventricular cavity and gradual thinning of the wall becomes apparent as this type of aneurysm is approached (Figure 20-3). Usually residual myocardial elements can be identified even in those cases where the wall consists predominantly of fibrous tissue. The cavity of these aneurysms is frequently lined by mural thrombus.[3,11] In contrast to a pseudoaneurysm, rupture of a true aneurysm is quite rare, because of the strength of the fibrotic aneurysmal wall and support of the thickened pericardium.[10] There is a propensity toward involvement of the apex and anterior segments of the left ventricle.[3,12] This relates to the high frequency of prior anterior myocardial infarction in patients with an aneurysm.[3,5,8]

In our series of 324 patients (mean age 55 ± 11 years; 61 females and 263 males) with a cineangiographically documented aneurysm of the left ventricle, 118 patients (74%) had anterior and/or lateral infarction implicating the left anterior descending artery and its major branches. Occlusion of the right or circumflex arteries may be responsible for the infrequent posterior basal aneurysms.

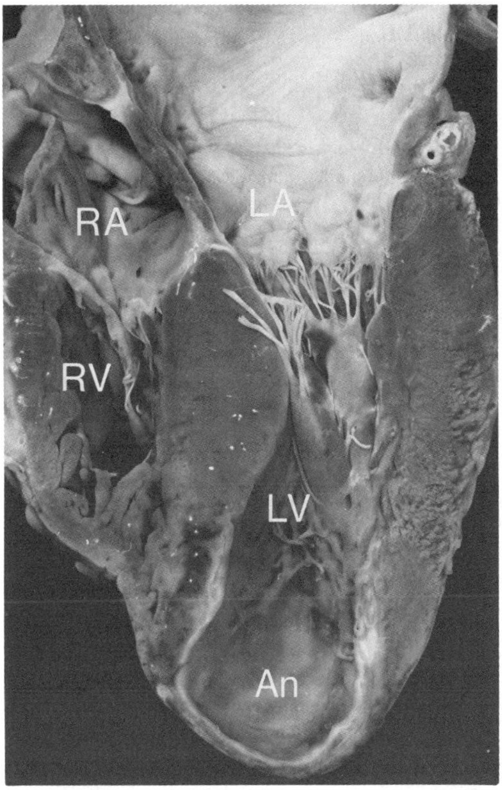

Figure 20-3 A four-chamber cross section through the heart which reveals a left ventricular apical aneurysm (An) as the end-stage of a previous transmural infarction. The cardiac contour is much distorted by this aneurysm. The wall is thin and composed of connective tissue. RA = right atrium, LA = left atrium, RV = right ventricle.

Usually patients with a left ventricular aneurysm have severe and extensive coronary artery disease.[5-7] In our series 44% had three-vessel disease, 30% two-vessel disease and 26% one-vessel disease. The left main artery was affected (more than 50% narrowing) in 3%. The extent of coronary artery disease was similar in patients aged 65 years or less (n = 277) and patients older than 65 years (n = 47).

Clinical Characteristics

The commonest clinical manifestations of a left ventricular aneurysm are congestive heart failure, angina pectoris, serious ventricular arrhythmias (ventricular tachycardia and ventricular fibrillation), and systemic emboli.[13] The large majority of our patients (77%, Table 20-1) had angina pectoris, a higher proportion than previously reported, although the demographic characteristics were about similar. This discrepancy is not surprising since in the last 5 years patients with angina pectoris are catheterized earlier. Congestive heart failure is reported to be present in 51% to 85% of patients with an aneurysm.[13] About half of the patients older than 65 years in our series had congestive heart failure in contrast to 31% of the patients aged 65 years or younger ($P<$ 0.012, Table 20-1). Serious ventricular arrhythmias were found in 25% of our patients. This is in keeping with other reports. The incidence was similar in both age groups. Clinically recognized systemic emboli are reported in up to 13%.[14-16] We did not evaluate this complication in our series because of the partly retrospective nature of our study.

Clinical Diagnosis

A successful clinical diagnosis of a postinfarction ventricular aneurysm based on physical examination, ECG and roentgenogram of the chest is usually made in 80% of patients. In our series an aneurysm was diagnosed correctly on physical examination in 32%.

The ECG, at rest and after exercise, was very helpful in our series in identifying an aneurysm. In 69% of our patients the presence of an aneurysm was diagnosed correctly. This is in keeping with other reports.[17] In our patients routine chest radiology in posteroanterior and lateral views revealed the presence of an aneurysm in 24%. The value of chest radiology is controversial. Mourdjinis et al[17] noted a high incidence of a localized protrusion along the left heart border, whereas others felt that routine chest film rarely led to the diagnosis of ventricular aneurysm.[6] It has previously been noted that aneurysms confined to the apical region can be completely obscured by the diaphragmatic shadows.[18] Since the large majority of aneurysms are located at the level of the cardiac apex[3] the limited value of routine chest films is therefore not surprising.

With the advent of radionuclide angiography and echocardiography the diagnostic accuracy has been significantly improved[19,20] (Figure 20-4). We recently found for two-dimensional echocardiography a sensitivity of 93% and a specificity of 94% in detecting a postinfarction aneurysm in a large prospective study including 422 patients with documented myocardial infarction. Furthermore, these technics are capable of differentiating true from false aneurysms.[21,22]

At present left ventricular cineangiography is still the gold standard in determining the nature and extent of left ventricular asynergy. It is largely on the basis of this test that one decides whether or not a patient will undergo ventricular aneurysmectomy.

Hemodynamic Findings

When the noncontractile area of the left ventricle is small the normal myocardium can maintain an overall ventricular function near normal by increased fiber shortening.[23] However, Johnston et al[6] reported that when the internal surface of the noncontractile region exceeds 20% to 25% of the left ventricular internal surface, increased fiber shortening of the normal residual or nonan-

Table 20-1
Most Common Clinical Manifestations in 324 Patients with Ventricular Aneurysm in Relation to the Age of 65 Years

	$\leqslant$65 Years (n = 291)			>65 Years (n = 47)	
	No.	*% of Total*		*No.*	*% of Total*
Angina pectoris	214	74	ns	36	77
Congestive heart failure	89	31	$P<0.012$	23	49
Ventricular arrhythmia	73	25	ns	9	19

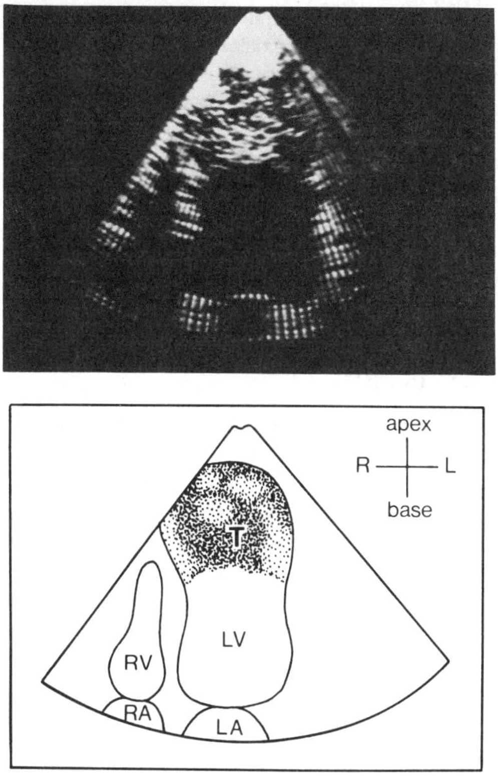

Figure 20-4 Apical four-chamber echocardiogram demonstrating a large apicoseptal aneurysm with a thrombus (T).

eurysmal myocardium cannot maintain a normal stroke volume. In such a patient the stroke volume may increase if the left ventricle enlarges.[24]

The disadvantage of ventricular enlargement according to the law of Laplace is that an augmented wall stress is required in order to generate the intraventricular pressure.[25] This results, however, in an increase in myocardial oxygen requirement and may provoke ischemic dysfunction in nonaneurysmal segments perfused by diseased coronary arteries. Further compromise of the nonaneurysmal myocardium may be caused by the impaired diastolic function of the ventricle, ie, a decreased compliance resulting in an elevated end-diastolic pressure, which is often present in patients with an aneurysm.[9,26] This was the case in 60% of our patients. The elevated end-diastolic pressure may decrease the perfusion of the residual myocardium. Thus, to improve cardiac performance in patients with an aneurysm, reduction of the end-diastolic volume of the left ventricle by removal of the noncontractile area is advocated.

INDICATIONS FOR SURGICAL TREATMENT

The decision to perform surgical therapy for left ventricular aneurysm should be predicated on the surgeon's ability to improve a patient's functional status and on the longevity relative to his prognosis without operation. This decision can be a difficult one inasmuch as the prognostic significance of an aneurysm has not yet been clearly defined. Schlichter[2] found in retrospective studies with autopsy-proven aneurysms a 5-year mortality rate of approximately 80%. The most common cause of death in these reports was not refractory heart failure but acute myocardial infarction. The same was found by Gorlin et al[27] in a prospective study with cineangiographically documented aneurysms.

In another prospective study[17] a five-year mortality rate of about 50% was found in patients with large aneurysms, and a less than 10% five-year mortality rate in patients with small aneurysms. Recently Proudfit et al[28] observed in their 10-year follow-up study of 601 patients with different cineangiographic findings that patients with an aneurysm defined as "definite paradoxical bulging during systole," had a five-year mortality rate of approximately 50%, and patients with a hypokinetic or akinetic segment a 30% five-year mortality rate. According to the more recent Coronary Artery Surgery Study (CASS)[29] the natural history of patients with an aneurysm is not as poor as suggested by earlier reports.

Congestive Heart Failure

Considering that removal of the noncontractile area relieves the heart of several mechanical disadvantages, Bailey successfully performed the first aneurysmectomy in 1955 in a patient with refractory congestive heart failure utilizing a special clamp without extracorporeal circulation.[30] A temporary cardiopulmonary bypass was used for the first time by Cooley in 1958.[31] The mortality rate of aneurysmectomy shortly after infarction is high, up to 50%, in contrast to elective or late surgery.[32] In the largest series of 400 patients, Loop et al[33] reported a mortality rate of 8.4% in isolated aneurysmectomy and 11% in aneurysmectomy with related surgical procedures such as revascularization and mitral valve replacement. In our series we found an overall mortality rate of 24% in patients aged 65 years and younger and of 31% in patients aged over 65 years. This difference was not significant. Our mortality rate is higher than recently reported[33] and reflects the large proportion of patients undergoing urgent ventricular reconstruction and myocardial revascularization.

It has been suggested recently that the contractility of the nonaneurysmal portion of the left ventricle and the extent of coronary artery disease is of great importance to the short- and long-term prognosis following aneurysmectomy.[34] Most patients with severe congestive heart failure improve in functional class (New York Heart Association) after aneurysmectomy.[32,35] Increase of exercise tolerance was observed by Cullhed et al.[36]

In contrast to the almost unanimously reported clinical improvement, the hemodynamic results following aneurysmectomy are controversial.[36,37] Significant improvement as well as no change or significant deterioration has been reported in ventricular performance. However, the large majority of these studies were not prospective, the number of patients was limited, and postoperative evaluation was not performed at the same time. Thus, hemodynamic improvement following aneurysmectomy remains as yet unsettled.

Ventricular Tachycardia

Since reentry is the mechanism of ventricular tachycardia following acute myocardial infarction,[38] several surgical procedures have been developed recently to interrupt the reentrant circuit in patients with medically refractory ventricular tachycardias.[39,40] Ventricular aneurysmectomy with or without coronary revascularization was the most commonly attempted surgical treatment employed to abolish these tachycardias. The success rate, however, was moderate and the mortality rate high, especially in patients with recent (within 1 month) infarction or severe myocardial dysfunction.[41] More recently, endocardial excision has been introduced and would seem to be an important adjunct to simple aneurysmectomy for the surgical treatment of ventricular tachyarrhythmias.[42]

Recurrent Angina Pectoris and Systemic Emboli

Both recurrent or persistent angina pectoris and systemic emboli are the least encountered primary indications for aneurysmectomy. Angina pectoris is almost always eliminated or improved following surgical therapy.[33] This might be explained by improved hemodynamics and/or revascularization of coexisting obstructive lesions in other coronary arteries.

Considering the high incidence of intraaneurysmal thrombi the rather rare occurrence of clinically recognized systemic emboli is surprising. The reported incidence is up to 13%.[2,14-16,43]

Although the influence of long-term use of anticoagulants in patients with an aneurysm and thrombi has not yet been settled, this therapy should be evaluated in the individual patient before cardiac surgery.[44] Two-dimensional echocardiography might be of help in this respect.

CONCLUSION

The clinical signs and symptoms of a left ventricular aneurysm in patients age 65 years or younger and aged over 65 years are almost similar, and so is the mortality rate of aneurysmectomy. Since the operative mortality of aneurysm resection with or without revascularization is significant, especially shortly after infarction, operation should only be performed in patients refractory to medical treatment. Moreover, aneurysmectomy should only be performed in patients with a well-delineated aneurysm with a good residual function.

REFERENCES

1. Hunter J: An account of the dissection of morbid bodies. Original manuscript in the library of the Royal College of Surgeons, 1757;32:30–34.
2. Schlichter J, Hellerstein HK, Katz LM: Aneurysm of the heart: A correlative study of 102 proved cases. *Medicine (Baltimore)*, 1954;33:43–47.
3. Saksena FB, Kramer ME, Towne WD, et al: Infective aneurysm of the left ventricle: Angiographic and electrocardiographic features. *Am Heart J* 1978;96:384–389.
4. Symbas PN, Baldwin BJ, Schlant RC, et al: Unusual complications of bacterial endocarditis. *Br Heart J* 1971;33:664–670.
5. Appelbaum E, Nicolson GHB: Occlusive disease of the coronary arteries; An analysis of the pathological anatomy in 168 cases with electrocardiographic correlation in 36 of them. *Am Heart J* 1935;10: 662–669.
6. Johnson JB, Lam ACH, Wright JS: Ventricular aneurysm after infarction: Pathological and surgical features. *J Thorac Cardiovasc Surg* 1969;58: 14–21.
7. Davies MJ, Robertson WB: Diseases of the coronary arteries, in Pomerance A, Davies MJ (eds): *The Pathology of the Heart*. London, Blackwell Scientific Publications 1975, p 81.
8. Chesler E: Aneurysms of the left ventricle. *Cardiovasc Clin* 1972;4:187–193.

9. Klein MD, Herman MV, Gorlin R: A hemodynamic study of left ventricular aneurysm. *Circulation* 1967;35:614–620.
10. Roberts WC, Morrow AG: Pseudoaneurysm of the left ventricle. An unusual sequel. *Am J Med* 1967; 43:639.
11. Cooley DA, Hallman GL, Henly WS: Left ventricular aneurysm due to myocardial infarction. *Arch Surg* 1964;88:114–119.
12. Phares WS, Edwards JE, Burchell H: Cardiac aneurysms: Clinicopathologic studies. *Mayo Clin Proc* 1954;28:264–268.
13. Douglas AH, Sferrazza J, Marici F: Natural history of aneurysm of ventricle. *NY State J Med* 1962;62: 209-215.
14. Cooley DA, Hallman GL: Surgical treatment of left ventricular aneurysm: Experience with excision of postinfarction lesions in 80 patients. *Prog Cardiovasc Dis* 1968;11:222–229.
15. Favaloro RG, Elfer DB, Groves LK, et al: Ventricular aneurysm; Clinical experience. *Ann Thorac Surg* 1968;6:227.
16. Klage TH, Ullal SR, Hill JD, et al: Dyskinesia and aneurysm of the left ventricle: Surgical experience in 36 patients. *J Cardiovasc Surg* 1971;12:273–277.
17. Mourdjinis A, Oben E, Raphael MJ, et al: Clinical diagnosis and prognosis of ventricular aneurysm. *Br Heart J* 1968;30:497–501.
18. Baron MG: Postinfarction aneurysm of the left ventricle. *Circulation* 1971;43:762–767.
19. Kraemer R, Kerber RE, Abboud FM: Ventricular aneurysm: Use of echocardiography. *J Clin Ultrasound* 1973;1:60–65.
20. Weyman AE, Peskoe SM, Williams ES, et al: Detection of left ventricular aneurysms by cross-sectional echocardiography. *Circulation* 1976;54: 936–941.
21. Gatewood RP, Nanda NC: Differentiation of left ventricular pseudoaneurysm from true aneurysm with two-dimensional echocardiography. *Am J Cardiol* 1980;46:869–875.
22. Catherwood E, Mintz GS, Kotler MN, et al: Two dimensional echocardiographic recognition of left ventricular pseudoaneurysm. *Circulation* 1980;2: 294–298.
23. Herman MV, Heinle RA, Klein MD, et al: Localized disorders in myocardial contraction; Asynergy and its role in congestive heart failure. *N Engl J Med* 1967;277:222–228.
24. Gorlin R, Rolett EL, Yurchak PM, et al: Left ventricular volume in man measured by thermodilution. *J Clin Invest* 1964;43:1203–1208.
25. Burch GE, De Pasquale NP, Cronvich JA: Influence of ventricular size on the relationship between contractile and manifest tension. *Am Heart J* 1965; 69:624–628.
26. Graber JD, Oakley CM, Pickering BN, et al: Ventricular aneurysm: An appraisal of diagnosis and surgical treatment. *Br Heart J* 1972;34:830–835.
27. Gorlin RM, Klein MD, Sullivan JM: Prospective correlative study of ventricular aneurysm: Mechanistic concept and clinical recognition. *Am J Med* 1967;42:512–519.
28. Proudfit WL, Bruschke AVG, Sones FM Jr: Natural history of obstructive coronary artery disease: A ten-year study of 601 nonsurgical cases. *Prog Cardiovasc Dis* 1978;21:53–58.
29. Prognostic significance of angiographically documented left ventricular aneurysm from the Coronary Artery Surgery Study (CASS). *Am J Cardiol* 1982;50:157–162.
30. Likoff W, Bailey CP: Ventriculoplasty: Excision of myocardial aneurysm: report of a successful case. *JAMA* 1955;158:915–922.
31. Cooley DA, Collins HA, Morris GC, et al: Ventricular aneurysm after myocardial infarction: Surgical excision with use of temporary cardiopulmonary bypass. *JAMA* 1958;167:557-562.
32. Kapelanski DP, Jafar Al-Sadir, Lamberti JL, et al: Ventriculographic features predictive of surgical outcome for left ventricular aneurysm. *Circulation* 1978;58:1167–1172.
33. Loop FD, Effler DB, Navia JA, et al: Aneurysms of the left ventricle: Survival and results of a ten-year surgical experience. *Ann Surg* 1973;178:399–404.
34. Chia-Sen Lee D, Johnson RA, Boucher CA, et al: Angiographic predictors of survival following left ventricular aneurysmectomy. *Circulation* 1977;56: (suppl 2):12–18.
35. Donaldson RM, Honey M, Balcon R, et al: Surgical treatment of postinfarction left ventricular aneurysm in 32 patients. *Br Heart J* 1976;38:1223-1227.
36. Cullhed I, Delius W, Björk L, et al: Resection of left ventricular aneurysm: Late results. *Acta Med Scand* 1975;197:241–245.
37. Kitamura S, Echevarria M, Kay JH, et al: Left ventricular performance before and after removal of the noncontractile area of the left ventricle and revascularization of the myocardium. *Circulation* 1972;45:1005.
38. Wellens HJJ, Lie KI, Durrer D: Further observations on ventricular tachycardia as studied by electrical stimulation of the heart: Chronic recurrent ventricular tachycardia during acute myocardial infarction. *Circulation* 1974;49:647–652.
39. Gallagher JJ, Oldham HN, Wallace AG, et al: Ventricular aneurysm with ventricular tachycardia: Report of a case with epicardial mapping and successful resection. *Am J Cardiol* 1975;35:696–701.
40. Giraudon G, Fontaine G, Frank R, et al: Encircling endocardial ventriculotomy: A new surgical treatment for life-threatening ventricular tachycardia resistant to medical treatment following myocardial infarction. *Ann Thorac Surg* 1978;26:438–442.
41. Ricks WB, Winkle RA, Shumway NG, et al: Surgical management of life-threatening ventricular arrhythmias in patients with coronary artery disease. *Circulation* 1977;56:38–44.
42. Horowitz LN, Harken AH, Kastor JA, et al: Ventricular resection guided by epicardial and endocardial mapping for treatment of recurrent ventricular tachycardia. *N Engl J Med* 1980;302:589.
43. Reeder GS, Lengyel M, Tajik AJ, et al: Mural thrombus in left ventricular aneurysm. Incidence, role of angiography and relation between anticoagulation and embolization. *Mayo Clin Proc* 1981;56: 77–81.
44. Simpson MT, Oberman A, Kouchoukos NT, et al: Prevalence of mural thrombi and systemic embolization with left ventricular aneurysm. Effect of anticoagulation therapy. *Chest* 1980;77:463–468.

CHAPTER 21
Diagnosis and Management of Arterial Occlusive Disease in the Elderly

Sandor A. Friedman

PERIPHERAL ARTERIAL DISEASE

Arterial occlusive disease of the lower extremities is a major cause of disability in the elderly. Since there has never been a thorough epidemiologic study of this problem based on complete clinical examination of the peripheral circulation, the true incidence and prevalence are not known. It is clear from routine medical practice, however, that a sizable proportion of the population over the age of 60 has at least asymptomatic peripheral arterial disease. The only available data grossly underestimate the incidence and prevalence of peripheral arteriosclerosis because they focus only on very limited aspects of the problem. In the Framingham study, the annual incidence of intermittent claudication was 2.6/1000 for men and 1.1/1000 for women.[1] There was a sharp increase in incidence with age, with most new cases occurring after the age of 50. Radiologically visible calcification of the aorta has been found in 10% of 40-year-old individuals.[2]

In the past, there has been a great deal of confusion about the criteria for diagnosis. The presence of one palpable foot pulse was considered normal. We now know, however, that a missing posterior tibial pulse is always indicative of arterial occlusion.[3] This fact was established in a study of over 800 small children. The dorsalis pedis pulse may be congenitally absent in a small percentage of the normal population, probably no more than 5%. The externally measured blood pressure in each of these peripheral arteries should never be lower than arm blood pressure but may appear higher because of cuff artifact induced by the wider girth of the lower extremity.

If one uses these more stringent criteria for diagnosis, peripheral arterial disease in asymptomatic form may be found quite often in individuals who have not yet had any clinical manifestations of atherosclerosis. In one study of patients entering a coronary care unit with their first symptoms of ischemic heart disease, 50% already had evidence on physical examination of peripheral arterial disease.[4] Thus routine examination of pulses in middle-aged and elderly individuals may be helpful in assessing the risk of developing serious ischemia elsewhere.

Risk Factors for Peripheral Arteriosclerosis

The known risk factors for atherosclerosis are virtually identical throughout the body, but their relative importance varies considerably among vascular beds. In the case of peripheral arterial disease, diabetes mellitus is clearly the most important predisposing condition. Since precise criteria for the diagnosis of diabetes mellitus are not available, estimates of its prevalence in patients with peripheral arteriosclerosis vary widely. Glucose tolerance decreases normally with aging, and one cannot apply the standard criteria based on normal individuals in the third decade to patients in the seventh decade. In one study, clinical evidence of peripheral arterial occlusion was found 11 times as frequently in diabetics as in normal individuals.[5] Other studies have suggested that at least 15% to 20% of patients with femoropopliteal occlusion have diabetes. With more liberal criteria, one can conclude that a much higher proportion of patients with femoropopliteal disease under the age of 60 have diabetes. A high but somewhat smaller proportion of patients with aortoiliac disease are also diabetic. These statements appear valid if the diagnosis of diabetes is based on at least one of the following criteria: (1) documentation of long-term treatment for diabetes mellitus, (2) persistent elevation of blood sugar levels above 180 mg/100 ml associated with intermittent glucosuria, (3) 2-hour postprandial blood sugar levels above 200 mg/100 ml, (4) 2-hour postprandial blood sugar levels above 180 mg/100 ml and a history of diabetes mellitus in a parent.

There is no correlation between the severity of glucose intolerance and the likelihood of a diabetic patient developing peripheral arterial disease, and treatment of hyperglycemia has no effect on the course of arteriosclerosis. This lack of correlation tends to obscure the close relationship between the two disorders. Careful testing of 2-hour postprandial blood sugar levels would be necessary to ascertain the true frequency of diabetes in these patients.

An even more striking correlation is found between diabetes mellitus and severe peripheral arterial disease. Although the incidence of arterial occlusion rises sharply over the age of 60, relatively few nondiabetics ever develop gangrene. Gangrene is reported to be 40 times as common in diabetics as in nondiabetic patients over the age of 50.[6] Arteriosclerotic gangrene in the presence of palpable peripheral pulses occurs almost exclusively in diabetic individuals. It is, therefore, apparent that diabetes mellitus is a major prognostic as well as etiologic factor in peripheral arteriosclerosis.

Unfortunately, the mechanism for premature arteriosclerosis in diabetes is not known. Many of these patients have associated hyperlipidemias which may lead independently to arterial damage, but arterial lesions are also very common in patients with normal plasma lipid levels. Some studies have shown enhanced platelet aggregability in patients with diabetes mellitus even in the absence of obvious arterial disease.[7] However, it has not been shown that these patients are more likely to manifest eventual arteriosclerosis than those with normal platelet function tests. Furthermore, since there are no data concerning the efficacy of antiplatelet drugs in preventing arterial lesions, we still do not know whether increased platelet aggregation is a cause of atherosclerosis or merely an effect of abnormal arterial intimal surfaces.

It is possible that diabetes mellitus is a marker for premature aging in general since it is associated with almost all degenerative changes. For example, severe osteoarthritis, loss of teeth due to resorption of the maxilla and mandible, aging of cartilage, loss of ankle reflexes and vibratory sensation on the feet, hearing loss,[8] and cataract formation all occur more frequently and earlier in the diabetic population. In this context, one might hypothesize that early arteriosclerosis is part of this accelerated aging process.

Cigarette smoking may be the second most important risk factor for peripheral arteriosclerosis. Every major health survey concerning smoking has shown a strong statistical association between smoking and coronary, cerebral, and peripheral arteriosclerosis. One study reported that only 2.5% of patients with peripheral arterial disease were nonsmokers in contrast to 25% of normal individuals.[9] Patients with peripheral arterial disease who stop smoking have a lower rate of limb amputation than those who continue.

The mechanisms of arterial injury in smoking have not been fully clarified, but several effects have been documented. Nicotine is a peripheral vasoconstrictor, which can compromise blood flow in an already ischemic limb. Smoking has been shown to increase platelet aggregation, which may cause an increased tendency to intraluminal thrombosis and subintimal damage.[10] In addition, smoking raises the level of carboxyhemoglobin in blood, and there is some evidence to suggest that this substance may damage arterial intima.[11] There may be many other products in tobacco smoke that are injurious to arterial walls, but relatively little investigation has been performed in this area.

Hyperlipidemia is also a major factor, particularly in relatively young individuals who develop peripheral arterial disease. In reviewing patients with hyperlipidemia, the classification of congenital hyperlipidemias by Fredrickson and Lee[12] is still useful. They recognized five broad categories based on lipoprotein analysis of serum: type I, hyperchylomicronemia (elevation of low molecular weight triglycerides); type II, beta-hyperlipoproteinemia; type III, broad-beta hyperlipoproteinemia; type IV, pre-beta-hyperlipoproteinemia; type V, type I plus type IV.

Types II through V are associated with premature atherosclerosis, and type IV is the most common. In type IV hyperlipoproteinemia, the serum cholesterol level may or may not be elevated, but the triglyceride concentration is disproportionately high. It is induced by a high carbohydrate intake and is strongly associated with diabetes mellitus and obesity. It can also be induced by alcohol and estrogen preparations. Treatment of this lipid abnormality is primarily a matter of weight loss and restriction of carbohydrate intake. People of normal weight may also require drug therapy. Clofibrate is effective in lowering serum triglyceride levels, but it is wise to avoid long-term continuous use if possible because it predisposes to cholelithiasis.

Even if a patient with type IV hyperlipoproteinemia does not appear to be grossly overweight, one should inquire about previous weights. Regardless of initial weight, there is good epidemiologic evidence to support a positive correlation between weight gain after age 25, hypertriglyceridemia, and premature atherosclerosis. Loss of 10 or 15 lb, therefore, may have a significant beneficial effect on the hyperlipidemia. The much rarer types III and V are also carbohydrate-dependent and associated with diabetes mellitus. In type III, both cholesterol and triglyceride levels tend to be high, but it may be confused with type IV.

Type II hyperlipoproteinemia is the second most common hyperlipidemia and is associated primarily with hypercholesterolemia. Xanthelasma and tendinous xanthomas are common and enhanced platelet aggregation has been noted. This is basically a fat-induced problem and more difficult to treat than the carbohydrate-dependent lipid abnormalities. A low saturated fat diet in combination with an agent that interferes with the enterohepatic circulation of bile is used for this problem. Agents such as cholestyramine and colestipol block the reabsorption of cholesterol and bile salts from the gut. Unfortunately, their use is frequently associated with abdominal discomfort, nausea, and bloating, and thus patient compliance is rather poor. Furthermore, although they rarely lead to frank malabsorption, one must make sure that they do not interfere with the absorption of important drugs that the patient may be taking, especially fat-soluble agents.

Another important facet of lipid metabolism is the apparent protective effect of high-density lipoproteins (HDL).[13] There is evidence that smoking lowers HDL levels and regular strenuous exercise raises them.[14] In order to assess accurately the lipid status of any patient, one should perform serum lipoprotein electrophoresis as well as cholesterol, triglyceride, and HDL levels after a 12-hour fast. A cholesterol level alone, although it is a useful screening tool for hyperlipidemia, may miss type IV hyperlipoproteinemia and does not distinguish between low-density and high-density lipoproteins, both of which contribute to the total cholesterol level.

Hypertension is synergistic with other factors in producing peripheral arterial disease but is probably not an independent cause. Although elevated blood pressure is frequently found in these patients, generally one also finds coexistent diabetes and often a history of smoking. This is in sharp contrast to the cerebral circulation where hypertension is the leading risk factor. Many patients, particularly the elderly, with peripheral arteriosclerosis have elevated systolic pressures and wide pulse pressures, but this is probably a reflection of arteriosclerotic changes and fibrosis in the media of large arteries rather than a cause of arteriosclerosis.

Another factor, which is probably equally important in all arterial beds, is whole blood viscosity. A high viscosity leads to intimal shearing and injury and predisposes to lipid deposition. Since the red cell concentration is the chief determinant of blood viscosity, one can use hematocrit to judge the magnitude of this risk. Blood viscosity rises steeply as hematocrit increases beyond 55%, but even a hematocrit of 50% is associated with a significantly higher viscosity than a hematocrit in the low 40s. The importance of hematocrit should be considered in several clinical situations: (1) A lower mean hematocrit secondary to menstrual bleeding may be one reason for a lower incidence of atherosclerosis in premenopausal women. The effects of this physiologic phlebotomy are offset by iron therapy; it is probably not advisable to attempt to restore iron stores to normal in an asymptomatic woman with mild iron deficiency. (2) Second, an additional deleterious effect of smoking is the production of significant polycythemia secondary to high blood levels of carbon monoxyhemoglobin and consequent tissue hypoxia. (3) Third, overzealous use of diuretic agents may also raise hematocrit. (4) Finally, chronic oxygen therapy in patients with severe chronic obstructive lung disease may prevent vascular thrombosis by eliminating secondary polycythemia.

One final factor to consider is the question of castration and estrogen replacement in women. It has been abundantly clear for many years that castration of premenopausal women is associated with accelerated atherosclerosis. In one series, a significant proportion of patients with aortoiliac occlusion had had early ovarectomies.[15] The earlier the castration, the more likely is atherosclerosis to develop. A more recent study demonstrated a higher incidence of premature atherosclerosis even in women having premenopausal hysterectomy without ovarectomy.[16] Whether this is due to loss of menstrual bleeding or other factors is not clear.

Attempts to replace normal ovarian function with synthetic estrogen replacement appear to increase the incidence of both arterial and venous thrombosis. Although the data from multiple studies are confusing, it is apparent that we do not know which hormones, if any, protect against arterial disease, and our understanding of the role of female reproductive organs in health maintenance is quite incomplete. It is certainly prudent at this time to take a very conservative approach to hysterectomy in premenopausal women, reserving it mostly for the treatment of cancer.

The roles of the known risk factors in the development of peripheral arterial disease are more apparent in younger than older individuals. It is rare to find a patient under the age of 55 with clinical evidence of arterial occlusion and none of these factors. Such a patient should be evaluated for other causes of arterial insufficiency such as collagen-vascular diseases and coagulopathies before an etiologic diagnosis of arteriosclerosis is made. On the other hand, patients over the age of 65 may have either symptomatic or asymptomatic disease without obvious risk factors. Even at advanced ages, however, gangrene and loss of limb are unusual in the absence of the above-mentioned factors.

Circulatory Physiology

In dealing with patients who have arterial insufficiency of the lower extremities, it is important to consider the physiology of limb circulation. There are really two rather separate components to blood flow in the extremities: the cutaneous and the muscle circulation. Each is modulated differently and may be independently involved as a result of arterial occlusion. Blood flow to skin is subject to enormous influences of vasoconstriction and vasodilatation. The former results mainly from stimulation of alpha-receptors of the sympathetic nervous system in response to such stimuli as cold, anxiety, and decreases in cardiac output. A cold environment also causes direct vasoconstriction. Vasodilatation is mostly a passive process, occurring in the absence of alpha-adrenergic stimulation. However, there are also some beta-adrenergic receptors which promote active vasodilatation. Blood flow to the skin of the feet and hands, on which limb survival depends, varies in the normal individual from moment to moment and ranges from clinically undetectable amounts under conditions of intense vasoconstriction to as much as 100 ml per 100 ml of tissue per minute in a state of total vasodilatation. It is, therefore, necessary to define the operative physiologic conditions in any discussion of cutaneous blood flow. It is appropriate to define blood flow capacity to the foot as the total cutaneous flow under conditions of maximal vasodilatation. One way to assess the circulation of the foot is to measure toe temperatures in a constant-temperature room.[17] At 20°C, toe temperature is directly related to mean blood flow. Body heating is used to promote maximal vasodilatation, and the highest recorded toe temperature represents maximum blood flow. In the normal individual, toe temperature reaches 32°C in a 20°C room, indicating a blood flow between 30 and 100 ml per 100 ml of tissue per minute. A final toe temperature below 26°C suggests severe arterial insufficiency.

The muscle circulation is under relatively little autonomic control and responds mostly to exercise. Muscle requires very little blood flow at rest, and even patients with moderately severe peripheral arterial disease have a normal or near normal resting blood supply. With ordinary walking, calf blood flow rises 500- to 1000-fold in the normal individual. It is the failure to increase muscle circulation adequately that leads to symptoms of ischemia. This principle is well demonstrated by procedures in which a radioactive compound such as sodium iodide I 131 is injected directly into calf muscle and its rate of disappearance measured.[18] Under standardized exercise conditions, the rate of disappearance of the isotope varies inversely with clinical symptomatology and directly with the length of time that a patient can walk on a treadmill and is remarkably reproducible from day to day. Plethysmographic studies in patients with chronic arterial occlusion have shown normal resting calf blood flow but an inadequate increase with exercise.[19]

Since exercising muscle requires more blood flow than skin, it is not surprising that the first symptoms of large vessel occlusion in the lower extremity in ambulatory patients relate to the muscle circulation. On the other hand, patients whose occlusive disease is only in distal vessels or who are quite sedentary may never notice muscle symptoms. Their first problem may be foot pain or gangrene. Since elderly people tend to be more sedentary, it is not unusual to see gangrene as the first clinical sign in the later decades.

SIGNS AND SYMPTOMS OF LOWER EXTREMITY ISCHEMIA

The cardinal and only specific symptom of arterial insufficiency of the lower extremities is intermittent claudication. Like its counterpart in the coronary circulation, angina pectoris, claudication is a result of muscle ischemia, and also like angina, its exact cause is not known. Metabolites of anaerobic metabolism have been suggested as the source of discomfort, but injection of these products does not reproduce the symptom. Claudication is a diagnosis of history and is much less variable than angina in its presentation. Unlike angina, it is always related to exercise and never occurs at rest. The symptom of claudication is usually a pressing or tightening sensation but may be sharp or dull pain or even a sense of overwhelming weakness. Intermittent claudication always forces the patient to stop walking after a certain distance, requiring seconds or minutes of rest before the patient can resume walking and generally continue a similar distance. In this discontinuous way, most patients can walk for miles if they have no other disabilities. The distance that a patient can traverse under standard conditions does not change appreciably from day to day. This has been documented by carefully performed treadmill studies.[20] Of course, increasing the speed of walking will decrease walking distance as will cold and windy weather. Claudication distances vary from a few yards in very severe cases up to about six blocks with very mild circulatory impairment. Most patients can walk one to three blocks before having to stop. People who walk more than six blocks before stopping probably do not have claudication since ischemia develops sooner even in mild arterial insufficiency.

There are occasional variations in the classical history of claudication. Some patients have a so-called warming-up effect and can walk longer distances after the first stop, but they still cannot walk indefinitely without pausing. Their walking distance may increase several blocks. A few others may describe decreasing distances after each stop. Rarely, patients with a high threshold for pain may walk through the discomfort to the point where they fall because of sudden loss of muscular function secondary to severe ischemia. Walking surface affects claudication. There are patients who can walk almost indefinitely on the springy surface of a boardwalk but must stop after a few blocks on a concrete sidewalk.

The location of claudication bears some relationship to the site of major artery occlusion. Patients with femoropopliteal disease always develop their claudication in the calves whereas patients with aortoiliac occlusion usually have buttock and upper thigh symptoms. Some of the latter, however, develop calf claudication, the reason for which is not clear. Occasional patients with posterior tibial artery occlusion complain of ankle and foot claudication.

There are a number of conditions that can easily be confused with claudication if a detailed history is not elicited from the patient. Lumbosacral spine disease is an example. With severe claudication, walking distance may be so short (less than 100 feet) that the exact relationship to walking may not be apparent. On the other hand, patients with spine problems may be thought to have claudication because their pain is aggravated by walking. However, it also occurs at rest and is aggravated by prolonged standing, coughing, and straining. Similarly, painful arthritis of the hip may simulate aortoiliac disease. Arthritis of the knee, if it causes calf pain, may be confused with femoropopliteal claudication, but isolated pain in the knee is never related to arterial disease. It is helpful to remember that claudicators, unlike patients with musculoskeletal complaints, never obtain relief from canes or other walking supports because muscle function is normal until ischemia develops.

Diabetic peripheral neuropathy, which is frequently coexistent in patients with peripheral arterial disease, may produce radiating or lancinating leg pains aggravated by walking, but they also appear at rest and are generally inconstant from day to day. Sedentary people may complain of leg fatigue when they are forced to walk several blocks. Usually, however, they are not forced to stop, and when they finish, relief comes only from sitting down for 5 to 10 minutes. This symptom is common in elderly people and is a definite source of over diagnosis of claudication.

Glycogen storage disease of skeletal muscle is the only disorder that completely mimics arterial claudication. Here the failure to break down glycogen and provide carbohydrate substrate for muscle cells leads to a "functional" ischemia. This rare and inborn error of metabolism begins early in life and can be diagnosed by demonstrating the failure of femoral vein lactate levels to rise during exercise.

All the other symptoms of arterial insufficiency relate to the cutaneous circulation and are much less specific. Numbness or paresthesia in an entire foot or toes is a common ischemic symptom but is even more frequently found in diabetic neuropathy. Since many elderly patients have both arterial occlusion and neuropathy, it may be difficult to assess accurately the relative roles of each in producing this symptom. Neuropathy tends to cause symmetrical involvement of feet and often the hands too. Numbness appearing or becoming exaggerated during walking and relieved by rest is more specific since it is really a claudication equivalent, representing a steal syndrome. Cutaneous blood flow is diverted through vasodilatation of muscle arterioles to ischemic calf muscle. One must always perform a careful neurologic evaluation to rule out not only diabetic neuropathy but also nerve root compression and vitamin B_{12} deficiency before ascribing numbness to peripheral arterial disease.

Another frequent symptom is coldness, which is even more nonspecific than numbness and is most often the result of vasoconstriction. Coolness becomes clinically relevant if it is of recent onset or unilateral. One can ask how the patient's feet feel to him when he awakens in the morning. People with high vasomotor tone may have cold feet when they go to bed at night, but they generally vasodilate during sleep, whereas the patient with peripheral arterial disease has persistently cold feet.

Ischemic rest pain is a dire symptom. It represents failure of collateral circulation to maintain adequate blood flow to the foot despite maximal vasodilatation. Since a foot requires relatively little flow to maintain its nutrition, rest pain signifies a severe deficit, corresponding to a blood flow capacity of less than 10% of normal and a maximal toe temperature of less than 24°C in a 20°C constant temperature room.

In a given patient, one cannot assume that foot pain is ischemic in nature merely because pulses are missing. Arteriosclerotic patients are subject to all the other causes of foot pain. In fact, elderly diabetics are particularly subject to osteoarthritis, bony spurs, tender callouses, and neuropathic pain. By misinterpreting the cause of foot pain, one may presume that a patient with mild arteriosclerosis has limb-threatening disease. True ischemic pain is a result of ischemic peripheral neuritis. For this reason, it tends to have paradoxically a burning as well as paresthetic quality even though the foot may actually be cold. Some patients may obtain partial relief by dangling their legs, perhaps through a gravitational increase in blood flow. The pain tends to appear first at night and to be most severe when the patient is in bed. Many patients sleep poorly or not at all and may resort to sleeping in a chair. Unfortunately, once this pain begins, it usually progresses inexorably over a period of weeks or months until either gangrene ensues or it becomes difficult to control even with narcotic analgesics.

Ischemic rest pain never occurs above the ankle because the blood flow requirement of resting muscle is very low, and calf and thigh skin have much better collateral circulation. Thus, nocturnal cramps, a frequent complaint at all ages but especially of older individuals, should never be confused with ischemic rest pain. They have no relationship to arterial insufficiency and are actually relieved by standing and walking. Nocturnal cramps can occur with diabetic and other neuropathies as well as electrolyte disorders, but the cause in most cases is unknown.

Physical diagnosis is the major key to diagnosis of peripheral arterial disease. The accessibility of the peripheral circulation allows the skilled observer to localize the site of obstruction and, in most cases, to assess its severity without resort to laboratory tests. The most important maneuver is careful palpation of pulses, since in the overwhelming majority of patients, at least some pulses are missing or attenuated. Unfortunately, relatively little emphasis is given to pulse palpation in medical schools and residency training programs, and consequently, many physicians are not skilled in this area. The two most difficult pulses to palpate are the popliteal and posterior tibial arteries, but even the dorsalis pedis pulse is often missed. In obese individuals, femoral pulses may be difficult to palpate when the abdomen protrudes over the inguinal area.

The popliteal pulse is best felt with the patient in the supine position and the examiner on the same side as the pulse he or she is palpating. With the leg relaxed and the knee flexed about 10° to 20°, one palpates with both hands under the knee laterally as well as medially since the position of the popliteal artery is variable. The posterior tibial pulse runs below the medial malleolus and is often hidden by the bony protuberance. Again with the patient supine and the examiner on the same side, one palpates carefully along the whole area under the malleolus. Often, extension and eversion of the foot make this pulse easier to feel. The dorsalis pedis is a continuation of the anterior tibial artery and usually runs along the medial side of the dorsum of the foot. In some patients the lateral tarsal branch of the anterior tibial artery can also be palpated lateral to the dorsalis pedis pulse.

As previously stated, failure of a skilled observer to find a posterior tibial pulse is tantamount to a diagnosis of peripheral arterial disease unless the effort is impeded by significant edema or bony abnormality of the ankle. Similarly, a missing dorsalis pedis, particularly if the finding is unilateral, strongly suggests the probability of arterial occlusion. A distinct weakness in a pulse as compared to its counterpart in the other leg is also evidence for arterial disease. Although a weak pulse in an asymptomatic individual may be considered early clinical disease, it represents a late stage in the pathologic process. Before there can be any fall in distal perfusing pressure an artery must have a stenosis of at least 65% to 70% of the cross-sectional area of its lumen.

In an effort to make clinical assessment of peripheral pulses more objective, the portable Doppler unit has been introduced. This machine, highly compact, is an ultrasound source and recorder. It records high-frequency sound waves beamed against a vessel and reflected back by the moving column of blood. The resulting sound and recorded vibrations take the shape of the peripheral pulse wave. It is often used to confirm the presence or absence of a pulse but is fraught with error. In the first place, the pulse may not be recorded if the transducer is not placed sufficiently close to the artery, and so it must be moved into multiple positions along the route of a vessel before one assumes that it is occluded. Furthermore, the Doppler technic is quite sensitive. An artery with a very severe stenosis and a mere trickle of blood flow (insufficient to make the pulse palpable) may yield an audible signal. Doppler ultrasound may also record flow in collateral vessels.

On the other hand, Doppler ultrasound is extremely useful in measuring systolic blood pressure in a limb, particularly when distal pulses are not palpable. One merely raises the pressure in a sphygmomanometer cuff applied around the calf until the recorded signal is obliterated. With this technic, one can compare blood pressure in the two legs and with upper extremity pressure. If blood pressures in the upper and lower extremities appear to be approximately equal, then one exercises the leg, either through walking or lifting and bending movements of the knee and ankle while the patient is supine. Distal to an arterial obstruction, systolic pressure falls during exercise because of vasodilatation of arterioles in the region of ischemic muscle.[21] Often a palpable pulse disappears during exercise. The magnitude of the fall in pressure and its duration after exercise are directly related to the blood flow deficit in the muscle circulation.

The other clinical signs involve the cutaneous circulation of the foot. One looks first for pallor either in the horizontal position or after 20° to 30° of elevation. If any degree of pallor is evident, there is at least some decrease in blood flow capacity. The degree of ischemia is directly related to the time required for color to come back to normal after the leg is lowered to the dependent position. With mild ischemia, color returns within 15 seconds; a delay beyond 45 seconds indicates very severe ischemia. A parallel observation is venous filling time. In the absence of varicose veins, which produce retrograde filling, the time required for filling of dorsal foot veins after the leg is lowered from the elevated to dependent position is also a reflection of cutaneous blood flow. Normally, the veins should fill within 10 to 15 seconds, but vasoconstriction may also slow venous filling. Comparison of filling time in the two feet is particularly helpful.

Foot temperature may be very misleading because it depends largely on ambient temperature. In a warm room, even a very ischemic foot may not feel cold. Conversely, vasoconstriction in a cool environment can reduce skin blood flow to unmeasurable levels. A difference in temperature between the two feet, however, is almost always significant. Since arterial insufficiency is worse in the most distal portion of the extremities, one should palpate the toes carefully. With experience, one can appreciate a difference of 1°C.

The most dire sign of foot ischemia is rubor on dependency. This is a homogeneous, violaceous color, appearing after pallor has disappeared and generally requiring 30 to 120 seconds to reach its full expression after the limb has been placed in a dependent position. The color is most marked in the toes and distal portions of the foot and may involve the whole foot. This rubor is the result of severe tissue hypoxia and anoxic capillary dilatation. Cyanotic blood remains pooled in capillaries after maximal tissue extraction of oxygen. Dependent rubor (and/or blanching persisting beyond 60 seconds) indicates that blood flow capacity is less than 10% of normal and is generally present when rest pain appears. Many patients with rubor, however, have no rest pain. This is particularly true of the elderly who may have severe diabetic neuropathy, cerebrovascular disease, or organic brain syndromes blunting sensory perception. In very ischemic feet, rubor may be present in the horizontal and even elevated position and mask any blanching that might otherwise appear. One must be careful not to confuse the homogeneous color of dependent rubor with the cyanotic, patchy discoloration that occurs on dependency in patients with venous insufficiency. The latter tends to develop almost immediately after the leg is made dependent and is not associated with blanching on elevation. It is also necessary to distinguish an erythematous color that occurs on dependency from true rubor. Erythema represents reactive hyperemia that may occur in response to even mild ischemia and does not have the grave implications of rubor.

Shortly after the onset of rubor, petechiae may appear, which are the result of capillary porosity secondary to ischemia. If rubor becomes intensely cyanotic, it is often followed by the appearance of gangrene and ischemic ulcers. Skin breakdown is most likely to occur on the toes, heel, and lateral malleolus. Ischemic ulcers are generally pale and often have a cyanotic border in contrast to the hyperemic venous ulcer, which usually develops just above the medial malleolus. If the ulcer becomes infected, it may be surrounded by signs of cellulitis. The degree of inflammatory reaction around an infected ulcer is a measure of the severity of ischemia and the prognosis for the foot. A "cold" cellulitis (erythema and purulent secretion without a significant increase in local temperature) is indicative of an extremely poor blood supply.

One does not always see sequential changes from mild blanching on elevation to dependent rubor to gangrene. Unfortunately, chronic or acute trauma, by increasing blood flow requirements, can lead quickly to unhealing tissue breakdown in a foot with relatively good circulation. This is particularly true of elderly patients who may not see well and are more likely to suffer from sensory deprivation secondary to diabetic neuropathy.

Treatment

Once the diagnosis of peripheral arterial disease is established, one must decide on appropriate therapy. Patients with arterial insufficiency can be placed into one of three broad categories: (1) asymptomatic disease with no signs of cutaneous ischemia; (2) intermittent claudication with no signs of cutaneous ischemia; (3) varying degrees of cutaneous ischemia with or without claudication.

Patients with asymptomatic disease, discovered through pulse palpation or routine physical examination, constitute the largest group. Most will never develop serious ischemia unless subject to unusual stress or trauma. No treatment is necessary, but careful surveillance by physician and patient is in order. Periodic examination two or three times a year is advisable, at which time one should re-evaluate pulses, look for signs of cutaneous ischemia, and check skin hydration. Particularly in elderly people, the skin of the lower legs and feet may become very dry in the winter and begin to crack. If there is even mild arterial insufficiency, frank ulceration may develop. Patients with dry skin should be given an emollient such as lanolin to apply once or twice a day. One also examines between the toes for scaling or maceration, which indicate the presence of superficial fungal infection. Even mild dermatophytosis may lead to ulceration. A topical antifungal medication should be prescribed for this. Toenails should also be examined carefully for in-curving under the skin and dystrophic thickening under the plate that may put pressure on the underlying skin. Thick callouses on the plantar surface and sides of the feet should be noted because these pressure points are areas of potential friction and ulceration.

The patient must be given very specific instructions about foot care. The following are the instructions given to patients in our vascular clinic:

Instructions for Care of the Feet for Patients with Poor Circulation of the Legs

1. Tobacco: Do not smoke.
2. Cold: Avoid extreme cold. Dress very warmly in winter. Do not bathe or swim in cold water.
3. Heat: Never apply heat or ice to the feet. Avoid exposure of feet or legs to the sun.
4. Position: Sleep with your legs in a level position. Never sit with legs crossed.
5. Cleanliness: Wash your feet with a mild soap in lukewarm water only. Dry feet carefully, especially between the toes.
6. Dry scaly skin: You may apply lanolin or cold cream to your feet; gently massage into the dry scaly areas.
7. Toenails: Should be cut by a podiatrist or a member of your family. Cut the toenails straight across and never cut in at the corners or too close to the skin.
8. Corns and callouses: Should be taken care of by a podiatrist.
9. Shoes and socks: Never walk in your bare feet. Wear only comfortable, properly fitting shoes and socks. Square or round-toed shoes are preferred. Wear a clean pair of socks each day. Do not wear circular garters or hose with elastic tops.
10. Local medication: Never use a strong antiseptic. Apply no corn remedies or corn plasters to your feet. Use only medications ordered by your physician.
11. Exercise: Walking is a good way to improve your circulation.
12. Injuries: Try to avoid even minor injuries to your feet by following these rules. Consult

your physician at the first sign of discomfort in your legs or any injury to your legs or feet.
13. Self-inspection: You may not be able to feel pain in your feet as well as you should. Therefore, examine your feet every week. If there are cracks or cuts in the skin or new color changes, consult your physician even if you have no pain.

In the second group of patients, one must also make a decision about intermittent claudication. There is basically no specific medical therapy for this symptom. Although vasodilating drugs are widely prescribed, there is no substantial evidence that they are effective. In fact, studies of calf blood flow before and after administration of these agents have shown only a modest increase, not nearly enough to meet the requirement for normal walking. Patients with claudication of less than three to four months' duration may improve spontaneously through development of collateral circulation, and this can be promoted through walking, cessation of smoking, and weight loss in the case of obese patients.

Beta-adrenergic blocking agents, which many of these patients receive for relief of angina, may aggravate claudication by blocking vasodilatation. One must assess the relative roles of angina and claudication in a patient's disability in deciding whether they should be continued.

For patients with chronic claudication, one must decide whether to pursue the possibility of surgical repair. Claudication is certainly not a fatal problem nor does it threaten the viability of a limb. Most individuals with this problem can learn to adjust to it. They should be encouraged to walk as much as possible, briefly stopping for rest when discomfort begins. Unless they are in occupations that require continuous walking for long distances, they are likely to lead reasonably normal lives. Claudicators, for example, almost never have difficulties in their home or while doing office work. Certainly, retired individuals and those accustomed to a relatively sedentary life style adjust quite well to claudication unless it is very severe, and so there is relatively little indication for arterial surgery in the elderly.

Those patients who are severely handicapped by their claudication must be evaluated very carefully before surgery is seriously contemplated. One must take into account a number of factors including claudication distance, general health, and presence or absence of other cardiovascular disease. One must recognize that even carefully planned arterial surgery is not always successful. If collateral vessels are severed to perform an arterial bypass that does not remain patent, arterial blood flow may decrease rather than increase. If a patient has angina pectoris after walking three blocks, eliminating two-block claudication is of little value. Furthermore, the presence of cardiac or cerebrovascular disease increases the morbidity and mortality rates of major surgery. The presence of a good popliteal pulse is a contraindication to surgery for claudication since it indicates that the major area of obstruction is in the tibial arteries, where the results of bypass are not good.

Only after the patient is identified as a candidate for bypass surgery should arteriography be performed. Although this invasive procedure is relatively safe, catheterization of an artery can cause intimal tears and thrombi and occasional perforations. It is unnecessary for diagnosis and assessment of arterial insufficiency and only justifiable if it influences therapy. The only purpose of the arteriogram is to assess the arterial tree (surgical run-off) beyond an obstruction that has already been diagnosed by clinical means (Figures 21-1 to 21-3).

The third group of patients, who have varying degrees of cutaneous ischemia, must also be managed on an individual basis. Ischemic rest pain, significant dependent rubor and/or prolonged pallor, gangrene, and ischemic ulcers are often pressing indications for arterial surgery. However, there are many exceptions, particularly for elderly people who tolerate major surgery less well and whose vessels are often more atherosclerotic and difficult to handle than those of younger individuals. An older person with dependent rubor but no rest pain who has chronic congestive heart failure, for example, may be best served by frequent surveillance and good foot care rather than perilous surgery as long as there is no skin breakdown. Even superficial, limited ulceration or gangrene can often be treated medically. Superficial necrotic tissue sloughs with healing beneath it. Dry gangrene of a toe often demarcates over a period of weeks, and one can wait for autoamputation. Superficial, ischemic ulcers can be treated with relief of pressure, body temperature soaks and debriding agents, and antibacterial substances for secondary infection. In an older individual with significant cardiopulmonary disease, this approach may be warranted if the foot as a whole does not appear very ischemic. In treating patients with ischemic feet medically, it is best to avoid beta-adrenergic blocking agents. Substitution of a calcium chan-

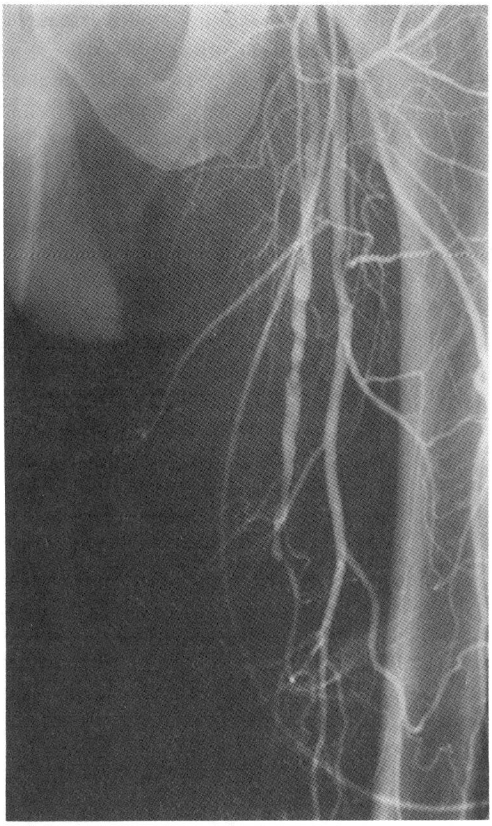

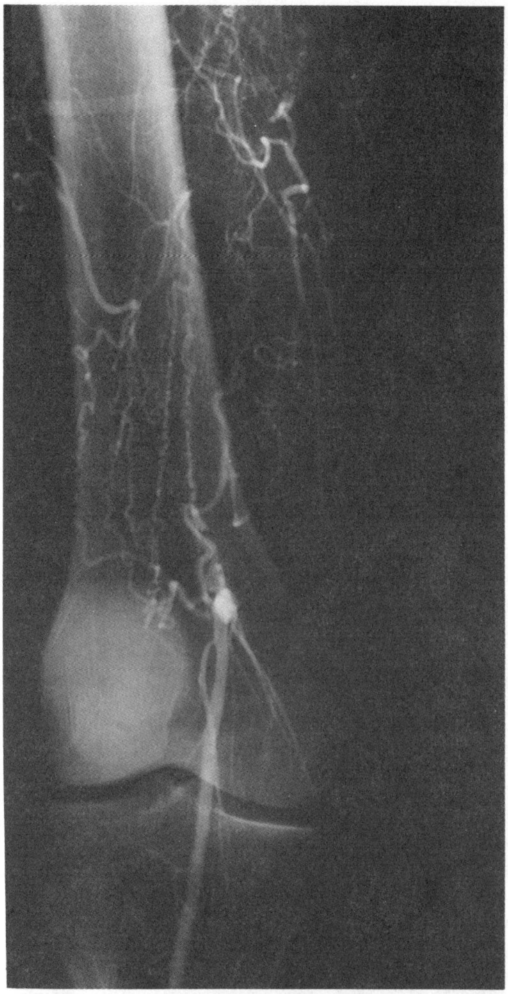

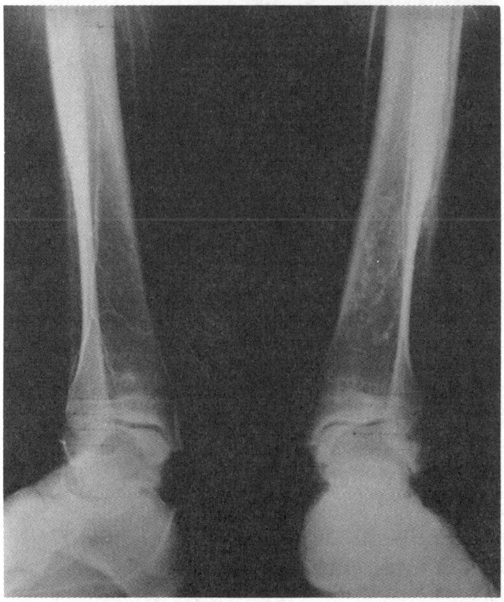

▲
Figure 21-1 Femoral artery occlusion with excellent surgical run-off. **A** Arteriography shows obstruction of a superficial femoral artery with collateral vessels from the profunda femoral artery extending distally in the thigh.

Figure 21-1B Reconstitution of the popliteal artery is seen. ►

Figure 21-1C Adequate distal run-off is present with a patent right posterior tibial artery in the region of the ankle and forefoot. ►

nel blocking agent may suffice for treatment of angina and lead to peripheral vasodilatation instead of constriction.

On the other hand, widespread gangrene or marked dependent rubor and gangrene is always an indication for surgery if feasible because the prognosis for survival of the foot is otherwise very poor.

The location of an arterial occlusion has a bearing on symptoms, prognosis, and appropriate treatment. One can categorize arterial insufficiency in the lower extremities as predominantly aortoiliac, femoropopliteal, or tibial.

Aortoiliac disease Aortoiliac occlusion, if it involves both common iliac or internal iliac

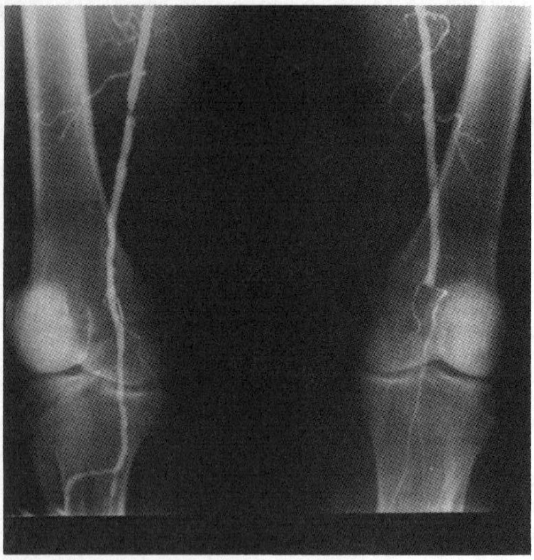

Figure 21-2A Arteriography shows abrupt occlusion of the left popliteal artery and arteriosclerotic narrowing of the right femoropopliteal axis.

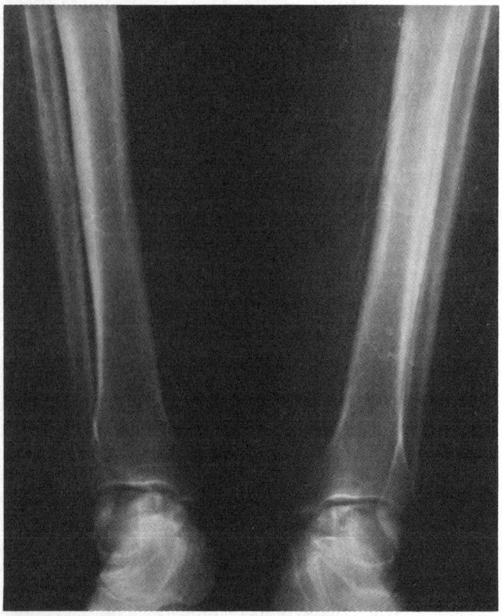

Figure 21-2B Distal film reveals extensive occlusion of the tibial arteries bilaterally with no evidence of a major patent vessel. Bypass surgery is not possible.

arteries, presents with impotence in the male as well as claudication, which is usually located in the hips and buttocks.

Arterial obstruction in this location develops much earlier (mean age 49) than in the femoropopliteal area (mean age 62). Since the obstruction is proximal, there is a great deal of potential for collateral circulation and so serious cutaneous ischemia is quite unusual. If pulses are palpable, one may require blood pressure measurements to make the diagnosis. Bruits over the femoral arteries at rest or after exercise also point to aortoiliac disease. In fact, if gangrene develops, one can safely assume that the patient also has femoropopliteal and or tibial artery involvement. The results of surgery for claudication are best in the aortoiliac area because of excellent run-off. For localized aortoiliac disease, both aortofemoral bypass grafting and thromboendarterectomy result in a five-year patency rate of approximately 90%.[22,23]

Unfortunately, the results of surgery for impotence are not sanguine. In fact, many patients have become impotent after aortoiliac surgery because of destruction of lower sympathetic ganglia. Although some impotent patients may benefit from aorto-to-internal iliac bypass, it is not a recommended procedure for the elderly in whom sexual dysfunction is often multifactorial.

In patients with multiple areas of obstruction who require surgical relief, the most proximal obstruction must be relieved first if any more distal bypass is to remain open, even if the proximal bypass is relatively mild. With combined aortoiliac and femoropopliteal disease causing severe ischemia, one usually performs only aortoiliac bypass first and then waits several weeks to determine whether this procedure has increased distal pressure sufficiently through collateral vessels to revascularize the foot. Often, a second procedure in the femoropopliteal area is unnecessary.[24] If the aortoiliac obstruction is mild and short, one can perform percutaneous transluminal angioplasty[25] and then femoropopliteal bypass as a single operative procedure.

For patients who are poor operative risks, there are two surgical alternatives to direct aortoiliac surgery which allow the surgeon to decrease operative time and avoid both laparotomy and general anesthesia. If iliac disease is unilateral, a femoro-femoral shunt across the pubis area can be performed. The five-year patency rate of this graft is only about 10% less than that of direct iliofemoral bypass.[26] Of course, subsequent development of peripheral arterial disease in the patent iliac system can threaten the viability of both legs. The second procedure is axillofemoral shunting in which a prosthesis is tunneled subcutaneously from the axillary to the femoral artery.[27] It is a limb-saving operation in many cases but has a two-year patency rate of no better than 50%. Both of these alternatives are especially suitable to elderly patients who have significant cardiopulmonary or cerebrovascular disease or are too debilitated for the rigors of major surgery.

Femoropopliteal disease Patients with femoropopliteal disease have good femoral pulses but weak or absent popliteal pulses. The results of surgery (femoropopliteal or femoroproximal tibial bypass) vary from series to series, depending on the type of referral center accumulating data. A group of relatively young patients with mild claudication and a single stenosis will tend to fare better than older patients with multiple occlusions and generalized arteriosclerosis, who are likely to have more rapid progression of degenerative arterial disease distal to a graft. In the former, the five-year patency rate may be as high as 75%,[28] but in the latter group fewer than 50% remain open for five years. Thus, the patients who are in greatest need of revascularization are the least likely to obtain long-term benefit from bypass surgery.

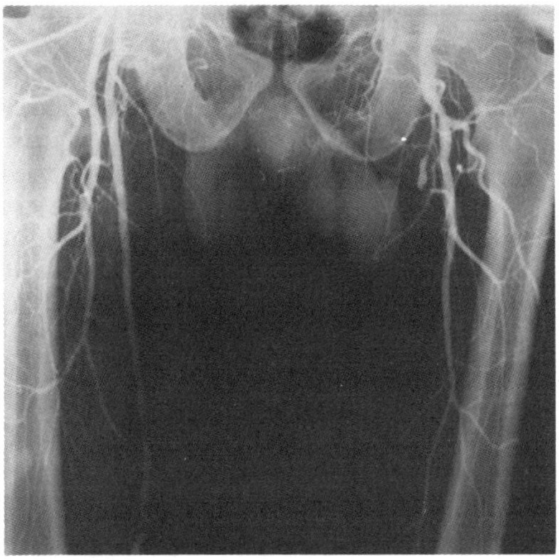

Figure 21-3A Arteriography reveals total occlusion of the left superficial femoral artery beginning at its origin from the common femoral artery. Only the profunda femoral artery is visualized on the left side.

Certainly, for an elderly, retired person with stable claudication, one is generally loathe to recommend arterial surgery. Furthermore, since the arteriosclerotic process tends to be symmetrical in distribution, many patients with unilateral claudication often have significant femoropopliteal stenosis in the contralateral leg. A successful bypass in the symptomatic limb is not of much help if the patient begins to have claudication in the other leg once he is able to walk a little further. Therefore, preoperative evaluation of the asymptomatic limb with blood pressures is quite important. If bilateral disease is present, physician and patient must be prepared for a possible second operation after a successful bypass.

Tibial artery disease Tibial artery disease is probably the most common pattern, and many of

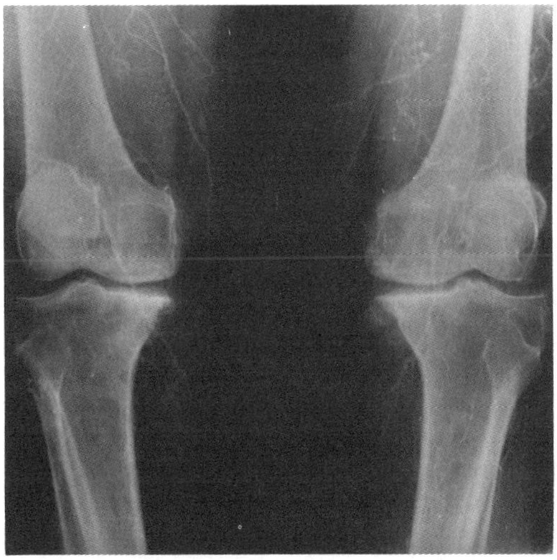

Figure 21-3B Extensive occlusion of both femoropopliteal segments is seen with partial patency of the right popliteal artery.

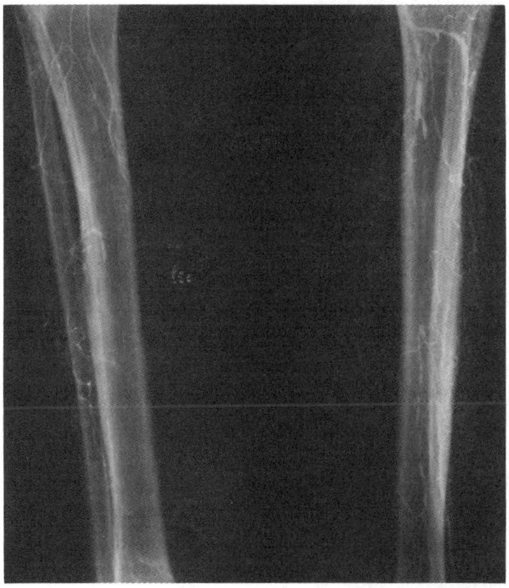

Figure 21-3C A distal film reveals distal tibial artery occlusion with marked stenosis of the proximal tibial arteries. Bypass grafting from the proximal right femoral artery to the popliteal artery is possible but very difficult. Since graft failure would be likely, surgery should be performed only for limb-threatening ischemia.

the asymptomatic elderly patients fall into this group. One never performs femoro–distal tibial bypass for claudication alone because the rate of failure is quite high and the two-year patency rate is less than 50%.[29] It is purely a salvage operation to prevent amputation.

For patients with severe ischemia and arterial obstruction that cannot be bypassed, two alternative procedures have enjoyed waves of popularity through the last few decades. If there is stenosis of the profunda femoral branch of the common femoral artery, one can perform an endarterectomy in an attempt to improve collateral circulation and increase distal perfusing pressure. Since the profunda femoral branches link up with geniculate vessels around the knee to provide the major collateral circulation in the presence of femoropopliteal occlusions, profundaplasty has a logical rationale. However, the results are usually disappointing. Lumbar sympathectomy is still performed by many surgeons with the hope of improving distal blood flow through maximal vasodilatation. Although this procedure has been employed for decades, there has never been evidence to support the notion that it is effective. The seriously ischemic limb is generally maximally vasodilated, and sympathectomy does not appreciably increase blood flow to the foot.

UPPER EXTREMITY ARTERIAL DISEASE

Arteriosclerosis is much less common in the upper than lower extremities, but a significant portion of the elderly population have asymptomatic involvement. This may take the form of a missing ulnar or radial pulse or difference in blood pressure between the two arms. In normal individuals, radial pulses are always present, and the ulnar pulse is missing in no more than 3% of cases.[30] When there is congenital absence of the ulnar pulse, it is usually a bilateral phenomenon.

One can confirm the absence of an ulnar or radial pulse by performing the Allen test. One compresses both wrist arteries and asks the patient to open and close his fist until the hand is pale. Then one releases each artery separately and watches for reactive hyperemia. Prolonged pallor after release of both arteries suggests either arteriospasm or diffuse arterial occlusion. An abnormal result with only one vessel, on the other hand, is strong evidence for arterial occlusion. Although each wrist artery ordinarily supplies the entire hand through the palmar arch that connects radial and ulnar arteries, some people have an incomplete arch. In that case, the Allen test shows reactive hyperemia of only half the hand when a single artery is released. The advent of arterial lines for blood pressure measurement in acute cardiovascular disorders has increased the importance of the Allen test. If the entire hand is not supplied by both wrist arteries, it is not wise to cannulate either artery because damage to the invaded artery can threaten the viability of the hand.

Patients with upper extremity arterial insufficiency rarely develop skin breakdown because collateral circulation is excellent. The appearance of gangrene in a hand or fingers suggests an etiology other than arteriosclerosis. One must then consider the possible presence of collagen-vascular diseases, coagulopathies, and arterial emboli.

Some patients with subclavian or axillary stenosis have significant fatigue of the arm on exertion. This may be severe enough to inhibit simple activities such as hair-brushing and carrying light packages, but in most cases, limits only heavy lifting and manual labor. Arterial bypass is rarely necessary.

If the subclavian artery is stenosed in its intrathoracic portion proximal to the origin of the vertebral artery, the patient may develop the subclavian steal syndrome[31] in addition to arm fatigue. Because of the low pressure in one vertebral artery, blood from the patent subclavian and vertebral axis, after reaching the proximal basilar artery, flows in retrograde fashion through the vertebral artery on the involved side and into the distal subclavian artery. As a result of this diversion of blood from the brain stem to the arm, the patient develops neurologic symptoms such as dizziness, syncope, diplopia, and dysarthria. These symptoms may be aggravated by exercise of the involved arm. The diagnosis is suspected clinically when a weak or absent subclavian pulse is found in the supraclavicular fossa associated with a blood pressure difference of at least 50 mmHg between the two arms. The diagnosis is corroborated by four-vessel cerebral angiography, demonstrating a subclavian stenosis and retrograde filling of the involved side after the normal subclavian and vertebral axis have filled in antegrade fashion. The steal can be eliminated by equalizing the blood pressure in both arms. This is most easily accomplished with an axillo-axillary graft tunneled in subcutaneous tissue across the chest. Dizziness and syncope are very common complaints in the elderly and should always prompt blood pressure determinations in both arms since subclavian steal syndrome is one easily treatable cause.

SMALL VESSEL SYNDROME

Whenever cutaneous ischemia develops in a hand or foot in the presence of at least one palpable distal pulse, one must assume that the patient has small vessel disease involving arterioles and/or small arteries such as digital arteries. Small vessel disease must also be suspected in a pulseless hand or foot if there are localized small infarcts without generalized ischemia. A foot with a gangrenous toe but no evidence of dependent rubor or pallor, for example, should raise this suspicion. Although diabetic patients may develop small vessel arteriosclerosis, this must be a diagnosis of exclusion. In any patient with the small vessel syndrome, the following entities must be considered: (1) thrombocytosis[32] and polycythemia, (2) emboli from arterial aneurysms, (3) cryoglobulinemia,[33] (4) cryofibrinogenemia, (5) disseminated intravascular coagulation (DIC),[34] (6) collagen-vascular diseases, (7) subacute bacterial endocarditis (SBE).

Essential thrombocytosis is a myeloproliferative disease involving megakaryocytic proliferation without leukemia or polycythemia. This disorder can present with purpura secondary to abnormal platelet function or small vessel occlusion. Digital gangrene and strokes are common. There may be splenomegaly and loss of pedal pulses. Thrombosis and hemorrhage can occur when the platelet count is above 800,000/μL. Platelet function tests usually show delayed platelet aggregation in response to epinephrine, and giant platelets may be seen on peripheral smear. Treatment with busulfan or hydroxyurea is usually quite successful, and platelet function returns to normal as the count falls below 700,000 μL. Prognosis is excellent if thrombocytosis is treated before there is irreversible vascular damage. Chemotherapy can usually be stopped after one to two months of therapy, but lifelong periodic surveillance of the platelet count is indicated. Some patients require intermittent courses of therapy. Essential thrombocytosis is a diagnostic consideration in any patient with unexplained gangrene or cerebrovascular symptoms in the absence of hypertension or diabetes.

Infarcts confined to one foot always suggest the possibility of a popliteal aneurysm. Careful palpation of this pulse and sonography can establish the diagnosis. With gangrene of the hand, one must consider a subclavian artery aneurysm.

Cryoglobulinemia, cryofibrinogenemia, and DIC are seen on a chronic basis secondary to malignancies, which may be quite occult, and also in collagen vascular diseases. In an elderly patient, they are much more likely to represent malignancy and require thorough investigation. Gangrene in association with cryofibrinogenemia and/or DIC is also seen in septic patients. Since septicemia can occur in the elderly without fever or leukocytosis, blood cultures are always indicated in the evaluation of patients with the small vessel syndrome.

With one exception, collagen-vascular diseases do not usually begin in the later decades. Elderly people frequently receive multiple medications and can develop drug-induced lupus erythematosus. Frequently incriminated drugs include hydralazine, procainamide, and phenytoin. A good drug history and an antinuclear antibody test are indicated in patients with unexplained small vessel disease.

RAYNAUD'S PHENOMENON

Raynaud's phenomenon is a syndrome of paroxysmal arteriospasm, which can affect the hands and/or feet and occasionally the ears and nose. In the classical case, the patient develops cold hands and feet with marked pallor on exposure to a cold environment or when emotionally upset. The phase of pallor is followed by intense cyanosis and then warmth and redness as blood flow returns. Raynaud's phenomenon may be asymptomatic or accompanied by pain and numbness in the arteriospastic phase or pain and a feeling of uncomfortable warmth during the stage of reactive hyperemia. The physiology of these color changes is not well understood. Although blood flow to the digits is not measurable during the arteriospastic phase, this is also true of any individual whose fingers are exposed to prolonged cold. In fact, many people without Raynaud's phenomenon have much more pain on exposure to intense cold. Nevertheless, the syndrome of color changes is distinct and can be a harbinger of systemic disease.

In the elderly, episodes of Raynaud's phenomenon are often less typical. Often only pallor occurs and reactive hyperemia may not be evident. Although most cases of Raynaud's phenomenon in young people are idiopathic (Raynaud's disease) patients who first notice this syndrome after the age of 40 usually have an underlying cause. The differential diagnosis includes: (1) collagen disease, particularly scleroderma; (2) cryoglobulinemia and cryofibrinogenemia; (3) cold hemagglutinin disease; (4) hypothyroidism; (5) use of beta-adrenergic blocking agents.

From this list, it is apparent that Raynaud's phenomenon can be a harbinger of occult malignancy. Hypothyroidism is also an important consideration since Raynaud's phenomenon may be its only obvious clinical manifestation in an elderly patient whose slow but progressive changes in mentation may have gone unnoticed or been ascribed to aging.[35]

In scleroderma (progressive systemic sclerosis), a disease that often begins in the fifth to seventh decade, Raynaud's phenomenon is almost always the first clinical manifestation and may precede other signs and symptoms by more than 10 years. The pathology consists of low-grade small vessel vasculitis and subcutaneous fibrosis, which eventually leaves the skin taut and inflexible with loss of wrinkles. Eventually subcutaneous calcification may occur. Visceral involvement may lead to dysphagia due to poor esophageal motility, cardiac conduction defects, interstitial lung disease, and renal failure. In order to make a diagnosis of scleroderma, one must find Raynaud's phenomenon in association with internal organ involvement or skin changes on the trunk or proximal to the wrists. Esophageal motility studies and determination of pulmonary diffusion capacity are sensitive tests for detecting early visceral involvement. Subcutaneous fibrosis in the digits (sclerodactyly) is nonspecific since it can occur in any patient with long-standing Raynaud's phenomenon. Patients with scleroderma tend to have small vessel occlusion as well as arteriospasm and are, therefore, subject to digital ulcers and gangrene.

Prognosis for scleroderma depends heavily on the presence or absence of internal organ involvement. In one large series, the 7-year cumulative mortality was 50% for patients with cardiac, pulmonary, or renal disease.[36] Women fared better than men. There is evidence that arteriospasm plays a role in visceral disease. Renal blood flow appears to decrease in scleroderma patients during attacks of Raynaud's phenomenon.[37] Patients seem to die more frequently during cold than warm seasons.

ACUTE ARTERIAL OCCLUSION

Acute arterial occlusion in an extremity classically presents with the sudden onset of severe sharp pain and a feeling of coldness, followed within hours by numbness. However, many elderly patients with diabetic neuropathy or organic brain syndrome may be asymptomatic and silently develop gangrene. Physical examination reveals well-demarcated coldness and cyanosis, mottling or pallor in the distal portion of the extremity. Extreme pallor, loss of sensation, and motor paralysis are poor prognostic signs.

The usual cause of acute arterial occlusion is systemic embolization, but a significant proportion of cases in the elderly occur secondary to sudden thrombosis in situ in the area of a large atheromatous plaque.

Emboli generally come from the heart or arterial aneurysms. Sources of cardiac emboli include:

1. Left atrium: (*a*) mitral stenosis, (*b*) mitral valve prolapse,[38] (*c*) atrial myxoma, (*d*) atrial fibrillation, (*e*) sick sinus syndrome[39]
2. Left ventricle: (*a*) myocardial infarction, (*b*) ventricular aneurysm
3. Mitral or aortic valve: (*a*) infective endocarditis, (*b*) prosthetic heart valve, (*c*) marantic endocarditis
4. Paradoxical emboli through a patent foramen ovale in patients with pulmonary hypertension

An echocardiogram to look for valvular pathology and vegetations[40] and blood cultures should always be obtained in acute arterial occlusion of unknown etiology. Elderly patients with atrial fibrillation may have occult mitral stenosis, which is easily diagnosed by echocardiography.[41] At least 20% of patients with mitral stenosis, if not anticoagulated, can be expected to have at least one arterial embolus.[42] Two-dimensional echocardiography or radionuclide angiography is needed if there is a suspicion of ventricular aneurysm.[43]

Except for infective endocarditis, anticoagulation is generally indicated in cases of arterial embolism. The duration of anticoagulation depends on the cause. If the embolus results from mitral stenosis or a ventricular aneurysm, lifelong therapy is advisable unless the patient develops a contraindication such as severe hypertension, stroke or gastrointestinal hemorrhage.

For an embolus after an acute myocardial infarct, one might treat for only six months if laboratory evaluation shows no evidence of a ventricular aneurysm at the end of the treatment period.

An antiplatelet agent is an alternative therapy when anticoagulation is contraindicated. Dipyridamole has been shown to be effective in preventing emboli from prosthetic heart valves, and sulfinpyrazone appears to be helpful in mitral stenosis.[44,45]

Arterial emboli, if discovered within the first 48 hours, usually can be removed with a Fogarty catheter. This catheter has an inflatable balloon and is inserted through an arterial cut-down with the balloon deflated. It can be passed in antegrade or retrograde direction past the embolus whereupon the balloon is inflated and the embolus pulled out of the vessel. Results are best if the procedure is performed in the first 24 hours. Since this embolectomy is simple and can be performed under local anesthesia, it is indicated in almost all cases of iliac and femoropopliteal emboli. In the case of tibial and upper extremity emboli, one can be guided by the clinical appearance of the extremity. Cyanosis or pallor persisting for several hours is certainly an indication for embolectomy, even in these locations.

It is not uncommon for elderly patients to present with severe limb ischemia of unknown duration and no obvious source of embolization. In this situation, it is often prudent to attempt an embolectomy although the results tend to be poor since, in most cases, thrombosis in situ has occurred. Even if emboli are present, they are often difficult to remove in the face of underlying, severe atherosclerosis.

REFERENCES

1. Kannel WB, Skinner JJ Jr, Schwartz MJ, et al: Intermittent claudication: Incidence in the Framingham study. *Circulation* 1970;4:875–878.
2. Schilling FJ, Christakis G, Hempel HH, et al: The natural history of abdominal aortic and iliac atherosclerosis as detected by lateral abdominal roentgenograms in 2663 males. *J Chronic Dis* 1974;27: 37–41.
3. Barnhorst DA, Barner HB: Prevalence of congenitally absent pedal pulses. *N Engl J Med* 1968;278: 264–269.
4. Friedman SA, Pandya M, Greif E: Peripheral arterial occlusion in patients with acute coronary heart disease. *Am Heart J* 1973;86:415–419.
5. Dry TJ, Hines EA, Jr: The role of diabetes in the development of degenerative vascular disease: With special reference to the incidence of retinitis and peripheral neuritis. *Ann Intern Med* 1941;14: 1893–1896.
6. Bell ET: Incidence of gangrene of extremities in nondiabetic and in diabetic persons. *Arch Pathol* 1950;49:469–471.
7. Sagel J, Colwell JA, Cook L, et al: Increased platelet aggregation in early diabetes mellitus. *Ann Intern Med* 1975;82:733–736.
8. Friedman SA, Schulman RH, Weiss S: Hearing and diabetic neuropathy. *Arch Intern Med* 1975; 135: 573–577.
9. Juergens JL, Barker NW, Hines EA Jr: Arteriosclerosis obliterans: Review of 520 cases with special reference to pathologic and prognostic factors. *Circulation* 1960;21:188–191.
10. Levine PH: An acute effect of cigarette smoking on platelet function: A possible link between smoking and arterial thrombosis. *Circulation* 1973;48:619–622.
11. Wald N, Howard S, Smith PG, et al: Association between atherosclerotic diseases and carboxyhaemoglobin levels in tobacco smokers. *Br Med J* 1973;1:761–766.
12. Fredrickson DS, Goldstein JL, Brown MW: The familial hyperlipoproteinemias, in Stanbury JB, Wyngaarden JB, Fredrickson DS (eds): *The Metabolic Basis of Inherited Disease.* New York, McGraw-Hill Book Company, 1977, pp 604, ed 4.
13. Gordon T, Castelli WP, Hjortland MC, et al: High density lipoprotein as a protective factor against coronary heart disease: The Framingham study. *Am J Med* 1977;62:707–709.
14. Hartung GH, Foreyt JP, Mitchell RE, et al: Relation of diet to high density lipoprotein cholesterol in middle-aged, marathon runners, joggers and inactive men. *N Engl J Med* 1980;302:357–358.
15. Friedman SA, Holling HE, Robert B: Etiologic factors in aortoiliac and femoropopliteal vascular disease: The Leriche syndrome. *N Engl J Med* 1964;271:1382–1385.
16. Gordon T, Kannel WB, Hjortland MC, et al: Menopause and coronary heart disease. The Framingham Study. *Ann Intern Med* 1978;89:157–160.
17. Felder D, Russ E, Montgomery H, et al: Relationship in the toe of skin surface temperature to mean blood flow measured with a plethysmograph. *Clin Sci* 1954;13:251–254.
18. Coffman JD, Mannick JA: A simple, objective test for arteriosclerosis obliterans. *N Engl J Med* 1965; 273:1297–1300.
19. Holling HE, Boland HC, Russ E: Investigation of arterial obstruction using mercury-in-rubber strain gauge. *Am Heart J* 1961;62:194–198.
20. Collens WS, Altman MA, Stern AB: A motorized treadmill. A method for quantitating intermittent claudication. *Am J Med Sci* 1955;230:190–195.
21. Skinner JS, Strandness DE Jr: Exercise and intermittent claudication. II. Effect of physical training. *Circulation* 1967;36:23–26.
22. Gomes MR, Bernatz PE, Juergens JL: Aortoiliac surgery: Influence of clinical factors on results. *Arch Surg* 1967;95:387–390.
23. Butcher HR Jr, Jaffe BM: Treatment of aortoiliac arterial occlusive disease by endarterectomy. *Ann Surg* 1971;173:925–928.
24. Szilagyi DE, Smith RF, Elmquist JG, et al: Angioplasty in the treatment of peripheral occlusive arteriopathy: A summary of 12 year's experience. *Arch Surg* 1965;90:617–621.
25. Gruntzig A, Kumpe DA: Technique of percutaneous transluminal angioplasty with the Gruntzig balloon catheter. *Am J Roentgenol* 1979;132:547–549.
26. Brief DK, Alpert J, Parsonnet V: Crossover femoro-femoral grafts. *Arch Surg* 1972;105:889–903.
27. Plecha FR, Pories WJ: Extra-anatomic bypasses for aortoiliac disease in high-risk patients. *Surgery* 1976;80:480–484.
28. Darling RC, Linton RR, Razzuk MA: Saphenous vein bypass grafts for femoropopliteal occlusive disease: A reappraisal. *Surgery* 1967;61:31–36.
29. Noon GP, Diethrich EB, Richardson, WP, et al:

Distal tibial arterial bypass. *Arch Surg* 1969;99: 770–773.
30. Friedman SA: Prevalence of palpable wrist pulses. *Br Heart J* 1970;32:316–320.
31. Fields WS, Lemark NA: Joint study of extracranial arterial obstruction. VII. Subclavian Steal – A review of 168 cases. *JAMA* 1972;222:1139–1141.
32. Hussain S, Schwartz JM, Friedman SA, et al: Arterial thrombosis in essential thrombocythemia. *Am Heart J* 1978;96:31–35.
33. Lerner AB, Barnum CP, Watson CJ: Studies on cryoglobulins II: The spontaneous precipitation of protein from serum at 5° C in various disease states. *Am J Med Sci* 1947;214:416–420.
34. Mosseson MW, Colman RW, Sherry S: Chronic intravascular coagulation syndrome. *N Engl J Med* 1968;278:815–819.
35. Shagan BP, Friedman SA: Raynaud's phenomenon and thyroid deficiency. *Arch Intern Med* 1980;140: 832–835.
36. Medsger TA Jr, Masi AT, Rodnan GP, et al: Survival with systemic sclerosis (scleroderma): A life-table analysis of clinical and demographic factors in 300 patients. *Ann Intern Med* 1971;75:369–373.
37. Kovalchik MT, Guggenheim SJ, Silverman MH, et al: The kidney in progressive systemic sclerosis: A progressive study. *Ann Intern Med* 1978:89: 881–886.
38. Barnett HJ, Jones MW, Boughner DR, et al: Cerebral ischemic events associated with prolapsing mitral valve. *Arch Neurol* 1976;33:777–780.
39. Fairfax AJ, Lambert CD, Leatham A: Systemic embolism in chronic sinoatrial disorder. *Am J Cardiol* 1975;35:872–875.
40. Dillon JC, Feigenbaum H, Knoecke LL, et al: Echocardiographic manifestations of valvular vegetations. *Am Heart J* 1973;86:698–701.
41. Cope GD, Kisslo JA, Johnson ML, et al: A reassessment of the echocardiogram in mitral stenosis. *Circulation* 1975;52:664–670.
42. Coulshed N, Epstein EJ, McKendrick CS, et al: Systemic embolism in mitral valve disease. *Br Heart J* 1970;32:26–30.
43. Borer JS, Bacharach SL, Green MV, et al: Real-time radionuclide cineangiography in the noninvasive evaluation of global and regional left ventricular function at rest and during exercise in patients with coronary artery disease. *N Engl J Med* 1977; 296:839–843.
44. Steele PP, Weily HS, Davies H, et al: Platelet survival in patients with rheumatic heart disease. *N Engl J Med* 1974;290:537–540.
45. Steele PP, Rainwater JO, Genton E: Favorable effects of sulfinpyrazone on thromboembolism in patients with rheumatic heart disease. *Clin Res* 1979; 27:205–209.

CHAPTER 22
Thyroid Heart Disease in the Elderly

James J. Leonard
William J. deGroot

CIRCULATION AND THE ALTERED THYROID STATE

Hyperthyroidism is a systemic illness in that almost all tissues of the body participate in the hypermetabolic state.[1] Since the circulation delivers the necessary nutrients to the tissues, it is not surprising that there is an increased cardiac output, but closer scrutiny of the circulatory changes in hyperthyroidism reveals that the increased cardiac output far outstrips the heightened oxygen consumption. The circulatory adjustment is quite unlike that of other hypermetabolic states. Similar increases in oxygen consumption resulting from salicylate ingestion in man or dinitrophenol administration in animals is accompanied by little or no increase in cardiac output.[1] The increased tissue needs for oxygen are satisfied in these conditions by increased extraction of oxygen from the capillary bed and, as a result, the arteriovenous oxygen difference is widened.

In this sense the circulation of hyperthyroidism resembles more closely the hyperkinetic syndromes seen in peripheral arteriovenous fistulas.[2] Regional distribution of flow is uneven with normal cerebral and hepatic flow but marked increase in coronary and muscle blood flow.

If one measures skin blood flow in hyperthyroidism it is impressive to find that when the cardiac output is increased 100%, the skin flow is increased over 200%.[3] This fact has led physiologists to speculate that the increased volume flow in hyperthyroidism is a homeostatic mechanism to dissipate heat and that cardiac output is set at the level necessary to deliver blood to the periphery. It may be that the discussion of total body oxygen consumption is a superficial and misleading way to look at the oxygen needs of tissues. There may be an impediment to oxygen utilization and electron transfer at the mitochondrial level in hyperthyroidism. Huckabee showed that poisoning the respiratory enzyme system of laboratory animals by the administration of cyanide resulted in tissue anoxia in spite of adequate circulatory delivery.[4] The cardiovascular response was an increased cardiac output with maximal delivery of blood to the tissues but the AV oxygen difference approached zero because the cells could extract little or none of the oxygen presented by the circulation.

A stimulus such as tissue anoxia or metabolic byproducts resulting in vasodilation may be the prime circulatory abnormality in hyperthyroidism. This cardiovascular response then is the normal reflex adjustment one would expect as the heart and circulation respond to the unloading effect of peripheral vasodilation and defend against hypotension. If this were true, then hyperthyroidism could be termed a hyperkinetic state similar to that seen in the large peripheral AV fistula. There is some experimental evidence to support this theory. Infusion of pressor amines such as methoxamine and phenylnephrine in normal man result in striking increases in blood pressure. If reflex bradycardia is blocked there is no change in cardiac output. Similar infusions in hyperthyroid patients result in little pressor effect but rather a

The opinions or assertions contained herein are the private views of the authors and are not to be construed as official or as reflecting the opinions of the Department of Defense.

dramatic decrease in cardiac output to normal levels.[5] These observations lead one to believe that the primary circulatory change is the peripheral vasodilation, and that the tachycardia and increased cardiac output are reflex in nature.

Increased contractility of the heart per se would not be expected to result in significant increases in cardiac output unless accompanied by other changes such as tachycardia and vasodilation.

THYROIDAL ADRENERGIC INTERRELATIONSHIPS

Every discussion of the circulation in hyperthyroidism requires a reference to the classical work of Brewster.[6] This group of investigators rendered a series of dogs hyperthyroid by feeding them thyroid extract. They then submitted these animals to complete epidural sympathectomy. This blockade resulted in a reversal of the hemodynamic and metabolic changes back to the control euthyroid level. It was concluded by these investigators that thyroid hormone acts exclusively by sensitizing the organism to its own endogenous catecholamines. Since that time a large body of information has built up on thyroidal adrenal and thyroid catecholamine interrelationship.[7] It seems imperative at this juncture to make the following point. Studies by excellent modern investigators have repeatedly shown that neither the heart nor the circulation of hyperthyroid laboratory animals[8,9] or man[10] is supersensitive to endogenous or exogenous catecholamines.

It continues to be stated that: "The administration of sympatholytic agents such as reserpine, guanethidine, or propranolol to patients with hyperthyroidism uniformly reduces heart rate, cardiac output, pulse pressure and oxygen consumption to nearly normal levels."[11] These agents uniformly decrease heart rate. On the other hand, repeated careful studies in a number of different laboratories failed to show a significant decrease or a normalization in the cardiac output or oxygen consumption using these agents.[12] On the other hand, administration of such drugs by slowing the pulse, sedating the patient, decreasing perspiration, and ameliorating the symptoms of palpitation and heart pounding create a syndrome not unlike "masked hyperthyroidism."

THE HEART AND THE ALTERED THYROID STATE

In hyperthyroid man, adrenergic blocking agents decrease heart rate both at rest and during exercise but carefully controlled studies by Wilson[13] indicate that the decrement in heart rate both at rest and exercise after beta-adrenergic blockade in hyperthyroidism is similar to the same decrement in euthyroid patients upon administration of adrenergic blocking agents.

Myocardial force velocity relationships in hyperthyroidism have been studied by the papillary muscle technic. Buccino showed that the rate of development of tension increased and the time to peak tension shortened in papillary muscles of cats rendered hyperthyroid.[8] The opposite effect occurred in the hypothyroid state. On the other hand, peak tension differed little between hyper-, hypo-, and euthyroid states. It is as if thyroid lubricates the system, speeding the velocity but not increasing the force of contraction. The maximum velocity of shortening at light loads is increased in hyperthyroidism and decreased in hypothyroidism. This alteration in the contractile state is one which is best suited for cardiac adaptation to volume overload at fast heart rates. These changes in the intrinsic contractile properties of the heart reflect the thyroid state independent of catecholamine stores since they persisted in the face of reserpine depletion of catechols.[8] The same force velocity changes were observed in the hearts of closed chest-sedated dogs.

These observations have been expanded to man using external indices of myocardial contractility such as systolic time intervals. It has been shown in man that there is an increase in ventricular systolic ejection rate and the myocardial contractile state.[14] In hypothyroidism the opposite occurs.[14]

THYROID HEART DISEASE

The question repeatedly arises as to whether or not there is a clinically significant anatomical alteration or mechanical impairment of cardiac function in thyroid disease.

In mild and moderate hyperthyroidism, the augmentation of cardiac output is primarily or exclusively the result of tachycardia and it is generally considered unlikely that tachycardia with increased minute output of the heart will lead to hypertrophy or impairment. But as the hyperthyroidism becomes more severe as evidenced by increasing levels of oxygen consumption, the stroke volume and stroke work begin to increase.[15] This may be the necessary stimulus to hypertrophy. Animal studies have shown an increase in left ventricular mass in experimental hyperthyroidism with complete regression upon stopping thyroid administration.[16,17] This work has been confirmed in man by Nixon et al.[18] Using echocardiographic technics, they showed that successful therapy for thyrotoxicosis resulted in a significant reduction in left ventricular mass. This increase in left ventricular mass occurred in the presence of increased myocardial contractility. This question has most recently been addressed by Forfar et al.[19] These authors studied left ventricular ejection fraction in a group of hyperthyroid patients at rest and during exercise and repeated the observations after pretreatment with propranolol and again after the patients became euthyroid. Using radionuclide ventriculography they showed that the left ventricular ejection fraction was enhanced at rest when the patient was hyperthyroid, but that upon exercise the ejection fraction fell. This is a distinctly abnormal response. This response to exercise persisted in spite of pretreatment with propranolol. After patients returned to the euthyroid state, the resting ejection fraction fell to normal values and the normal expected augmentation of ejection fraction on exercise returned. From these observations, they concluded that a reversible functional cardiomyopathy independent of beta-adrenoreceptor activation existed in these patients, presumably a direct effect of an excess in circulating thyroid hormones.[19]

The myocardial abnormality uncovered by this study has been postulated to represent an intermediate state between normal left ventricular function and obvious dysfunction at rest which might be expected to appear in severe longstanding hyperthyroidism. This comment is important since the time lag between the onset of hyperthyroidism and its clinical diagnosis is much longer in the elderly patient than in the young.

CARDIAC AND NONCARDIAC CIRCULATORY CONGESTION IN ALTERED THYROID STATES

Although thyroid hormone increases myocardial contractility in a way to enhance adaptation to a large volume overload at a fast heart rate, nevertheless on occasion the volume load is so great that circulatory congestion results. At this point the cardiac output is very high and the resulting clinical picture has been labeled noncardiac circulatory congestion simulating congestive failure. Contractility is enhanced but the load is overwhelmingly high and circulatory failure ensues. In hypothyroidism contractility is decreased but the cardiac output decreases much more dramatically than the oxygen consumption and the myxedematous heart can still function at a level satisfactory to cope with the reduced volume load. As a result, pure hypothyroid heart disease is quite rare.

In view of the recent observations of a cardiomyopathy in hyperthyroidism, the previous work of Graettinger et al on high-output heart failure in this condition is worthy of review.[20] Graettinger et al made observations at rest and during exercise on a group of hyperthyroid patients. All had signs suggestive of circulatory congestion. Although both groups had high output at rest, one of these groups was unable to augment cardiac output in a normal manner in response to exercise. Graettinger felt that this subnormal or absent response to exercise defined the high cardiac output *heart* failure group. These observations are consonant with the recent description of a functional myopathy which is unmasked by exercise.

HEART FAILURE IN THE PRESENCE OF THYROID DISEASE

Although the circulatory load or the thyroid myocardiopathy may be the cause of failure in the presence of hyperthyroidism, the most common cause of heart failure in this setting is the presence of atrial fibrillation with an uncontrolled ventricular rate or the presence of an independent form of heart disease which is aggravated by the thyroid dysfunction.

Atrial Fibrillation

Hyperthyroidism, especially Graves' disease, is primarily a disease of young women. The appearance of atrial fibrillation as a presentation or complication of thyrotoxicosis in this group is indeed rare. On the other hand, atrial fibrillation as a presenting or dominant feature of hyperthyroidism in older patients, particularly in the 50- to 70-year age group is quite frequent. This fact had led clinicians to favor the view that the presence of atrial fibrillation in patients with hyperthyroidism signifies complicating underlying heart disease which is either obvious or occult. The occult disease has been presumed to be coronary atherosclerosis. This conclusion has not been confirmed by laboratory observation. In fact, atrial fibrillation as a presenting complaint in coronary artery disease uncomplicated by myocardial infarction is quite unusual, occurring in less than 5% of the cases. In addition, although it was previously considered that atrial fibrillation per se represented organic heart disease, it is now recognized that over 10% of the patients with paroxysmal atrial fibrillation or permanent atrial fibrillation have no known organic heart disease. We also now recognize the fact that in the older age group, abnormalities of SA node impulse formation or propagation occurs as part of an aging process of the conduction tissue independent of hypertension or arteriosclerotic heart disease and accounts for many instances of arrhythmia or conduction abnormalities.

The atrial fibrillation of hyperthyroidism may be paroxysmal or fixed and in general the ventricular response is quite fast in the range of 140 to 170 bpm. Although the ventricular response for a group of hyperthyroid patients may be faster than patients with atrial fibrillation who are not hyperthyroid, the overlap is too great for this phenomena to be of any diagnostic value in an individual case. While the patient is still thyrotoxic the therapeutic goal in the presence of atrial fibrillation is to control the excessive rate rather than attempt reversion or cardioversion to normal sinus rhythm. Satisfactory control of the heart rate during atrial fibrillation may be difficult to obtain in this setting. At any given dose of digitalis, the blood levels will be lower because of a difference in the space of distribution of the drug.[21] As a result, such patients will tolerate increased dosage of the drug. The most effective way to control the ventricular rate after full doses of digitalis have been given is to add a drug such as propranolol hydrochloride to the regimen. Although there is theoretical concern that the beta blockade in this setting may precipitate or aggravate congestive heart failure, experience has shown that this drug is well tolerated, especially if it slows the rate significantly. Since the purpose of its use in this setting is to control the ventricular rate, the dosage should be adjusted to this end-point. As little as 10 mg four times a day may slow the rate to a tolerable level. Hyperthyroid patients with normal sinus rhythm have resting pulses in the range of 110 to 115 bpm. To slow the heart rate to about 100 bpm in the presence of atrial fibrillation seems to represent satisfactory control until the effect of specific thyroid medications takes place.

After the patient becomes euthyroid the paroxysms of atrial fibrillation usually disappear. On the other hand, fixed atrial fibrillation may persist. This fact has also been used for evidence for underlying heart disease. If such patients are returned to normal sinus rhythm by drugs such as quinidine or with cardioversion, the majority will remain in normal sinus rhythm for long periods of time. Those who repeatedly return to atrial fibrillation have been considered to be suffering from the chronic effect of long-standing thyrotoxicosis with complicating cardiomyopathy. There is little clear evidence in man to support this theory. In thyrotoxic patients over the age of 60, the incidence of atrial fibrillation approaches 40%.[22] Although these patients may have the usual fast ventricular response, they frequently have a slower ventricular rate. In the apathetic hyperthyroid, this is considered to be caused by some central block or end-organ resistance to changes in autonomic tone. In others it is probably indicative of disease of the AV conduction system. Impaired AV conduction on the basis of degenerative changes in specialized conduction tissue is not uncommon in the older age group.

In summary, atrial fibrillation, paroxysmal or fixed, may be a presenting or complicating feature of hyperthyroidism. It rarely if ever occurs in young women; it may be seen quite frequently in the older age group, both men and women. There is no direct evidence to support the concept that atrial fibrillation in a patient with hyperthyroidism necessarily means underlying heart disease. It is frequently difficult to effectively slow the ventricular rate in thyrotoxic patients with atrial fibrillation using digitalis alone. The addition of propranolol in moderate doses may result in satisfactory control with little risk of aggravating failure as a result of beta-adrenergic blockade. When the patient becomes euthyroid the dysrhythmia may disappear spontaneously. If it does not, pharmacologic or electrical reversion is indicated. Many patients return to normal sinus rhythm in this fashion and remain so for indefinite periods of time.

HYPERTHYROIDISM IN THE ELDERLY

The clinical picture of thyroid overactivity is highly variable in the older age group. Cardiovascular symptoms frequently dominate. Levine in 1924 called attention to hyperthyroidism "masked" as heart disease.[23] Failure to recognize the role of the overactive thyroid in precipitating or aggravating symptoms of underlying organic heart disease results in the loss of an opportunity to treat a curable component of the cardiac condition. In 1931, Lahey pointed out a form of thyrotoxicosis which he termed "apathetic" hyperthyroidism.[24] This condition is seen much more frequently but not exclusively in the elderly and is considered by some to be a distinct clinical entity with the following features: (*a*) an elderly patient with a thoroughly typical placid apathetic face, quite different from the usual hyperkinetic thyrotoxic patient; (*b*) a small goiter; (*c*) the presence of depression, lethargy or apathy; (*d*) absence of ocular manifestations usually associated with hyperthyroidism; (*e*) substantial muscular weakness and wasting; (*f*) excessive weight loss; and (*g*) cardiovascular dysfunction with atrial fibrillation. Most such patients are diagnosed in the hospital having been admitted as organic heart disease, usually hypertension, or arteriosclerotic heart disease with atrial fibrillation. The diagnosis of hyperthyroidism may be serendipitous in that it is made only after thyroid function studies are returned, having been drawn as a result of policy to request such studies on all patients with atrial fibrillation. The apathetic hyperthyroid patient frequently has a heart rate in the range of 80 to 100 bpm with or without atrial fibrillation and this slow rate draws attention away from the thyroid overactivity to the underlying cardiovascular disease as the exclusive cause of congestive heart failure, cardiovascular dyspnea, and atrial fibrillation.

ANGINA PECTORIS AND THYROID DISEASE

Overactivity of the thyroid gland increases myocardial oxygen demand. The most obvious mechanism is that of tachycardia but in addition, the increased rate of development of tension seen in the hyperthyroid heart increases myocardial oxygen consumption. These factors in the clinical setting of hyperthyroidism may result in the onset of angina pectoris in a previously asymptomatic individual, or may increase the frequency and severity of angina in a given patient, especially in the older age group. The implication in both instances is that there is underlying coronary atherosclerosis and statistically this is overwhelmingly the most likely explanation. However, Resnekov[25] has reported chest pain accompanied by coronary sinus lactate production in a small group of three young women found to have normal coronary arteries at the time of coronary angiography. The role of spasm or coronary embolism secondary to atrial fibrillation was not investigated in these cases and the relationship between hyperthyroidism and coronary spasm has not been reported.

Slowing the resting heart rate as well as the heart rate at any level of exercise is the most effective way to alleviate angina pectoris in hyperthyroidism. This usually can be accomplished quite readily by propranolol or some other beta-adrenergic blocking agent. On the other hand, the increased contractility of the myocardium seen in hyperthyroidism persists unchanged after treatment with beta-adrenergic blockade. But this component of angina is of less importance and therefore the relief of tachycardia is paramount.

Conversely, hypothyroidism may mask the presence of coronary atherosclerosis and ischemic heart disease because the slow heart rate and the diminished contractility lessens the demand on the coronary circulation. It is quite rare for hypothyroid patients to have complicating angina pectoris while severely myxedematous. When the combination is present it poses a severe therapeutic dilemma. Although with treatment of the myxedema the angina pectoris is likely to become more severe, nevertheless in a minority of cases the angina pectoris actually improves. The basis of this observation is not clear. The most prudent approach is to seek the middle road and attempt to alleviate the less tolerable symptoms of myxedema while at the same time treating the angina with the usual cardiac medications. Treatment of the hypothyroidism should proceed slowly and one should undershoot the usual therapeutic goals of rendering the patient completely euthyroid. Part of the approach is to improve the patient's thyroid status to the point where further diagnostic studies can be safely tolerated. This same approach should be taken with all profoundly myxedematous patients in the older age group since as many as one third will develop angina for the first time during or within one year of the institution of therapy. There is reason to believe that the severe hypertension seen in some patients with myxedema will partially ameliorate after successful thyroid administration. This reasoning is based on the fact that a significant number of patients rendered hypothyroid as a result of treatment for thyrotoxicosis develop hypertension not previously present.

ELECTROCARDIOGRAPHY

The ECG findings in hyperthyroidism are for the most part nonspecific and offer little help in diagnosis. The PR interval is frequently long, especially when adjusted for heart rate. Abnormalities of the QRS complex are most likely incidental or due to complicating independent heart disease. The T waves are frequently flat and the QT interval is short. Major AV conduction disturbances or intraventricular conduction abnormalities are unusual and, when present, are difficult to establish as being secondary to the thyroid disease.

The obvious rhythm abnormality seen, especially in the older age group, is atrial fibrillation. The characteristics and the management of this dysrhythmia are discussed under the section on atrial fibrillation.

In hypothyroidism the heart is slow, the QT interval is long, and the T waves are flat or inverted. A decrease in the electromotive force of the T vector is almost always present whether or not there is low voltage of the QRS complex, which also occurs quite frequently. Although the presence of pericardial effusion may explain in part the low voltage seen on the ECG, nevertheless this finding frequently exists when the effusion is small or persists after pericardial tap with removal of the fluid.

CHEST ROENTGENOLOGY

In hyperthyroidism the cardiac silhouette is usually on the full side and may at times exceed the upper limit for normal without specific chamber enlargement. Massive enlargement is not seen without complicating heart disease. Radionuclide studies have shown an increase in left ventricular mass as has been previously mentioned. This increase is in the range of 20% and as such cannot be anticipated to cause a significant change on the roentgenogram. It is known that mild or moderate increase in left ventricular volume in other types of heart disease cannot be demonstrated on chest films but can be diagnosed by ultrasound.

The most frequent abnormality of the chest film in these patients is prominence of the pulmonary artery, which occurs in about 30% of patients. The cause of the pulmonary artery dilatation is not clear.

The classical roentgenographic finding in myxedematous heart is the so-called ham-shaped heart characteristic of pericardial effusion. Pericardial effusion of varying amounts is almost always present in myxedema. It disappears with thyroid replacement and the cardiac silhouette returns to normal. In the past these changes in the cardiac silhouette were frequently misinterpreted as cardiac enlargement followed by regression on therapy and considered diagnostic of myxedematous heart disease with failure. Much of the confusion concerning myxedematous heart disease is centered around this finding. It is well to remember that this is not a pericarditis but rather an accumulation of fluid. This effusion leads neither to tamponade or constrictive pericarditis and although the fluid has a rich protein content, it does not represent a true exudate with inflammatory cells.

CLINICAL FEATURES

Patients with hyperthyroidism often complain of palpitation which is caused by forceful heart action. The tachycardia coupled with the wide pulse pressure makes the patient aware of his or her own cardiac activity and even more keenly aware of any irregularity—an awareness similar to that of patients with aortic insufficiency.[1] As a result, paroxysmal atrial fibrillation, frequent atrial extrasystoles, or ventricular extrasystoles cause intense anxiety and discomfort.

The patient with hyperthyroidism also frequently complains of breathlessness or difficulty in breathing. Dyspnea occurs principally on exertion and is seen in over 75% of cases. Patients with hyperthyroidism have definite weakness of the respiratory muscles and this fact coupled with a diminished lung compliance of unknown cause may be responsible for the symptoms. In addition, just as the heart rate response to exercise is exaggerated, so the minute ventilation response to exertion is also excessive with respiratory rates reaching 45/min at moderate levels of exercise. The result is that a large proportion of the minute volume is expended uselessly in ventilating dead space.[26]

It is the hemodynamic change occurring in thyrotoxicosis which is responsible for the striking features. The fast bounding pulse; the conspicuous precordial activity; warm, moist, flushed skin as a result of increased cutaneous flow, are prominent features. Superficial veins are prominent which suggests augmented blood volume from the periphery. Veins appear abnormally full and the venous pressure is at the upper limits of normal in the absence of congestive failure. With few exceptions a continuous bruit or venous hum is audible on auscultation in the supraclavicular fossa. This sound is best heard on the right side with the patient standing or sitting and may be accompanied by a thrill.[27] Transmission to the precordium occurs occasionally. In patients with severe thyrotoxicosis, the murmur frequently persists when the patient lies down. In the absence of severe anemia, the presence of a venous hum, particularly in an adult or patient in the older age group, should immediately suggest the diagnosis of hyperthyroidism. Definitive identification of this murmur is easily made by demonstrating its disappearance with jugular venous compression. The typical thyroid bruit is actually heard less frequently. This murmur is usually systolic in time and if the bruit spills over into diastole, it signifies relative compression of the vessel by the enlarged thyroid.

CARDIAC AUSCULTATION[27]

Cardiac auscultation usually reveals a number of sounds which may cause consternation. The occasional transmission of the venous hum to the high precordium may be misinterpreted as a heart murmur. The first heart sound is loud and this increase in intensity is present independently of a short or long PR interval and is undoubtedly a manifestation of the increased rate of development of tension and pressure in the ventricle. An early systolic ejection sound followed by an ejection murmur can be heard in most patients. The murmur is usually louder at the base of the heart and occasionally it may have a scratching quality which suggests the systolic component of a friction rub. This is the sound which Means and Lerman described.[27] These authors felt that the sound was caused by an enlarged pulmonary artery rubbing against adjacent structures. There are really no data to support this theory nor is there any reason to believe that the "scratch" is any different in etiology than the more commonly elicited ejection murmur heard in the pulmonic area which in turn frequently has a scratchy characteristic. Most thyrotoxic patients will have a prominent S_3 as is true in other hyperkinetic states such as severe anemia and AV fistula. As such, this sound is indicative of an increased rate of filling of the left ventricle and not intrinsic myocardial disease. In addition, an S_4 is heard in over two thirds of hyperthyroid patients. It is likely that this sound occurs in that subset of patients with an increased stroke volume with the ventricle operating closer to the steep part of the filling curve. Again, this sound does not infer cardiac muscle disease but merely the high volume preload that occurs in hyperthyroidism with a large stroke volume in the face of fast heart rates. Since most such patients have rapid heart rates, there may be a loud sound in diastole which represents a summation gallop. With the presence of both an S_3 and an S_4 such patients have a so-called quadruple rhythm. Incomplete summation of these diastolic sounds is the usual source of the so-called mid-diastolic rumbling murmur heard in patients with hyperthyroidism. At times a true mitral diastolic rumble may occur. Evidence to support this assumption can be gleaned from the fact that phono catheters placed in the left ventricular inflow tract of patients with hyperthyroidism occasionally pick up diastolic rumbling murmurs.[27]

TREATMENT

The definitive treatment of hyperthyroidism in the older age group is the administration of radioiodine. Although this mode of therapy is generally agreed upon by clinicians, it is recognized that the full effect of radioiodine is not reached until six to 12 months after initiation of therapy. When more prompt control of thyroid activity is required, antithyroid drugs and potassium iodide must be added as soon as a therapeutic dose of radioiodine has been administered.

The addition of these drugs will usually bring the patient under control in one to four weeks. This may be sufficiently rapid if the cardiovascular symptoms are mild or moderate in nature.

As previously stated, angina is best controlled by slowing the heart rate. Careful administration of beta-adrenergic blocking agents such as propranolol may result in sufficient slowing of the pulse to relieve angina at relatively low dosage. One may start with 10 mg four times a day and find that the heart rate is under satisfactory control before a dose of 40 mg four times a day is reached.

The management of atrial fibrillation has been discussed previously. Severe congestive heart failure in a thyrotoxic patient in the face of normal sinus rhythm is in reality a more difficult management problem than the patient with atrial fibrillation at an excessively fast ventricular rate. In the latter, drugs are usually successful in creating the AV block necessary to control the rate. It is more difficult to slow the heart rate if the mechanism is sinus tachycardia. The signs and symptoms of heart failure in the face of hyperthyroidism are not dramatically improved with digitalis. Nevertheless, the drug should be administered in the usual fashion. Laboratory studies have shown that the heart in hyperthyroidism is less responsive to digitalis in terms of augmentation of myocardial contractility but since digitalis and the thyroid hormone act on the myocardium in a fundamentally different manner, the drug should be administered together with diuretics. Although serum levels of digitalis may be lower at any given dose in the hyperthyroid patient due to an increased volume of distribution, nevertheless the relative ineffectiveness of digitalis in this setting makes pushing the drug dosage to potentially toxic levels unwarranted. Once the patient is digitalized, the careful addition of propranolol in doses starting at 10 mg four times a day, may slow the heart rate and improve the general cardiovascular status of the patient.

The treatment of an elderly patient with myxedema requires careful thyroid replacement starting with doses as low as 0.0125 mg daily. The dose can then be doubled every two weeks but only under careful surveillance looking for the onset of or worsening of angina pectoris. The first plateau of definitive therapy is to get the patient under partial control so that diagnostic studies relative to more specific therapy can be carried out safely.

The myxedematous patient with valvular heart disease may suddenly decompensate during thyroid replacement. Even with interruption of the medication the therapeutic effect will last a number of weeks during which time the management of the patient's cardiovascular status can be quite difficult.

REFERENCES

1. Leonard JJ, deGroot WJ: The thyroid state and the cardiovascular system. *Mod Concepts Cardiovasc Dis* 1969;38:23-27.
2. deGroot WJ, Leonard JJ: Hyperthyroidism as a high cardiac output state. *Am Heart J* 1970;79: 265-275.
3. Kontos HA, Shapiro W, Mauch HP, et al: Mechanism of certain abnormalities of the circulation to the limbs in thyrotoxicosis. *J Clin Invest* 1965; 44:947–956.
4. Huckabee WE: Circulatory response to cytochrome oxidase inhibition in vivo abstracted. *Fed Proc* 1960;19:119.
5. Theilen EO, Wilson WR: Hemodynamic effects of peripheral vasoconstriction in normal and thyrotoxic subjects. *J Appl Physiol* 1967;22:207–210.
6. Brewster WR Jr, Isaacs JP, Osgood PF, et al: Hemodynamic and metabolic interrelationships in the activity of epinephrine, norepinephrine and the thyroid hormones. *Circulation* 1956;13:1-20.
7. Harrison TS: Adrenal medullary and thyroid relationships. *Physiol Rev* 1964;44:161–185.
8. Buccino RA, Spann JF Jr, Pool PE, et al: Influence of thyroid state on the intrinsic contractile properties and energy stores of the myocardium. *J Clin Invest* 1967;46:1669–1682.
9. Cairoli VJ, Crout JR: Role of the autonomic nervous system in the resting tachycardia of experimental hyperthyroidism. *J Pharmacol Exp Ther* 1967;158:55-65.
10. Aoki VS, Wilson WR, Theilen EO, et al: The effects of triiodothyronine on hemodynamic responses to epinephrine and norepinephrine in man. *J Pharmacol Exp Ther* 1967;157:62–68.
11. Skelton CL: The heart and hyperthyroidism, editorial. *N Engl J Med* 1982;307:1206–1208.
12. Theilen EO, Wilson WR, Tutunji FJ: Acute hemodynamic effects of alpha-methyldopa in thyrotoxic patients and normal subjects. *Metabolism* 1963;12: 625–630.
13. Wilson WR, Theilen EO, Fletcher FW: Pharmacodynamic effects of beta-adrenergic receptor blockade in patients with hyperthyroidism. *J Clin Invest* 1964;43:1697–1703.
14. Amidi M, Leon EF, deGroot WJ, et al: Effect of the thyroid state on myocardial contractility and ventricular ejection rate in man. *Circulation* 1968; 38:229–239.
15. Kroetz F, deGroot WJ, Leonard JJ, et al: Relationship of oxygen consumption to hemodynamic response in hypermetabolic states abstracted. *Clin Res* 1962;10:19.
16. Sandler G, Wilson GM: Production of cardiac hypertrophy by thyroxine in the rat. *Q J Exp Physiol* 1959;44:282–289.
17. Beznak M: Cardiovascular effects of thyroxine treatment in normal rats. *Can J Biochem* 1962;40: 1647–1654.
18. Nixon JV, Anderson RJ, Cohen ML: Alterations in left ventricular mass and performance in patients treated effectively for thyrotoxicosis: A comparative echocardiographic study. *Am J Med* 1979;67:268–276.
19. Forfar JC, Lever AL, Sawers SA, et al: Abnormal left ventricular function in hyperthyroidism: Evidence for a possible reversible cardiomyopathy. *N Engl J Med* 1982;307:1165–1170.
20. Graettinger JS, Muenster JJ, Selverstone LA, et al: Correlation of clinical and hemodynamic studies in patients with hyperthyroidism with and without congestive heart failure. *J Clin Invest* 1959;38: 1316–1327.
21. Doherty JE, Perkins WH: Digoxin metabolism in hypo- and hyperthyroidism: Studies with tritiated digoxin in thyroid disease. *Ann Intern Med* 1966; 64:489–507.
22. Davis PJ, Davis FB: Hyperthyroidism in patients over the age of 60 years. *Medicine* 1974;53:161–181.
23. Levine SA, Sturges CC: Hyperthyroidism masked as heart disease. *Boston Med Surg J* 1924;190:233–237.
24. Lahey FH: Non-activated (apathetic) type of hyperthyroidism. *NEJM* 1931;204:747–748.
25. Resnekov L, Falicov RE: Thyrotoxicosis and lactate-producing angina pectoris with normal coronary arteries. *Br Heart J* 1977;39:1051–1057.
26. Stein M, Kimbe P, Johnson RL: Pulmonary function in hyperthyroidism. *J Clin Invest* 1961;40:348–363.
27. Leonard JJ, Renfro NL, deGroot WJ, et al: The auscultatory diagnosis of the hyperkinetic state, in Segal BL, Likoff W, Moyer JH (eds): *The Theory and Practice of Auscultation*. Philadelphia, FA Davis Company, 1964, pp 180–190.
28. Lerman J, Means J: Cardiovascular symptomatology in exophthalmic goiter. *Am Heart J* 1932; 8:55–65.

CHAPTER 23
Arterial Embolism: Diagnosis and Management

David C. Brewster

Despite tremendous advances in the management of cardiovascular diseases, arterial embolism remains a common and important cause of limb-threatening ischemia or loss of vital organ function, particularly in the older patient population. The morbidity and mortality of embolic events remains significant, with reported mortality in the range of 15% to 25%, even in recently reported series from large institutions. The overall frequency of arterial embolism also appears to be increasing. This may, in part, be due to better diagnosis and recognition, but there is little doubt that an aging patient population, longer survival of patients with advanced cardiac disease, and greater use of cardiac and vascular prosthetic devices all contribute to a rising incidence of thromboembolic problems particularly likely to affect the elderly.

Optimal treatment is based upon prompt recognition of acute arterial insufficiency of a limb or organ, and identification of an embolic rather than thrombotic etiology of such ischemia. Diagnosis must often be based upon a high index of suspicion in the embolus-prone patient. Best results follow expeditious treatment to alleviate the ischemia, usually by surgical removal of the embolus.

CHANGING CLINICAL POPULATION

Over the past three to four decades, definite shifts in the characteristics of the patient population with arterial emboli have occurred. Several decades previously, patients were most often in the 40- to 50-year age group, with rheumatic heart disease the most common cause of an embolus. In contrast, the majority of patients today are over 65 years of age, with arteriosclerotic heart disease and its complications by far the most frequent etiology of an arterial embolus. Many patients currently are in or beyond their eighth decade of life, with widespread coronary artery, cerebrovascular, and peripheral occlusive disease, all significant contributing factors to the persistent high mortality of arterial embolic disease.

Such trends have been clearly documented over a 40-year time frame by a series of previous reports of experience with arterial embolism at the Massachusetts General Hospital, Boston.[1–4] As indicated in Table 23-1, during the four decades spanned by the different series the incidence of rheumatic heart disease was cut in half, while the frequency of emboli attributable to arteriosclerotic heart disease and associated atrial fibrillation or myocardial infarction almost doubled. During this period, average age of patients rose from 52 to 69 years. Similar changes in the patient population have been reported from other institutions by other investigators.[5]

PATHOPHYSIOLOGY

An embolus is defined as a blood clot or other foreign body, formed in one location and carried by blood flow to another site, where it produces occlusion of the more distal vessel. Thrombus causing embolic occlusion of major arteries may accumulate in the heart, diseased great vessels, or upon vascular prosthetic valves or grafts. Rarely, foreign bodies such as bullets, fragments of medical diagnostic devices, etc, may gain access to the circulation and subsequently embolize to distal segments of the arterial tree. Clinical manifestations produced depend upon several factors, including the site of occlusion, length of the occluded segment, availability of collateral

Table 23-1
Cardiac Disease in Patients with Arterial Emboli
Massachusetts General Hospital, 1937–1980

	1937–1946[1]	1947–1953[2]	1954–1963[3]	1964–1980[4]
Rheumatic heart disease	42%	49%	36%	20%
Arteriosclerotic heart disease	34%	42%	51%	66%
Other	24%	9%	13%	14%

circulation, subsequent propagation of clot, and duration of ischemia.

Sources of Emboli

While characteristics of the patient population have changed, the heart remains the source of thrombus causing emboli in 85% to 90% of cases (Table 23-2). Clot forming in the left atrium secondary to atrial fibrillation continues to represent the most common cause of systemic arterial emboli, responsible for 50% to 75% of emboli in various reported series. As already noted, the underlying cardiac abnormality leading to atrial fibrillation has shifted from rheumatic heart disease to coronary artery disease in the majority of patients.

Within the left ventricle, thrombus forms most commonly as a sequel to myocardial infarction. Mural thrombus, most frequently at the apex of the left ventricle, was found at autopsy in 44% of patients with fatal myocardial infarctions.[6] In Darling's report from the Massachusetts General Hospital, more than one half of patients presenting without atrial fibrillation were found to have myocardial infarction as the source of their arterial embolus. Of all patients with a systemic arterial embolus, acute myocardial infarction was found to precede the embolus in one out of every seven patients, or 14.2%. Myocardial infarction had occurred from three to 28 days prior to the embolic episode, with an average of 14 days.[3]

An arterial embolus, on occasion, may be the initial manifestation of a "silent" myocardial infarction. For this reason, careful evaluation of the ECG is essential in patients presenting with an acute embolus, especially if they are not in atrial fibrillation. Left ventricular clot may also form in ventricular aneurysms secondary to more remote myocardial infarctions.

Another cardiac source of arterial emboli stems from the increasingly frequent implantation of prosthetic valves or other devices. This growing problem is especially common when postimplantation anticoagulation is inadequate or discontinued.

Although rare, intracardiac tumors such as atrial myxoma may give rise to tumor emboli sufficiently large to occlude major vessels, and occasionally vegetations from mitral or aortic valve leaflets in patients with bacterial endocarditis may cause recognizable arterial embolic events. For these reasons, careful pathologic and bacteriologic examination of thrombus removed at the time of surgical embolectomy is advisable in all cases.

Noncardiac sources of emboli are responsible for approximately 10% to 15% of cases. In half of such noncardiac etiologies, abnormalities of proximal vessels cause thrombus formation and subsequent peripheral embolization. Aneurysms of the aorta, iliac, femoral, or popliteal arteries are perhaps the most common arterial sites associated with downstream emboli. Subclavian aneurysms, often due to unsuspected cervical rib or thoracic outlet compression, may give rise to upper extremity or digital emboli. Ulceration of

Table 23-2
Sources of Arterial Embolism

Cardiac	
Rheumatic heart disease with atrial fibrillation	20%
Arteriosclerotic heart disease with atrial fibrillation	30%
Arteriosclerotic heart disease with myocardial infarction, +/− atrial fibrillation	25%
Prosthetic heart valves, unusual cardiac sources	10%
	85%
Noncardiac	
Proximal arterial aneurysm, prosthetic graft, ulcerated plaque, false aneurysm, paradoxical embolus	7.5%
Undetermined sources	7.5%
	15.0%

atheromatous plaques may serve as a nidus for surprisingly large thrombi leading to embolic events. These are most common in the thoracic or abdominal aorta. Thrombus or bits of poorly aherent fibrin from the pseudointima of prosthetic grafts implanted for arterial reconstruction are an increasingly frequent source of a peripheral embolus. Similarly, iatrogenic or traumatic injuries to major vessels, resulting in intraluminal clot or associated false aneurysms, may be an unsuspected cause of a peripheral arterial embolus.

In the remaining cases (approximately 7.5%), the specific source of an embolus cannot be determined either clinically or even at autopsy. As diagnostic procedures continue to improve, however, this percentage appears to be declining.

Sites of Embolism

While the nature of associated diseases leading to arterial embolism has undergone changes within the past three decades, anatomical sites of embolic occlusions have remained relatively constant.

The term embolus is derived from the Greek *embolos*, meaning a plug or stopper, and was first introduced by Virchow in 1854. Because vessel diameters change most abruptly at points of arterial branching, sites of embolic occlusion are most often related to major arterial bifurcations. In approximately two thirds of clinically detected embolic episodes, embolic occlusion involves major limb vessels. This is indeed fortunate, as such locations are most amenable to surgical embolectomy.

As seen in Figure 23-1, the lower extremities are the site of embolic occlusion in approximately 50% of all clinically detectable emboli, or 75% of all limb emboli. The common femoral bifurcation is the most common site for an embolus to lodge, and is the site most readily approached surgically, often with simple local anesthesia. Together, the femoral and popliteal arteries are involved more than twice as frequently as the aorta and iliac vessels, probably reflecting the simple mechanical fact that only a thrombus of considerable size will impact at the aortic or common iliac bifurcations unless they are narrowed by pre-existent occlusive disease.

Approximately 20% of arterial emboli involve the carotid vessels, and about 10% the visceral organs. Both categories are much more difficult to treat surgically, and consequently continue to be associated with considerable morbidity and mortality. Concomitant or subsequent mesenteric emboli are the cause of death in approximately 20% of patients with arterial emboli.[3] In addition, it should be emphasized that many visceral emboli may go undetected. If small, little physiologic disturbance may be present to indicate their occurrence, whereas if large they may prove rapidly fatal and are perhaps frequently confused with other causes of sudden death such as myocardial infarction, pulmonary embolus, etc.

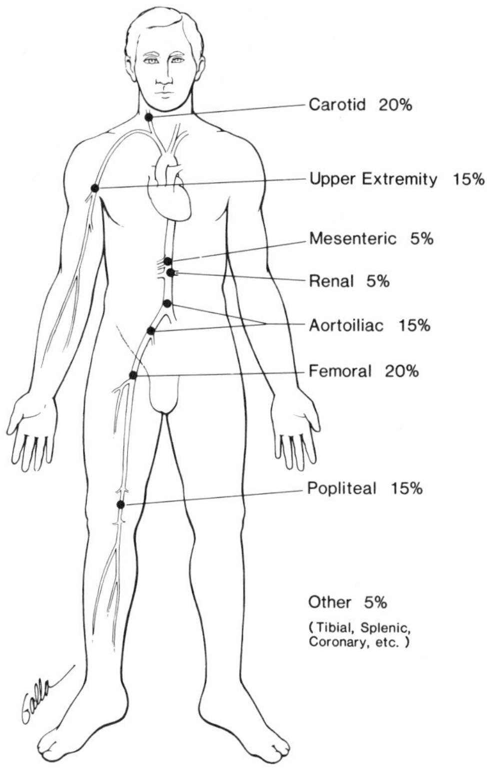

Figure 23-1 Sites of embolism.

Effects of an Embolus

Local manifestations of an acute arterial occlusion by an embolus obviously relate to the ischemic effects upon the limb or organ involved. Generalized systemic sequelae may follow later if the local ischemia is profound or neglected. Such systemic effects relate to the toxic products of ischemic tissue breakdown of the involved area, leading potentially to acidosis, hyperkalemia, hypotension, myoglobinuria, renal failure, and possible septicemia.[7] These potentially disastrous problems are major causes of the significant mortality associated with advanced prolonged ischemia frequently seen in patients treated late in the course of embolic occlusion and have led some authorities to advocate primary amputation for such advanced cases.

In general, the natural clinical course of any embolic event depends upon the location of the occlusion, the organ involved, the size of the vessel, the degree of completeness of obstruction, and most importantly, the amount of collateral circulation available. The adequacy of collateral flow around the site of acute embolic occlusion is the chief determinant of the severity and outcome of the event.

Formerly, much emphasis was placed upon the necessity to intervene therapeutically within a 4- to 6-hour period, as it was felt that this usually represented the maximum period of tolerable ischemia. While this may be true in most instances, it is now well recognized that no arbitrary time limit can be applied to all cases, and that the physiologic state of the limb rather than elapsed time from the onset of occlusion best determines operability and salvagability. In many instances, enough collateral circulation may be present to allow survival of the ischemic limb or organ, although its function may be severely impaired. Nonetheless, many reported instances of delayed embolectomy, carried out as late as weeks after the initial embolic event, have been described with successful restoration of normal function to a limb or organ.

Following initial arterial occlusion by the embolus, several possible events may occur to aggravate the severity of ischemia. Impairment of collateral circulation by propagation of clot, which tends to occur most often distal to the site of embolic occlusion, is the major secondary factor leading to worsening of ischemia following an embolus. Prevention of such secondary clot propagation is the basis for the importance of immediate therapy with full-dose heparin once a diagnosis of acute arterial insufficiency is made, as discussed below.

Associated venous thrombosis may also occur with prolonged severe arterial ischemia, probably due to a combination of sluggish flow and ischemic injury to the intima of veins in the involved area. Such venous thrombosis may further aggravate limb ischemia, or lead to pulmonary embolism, a major cause of death in neglected cases of severely ischemic limbs.

Fragmentation of an embolus and subsequent migration to distal vessels beyond collateral sources may on occasion be another secondary factor in later worsening of ischemia. Conversely, embolus lysis and fragmentation may sometimes be responsible for spontaneous clinical improvement noted in some cases.

CLINICAL MANIFESTATIONS

Most frequently, an arterial embolus is associated with the sudden onset of arterial ischemia. The cardinal signs and symptoms are classically classified by the mnemonic for acute arterial insufficiency, the "five *p*'s"; pulselessness, pain, pallor, paresthesia, and paralysis.

Sudden loss of a previously present pulse is the hallmark of an embolic occlusion. Recognition is easiest when previous known pulses existed at a particular site, and obviously more difficult if the prior pulse status of a limb was unknown or already abnormal due to associated arteriosclerotic occlusive disease. It is also important to emphasize that a normal or even bounding pulse may often be felt initially at the actual site of embolic impaction, representing transmitted pulsations through the fresh clot. Occasionally, tenderness can be noted over a deep vessel with acute embolic occlusion, clearly defining the point of obstruction.

Pain and pallor are well-known classical symptoms of acute arterial insufficiency. The pain is characteristically a severe and steady ache, involving major muscle groups below the level of obstruction, and usually progressively worse at locations increasingly distal to the point of occlusion. Occasionally, however, sensory disturbances predominate and may mask primary complaints of pain. In such instances, the patient may complain primarily of numbness or paresthesias. The color of the limb distal to the occlusion is initially white and "waxy"—often termed "cadaveric." Subsequently, blotchy mottled areas of cyanosis may appear and eventually blistering and the deeper discoloration typical of early gangrene.

Advanced ischemia is characterized by diminished to absent motor and sensory function, reflecting ischemia to both muscles and nerves distal to the arterial occlusion. The extent of anesthesia and motor paralysis of a limb is a good index of the degree of tissue anoxia and correlates well with the ultimate prognosis. Preservation of sensitivity to light touch is often the best guide to viability. Its absence demands surgical intervention if at all possible. Paralysis is similarly a grave sign. Frank muscle rigidity is often considered a sign of irreversibility, although the limb may still be salvaged by prompt intervention in some cases. Ultimate function of such limbs is often permanently compromised, however, and the metabolic effects of revascularization may be profound and sometimes lethal.

Topographic localization of the site of occlusion is often possible based upon careful physical examination. Aside from noting the site of pulse disappearance, typically a level of temperature demarcation can be noted approximately "one joint" distal to the point of occlusion. That is, a temperature level just above the ankle often denotes occlusion at the popliteal bifurcation, while a level at or just above the knee suggests blockage at the femoral bifurcation. Similarly, changes to the upper thigh on one side suggests an iliac embolus, while involvement of both thighs to the groins or lower abdomen or buttocks suggests an aortic bifurcation "saddle" embolus. In the latter case, one must be aware of possible associated renal, visceral, or spinal cord ischemia.

DIFFERENTIAL DIAGNOSIS

Acute arterial occlusion due to an embolus is often difficult to distinguish clinically from in situ thrombosis of a diseased and stenotic artery involved with occlusive disease. Occasionally, sudden thrombosis may also occur in a vessel with pre-existent aneurysmal disease. Distinction between embolic and thrombotic occlusion is becoming increasingly difficult due to the advancing age and frequency of associated arteriosclerotic vascular disease present in patients with arterial emboli.

Differentiation is of significant clinical importance, as a decision to proceed with surgical intervention is often markedly different for the two conditions. Whereas embolectomy is often successful and the surgical procedure usually limited, attempts at thrombectomy for thrombosis in situ will often fail. In many cases, it may make matters worse and lead to the necessity of a major arterial reconstruction on an emergency basis in a poorly prepared patient. For these reasons, most vascular surgeons prefer to manage acute arterial thrombosis (vs embolus) nonoperatively in its initial stages, if feasible.

As indicated in Table 23-3, several clues may be obtained from a careful history and physical examination. Typically, patients with an embolus have a very sudden onset of symptoms, and usually have a recognizable source for an embolus, most often cardiac disease with atrial fibrillation. As many as one third of patients will have a history of a prior embolic episode. A history of prior claudication is usually absent in the patient with an embolus, with no evidence of occlusive disease present in the contralateral limb on pulse examination. The level of temperature demarcation is often quite sharp in embolic occlusions, in contrast to the patient with pre-existent occlusive disease and better developed collateral networks.

Arteriography may also be useful. In the patient with an embolus, a sharp cutoff in an otherwise fairly normal vessel without extensive collateral development is seen. In contrast, patients with acute thrombosis have more obvious and diffuse atheromatous changes and better developed collaterals. In general, most surgeons proceed with embolectomy without arteriography if the diagnosis and site of obstruction seem well-established clinically. Postembolectomy intraoperative arteriograms can then the utilized as indicated. On the other hand, if the diagnosis is unclear and inordinate time delay can be avoided, arteriography may be helpful in diagnostic and management decisions.

Acute aortic dissections may cause sudden limb or organ ischemia, abrupt loss of pulses, and other signs of sudden acute ischemia. However,

Table 23-3
Differentiation of Embolus from Thrombosis

	Embolus	Thrombosis
Onset	Sudden	More gradual
Identifiable source for embolus	Usual	Less common
History of claudication	Rare	Common
Physical findings suggestive of vascular disease	Few	Often present
Temperature level demarcation	Sharp	Less well defined
Arteriogram	Minimal atherosclerosis, few collaterals	Diffuse atherosclerosis, well-developed collaterals

recognition and differentiation from an acute embolic occlusion is usually possible by a classic history of hypertension and chest or intrascapular back pain radiating downward. A murmur of aortic insufficiency may be noted or a difference in the strength or character of carotid or upper extremity pulses between the right and left sides may be detected. Widening of the mediastinum may be appreciated on chest film. The diagnosis may usually be confirmed by aortography or computed tomography (CT) scan. Sometimes limb or visceral ischemia may be transient if spontaneous re-entry of the aortic dissection occurs. In some instances, the actual pathologic problem may not be appreciated until the time of embolectomy. The surgeon notes that a Fogarty balloon catheter will either not pass beyond the point of occlusion, or if it does no clot is retrieved or blood flow restored. In such instances, the possibility of aortic dissection must be immediately suspected and pursued by further arteriographic evaluation or surgical exploration.

Several other conditions are occasionally confused with lower extremity emboli. Phlegmasia cerulea dolens due to massive ileofemoral deep venous thrombosis may present with a suddenly painful leg. Indeed, swelling often makes pulses difficult to feel, and in its late stages secondary arterial insufficiency may in fact develop. However, it is usually differentiated initially by the sudden acute swelling of the limb always present at the onset, very atypical for the initial presentation of an acute arterial occlusion. In addition, the intense cyanotic congestion of the limb with deep venous thrombosis and phlegmasia is in distinct contrast to the typical pallor and collapsed superficial veins seen with acute arterial insufficiency.

On occasion, aortic saddle emboli may present primarily with sudden onset of bilateral lower extremity weakness and sensory loss, progressing rapidly to a paraplegic-like state. Care must be taken to avoid initial confusion with acute neurologic problems, leading to time-consuming and misdirected diagnostic and therapeutic efforts.

MANAGEMENT

Today, optimal therapy is prompt surgical removal of the embolus in most instances. This requires an expeditious diagnosis of acute arterial occlusion and recognition of a probable embolic etiology. Initial evaluation and treatment should also aim to define the degree of ischemia and thereby indicate the urgency of surgical intervention.

Although difficulty may exist in initial differentiation of embolic vs thrombotic occlusion, intravenous heparin should be administered as soon as the diagnosis of acute arterial occlusion is made. This is intended to prevent propagation of clot and stabilize the situation long enough to allow consideration of diagnostic possibilities and, most importantly, evaluation and initial treatment of the cardiac abnormality usually present with embolic disease. Overt or subtle cardiac failure, myocardial ischemia, arrhythmias, electrolyte disturbances, or similar problems are promptly corrected to the best extent possible by the usual maneuvers.

Heparin sodium should be administered in full dosage. We generally prefer an initial bolus of 10,000 units, approximating 1–2 mg of heparin per kilogram of body weight. This can then be followed by subsequent continuous intravenous infusion of approximately 1000 units/h. Heparin should be administered promptly even if a decision to proceed with immediate surgical embolectomy is made.

After initial heparinization and evaluation of the patient's cardiac status, a decision must be reached regarding surgical intervention. In general, the proper treatment of an embolus is prompt surgical removal, while acute arterial thrombosis is best managed initially in most instances if feasible by nonoperative measures. As discussed above, arteriography may be helpful in making such a therapeutic decision. If the diagnosis and site of embolic occlusion are fairly well-established, most feel it unnecessary, however.

The location of the embolus will obviously play a role. Most cerebral emboli are intracranial and not accessible to the usual methods of surgical embolectomy. However, sudden onset of cerebrovascular ischemia in a fibrillating patient with concomitant loss of the superficial temporal pulse in the preauricular region may indicate lodging of an embolus at the surgically accessible carotid bifurcation in the neck rather than intercranial branches of the internal carotid artery, and may suggest the advisability of immediate surgical exploration or angiography.

Development of the balloon-tipped embolectomy catheter by Fogarty and associates in 1963 has greatly simplified surgical therapy, often allowing treatment with limited incisions, often under local anesthesia, at a distance from the embolus which may be lodged at more inaccessible locations.[8] These are frequently vital considerations in the often poor-risk elderly patients with severe cardiac problems. Use of the balloon catheter is obviously not feasible in surgical management of all emboli, however, and emboli to the mesenteric or renal circulation usually still require laparotomy. However, limb emboli account for approximately two thirds of clinically recognizable arterial embolic episodes and are generally managed quite effectively by use of the balloon catheter.

The place of thrombolytic therapy in the management of embolic occlusions remains unsettled. Insufficient experience exists to provide definitive information. Systemic use of agents such as streptokinase may be useful, but may have a significant incidence of systemic side-effects and bleeding disturbances. More precise local delivery of thrombolytic agents, via an arterial catheter placed at or near the site of occlusion, seems more logical, and we have had some success with such therapy. It appears best suited, however, to management of acute thrombotic occlusions, whereas an embolus is usually best removed surgically if accessible to a balloon catheter.

Surgical Embolectomy

The first reported successful surgical removal of an arterial embolus was performed in 1911. Treatment of arterial emboli remained nonsurgical in many instances, however, until more recent years. With availability of anticoagulants, improvements in vascular surgical technics, and particularly with the development of the Fogarty balloon embolectomy catheter, there has been a dramatic trend toward surgical treatment over the past three decades; whereas only 23% of emboli were treated by embolectomy in the years 1937–1946 at Massachusetts General Hospital, 88% underwent surgical embolectomy in the most recent era reviewed, 1964–1980.[4]

The Fogarty catheter is a flexible, hollow catheter available in varying lumen sizes and lengths, with a soft distensible balloon at its tip. This balloon is connected to a port at its opposite end to which a syringe filled with either air or fluid may be connected to distend the balloon.

The catheter is inserted through a small arteriotomy and passed beyond the occlusion. It usually has no difficulty traversing soft clot of a fresh embolus. Once beyond the point of occlusion, the balloon is partially inflated and as the catheter is withdrawn the balloon forces the clot proximal to it and eventually out the arteriotomy site. The operator maintains uniform contact with the arterial wall during withdrawal, and any deformity of the arterial wall due to an arteriosclerotic plaque, etc, is mostly accommodated for by distortion of the balloon. However, it is mandatory that the same surgeon manipulate both the catheter and the syringe during withdrawal, so that changes in resistance can be appreciated and balloon volume altered appropriately. Inappropriate use of the catheter may lead to perforation, intimal dissection and thrombosis, avulsion of arteriosclerotic plaques, and a variety of other potentially troublesome technical complications.

Most lower-extremity emboli (approximately one half of all clinically recognizable arterial emboli) can be approached via a groin incision and limited arteriotomy in the common femoral artery. Local anesthesia may often be utilized, if advisable, making the technic particularly valuable in the unstable cardiac patient in whom any form of general or regional anesthesia may be hazardous. Such an approach has greatly simplified management of emboli to the aortic and iliac bifurcation which formerly required a major transperitoneal or retroperitoneal open operation. Popliteal emboli may often be approached initially via a femoral arteriotomy, but if clot is present beyond the popliteal bifurcation a direct surgical approach to the politeal artery is often preferable, allowing extraction selectively from each tibial vessel.

Upper-extremity emboli are usually readily managed by similar technics via a brachial arteriotomy. Again, embolectomy can most often be simply accomplished under local anesthesia.

Management of renal or visceral arterial emboli usually involve more extensive surgical technics beyond the scope of this discussion. Fortunately, they account for no more than approximately 10% of arterial embolic events.

Following clot removal, the surgeon should ensure the adequacy of peripheral circulation by restoration of palpable distal pulses. If not, intraoperative arteriography or one of several methods of intraoperative monitoring with a Doppler or pulse volume recorder should be utilized to document a satisfactory outcome.[9]

Continuation of anticoagulation postoperatively is important to prevent recurrence of emboli. Untreated, patients with an arterial embolus have approximately a 30% chance of recurrence. Recurrent emboli are often multiple, and carry an increasingly grave prognosis, with steep increase in mortality rates with each subsequent event. Darling et al[3] found that 102 of 224 patients who survived an initial embolic episode demonstrated a recurrence at some point in the follow-up period. Most recurrent emboli, especially in patients with atrial fibrillation, were noted to occur early. In Darling's report, the number of recurrences in the first two weeks equaled that seen in the subsequent two years. Two thirds of recurrences occurred within six months.

The vast majority of patients with recurrent emboli are inadequately anticoagulated, due to poor patient compliance or insufficient dosage, or untreated. This reemphasizes the importance of careful and full therapeutic anticoagulation of these patients postoperatively. We generally prefer to wait approximately 6 to 12 hours, however, to minimize the incidence of wound bleeding and hematoma formation which otherwise is unacceptably high. Heparin by continuous infusion may then be reinstituted, and warfarin sodium begun at the same time by mouth. Lifelong anticoagulation is generally indicated, unless the source of an embolus can be eradicated. Examples of such risk elimination of recurrent emboli would be resection of a proximal aneurysm which had been responsible for a peripheral arterial embolus, cardioversion of a patient previously in atrial fibrillation, etc. Since recurrent emboli are unusual after 12 to 14 weeks in patients with an acute myocardial infarction, uncomplicated by ventricular aneurysm or atrial fibrillation, it may be possible to stop anticoagulation after six months in these patients.

The value of anticoagulation in minimizing the chances of recurrent embolic events is illustrated by the experience reported by Green et al,[10] who found that the in-hospital embolic recurrence rate in anticoagulated patients was 9%, which compared very favorably to a 31% incidence of recurrence for those patients not anticoagulated.

If clearly advanced ischemia is present, or treatment has been unduly delayed, one must anticipate the systemic effects of revascularization of the severely ischemic limb.[7] Hyperkalemia, acidosis, hypotension, myoglobinuria, and possible renal failure are among the most common abnormalities encountered. In such settings, intravenous mannitol by bolus or drip infusion may often help reduce the incidence of renal failure and promote clearing of myoglobin by inducing brisk diuresis. Alkalinization of the urine is also probably advisable. Use of sodium bicarbonate to correct acidosis, aggressive treatment of hyperkalemia, and maintenance of cardiac output by optimal fluid therapy and use of cardiotonic drugs are all of importance.

The increased hazards of revascularization of the limb with advanced ischemia, leading to metabolic derangement and perhaps significantly increased mortality rates, had led some authorities such as Blaisdell et al to recommend avoidance of surgical embolectomy in many patients with acute arterial insufficiency.[11] Blaisdell et al reported a 7.5% mortality in patients with acute arterial ischemia who were treated with either high-dose heparin therapy alone, or immediate amputation. This compares favorably with their previous mortality experience for embolectomy or thrombectomy, and with the average mortality rates reported in previous studies in the surgical literature. These authors emphasized that the significant mortality commonly associated with embolectomy is related to the metabolic factors released from the ischemic limb with revascularization, which may precipitate or aggravate cardiac difficulties, acute pulmonary problems, etc. A lower mortality may be achieved by high-dose heparin therapy alone or primary amputation, although obviously at the expense of a lower rate of limb salvage. While we would agree that such metabolic derangements must be anticipated, and that surgery should be avoided in some particularly advanced cases, we continue to favor embolectomy in most instances. Careful clinical judgment remains paramount however.

RESULTS

Despite advances in surgical technics, anesthesia, and postoperative care, the mortality associated with arterial emboli remains formidable, in the range of 15% to 25% even in the most recently reported experience. Several factors contribute to this continuing significant mortality. First, most patients with arterial emboli are older, with frequently associated generalized arteriosclerosis. Co-existent cerebral, renal, and pulmonary disease is often present. Secondly, the majority of deaths are still due to the underlying cardiac problem that led to the embolus, such as those emboli associated with acute transmural myocardial infarction, severe cardiac decompensation, etc. Finally, metabolic complications or pulmonary emboli, most often occurring in advanced or neglected cases, account for most of the remaining deaths.

In addition, it is important to know whether mortality figures include cases of cerebral and visceral emboli. Both cerebral emboli, usually inaccessible surgically, and mesenteric/visceral emboli continue to be associated with high mortality, perhaps greater than 25% for the former and from 50% to 75% for the latter, even in experienced hands. In contrast, uncomplicated limb emboli without severe precipitating cardiac problems generally do well, with modern therapy now yielding low mortality rates approximating 5%.

Recurrent emboli are also a contributing factor. Mortality associated with recurrent embolic events rises steeply, almost doubling that associated with a primary event.

Using modern surgical technics of embolectomy, a high success rate in limb salvage is generally possible. Most current series report limb salvage in about 90% of cases. If the patient with a surgically accessible embolus without widespread associated occlusive disease is seen and treated early, almost uniform success should be obtained in restoring normal function to the limb that might otherwise be lost. Even if the above optimal conditions are not present, a high limb salvage rate with reasonable mortality should be obtainable. Operation carried out after 12 hours is associated with a significant reduction in the chances of full functional recovery of a limb in most series. In the most recent report of experience at the Massachusetts General Hospital, the survival rate was 81% and limb salvage rate 93% in patients with noncerebral emboli whose treatment began less than 12 hours after onset. In contrast, in patients in whom there was a delay of greater than 12 hours, only 69% survived and 78% achieved limb salvage.[4] Nonetheless, delayed embolectomy may often be feasible and beneficial in properly selected patients.[12] In our opinion, the only absolute contraindication to surgical intervention is an obviously nonviable limb or a patient totally unfit for any form of surgical procedure.

Arterial embolism remains a frequent and important clinical problem. However, prompt diagnosis, immediate use of intravenous heparin, and expeditious surgical treatment by an experienced surgeon should result in a gratifying salvage of life and limb in most instances.

REFERENCES

1. Warren R, Linton RR: The treatment of arterial embolism. *N Engl J Med* 1948;238:421–429.
2. Warren R, Linton RR, Scannell JG: Arterial embolism; Recent progress. *Ann Surg* 1954;140:311–317.
3. Darling RC, Austen WG, Linton RR: Arterial embolism. *Surg Gynecol Obstet* 1967;124:106–114.
4. Abbott WM, Maloney RD, McCabe CC, et al: Arterial embolism: A 44 year perspective. *Am J Surg* 1982;143:460–464.
5. Hight DW, Tilney NL, Couch NP: Changing clinical trends in patients with peripheral arterial emboli. *Surgery* 1976;79:172–176.
6. Hellerstein HK, Martin JW: Incidence of thromboembolic lesions accompanying myocardial infarction. *Am Heart J* 1947;33:443–452.
7. Haimovici H: Myopathic-nephrotic-metabolic syndrome associated with massive acute arterial occlusions. *J Cardiovasc Surg* 1973;14:589–600.
8. Fogarty T, Cranley JJ, Krause RJ, et al: A method for extraction of arterial emboli and thrombi. *Surg Gynecol Obstet* 1963;116:241–244.
9. O'Hara PJ, Brewster DC, Darling RC, et al: The value of intraoperative monitoring using pulse volume recording during peripheral vascular reconstructive operations. *Surg Gynecol Obstet* 1981; 152:275–281.
10. Green RM, DeWeese JA, Rob CG: Arterial embolectomy before and after the Fogarty catheter. *Surgery* 1975;77:24–33.
11. Blaisdell FW, Steele M, Allen RE: Management of acute lower extremity arterial ischemia due to embolism and thrombosis. *Surgery* 1978;84:822–834.
12. Jarrett F, Dacumos GC, Crummy AB, et al: Late appearance of arterial emboli: Diagnosis and management. *Surgery* 1979;86:898–906.

CHAPTER 24
Mitral Valve Prolapse Syndrome in the Elderly Population

Albert J. Kolibash
Charles F. Wooley

The diagnosis and classification of diseases are in constant evolution. The terms *mitral valve prolapse* and the *mitral valve prolapse syndrome* were introduced into the medical literature during the past two decades.[1-4]

Mitral valve prolapse (MVP), a common mitral valvular abnormality, refers to an anatomical entity. Alterations in the substance of the mitral valve include expansion of the cusp area and elongation of chordae, producing a "floppy" mitral valve.[5,6] The resultant changes in valve structure affect valve function, allowing prolapse of the floppy mitral valve into the left atrium in ventricular systole.[4,7] This is quite likely a hereditable disorder of connective tissue, since the specific histopathologic change of collagen dysruption or dysfunction has been observed in genetically inherited diseases such as the Marfan's syndrome[8] and the Ehlers-Danlos syndrome.[9] A recent study by Devereux et al provides additional confirmatory evidence of the autosomal dominant inheritance of this isolated, valvular abnormality.[10] Thus defined, anatomical mitral valve prolapse refers to a spectrum of valvular abnormalities which form the basis for a correspondingly broad spectrum of clinical manifestations ranging from (*a*) asymptomatic auscultatory[2,3] (isolated, nonejection systolic click), echocardiographic[11-13] or angiographic findings,[7,14] to (*b*) mild mitral regurgitation,[2,4,15] to (*c*) progressive and severe acute or chronic mitral regurgitation with resulting consequences.[2,6,16]

A precise definition of the mitral valve prolapse syndrome (MVPS) remains to be formulated, but in general the term refers to anthropometric[17] and symptomatic profiles[2,3] occurring in individuals with anatomical MVP. Broader concepts have been necessary to invoke a constitutional, neuroendocrine-cardiovascular process as a pathophysiologic explanation of the clinical symptoms and manifestations.[18,19] According to this schema, the heart and, in fact, the entire cardiovascular system, may be considered as target organs, and the anatomical MVP may be a marker of a hereditable phenomenon closely related to centrally mediated autonomic, adrenergic disorders.

The clinical expression of MVP and the MVPS changes with age.[10] Our long-term studies of MVPS patients include a group in the seventh to ninth decades.[20]

CLINICAL STUDY

Sixty-two patients 60 to 81 years of age were diagnosed as having the MVPS. Twenty-five patients were between the ages of 60 and 64 years, 22 patients between 65 and 69 years, 6 patients between 70 and 74 years, and 9 patients were 75 years old or more. These 62 patients, evaluated at University Hospital (Columbus, Ohio) because of debilitating cardiac symptoms (Table 24-1), included 20 patients (5 male, 15 female) with disabling chest pain, 16 patients (4 male, 12 female) with symptoms suggestive of arrhythmias, and 26 patients (16 male, 10 female) with symptoms of congestive heart failure and a murmur of mitral regurgitation.

The diagnosis of MVP was made on the basis of (1) classic auscultatory findings of midsystolic clicks and/or a late systolic or holosystolic murmur with typical postural variations,[2,3] (2) M-mode echocardiographic presence of mid- to

Table 24-1
Clinical Data of Elderly Patients with Mitral Valve Prolapse Syndrome

Clinical Presentation	No. Patients	Mean Duration of Symptoms/Murmur	Mean Age	Male	Female
Chest pain	20	4 yr	64	5	15
Palpitations/syncope	16	12 yr	66	4	12
Congestive heart failure/murmur	26	30 yr	68	16	10

late posterior systolic motion of the posterior mitral valve leaflet,[11-13] and (3) left ventricular angiographic demonstration of motion of the mitral valve leaflets into the left atrium beyond the mitral valve annulus in systole.[7,15] Each patient had at least two of these three clinical findings as the basis of the diagnosis of MVP. Fifty-two patients had adequate M-mode echocardiograms and 56 patients underwent cardiac catheterization which included coronary angiography. Significant coronary artery disease was defined as greater than 50% transluminal narrowing of at least one major coronary vessel.

Clinical Findings

The 62 patients in our study represented 3.7% of all patients 60 years of age or more who had a cardiac catheterization during the same time period in our catheterization laboratories. The presence of MVP as detected by each method used are shown in Figure 24-1. Auscultatory evidence of mitral valve prolapse was present in 61 patients. Thirty-five of the 36 patients with chest pain and symptoms of arrhythmia had abnormal cardiac physical findings. Thirty patients in this group had a midsystolic click and late systolic murmur whereas five patients demonstrated a midsystolic click only. All 26 patients with symptoms of congestive heart failure had a holosystolic murmur. Forty-five of the 52 patients with adequate M-mode echocardiograms had evidence of mitral valve prolapse. Angiographic mitral valve prolapse was seen in 55 of the 56 patients having left ventricular angiograms. Mitral regurgitation was present in 44 of these patients.

The various combinations by which the diagnosis of mitral valve prolapse was made in each of the patients are shown in Figure 24-2. MVP was evident by all three methods in 37 patients. The diagnosis was apparent in 17 patients by auscultation and left ventricular angiography, in seven patients by auscultation and echocardiography, and in the one remaining patient by echocardiography and angiography.

Patients with Chest Pain and Mitral Valve Prolapse

Twenty patients (5 male and 15 female) presented with disabling chest pain, only one of whom had previously sustained a documented

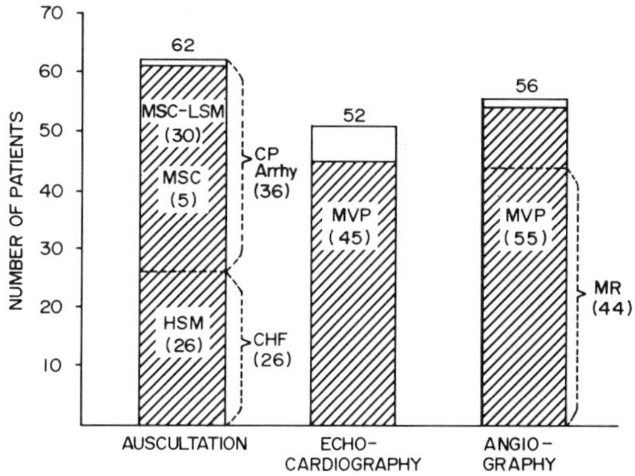

Figure 24-1 Clinical findings of various methods employed in diagnosing mitral valve prolapse. Hatched areas indicate numbers of patients with evidence of mitral valve prolapse with each method used. Arrhy = arrhythmias, CHF = congestive heart failure, CP = chest pain, HSM = holosystolic murmurs, MR = mitral regurgitation, MSC-LSM = midsystolic click-late systolic murmur, MVP = mitral valve prolapse.

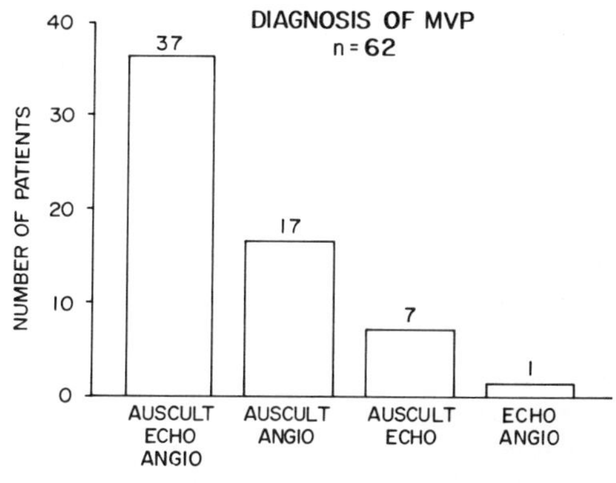

Figure 24-2 Various combinations of methods demonstrating MVP in individual patients.

myocardial infarction. The average duration of chest pain prior to admission was four years and the ages of these patients varied from 60 to 82 years with an average age of 64 (Table 24-1). The characteristics of the chest pain in most cases were suggestive of ischemic pain. Multiple noninvasive studies failed to differentiate those patients with coronary disease co-existent with MVP. The ECGs were abnormal in 16 of 20 patients. The abnormalities included 5 left anterior hemiblock, 4 subendocardial ischemia, 1 intraventricular conduction delay, 2 ventricular premature contractions (PVCs), 1 inferior myocardial infarction, and 3 nonspecific changes. These abnormalities occurred with equal frequency in patients with or without coronary artery disease.

Adequate treadmill stress tests using the Bruce protocol were obtained in seven patients. Four patients developed ST segment changes suggestive of ischemia (>1 mm ST depression 0.08 s after the J-point). Two of these patients had significant coronary artery disease and two had normal coronary anatomy on angiography.

Twenty-four-hour Holter monitoring performed in 10 patients revealed arrhythmias in all 10. These rhythm disturbances were of atrial origin in 3 (atrial fibrillation in 2 and atrial premature contractions [PACs] in 1) and of ventricular origin in 7 (PVCs in 6 and ventricular tachycardia in 1). The incidence and types of arrhythmias were similar in patients with and without coronary artery disease.

The echocardiogram demonstrated mitral valve prolapse in 14 of the 17 patients in whom adequate studies were obtained. Five of the 6 patients had coronary artery disease and 9 of the 11 had normal coronary arteries. The disabling chest pain, suggestive of ischemia, led to cardiac catheterization and coronary angiography in all 20 patients.

The data are shown in Table 24-2. The 7 patients with significant coronary artery disease included 1 with single vessel disease, 4 with double vessel disease, and 2 with triple vessel disease. Left ventricular ejection fraction and left ventricular end-diastolic volume were normal in all patients. Five patients with coronary artery disease and seven patients with normal coronary arteries had abnormally elevated postangiographic left ventricular end diastolic pressures. Angiographic mitral valve prolapse was seen in all 7 patients with coronary disease and 12 of 13 patients without coronary disease. Figure 24-3 is an angiographic demonstration of a prolapsing mitral valve in a patient with chest pain and normal coronary anatomy. Thus, in this elderly group of patients with disabling chest pain and MVP, left ventricular function remained well preserved and coronary artery disease, when present, had no influence on hemodynamics or the presence of angiographic MVP.

Patients with Arrhythmias and Mitral Valve Prolapse

Sixteen patients (4 male, 12 female) 60 to 90 years of age (mean age 66 years) with symptoms of arrhythmias complained primarily of palpitations and syncope. The average duration of symptoms prior to admission was 12 years (Table 24-1). Two patients with syncope had prehospital "sudden death" and required cardiopulmonary resuscitation. Two complained of visual blurring, had visual field defects suggesting systemic embolization, and did not have evidence of cerebral vascular disease. None of the patients in this group had a history of myocardial infarction, although two did complain of chest pain. Eleven of the 13 adequate echocardiograms in this group demonstrated mitral valve prolapse.

Table 24-2
Cardiac Catheterization Data in Elderly Patients with Mitral Valve Prolapse Syndrome

Patient Groups (No.)	Ejection Fraction	LVEDV (cc/m^2)	Abnormal Postangiography LVEDP (No. Patients)	Angiography MVP/MR
Chest Pain (20)	.69	70	12	19
CAD (7)	.70	72	5	7
No CAD (13)	.69	67	7	12
Arrhythmias (10)	.64	70	5	10
Mitral Regurgitation (26)	.67	119	12	26
MVR (21)	.68	125	9	21
No MVR (5)	.63	90	3	5

CAD = coronary artery disease; LVEDP = left ventricular end-diastolic pressure; LVEDV = left ventricular end-diastolic volume; MVP = mitral valve prolapse; MVR = mitral valve replacement; MR = mitral regurgitation.

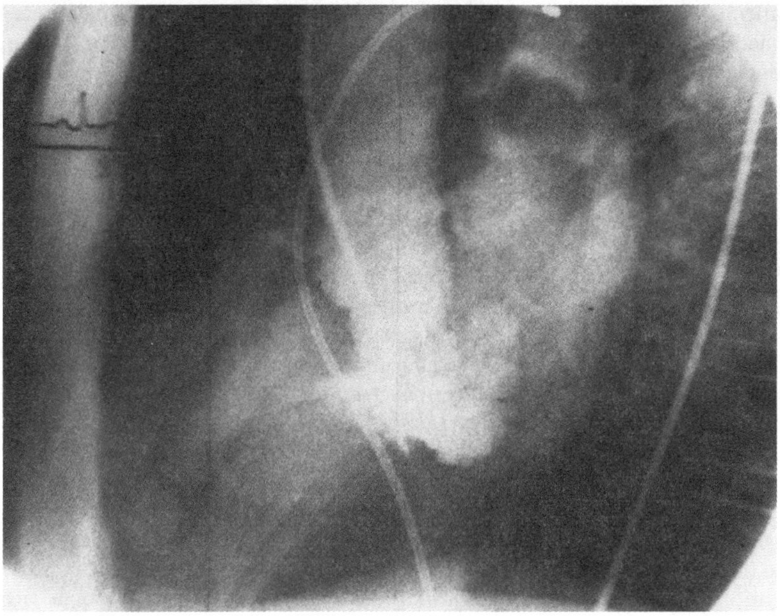

Figure 24-3 Cineangiographic demonstration of mitral valve prolapse without mitral regurgitation in a patient with chest pain and normal coronary arteries (left lateral projection).

Each patient was demonstrated to have significant cardiac arrhythmias as a basis for the clinical symptoms. Diagnostic methods and types of arrhythmias are shown in Figure 24-4. Fifteen of the 16 resting ECGs demonstrated a vast spectrum of abnormalities including atrial flutter, ventricular arrhythmias, intraventricular conduction delays, and nonspecific ST and T wave changes. The ventricular arrhythmias consisted of frequent PVCs (> 10/min), ventricular bigeminy, and ventricular tachycardia.

Twenty-four-hour Holter ambulatory ECG monitoring in 11 patients further defined the multiple rhythm disorders. Supraventricular tachyarrhythmias in three patients included paroxysmal atrial fibrillation, paroxysmal atrial tachycardia, and frequent PACs. Two patients had frequent PVCs only. Six patients showed rhythm disorders of both atrial and ventricular origin with combinations of frequent PVCs, ventricular bigeminy, and atrial tachycardia.

Electrophysiologic studies performed in 4 patients included 1 normal study and 3 patients with significant rhythm disorders. These included the development of atrial flutter with rapid atrial stimulation, supraventricular and ventricular tachycardia following provocative atrial and ventricular stimulation, and one patient with evidence of sick sinus syndrome.

Ten patients in this group underwent cardiac catheterization including coronary angiography (Table 24-2) and angiographic mitral valve prolapse was seen in all 10. All patients had normal ejection fractions and left ventricular end-diastolic volumes. The postangiographic left ventricular end-diastolic pressures were elevated in five patients, and two patients had single vessel coronary artery disease.

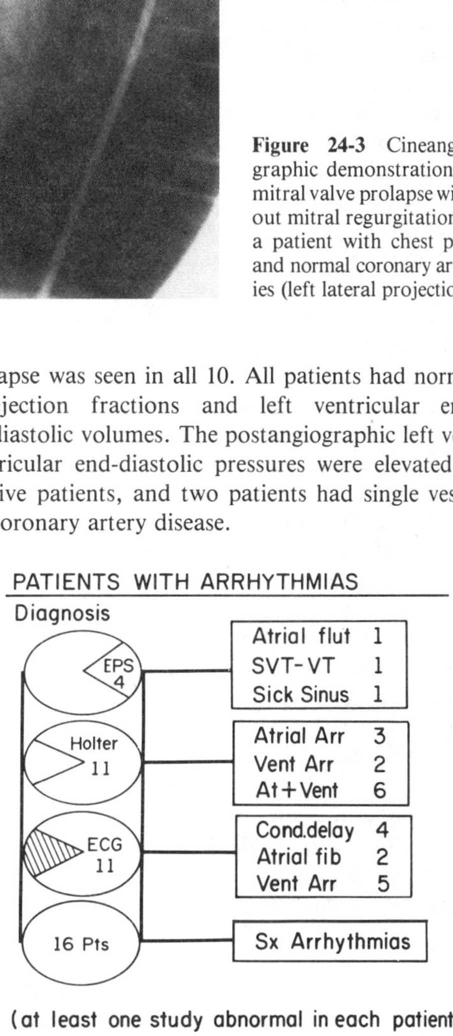

Figure 24-4 Methods used in diagnosing arrhythmias in 16 patients with palpitations and syncope and the specific types of arrhythmias detected. Arryh = arrhythmias, At = atrial, Atrial fib = atrial fibrillation, Atrial flut = atrial flutter, cond. delay = intraventricular conduction delay, Holter = Holter monitoring, ECG = electrocardiogram, EPS = electrophysiologic study, Pts = patients, SVT = supraventricular tachycardia, SX = symptoms, Vent = ventricular, VT = ventricular tachycardia.

This group of elderly patients with MVP and symptoms of arrhythmias had clinically defined significant rhythm disturbances which explained their symptoms. Left ventricular hemodynamics were normal and the incidence of significant coronary artery disease was low, so that neither left ventricular dysfunction nor coronary artery disease appeared to be a major factor in the pathogenesis of the arrhythmias.

Patients with Congestive Heart Failure, Heart Murmurs, Mitral Regurgitation, and Mitral Valve Prolapse

Twenty-six patients (16 male, 10 female) had symptoms of congestive heart failure and the murmur of mitral regurgitation. The mean age of these patients was 68 with a range of 60 to 81 years (Table 24-1). The average duration of a known heart murmur was 30 years. Twelve patients had known of a heart murmur prior to the age of 30 and seven others before the age of 60.

This group of patients was more severely ill than the patients with chest pain and arrhythmias. Twenty had radiographic left ventricular enlargement. Twenty-five had abnormal resting ECGs (atrial fibrillation in 13, left ventricular hypertrophy in 5). MVP was present on the echocardiogram in 20 patients, 5 of whom also had evidence of a flail mitral valve leaflet.

Cardiac catheterization data are presented in Table 24-2. Although the left ventricular volumes were increased, averaging 119 cc/mm^2, left ventricular function remained well-preserved with the average ejection fraction being 67%. Twelve patients had abnormally elevated postangiographic left ventricular end-diastolic pressures. The mean pulmonary capillary wedge pressure was 18 mmHg with an average V wave amplitude of 34 mmHg. Angiographic MVP and/or mitral regurgitation was present in all 26 patients.

Right ventricular angiography was performed in 12 patients, 6 of whom were shown to have tricuspid valve prolapse. Significant coronary artery disease was present in 4 patients, none of whom had either a totally occluded vessel or evidence of a myocardial infarction.

Twenty-one patients with progressive clinical deterioration had mitral valve surgery. The hemodynamic data from these patients are shown in Table 24-2. These patients tended to have the largest left ventricular volumes, the average being 125 cc/mm^2. However, the left ventricular ejection fraction was 68%. The postangiographic left ventricular end diastolic pressures were abnormally elevated in nine patients. The mean pulmonary capillary wedge pressure was 19 mmHg with an average V wave amplitude of 38 mmHg. Angiographic MVP and severe mitral regurgitation were seen in all 21 patients. Figure 24-5 is an angiographic example of a severely regurgitant prolapsing mitral valve in a patient who presented with congestive heart failure and the murmur of mitral regurgitation.

Two of the 21 surgical patients died in the perioperative period. The remaining 19 patients were discharged in an improved symptomatic state, all being either New York Heart Association functional classes I or II. The 19 surgically excised valves were described as enlarged and floppy with redundancy of the mitral valve leaflets and had an average mitral valve diameter of 4.5 cm. Histologically, all valves showed myxomatous degeneration and disarray of collagen throughout the valve leaflets.

These older patients with MVPS, congestive heart failure, and mitral regurgitation tended to be more ill, had left ventricular enlargement, and frequent ECG abnormalities. Despite left ventricular enlargement the left ventricular ejection fraction remained normal and the presence of significant coronary artery disease was low. Mitral regurgitation was a progressive lesion in this group and led to surgery, which was successful in 19 of 21 patients.

DISCUSSION

Pathologic Findings at Necropsy

Pomerance has described the changes present in the aging heart.[21] Mucoid degeneration, one of the several changes noted in the mitral valve, occurred with varying degrees of severity from localized ballooning to gross ectasia with voluminous cusps associated with gross mitral incompetence. The incidence of these changes increased to age 64 years in males and 74 years in females. Pomerance suggested that these findings were likely an expression of a disease rather than an involutional process, based on their extent and the fact that such changes were described in younger patients. Extensive ballooning deformities of the mitral valve accounted for 5% of systolic murmurs in 173 patients above the age of 70 years.[22]

Ballooning deformities of the mitral valve comprised 1% of all autopsies in another study by Pomerance;[23] 30 patients were 51 to 78 years of age with a mean age of 73.6 years. Their mitral

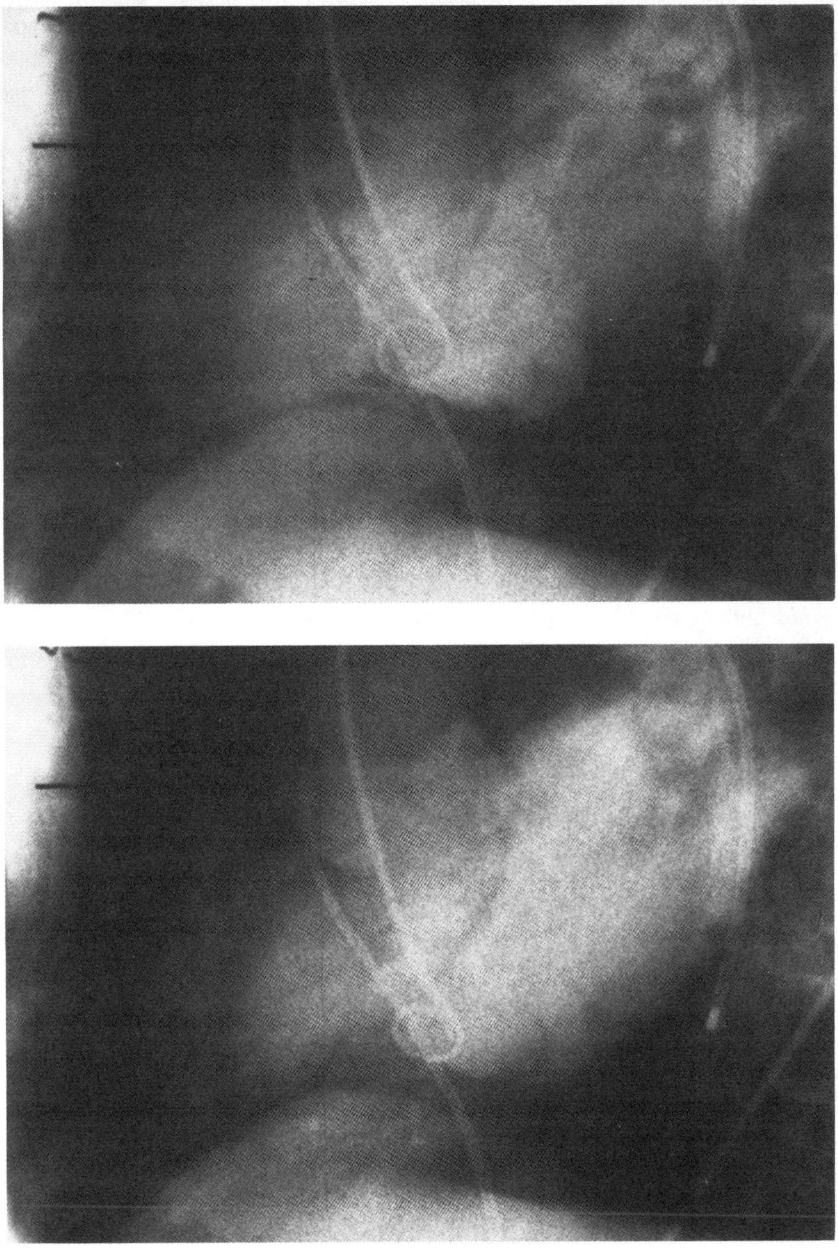

A

B

Figure 24-5 Cineangiographic views in lateral projections showing mitral valve prolapse (A) in early phase of contrast injection and mitral valve prolapse with severe mitral regurgitation during later phase of contrast injection (B). Patient had congestive heart failure and required mitral valve surgery. Ruptured chordae were found at the time of mitral valve replacement.

valves were voluminous, thickened, and involved with myxomatous changes. Significantly, 24 patients had a documented cardiac murmur, some at least 25 years prior to death.

Davies et al reported an important pathologic study with clinical relevance in which they described the nature and occurrence of floppy mitral valves in 44 surgically excised mitral valves, in 1984 necropsy studies, and 13 mitral valves obtained from forensic materials.[5] Mitral valves in the necropsy study were graded on a scale of 0 to 4 based upon the degree of cusp expansion, chordal elongation, the presence or absence of chordal rupture, and chordal fusion. The most severely involved valves (grade 2 or higher) were described as having expansion of cusp area and elongated chordae, some of which were ruptured and others of which were fused.

Minor degrees of floppy mitral valves (grade 1) were common but not clinically significant. On the other hand, 90 hearts had floppy mitral valves of significant degrees (grades 2 to 4). Grade 2 valves were usually associated with auscultatory findings and contributed to heart failure in some cases. Significantly, the grade 3 and 4 floppy valves were attributed as direct causes of death because of "bacterial endocarditis and/or mitral regurgitation."

The overall incidence of severely floppy valves (grades 2 to 4) was 3.9% in males and 5.2% in females, most of whom were above the age of 60. The frequency of these severely floppy mitral valves increased with age to a maximum of 5.5% in males in the eighth decade and 10% in females above 90 years. This incidence, higher than that reported by Pomerance who described only valves with the most extensive degrees of mucoid degeneration, included floppy mitral valves with less extensive but nevertheless significant degrees of abnormalities (grades 2 to 4). Interestingly, the incidence in the series of Davies et al (3.7% in males, 5.2% in females) is similar to the incidence of MVP in older patients coming to cardiac catheterization in our institution (3.7% overall).

Finally, it is noteworthy that only 15% of patients with grade 1 floppy mitral valves had a preceding history of a documented heart murmur whereas 80% of patients with severely floppy valves had a murmur documented in the past. In some instances the murmur had been recorded 48 years prior to death. A history of a heart murmur was more likely to be associated with more severe floppy valves as was a cardiac cause of death.

In summary, Pomerance and Davies et al have documented the presence of floppy mitral valves in their necropsy series. Severely floppy mitral valves with extensive mucoid degeneration were seen with increasing frequency with aging, and were often attributed as the direct cause of death in these patients.

Pathologic Findings in Surgically Excised "Myxomatous" Mitral Valves—Clinical Correlations

The studies by Pomerance[21–23] and by Davies[5] emphasized the pathologic findings in necropsy specimens. Surgically excised floppy mitral valves provide pertinent clinical information from a living population.

The gross morphologic and histologic characteristics of surgically excised prolapsing "myxomatous" mitral valves from 12 patients with severe mitral regurgitation were compared to 13 mitral valves from normal control individuals.[23a] Gross morphology (increased surface area, increased diameter, and decreased density) and histologic characteristics (collagen dissolution with myxomatous degeneration) allowed clear separation between control valves and "myxomatous" mitral valves that produced severe mitral regurgitation. Collagen dissolution in the pars fibrosa and chordae was present only in the "myxomatous" mitral valves which suggested the primacy of collagen dissolution in mitral valves of patients with severe mitral regurgitation complicating the MVPS. These findings led us to consider the basic process to be a disorder of collagen synthesis, content, or organization, ie, a "dyscollagenosis."

Studies support the theory that collagen dissolution involving the chordae and pars fibrosa, the main support structures of the mitral valve, may well be the basic pathologic process of MVP.

The increasing number of older patients undergoing mitral valve surgery for severe mitral regurgitation provides a link between the previously discussed pathology studies and clinical studies of the MVPS. Table 24-3 cites nine reports related to elderly patients undergoing mitral valve surgery because of progressive mitral regurgitation.[2,5,6,20,24–28] In every instance the mitral valves were described as being grossly enlarged and floppy. The histologic studies of these valves all showed extensive myxomatous changes. A high incidence of chordal rupture was also observed: 31/44 (70%) in Davies' series[5] and 41/66 (62%) in Salomon's study.[27]

Perhaps of greater significance is the fact that the vast majority of these patients were adults, many in their 50s or older. A history of a known heart murmur was also present in many of these patients. The known duration of a heart murmur varied greatly: from one to over 50 years. The presence of these previously described murmurs in asymptomatic patients who then developed symptoms of congestive heart failure secondary to worsening mitral regurgitation strongly implies a progressive process. More importantly, the fact that all surgically excised mitral valves showed extensive myxomatous changes suggests these patients may have had the MVPS.

Clinical Studies

The data presented in our study of 62 patients above the age of 60 years suggest that the MVPS is a distinct clinical entity in the elderly population.[20] Two other studies utilizing auscultatory findings and echocardiography considered the MVPS in older patients. Tresch et al[28] reported on 40 patients above the age of 60 including 29 symptomatic patients: ten patients with congestive heart failure, five of whom required mitral valve surgery. Higgins et al[29] studied 40 men 50 years old or more, 25 of whom were symptomatic. Twenty-one patients had radiographic cardiomegaly and 14 patients had atrial fibrillation. Thus, several clinical studies support the fact that many elderly patients have MVP and the MVPS.

Clinical Findings in Elderly vs Young Population

Table 24-4 lists six clinical studies of the MVPS: three describe clinical findings in younger patients whose mean ages are approximately 40 years and three describe similar findings in older patients whose mean ages are 66 years. These studies indicate that both younger and older individuals with the MVPS frequently present with symptoms of chest pain or arrhythmias in the presence of a nonejection click and/or systolic murmur. A total of 142 patients are included in three studies of elderly patients with the MVPS (Table 24-4).[20,28,29] Abnormal auscultatory events were present in 127 patients (89%), chest pain in 35 patients (25%), and symptoms of arrhythmias in 45 patients (32%). Females predominated in both the young and older populations with chest pain and symptoms of arrhythmias. Thus, abnormal auscultatory events, chest pain, and symptoms of arrhythmias occur frequently in both younger and older patients with the MVPS.

Chest Pain

The co-existence of coronary artery disease and MVP has been described.[30] The etiology of chest pain in the MVPS is not known[31] and one might naturally consider coronary artery disease to be a common cause of chest pain in the elderly population. However, this did not appear to be the case in the majority of our patients since 13 elderly patients with MVP and chest pain had normal coronary arteries.

The hemodynamic findings including the ejection fraction and left ventricular end-diastolic volume were normal in the MVP–chest pain patients with or without co-existent coronary

Table 24-3
Patients with Mitral Valve Prolapse Syndrome, Severe Mitral Regurgitation, Mitral Valve Replacement

Study	No. Patients	Ages (Mean)	Known Murmur Years (Mean)
Jerasaty[2]	5	26,44,59,69,56 (51)	–
Davies et al[5]	44	32–69 (51.4)	1–48
Bittar and Sosa[6]	3	57,53,43 (51)	5–24 (15)
Kolibash et al[20]	21	60–82 (68)	1–57 (30)
Read et al[24]	5	15,17,23,35,48 (27.5)	– (10)
Davis et al[25]	5	52,65,60,53,44 (55)	1–25 (9)
Rippe et al[26]	2	57,57 (57)	–
Salomon et al[27]	66	11–80 (58)	– (14)
Tresch[28]	4	62,63,66,67 (64.5)	– (–)

Table 24-4
Clinical Findings in Younger and Elderly Patients with Mitral Valve Prolapse Syndrome

Study	No. Patients	Ages (Mean)	Abnormal Cardiac Examination	Chest Pain	Symptoms of Arrhythmias
Jerasaty[2]	100	2–84 (41)	88	61	46
Fontana et al[3]	30	14–74	30	8	19
Hancock and Cohn[40]	40	8–73 (40)	40	14	19
Tresch et al[28]	40	61–81 (67)	39	9	14
Higgins et al[29]	40	50–90 (66)	27	6	15
Kolibash et al[20]	62	60–81 (67)	61	20	16

disease. Thus, in the elderly patient with the MVPS and chest pain, obstructive coronary disease was not usually the cause of the chest pain and, if present, coronary angiography was required to detect co-existing coronary artery disease.

Arrhythmias

The presence or co-existence of arrhythmias in the MVPS is well recognized and may contribute to significant morbidity.[32,33] The multiple types of arrhythmias include rhythm disturbances of both supraventricular and ventricular origin. An excellent review of arrhythmias in the MVPS by Swartz et al[33] included 589 patients from multiple studies with an average age of 37.8 years and a range from 2 to 84 years. The most common arrhythmias were atrial premature contractions (54.8% of patients) and ventricular premature contractions (44.9% of patients). More serious arrhythmias such as supraventricular tachycardia and ventricular tachycardia occurred in 6.1% and 6.3% respectively. Eight patients (1.4%) died suddenly.

The arrhythmias noted in our elderly patients with the MVPS[20] were very similar to those described by Swartz et al.[33] Atrial and ventricular premature contractions occurred quite frequently. Supraventricular and ventricular tachycardias also occurred but with less frequency; two of our patients were successfully resuscitated during prehospital episodes of "sudden death."

The etiology of arrhythmias in the MVPS is unknown. Proposed hypotheses include abnormal stress on the mitral valve leaflets as they balloon into the left atrium during systole,[34] a local cardiac or systemic role for catecholamines,[32] a primary myocardial disorder,[35] anomalous conduction pathways,[36] or a combination of these factors.

A reasonable explanation for the arrhythmias in the older patients with the MVPS might be coronary artery disease. Although abnormalities of the circumflex coronary artery in younger patients had been proposed by Gentzler et al,[37] subsequent studies failed to demonstrate consistent abnormalities of the circumflex artery.[2] Similarly, coronary artery disease was not responsible for the arrhythmias seen in the elderly patients with the MVPS reported in our study. Ten of our 16 patients with arrhythmias had coronary angiography and only two had significant coronary artery disease, both with single vessel disease. None of the MVPS patients with significant arrhythmias had a history of myocardial infarction, nor were ventricular contraction abnormalities detected. The six patients who did not undergo coronary angiography had no angina and no history of myocardial infarction.

Two of the 16 patients in our study with documented arrhythmias had visual field defects and their presentations were quite suggestive of systemic embolization. There appears to be an association between MVP and systemic emboli, but the pathogenesis remains to be explained.[38,39] Both of our patients with apparent systemic emboli had a history of atrial fibrillation which might have played a contributing role, but neither patient had a history or evidence of cerebral vascular disease.

Elderly patients with the MVPS may present with cardiac arrhythmias with incidence and types of arrhythmias similar to those noted in younger MVPS patients. Significant morbidity may be associated with these arrhythmias such as sudden death and systemic embolization. Coronary artery disease did not play a major contributing role in this subset of elderly MVPS patients.

Patients with Mitral Regurgitation and Congestive Heart Failure

The clinical hallmark of mitral valve prolapse is the presence of a nonejection click and late systolic murmur. These late systolic murmurs have been associated with mitral regurgitation, but in the vast majority of studies the degree of mitral regurgitation is usually minimal or mild and of little hemodynamic significance.[2,4,15] Severe mitral regurgitation is not a common clinical problem in younger patients with the MVPS but when present has been the cause of holosystolic murmurs and symptoms of congestive heart failure.[2]

The largest series of patients requiring mitral valve surgery for severe mitral regurgitation was reported by Salomon et al and included 66 patients.[27] The youngest patient in this group was 11 years of age. However, the mean age of Salomon's patients was 58 years.

These clinical studies demonstrate that progressive mitral regurgitation with congestive heart failure does exist in the younger MVP population, but is not a significant problem. However, it does appear to be a significant problem in the elderly patient. Ten of 40 patients (25%) in the series of Tresch et al had congestive heart failure, 4 of whom had mitral valve replacement.[28] Twenty-six of the 62 patients in our study had symptoms of congestive heart failure attributed to mitral regurgitation.[20] The mitral regurgitation in 21 of these patients had progressed to such an extent that mitral valve surgery was performed. Whether or not these older patients with severe mitral regurgitation who require mitral valve surgery represent the natural progression of a subset of younger MVP patients with mild mitral regurgitation associated with midsystolic clicks and late systolic murmurs is unknown. However, the previous existence of a heart murmur in many of these patients and the broadening of our understanding of the pathologic findings of floppy or "myxomatous" valves strongly suggest that the severe mitral regurgitation in these older patients is the end result of a lifelong progressive process.

Sixty-two percent (16/26) of our patients with severe mitral regurgitation and congestive heart failure were male.[20] Davies also reported a preponderance of males in his surgical series (31/44 or 70%). This preponderance of males with severe mitral regurgitation is in contrast to the female predominance seen in our patients with chest pain and arrhythmias and in the clinical studies of younger patients with MVP and the MVPS.[2]

Clinically, the elderly MVP patients with mitral regurgitation and congestive heart failure had a high incidence of atrial fibrillation,[20] a finding also described in several other studies involving patients with mitral valve prolapse and severe mitral regurgitation.[29] Tricuspid valve prolapse was also documented in six of our patients undergoing mitral valve surgery,[20] none of whom required tricuspid valve replacement. Tricuspid valve prolapse has been previously documented in younger patients with mitral valve prolapse.[26]

Coronary artery disease did not play a significant role in the etiology of mitral regurgitation in these older patients.[20] Although four patients had significant obstructive lesions of the coronary arteries, none had angina, a history of myocardial infarction, or segmental contraction abnormalities on the left ventricular angiogram. The remaining 22 patients had normal coronary arteriograms.

Thus, progressive mitral regurgitation leading to severe congestive heart failure requiring mitral valve surgery was a significant problem in the older patients with the MVPS. A large number of these patients had a heart murmur noted many years previously, which suggests a progressive process. Atrial fibrillation was common and associated abnormalities of the tricuspid valve were also noted. Coronary artery disease was not a significant factor in the etiology or pathogenesis of the mitral regurgitation in this patient subset.

Implications of MVPS

The natural history of the MVPS has not been well defined. The few published studies have suggested that mitral valve prolapse is a benign entity and that the majority of patients with MVP or the MVPS have a good prognosis. These conclusions do not seem warranted until multiple, long-term, studies are performed over the life span of the patients. It is apparent, even in these published studies, that certain patients with MVPS may be at risk to develop complications. These include endocarditis, chordal rupture, stroke, systemic embolism, heart failure, and progressive mitral insufficiency.

SUMMARY

The MVPS has been defined as a distinct clinical entity in patients above the age of 60 years and should be considered as a cause of symptomatic heart disease in the elderly population. Elderly patients with the MVPS presented in a clinically predictable manner with disabling chest pain, symptomatic arrhythmias, sudden death, systemic embolization, and progressive mitral regurgitation with severe congestive heart failure which usually required medical therapy and/or mitral valve surgery.

The clinical presentation of these patients was similar to younger patients with the MVPS in that the incidence of chest pain and symptomatic arrhythmias was high. The types of arrhythmias were also similar in the younger and older patients with the MVPS. However, progressive mitral regurgitation with severe congestive heart failure requiring mitral valve surgery was a more significant problem in the older population. Mitral valve surgery, when necessary, was performed with an acceptable risk and with good clinical results.

Although significant coronary artery disease was present in the elderly patients with the MVPS, coronary disease was not a major factor with respect to the etiology of chest pain, arrhythmias, or the pathogenesis of severe mitral regurgitation. The elderly female patients frequently experienced chest pain and arrhythmias, while progressive mitral regurgitation occurred more frequently in the males.

The present study was not a natural history study, but rather a study which identified the clinical characteristics of a group of elderly patients with MVP and the MVPS. While certain of the clinical characteristics in the elderly were similar to those seen in younger patients with the

MVPS, certain age-related differences were identified. These observations suggest that certain younger patients with MVP and the MVPS are at risk to develop complications later in life. Further long-term studies will be necessary to determine which patients are at risk.

ACKNOWLEDGMENT

The authors thank Miss Tami West for her time and secretarial efforts toward the preparation of this chapter.

REFERENCES

1. Barlow JB, Bosman CK: Aneurysmal protrusion of the posterior leaflet of the mitral valve. *Am Heart J* 1966;71:166-178.
2. Jerasaty RM: Mitral valve prolapse-click syndrome. *Prog Cardiovasc Dis* 1973;15:623-651.
3. Fontana ME, Pence HL, Leighton RF, et al: The varying clinical spectrum of the systolic click-late systolic murmur syndrome: A postural auscultatory phenomenon. *Circulation* 1970;41:807-816.
4. Fontana ME, Wooley CF, Leighton RF, et al: Postural changes in left ventricular and mitral valvular dynamics in the systolic click—Late systolic murmur syndrome. *Circulation* 1975; 51:165-173.
5. Davies MJ, Moore BP, Braimbridge MV: The floppy mitral valve: Study of incidence, pathology, and complications in surgical, necropsy, and forensic material. *Br Heart J* 1978;40:468-481.
6. Bittar N, Sosa JA: The billowing mitral valve leaflet: Report on fourteen patients. *Circulation* 1968;38:763-770.
7. Jerasaty RM: Ballooning of the mitral valve leaflets: Angiographic study of 24 patients. *Radiology* 1971;100:45-52.
8. Wagenvoort CA, Newfield HN, Edward JE: Cardiovascular system in Marfan's syndrome and in idiopathic dilatation of the ascending aorta. *Am J Cardiol* 1962;9:496-507.
9. Leier CV, Call T, Fulkerson PK, et al: The spectrum of cardiac defects n the Ehlers-Danlos syndrome. Types I and III. *Ann Intern Med* 1980; 92:171-178.
10. Devereux RB, Brown WT, Kramer-Fox R, et al: Inheritance of mitral valve prolapse: Effect of age and sex on gene expression. *Ann Intern Med* 1982; 97:826-832.
11. Popp RL, Brown OR, Silverman JF, et al: Echocardiographic abnormalities in the mitral valve prolapse syndrome. *Circulation* 1974;49:428-433.
12. DeMaria AN, King JF, Bogren HG, et al: The variable spectrum of echocardiographic manifestations of the mitral valve prolapse syndrome. *Circulation* 1974;50:33-41.
13. Kerber RE, Isaeff DM, Hancock EW: Echocardiographic patterns in patients with the syndrome of systolic click and late systolic murmur. *N Engl J Med* 1971;284:691-693.
14. Smith ER, Fraser DB, Purdy JW, et al: Angiographic diagnosis of mitral valve prolapse: Correlation with echocardiography. *Am J Cardiol* 1977; 40:165-170.
15. Ranganathan N, Silver MD, Robinson TI, et al: Idiopathic prolapsed mitral leaflet syndrome: Angiographic-clinical correlations. *Circulation* 1976; 54:707-716.
16. Fernex M, Fernex C: La dégénérescence mucoide des valvules mitrales: Ses répercussions fonctionnelles. *Helv Med Acta* 1958;25:694-705.
17. Bon Tempo CP, Ronan JA, de Leon AC Jr, et al: Radiographic appearance of the thorax in systolic click-late systolic murmur syndrome. *Am J Cardiol* 1975;36:27-31.
18. Gaffney FA, Karlsson ES, Campbell W, et al: Autonomic dysfunction in women with mitral valve prolapse syndrome. *Circulation* 1979;59:894-901.
19. Coghlan HC, Phares P, Cowley M, et al: Dysautonomia in mitral valve prolapse. *Am J Med* 1979; 67:236-244.
20. Kolibash AJ, Bush CA, Fontana ME, et al: Mitral valve prolapse syndrome; Analysis of 62 patients aged 60 years and older. *Am J Cardiol* 1983;52: 534-539.
21. Pomerance A: Ageing changes in human heart valves. *Br Heart J* 1967;29:222-231.
22. Pomerance A: Cardiac pathology and systolic murmurs in the elderly. *Br Heart J* 1968;30:687-689.
23. Pomerance A: Ballooning deformity (mucoid degeneration) of atrioventricular valves. *Br Heart J* 1969;31:343-351.

23a. King BD, Clark MA, Baba N, et al: "Myxomatous" mitral valves: Collagen dissolution as the primary defect. *Circulation* 1982;66:288-296.

24. Read RC, Thal AP, Wendt VE: Symptomatic valvular myxomatous transformation (the floppy valve syndrome): A possible forme fruste of the Marfan syndrome. *Circulation* 1965;32:897-910.
25. Davis RH, Schuster B, Knoebel SB, et al: Myxomatous degeneration of the mitral valve. *Am J Cardiol* 1971;28:449-455.
26. Rippe JM, Angoff G, Sloss LJ, et al: Multiple floppy valves: An echocardiographic syndrome. *Am J Med* 1979;66:817-824.
27. Salomon NW, Stinson EB, Griepp RB, et al: Surgical treatment of degenerative mitral regurgitation. *Am J Cardiol* 1976;38:463-468.
28. Tresch DD, Siegel R, Keelan MH, et al: Mitral valve prolapse in the elderly. *J Am Geriatr Soc* 1979;27:421-424.
29. Higgins CB, Reinke RT, Gosink BB, et al: The significance of mitral valve prolapse in middle-aged and elderly men. *Am Heart J* 1976;91:292-296.
30. Steelman RB, White RS, Hill JC, et al: Midsystolic clicks in arteriosclerotic heart disease: A new facet in the clinical syndrome of papillary muscle dysfunction. *Circulation* 1971;44:503-514.
31. Boudoulas H, Wooley CF: Chest pain associated with mitral valve prolapse. *Chest Pain* 1979;5:1-8.
32. Winkle RA, Lopes MG, Fitzgerald JW, et al: Arrhythmias in patients with mitral valve prolapse. *Circulation* 1975;52:73-81.
33. Swartz MH, Teichholz LE, Donoso E: Mitral valve prolapse: A review of associated arrhythmias. *Am J Med* 1977;62:377-389.
34. Criley JM, Zeilenga CW, Morgan MT: Mitral dysfunction: A possible cause of arrhythmias in the

prolapsing mitral leaflet syndrome. *Trans Am Clin Climatol Assoc* 1973;85:44–53.
35. Gulotta SD, Gulco L, Padmanabhan V, et al: The syndrome of systolic click, murmur, and mitral valve prolapse-A cardiomyopathy. *Circulation* 1974;49:717–728.
36. Gallagher JJ, Gilbert M, Swenson RH, et al: Wolff-Parkinson-White syndrome. The problem, evaluation, and surgical correction. *Circulation* 1975;51: 767–785.
37. Gentzler RD, Gault JH, Liedtke AJ, et al: Congenital absence of the left circumflex coronary artery in the systolic click syndrome. *Circulation* 1975;52:490–496.
38. Steele P, Weily H, Rainwater J, et al: Platelet survival time and thromboembolism in patients with mitral valve prolapse. *Circulation* 1979;60:43–45.
39. Cheitlin MD: Thromboembolic studies in the patient with the prolapsed mitral valve: Has Salome dropped another veil, editorial. *Circulation* 1979; 60:46–47.
40. Hancock EW, Cohn K: The syndrome associated with late systolic click midsystolic murmur. *Am J Med* 1966;41:183–196.

CHAPTER 25
Hypertrophic Cardiomyopathy in the Elderly

William J. McKenna
Angelika Kleinebenne

Early reports of hypertrophic cardiomyopathy described young and middle-aged patients with a high incidence of sudden death.[1-3] Recent reports, however, indicate that hypertrophic cardiomyopathy is not uncommon in the elderly.[4-12] Are these patients lifelong survivors with a benign form of the condition? Or did their disease develop in middle or old age or indeed do they have the same form of hypertrophic cardiomyopathy which has been associated with a high risk of sudden death?[3] We will examine these questions with a particular emphasis on diagnosis and management of elderly patients with hypertrophic cardiomyopathy.

HISTORICAL BACKGROUND

What is hypertrophic cardiomyopathy? While German workers at the beginning of this century described patients who undoubtedly had hypertrophic cardiomyopathy,[13] the first detailed characterization of patients was in 1958 when Teare[14] described asymmetrical septal hypertrophy in the hearts of young siblings who had died suddenly. In the early 1960s Goodwin et al,[15,16] Braunwald et al,[17] and Wigle et al[18] characterized the clinical aspects of hypertrophic cardiomyopathy and emphasized features of hyperdynamic systolic function, notably high ejection fractions with left ventricular outflow tract gradients. The detection of an inflow tract murmur, a 4th heart sound, a palpable atrial beat,[16] and documentation of a raised filling pressure in the absence of left ventricular failure or obstruction[19] suggested diastolic abnormalities were also important, but these have only more recently been emphasized since the development of noninvasive methods of quantitation[20-22] and their use in the assessment of pharmacologic agents which alter diastolic function.[23-25] The diagnosis was based on the demonstration of clinical and hemodynamic features of a left ventricular outflow tract gradient. A resting gradient which disappears after the administration of phenylephrine (Figure 25-1) differentiates the functional gradient of hypertrophic cardiomyopathy from the fixed obstruction of valvar aortic stenosis and was considered to be the classical presentation of the disease. The significance of such a gradient in hypertrophic cardiomyopathy is still a source of great controversy. Those who consider the gradient to represent true obstruction to left ventricular outflow[26] point out the beneficial symptomatic results which are associated with reduction in left ventricular gradients following surgical myectomy.[27] Other investigators, however, have demonstrated that patients with hypertrophic cardiomyopathy and hyperdynamic left ventricular function eject 90% of stroke volume in the first half of systole, regardless of the presence or absence of left ventricular gradients.[28-33] They contend that most left ventricular gradients are due to elimination of the left ventricular cavity with consequent entrapment of the catheter and that true obstruction is seldom, if ever, present.[33] The practical message from this ongoing debate is that in certain centers good surgical results are achieved for reasons that may be unrelated to "relief of obstruction."

The availability of M-mode echocardiography in the 1970s permitted noninvasive assessment of the upper anterior ventricular septum, the upper left ventricular posterior wall, and the mitral and aortic valves.[34] The association of asymmetrical

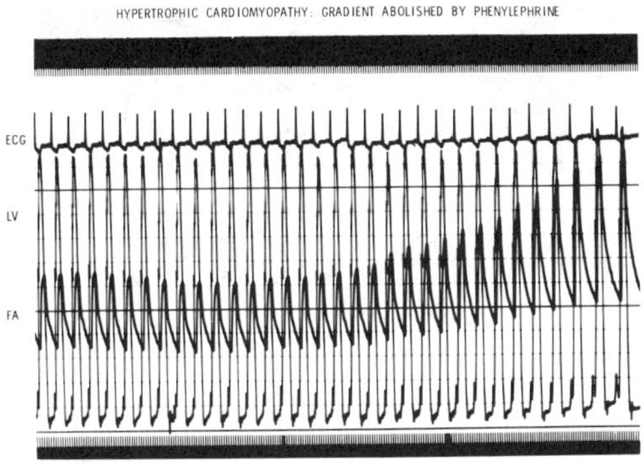

Figure 25-1 Tracings show simultaneous measurement of left ventricular (LV) and femoral artery (FA) pressure. There is a resting gradient of approximately 100 mmHg which is abolished following administration of the vasoconstrictor, phenylephrine. This is characteristic of the functional left ventricular gradient of hypertrophic cardiomyopathy.

septal hypertrophy, systolic anterior motion of the mitral valve, and early systolic closure of the aortic valve with left ventricular gradients was made[35-37] and some workers considered asymmetrical septal hypertrophy to be the pathognomonic feature of the condition.[38] Since the advent of cross-sectional echocardiography, however, a wider spectrum of hypertrophic cardiomyopathy has become apparent.[39,40] Left ventricular hypertrophy may be symmetrical, asymmetrical predominantly involving areas of the septum, or be localized in the distal ventricle.[41,42] The earlier experience of hypertrophic cardiomyopathy can then be seen in relation to the existing method of assessment; our understanding of the condition has been biased by patients with asymmetrical septal hypertrophy who were more readily identified.

The true incidence of hypertrophic cardiomyopathy is uncertain. It has been considered to be a rare disease with a poor prognosis. Recent blood pressure and echocardiographic evaluation of a large cohort from the Framingham study, however, suggests that unexplained left ventricular hypertrophy is much more common than has been previously recognized and that abnormal patterns of hypertrophy are present in approximately 2% of normotensive elderly patients.[43] It is probable that hypertrophic cardiomyopathy is more common but carries a less ominous prognosis than previous information would have led us to believe.

DIAGNOSIS

The World Health Organization defines hypertrophic cardiomyopathy to be a heart muscle disorder of unknown etiology which is characterized by unexplained left ventricular hypertrophy. This definition has received acceptance on both sides of the Atlantic.[44,45] Its limitation, however, is highlighted by the interpretation by some authors that the diagnosis of hypertrophic cardiomyopathy cannot be sustained in the presence of any other cause for left ventricular hypertrophy. Does a middle-aged or elderly patient with severe concentric left ventricular hypertrophy and mild systemic hypertension or a small aortic valve gradient also have hypertrophic cardiomyopathy? Other workers prefer to interpret the definition of hypertrophic cardiomyopathy as unexplained left ventricular hypertrophy or hypertrophy which is inappropriate to the stimulus, the severity of which may not always be easy to determine. Such then are the current limitations and a more precise definition of hypertrophic cardiomyopathy will require the determination of specific metabolic or genetic markers or identification of the cause of this condition.

Hypertrophic cardiomyopathy in old age often does not differ clinically from hypertrophic cardiomyopathy at any other age; however, as heart disease becomes increasingly common with advancing age, other diagnoses tend to be preferred. A loud late systolic murmur stopping before the aortic closure sound with a palpable atrial beat should give rise to suspicion of hypertrophic cardiomyopathy, particularly if the ECG shows marked evidence of left ventricular hypertrophy and the blood pressure is normal. Clinical recognition of hypertrophic cardiomyopathy in the elderly, however, may be difficult. Arterial pulses tend to be of higher volume and more rapidly rising because of inelastic arteries so that the character of the arterial pulses may not be helpful. Systolic murmurs due to sclerosis and stenosis of the aortic valve or to mitral regurgitation are common, and mitral leaflet prolapse from chordal lengthening or from papillary muscle dysfunction can give rise to late systolic murmurs very similar to those common in hypertrophic cardiomyopathy. In addition, elderly people with hypertrophic cardiomyopathy may have no murmurs attributable to the condition while having murmurs caused by degenerative aortic and mitral valve changes. The typical systolic murmur of hypertrophic cardiomyopathy is caused by turbulence in the left ventricular outflow tract often with mild late systolic mitral regurgitation. During the later period of ejection, both the outflow tract murmur and gradient are attributable to cavity elimination. The patients with hypertrophic cardiomyopathy who survive over a long period of time may spontaneously lose these murmurs. The cause is deterioration in left ventricular systolic function so that the left ventricle develops a larger residual volume, cavity elimination and gradients no longer occur, and the murmur disappears. It is for this reason that some elderly patients with hypertrophic cardiomyopathy are murmur-free but give a history of having had a murmur for many years when they were younger.

With deterioration in left ventricular function, the left ventricular diastolic pressure tends to rise because left ventricular compliance does not increase and the increased left ventricular diastolic volume is accommodated at a higher diastolic pressure. Left atrial volume also tends to rise due to incomplete emptying, and pulmonary venous congestion may occur. A murmur-free patient with radiologic evidence of left ventricular failure may not easily be recognized as having hypertrophic cardiomyopathy and if in addition atrial fibrillation has developed as is common, another clinical sign, the palpable atrial beat, disappears leaving a very nonspecific picture of left ventricular disorder. The chest film provides no particular help, usually showing a somewhat enlarged heart, perhaps with a left ventricular contour, some atrial distention, and pulmonary venous congestion. In such patients the ECG and echocardiography become very important.

When sinus rhythm is present the ECG may show marked changes of left or biatrial hypertrophy but heart failure is often precipitated by the onset of atrial fibrillation and these clues then vanish. Evidence of a marked left ventricular disorder is nearly always present in the elderly with hypertrophic cardiomyopathy whether or not they are in heart failure. Left anterior hemiblock is common (20%) but left or right bundle-branch block is rare. The QRS complex is often widened and if there is left anterior hemiblock midseptal V leads show qS waves suggestive of previous infarction, except that T waves are upright and this is unusual with previous infarction. Atrioventricular (AV) block has been described in hypertrophic cardiomyopathy but this is unusual and probably the result of chance rather than as one of the complications of hypertrophic cardiomyopathy. Other patients may show a nonspecific picture of left ventricular disorder with absent Q waves in leads 1, aA_L, V_5, and V_6, a slightly broadened QRS complex, and minor repolarization changes in left ventricular leads. It is very rare for the ECG to be normal in hypertrophic cardiomyopathy in old age, though this may occur in children.

The diagnosis of hypertrophic cardiomyopathy relies upon the demonstration of unexplained left ventricular hypertrophy. In the elderly as in the young this tends to depend very much on echocardiography. M-mode echocardiography can be diagnostic of hypertrophic cardiomyopathy but only when all or nearly all of the characteristics are present.[36] It has been stated already that left ventricular cavity elimination and outflow tract gradients often tend to disappear with increasing age and this removes two of the most important echocardiographic featues of the disease, systolic anterior motion of the mitral valve and systolic closure of the aortic valve. To be of diagnostic help systolic anterior motion of the mitral valve must be seen as a definitive midsystolic forward movement of the mitral valve onto the septum which precedes the forward movement of the posterior wall and which returns prior to the opening of the mitral valve. Minor anterior movement of the mitral valve in systole is common to a number of disorders, particularly those with hyperkinetic left ventricle function, as in systemic hypertension or mitral leaflet prolapse. In such conditions pseudosystolic anterior motion may occur in which the anterior motion reaches its peak at end systole and in parallel with the posterior wall.[46] Midsystolic closure of the aortic cusps is also nonspecific, occurring in mitral valve prolapse, and like mitral systolic anterior motion it tends to disappear in hypertrophic cardiomyopathy with diminishing left ventricular systolic function and loss of cavity elimination. This may leave the M-mode echocardiographic diagnosis of hypertrophic cardiomyopathy dependent upon abnormalities in left ventricular wall thickness and this means technically high-quality echocardiograms, which may be difficult to obtain in this age group. It is easy to record a spurious increase in septal thickness by incorporating tricuspid papillary muscle and the error may be missed if either technic or quality of record are imperfect. The thickness of the posterior left ventricular wall may be normal or increased in hypertrophic cardiomyopathy. The major limitation of the M-mode technic in hypertrophic cardiomyopathy, however, is that it visualizes only a single slice through the upper (and perhaps mid-) anterior septum and posterior wall. The mid- and distal portion of the left ventricle as well as the entire posterior septum and free wall are not visualized. In addition, accurate measurement of wall thickness can only be made if the transducer beam is at right angles to the myocardium and this may be difficult to assess.

Cross-sectional or two-dimensional echocardiography is currently the best available means to detect and to assess the distribution of left ventricular hypertrophy. Reliable measurements of myocardial wall thickness can be made in the anterior and posterior septum and in the left ventricular free and posterior wall in both the upper and the lower left ventricle.[42] The myocardial area at the true apex of the heart can only be assessed using long axis two- and four-chamber views and measurements of wall thickness from these views are less reliable. The diagnosis of hypertrophic cardiomyopathy is made by the demonstration of an unexplained increase in myocardial thickness greater than two standard deviations from the mean of a normal population, ie, >1.5 cm. Recent reports which suggest an increased incidence of hypertrophic cardiomyopathy in the elderly may reflect the application of this more sensitive technology to asymptomatic patients who have been undetected all their lives. Alternatively, elderly patients with unexplained left ventricular hypertrophy may have had systemic hypertension which is no longer present. In hypertensive heart disease without ventricular dilatation, blood pressure is usually high, the onset of left ventricular failure with dilatation usually being associated with a fall in blood pressure. This diagnostic dilemma may be solved if there is renal or ocular evidence of systemic hypertension, or when the myopathic process is detected in family members. Another diagnostic difficulty is posed by the patient who presents with mild elevation in blood pressure but with moderate or severe left ventricular hypertrophy in the absence of other target organ manifestations of severe systemic hypertension. Should one or two diagnoses be made? The relevance of the diagnosis of hypertrophic cardiomyopathy in such a patient relates strictly to prognosis and to the possibility of other family members being affected. If family studies are negative we would not diagnose hypertrophic cardiomyopathy in such a patient but we would search for arrhythmias as they may be occult yet of prognostic importance.

Older patients with hypertrophic cardiomyopathy may present murmur-free with left ventricular failure and may have echocardiographic left ventricular hypertrophy without dilatation. In such patients a differential diagnosis from amyloid heart disease may be difficult. There are no echocardiographic features which are specific to amyloid heart disease. Although a characteristic "granular sparkle" has been emphasized, a similar pattern may be seen to a more limited degree in hypertrophic cardiomyopathy and has been attributed to the excess of fibrous tissue. In most cases of amyloid heart disease, the ECG is of unusually low voltage whereas the converse is true in hypertrophic cardiomyopathy and this possibly provides the best differentiating clue to the diagnosis. The literature suggests that the pattern of hypertrophy may be helpful and that asymmetrical septal hypertrophy is more likely to be associated with hypertrophic cardiomyopathy whereas symmetrical or concentric hypertrophy is more common in secondary forms of left ventricular hypertrophy. This remains to be fully tested but there is sufficient anecdotal evidence to suggest that the pattern or distribution of left ventricular hypertrophy is of minimal diagnostic specificity.

NATURAL HISTORY

The available information on patients who were diagnosed prior to 60 years of age indicates that hypertrophic cardiomyopathy is associated with poor prognosis.[47] In our series of 254 patients 58 died during a six-year follow-up; of these deaths 32 were sudden and unexpected. The majority of these had minimal or no symptoms. A stepwise discriminate analysis revealed that young age at diagnosis, a family history of hypertrophic cardiomyopathy, and sudden death and previous history of syncopal episodes best predicted those patients at particular risk of sudden death. In a separate study we reviewed the clinical outcome of 37 patients who presented in childhood because of symptoms or an abnormality on physical examination. The five patients who presented with or developed severe symptoms died within three years after diagnosis in cardiac failure or in the perioperative period following myectomy. Of the remaining patients none had significant limitation of exercise tolerance, nevertheless 50% died suddenly during the nine years following diagnosis.[48] Hypertrophic cardiomyopathy in young patients can thus be viewed as a condition in which symptoms are usually mild and progress slowly; the most worrisome and important problem related to the condition is the risk of sudden death.

The natural history of hypertrophic cardiomyopathy in the elderly, however, is unknown. The available literature presents a total of less than 150 patients who were diagnosed after the age of 60. Symptoms of dyspnea, chest pain and syncope appear to be more common in the elderly (Table 25-1). In younger patients progressive symptoms occur in less than 20% but may improve spontaneously or in association with treatment[3]; the symptomatic course of elderly patients is uncertain. In younger patients the risk of sudden death is the most important problem related to the condition with a 6% annual mortality in children; the annual mortality from sudden death in elderly patients is not known but postmortem studies suggest that sudden death may be the commonest mode of death as in younger patients.[49] Features of interest in the elderly which differ from the experience in younger patients are the high incidence of female patients and the likelihood of an incorrect clinical diagnosis prior to echocardiography.[5] This is highlighted by the postmortem series of Pomerance and Davies in which 7 of 15 elderly patients with hypertrophic cardiomyopathy were not diagnosed antemortem.[49] This is consistent with Savage et al's finding of an increased incidence of left ventricular hypertrophy in normotensive elderly patients[43] and suggests that hypertrophic cardiomyopathy is even more common than was previously suspected. The higher incidence of female patients and the increased incidence of sudden death in young males[47] suggests that females with hypertrophic cardiomyopathy may have better prognosis.

ARRHYTHMIA

Arrhythmias are common in hypertrophic cardiomyopathy,[50,51] and are of similar incidence in the middle-aged and the elderly (Table 25-2). More than one quarter of patients will have ventricular tachycardia of three beats or more during 48-hour ambulatory ECG monitoring. Such episodes are invariably asymptomatic, but their presence is associated with subsequent sudden death.[51,52] In particular, ventricular tachycardia has been shown to be a sensitive but nonspecific marker of those patients who are at particular risk of sudden death.[53] An improved prognosis following abolition of ventricular tachycardia in hypertrophic cardiomyopathy has not yet been demonstrated. Nevertheless the association is sufficiently strong to warrant therapy. In this respect beta-adrenergic blocking agents[54] and verapamil[55] have been shown to be ineffective and other conventional agents (quinidine, disopyramide, mexiletine) are not usually successful at suppressing serious ventricular arrhythmias in patients with hypertrophic cardiomyopathy.[51]

Recently, the benzfuran derivative, amiodarone, has been used in patients with refractory ventricular arrhythmia. Ventricular tachycardia was suppressed in 18 of 19 patients after a loading dose of 800 to 1200 mg daily for one week followed by a maintenance dose of 400 mg daily for one month.[53] In such patients it is our practice to reduce the amiodarone to a minimum effective maintenance dose. This is monitored by ambulatory ECG monitoring 3 to 4 months after dose reduction when plasma and myocardial levels of amiodarone are probably at a steady state. Approximately half of our patients are eventually controlled on 200 mg daily and the remainder require 400 mg daily; during the two-year period on such doses no serious side-effects developed. An exception was the one patient who received 600 mg daily for one year: his ventricular tachycardia was never completely suppressed and he developed dermatologic side-effects which required discontinuation of the amiodarone. None of the patients with hypertrophic cardiomyopathy and

Table 25-1
Relation of Age and Clinical Features at Diagnosis

	Age at Diagnosis (yr)				
	≤14 *n=27*	*15–30* *n=67*	*31–45* *n=69*	*46–60* *n=64*	*>60* *n=121*
Syncope	9 (33%)	10 (15%)	8 (12%)	4 (7%)	28 (23%)
Exertional chest pain	5 (19%)	17 (25%)	20 (29%)	24 (38%)	70 (58%)
Dyspnea class II	12 (44%)	21 (31%)	22 (32%)	22 (34%)	68 (56%)
Classes III–IV	0	3 (5%)	5 (7%)	6 (9%)	

Patients aged ≤60 years are from the Hammersmith Hospital series.[47]
The symptoms at diagnosis in patients of more than 60 years have been summarized from references 4–12.
The characteristics of chest pain were not always described and it is possible that the greater incidence of exertional chest pain in the elderly may represent the inclusion of patients with chest pain which was not primarily exertional.

Table 25-2
The Incidence of Arrhythmia in Relation to Age in 135 Patients with Hypertrophic Cardiomyopathy

	Age (yr)				
	15 *n=3*	*16–30* *n=25*	*31–45* *n=32*	*46–60* *n=52*	*>60* *n=23*
Atrial fibrillation	0	0	2 (6%)	4 (8%)	2 (9%)
Supraventricular tachycardia	0	6 (24%)	12 (40%)	17 (35%)	8 (38%)
Ventricular tachycardia	0	4 (16%)	10 (31%)	14 (27%)	6 (26%)

ventricular tachycardia who have been treated with amiodarone died during two years. Nevertheless, longer follow-up of a larger number of patients is required to determine whether amiodarone treatment of patients with hypertrophic cardiomyopathy and ventricular tachycardia will improve prognosis.

Supraventricular arrhythmias are also common[50,51] and have an increased incidence in the middle-aged and elderly (Table 25-2). Approximately 10% of patients are in established atrial fibrillation and an additional 30% to 35% have paroxysmal atrial fibrillation or supraventricular arrhythmias during 48-hour ECG monitoring. Although AV nodal blocking drugs (digoxin, beta-blockers, verapamil) may control the ventricular response during supraventricular tachycardia they do not significantly reduce their incidence. In contrast, amiodarone will suppress paroxysmal supraventricular tachycardia[53] and restore sinus rhythm in approximately one third of patients with chronic atrial fibrillation.[55] These effects of amiodarone may suppress an otherwise troublesome therapeutic problem and if sustained control is demonstrated may obviate the need for anticoagulants. Since amiodarone potentiates the effect of warfarin, in patients who require anticoagulants careful monitoring of prothrombin time must be performed until steady-state amiodarone is achieved.[56] The final warfarin requirement is usually reduced by approximately 50%. Amiodarone also interacts with digoxin, increasing digoxin plasma levels. Approximately 15% of our patients with hypertrophic cardiomyopathy received digoxin for the treatment of cardiac failure or for the control of ventricular response in atral fibrillation, complications which are both more common in the elderly. The concomitant administration of amiodarone and digoxin should lead to the reduction of the latter by approximately half.[56] Many of the unwanted effects of amiodarone therapy are related to dose and duration of therapy but do not appear to have a higher incidence in the elderly.[57] One possible exception is hypothyroidism which is seen in approximately 1% to 2% of elderly patients receiving amiodarone. This may not represent an increased incidence of hypothyroidism in the elderly;[56,57] nevertheless vigilance for evidence of myxedema in elderly patients is warranted.

INVESTIGATIONS AND TREATMENT

Left ventricular angiography and invasive hemodynamic measurements are not necessary for the diagnosis or the characterization of young or elderly patients with hypertrophic cardiomyopathy. All patients should, however, undergo cross-sectional echocardiography to evaluate the extent and pattern of left ventricular hypertrophy as well as noninvasive assessment of left ventricular function using radionuclide cineangiography. The measurements of left ventricular wall thickness and the derived indices of left ventricular function provide a base line for subsequent comparison. All patients should also undergo 48-hour ECG monitoring at the time of diagnosis and at least annually thereafter. Serious ventricular arrhythmias are invariably asymptomatic and may develop despite the absence of change in symptoms, hypertrophy, or left ventricular function. Although paroxysmal or mild symptoms are common in elderly patients with hypertrophic cardiomyopathy, severe symptoms appear to be rare (approximately 20%). Significant limitation of exercise tolerance from dyspnea may be due to impaired systolic or diastolic function or less commonly from true left ventricular outflow tract obstruction. In addition, elderly patients who survive through middle age tend to develop degenerative changes on the mitral valve caused by turbulence in the narrow outflow tract at the point of apposition of the mitral valve with the septum during ejection. This can give rise to a fixed deformity of the mitral valve causing either regurgitation or stenosis or a mixture of both, and the mitral valve may actually become calcified. Such patients may develop severe symptomatic mitral regurgitation which is benefited by a mitral valve replacement with a low profile prosthesis. The five patients who have had this carried out in our institution have all been over the age of 60 and all have done well. Troublesome chest pain may also be caused by abnormalities of contraction, relaxation/filling, or associated coronary artery disease. When significant symptoms are present in patients with hypertrophic cardiomyopathy, left ventricular angiography, coronary arteriography and full hemodynamic assessment are warranted in order to determine appropriate therapy.

Propranolol is the treatment of choice for dyspnea and exertional or atypical chest pain. If the predominant hemodynamic abnormality is impaired relaxation or filling, combined use of propranolol and nifedipine,[58] or verapamil alone may be effective.[23,24] True left ventricular outflow tract obstruction may be defined as a significant left ventricular to ascending aortic pressure difference with a residual end-systolic cavity distal to the site of obstruction. Surgical myectomy should be reserved for patients with obstruction who have symptoms that have not been significantly improved by propranolol or verapamil; a good surgical result should be achieved in such patients. Approximately 10% to 15% of patients with hypertrophic cardiomyopathy will have impaired systolic function. Management of these patients is more difficult as they are prone to cardiac failure following the administration of negative inotropic agents such as propranolol, verapamil, or nifedipine; these drugs must be administered cautiously, often with concomitant antifailure medication (digoxin, diuretics). If stenotic coronary artery lesions are associated with severe refractory symptoms coronary artery bypass grafting is indicated.

Though amiodarone was originally developed and marketed in Belgium and France as an antianginal agent, we have observed no consistent symptomatic effect in patients with hypertrophic cardiomyopathy and chest pain. When dyspnea or chest pain coexist with refractory arrhythmia we have used amiodarone and propranolol together without complication. This combination, however, must be used cautiously in patients with sinoatrial or atrioventricular node disease, both of which are common in the elderly. The same constraint also applies to the combination of verapamil and amiodarone.

The follow-up of patients with hypertrophic cardiomyopathy should be directed at the prevention of complications, particularly endocarditis, embolic events, and sudden death. Antibiotic prophylaxis of all patients undergoing invasive dental or other procedures is warranted. Patients in established atrial fibrillation and those patients with a high incidence of supraventricular arrhythmias are prone to the development of emboli and should be anticoagulated. This underscores the need for regular (at least annual) ECG monitoring.

REFERENCES

1. Frank S, Braunwald E: Idiopathic hypertrophic subaortic stenosis. Clinical analysis of 126 patients with emphasis on the natural history. *Circulation* 1968;37:759–788.
2. Hardarson T, de la Calzada CS, Curiel R, et al: Prognosis and mortality of hypertrophic obstructive cardiomyopathy. *Lancet* 1973;2:1462–1467.
3. McKenna WJ, Goodwin JF: The natural history of hypertrophic cardiomyopathy, in Harvey P (ed): *Current Problems in Cardiology*. Chicago, Yearbook Medical Publishers, 1981; vol 6, pp 5–26.
4. Whiting RB, Powell WJ, Dinsmore RE, et al: Idiopathic hypertrophic subaortic stenosis in the elderly. *N Engl J Med* 1971;285:196–200.
5. Krasnow N, Stein RA: Hypertrophic cardiomyopathy in the aged. *Am Heart J* 1978;96:326–336.
6. Hamby RI, Aintablian A: Hypertrophic subaortic stenosis is not rare in the eighth decade. *Geriatrics* 1976;31:71–74.
7. Petrin TJ, Tavel ME: Idiopathic hypertrophic subaortic stenosis as observed in a large community hospital: Relation to age and history of hypertension. *J Am Geriatr Soc* 1979;27:43–46.
8. Berger M, Rethy C, Goldberg E: Unsuspected hypertrophic subaortic stenosis in the elderly diagnosed by echocardiography. *J Am Geriatr Soc* 1979;27:178–182.
9. Albin EL, Chandraratna PAN, Littleman BB, et al: Idiopathic hypertrophic suabortic stenosis in the elderly. *J Am Geriatr Soc* 1977;274:163–167.
10. Alday LE, Moreyra E, Amuchastegui IM, et al: Recognising and treating muscular subaortic stenosis. *Geriatrics* 1973;28:74–76.
11. Battle WE, Siegel FA, Fox IM: The older patient with idiopathic hypertrophic subaortic stenosis. *Geriatrics* 1977;32:61–69.
12. David M, Sestier F, Hamel D, et al: La stenose musculaire sousaortique chez la personne agee. *Union Med Can* 1981;110:132–137.
13. Liouville H: Recissement cardiaque sous aortique. *Gazette Medicale* (Paris) 1869;24:161–163.
14. Teare D: Asymmetrical hypertrophy in the heart in young adults. *Br Heart J* 1958;20:1–8.
15. Goodwin JF, Hollman A, Cleland WP, et al: Obstructive cardiomyopathy simulating aortic stenosis. *Br Heart J* 1960;22:403–414.
16. Cohen J, Effat H, Goodwin JF, et al: Hypertrophic

obstructive cardiomyopathy. *Br Heart J* 1964;26: 16–32.
17. Braunwald E, Morrow AS, Cornell WP, et al: Idiopathic hypertrophic subaortic stenosis: Clinical, hemodynamic and angiographic manifestations. *Am J Med* 1960;29:924–945.
18. Wigle ED, Heinbecker RO, Gunton RW: Idiopathic ventricular septal hypertrophy causing muscular subaortic stenosis. *Circulation* 1962;26:325–340.
19. Stewart S, Mason DT, Braunwald E: Impaired rate of left ventricular filling in idiopathic hypertrophic subaortic stenosis and valvular aortic stenosis. *Circulation* 1968;37:8–14.
20. Sanderson JE, Traill TA, St John Sutton MG, et al: Left ventricular relaxation and filling in hypertrophic cardiomyopathy: An echocardiographic study. *Br Heart J* 1978;40:596–601.
21. St John Sutton MG, Tajik AJ, Gibson DG, et al: Echocardiographic assessment of left ventricular filling and septal and posterior wall dynamics in idiopathic hypertrophic subaortic stenosis. *Circulation* 1978;57:512–520.
22. Hanrath P, Mathey DG, Siegert R, et al: Left ventricular relaxation and filling in different forms of left ventricular hypertrophy: An echocardiographic study. *Am J Cardiol* 1980;45:15–23.
23. Bonow RO, Rosing DR, Bacharach SL, et al: Effects of verapamil on left ventricular systolic function and diastolic filling in patients with hypertrophic cardiomyopathy. *Circulation* 1981;64:787–796.
24. Hanrath P, Mathey DG, Kremer P, et al: Effect of verapamil on left ventricular isovolumic relaxation time and regional left ventricular filling in hypertrophic cardiomyopathy. *Am J Cardiol* 1980;45: 1258–1264.
25. Lorell BH, Paulus WJ, Grossman W, et al: Modification of abnormal left ventricular diastolic properties by nifedipine in patients with hypertrophic cardiomyopathy. *Circulation* 1982;65:499–507.
26. Kuhn H, Krelhaus W, Bircks W, et al: Indication for surgical treatment in patients with hypertrophic obstructive cardiomyopathy, in Kaltenbach M, Loogen F, Olsen EG (eds): *Cardiomyopathy and Myocardial Biopsy*. Berlin, Springer-Verlag, 1978, pp 308–315.
27. Maron BJ, Merrill WH, Freier PA, et al: Longterm clinical course and symptomatic status in patients after operation for hypertrophic subaortic stenosis. *Circulation* 1978;57:1205–1213.
28. Hernandez RR, Greenfield JC Jr, McCall BW: Pressure-flow studies in hypertrophic subaortic stenosis. *J Clin Invest* 1964;43:401–407.
29. Pierce GE, Morrow AG, Braunwald E: Idiopathic hypertrophic subaortic stenosis. III. Intraoperative studies of the mechanism of obstruction and its hemodynamic consequences. *Circulation* 1964;29, 30:(suppl 4):152–213.
30. Wilson WS, Criley JM, Ross RS: Dynamics of left ventricular emptying in hypertrophic subaortic stenosis: A cineangiographic and hemodynamic study. *Am Heart J* 1967;73:4–16.
31. Murgo JP, Alter BR, Dorethy JF, et al: Dynamics of left ventricular ejection in obstructive and nonobstructive hypertrophic cardiomyopathy. *J Clin Invest* 1980;66:1369–1382.
32. Criley JM, Lewis KB, White RI Jr, et al: Pressure gradients without obstruction: A new concept of "hypertrophic subaortic stenosis." *Circulation* 1965; 32:881–887.
33. Goodwin JF: The frontiers of cardiomyopathy. *Br Heart J* 1982;48:1–18.
34. Tajik AJ, Giuliani ER: Echocardiographic observations in idiopathic hypertrophic subaortic stenosis. *Mayo Clin Proc* 1974;49:89–97.
35. Henry WL, Clark CE, Glancy DL, et al: Echocardiographic measurement of the left ventricular outflow gradient in idiopathic hypertrophic subaortic stenosis. *N Engl J Med* 1973;288:989–993.
36. Doi YL, McKenna WJ, Gehrke J, et al: M-mode echocardiography in hypertrophic cardiomyopathy: Diagnostic criteria and prediction of obstruction. *Am J Cardiol* 1980;45:6–14.
37. Gilbert BW, Pollick C, Adelman AG, et al: Hypertrophic cardiomyopathy: Subclassification by M-mode echocardiography. *Am J Cardiol* 1980; 45:861–873.
38. Henry WL, Clark CE, Epstein SE: Asymmetric septal hypertrophy. Echocardiographic identification of the pathognomonic anatomic abnormality of IHSS. *Circulation* 1973;47:225–233.
39. Maron BJ, Gottdiener JS, Bonow RO, et al: Hypertrophic cardiomyopathy with unusual locations of left ventricular hypertrophy undetectable by M-mode echocardiography. *Circulation* 1981;63:409–418.
40. Maron BJ, Gottdiener JS, Epstein SE: Patterns and significance of distribution of left ventricular hypertrophy in hypertrophic cardiomyopathy. *Am J Cardiol* 1981;48:418–428.
41. Maron BJ, Bonow RO, Seshagiri TNR, et al: Hypertrophic cardiomyopathy with ventricular septal hypertrophy localized to the apical region of the left ventricle (apical hypertrophic cardiomyopathy). *Am J Cardiol* 1982;49:1838–1848.
42. Shapiro IM, McKenna WJ: Distribution of left ventricular hypertrophy in hypertrophic cardiomyopathy: A two-dimensional echocardiographic study. *J Am Coll Cardiol* 1983;2(3):437–444.
43. Savage DD, Kannel WB, Garrison RJ, et al: Longterm retrospective blood pressure correlates of various forms of left ventricular hypertrophy—Preliminary findings. *J Am Coll Cardiol* 1983;1(2): 622.
44. Maron BJ, Epstein SE: Hypertrophic cardiomyopathy. Recent observations regarding the specificity of three hallmarks of the disease: Asymmetric septal hypertrophy, septal disorganization and systolic anterior motion of the anterior mitral leaflet. *Am J Cardiol* 1980;45:141–153.
45. Goodwin JF: Prospects and predictions for the cardiomyopathies. *Circulation* 1974;50:210–219.
46. Doi YL, McKenna WJ, Oakley CM, et al: "Pseudo" systolic anterior motion in patients with hypertensive heart disease. *Eur Heart J* 1983;4:838–845.
47. McKenna WJ, Deanfield J, Faruqui A, et al: Prognosis in hypertrophic cardiomyopathy: Role of age and clinical, electrocardiographic and hemodynamic features. *Am J Cardiol* 1981;47:532–538.
48. McKenna WJ, Deanfield JE, England D, et al: The prognostic implication of a clinical presentation with hypertrophic cardiomyopathy in childhood. *Br Heart J* 1983;49:290.
49. Pomerance A, Davies MJ: Pathological features of hypertrophic obstructive cardiomyopathy (HOCM) in the elderly. *Br Heart J* 1975;37:305–312.

50. Savage DD, Seides SF, Maron BJ, et al: Prevalence of arrhythmia during 24 hour electrocardiographic monitoring and exercise testing in patients with obstructive and nonobstructive hypertrophic cardiomyopathy. *Circulation* 1979;59:866–875.
51. McKenna WJ, England D, Doi YL, et al: Arrhythmia in hypertrophic cardiomyopathy: I. Influence on prognosis. *Br Heart J* 1981;46:168–172.
52. Maron BJ, Savage DD, Wolfson JK, et al: Prognostic significance of 24 ambulatory electrocardiographic monitoring in patients with hypertrophic cardiomyopathy: A prospective study. *Am J Cardiol* 1981;48:252–257.
53. McKenna WJ: Arrhythmia and prognosis in hypertrophic cardiomyopathy. *Eur Heart J* 1983;4:225–234.
54. McKenna WJ, Chetty S, Oakley CM, et al: Arrhythmia in hypertrophic cardiomyopathy: Exercise and 48 hour ambulatory electrocardiographic assessment with and without beta adrenergic blocking therapy. *Am J Cardiol* 1980;45:1–5.
55. McKenna WJ, Harris L, Perez G, et al: Arrhythmia in hypertrophic cardiomyopathy: II. Comparison of amiodarone and verapamil in treatment. *Br Heart J* 1981;46:173–178.
56. McKenna WJ, Rowland E, Kirkler DM: Amiodarone—The experience of past decade. *Br Med J* 1983;287:1654–1656.
57. Harris L, McKenna WJ, Rowland E, et al: Side effects of longterm amiodarone therapy. *Circulation* 1983;67:45–51.
58. Landmark K, Sire S, Thaulow E, et al: Haemodynamic effects of nifedipine and propranolol in patients with hypertrophic obstructive cardiomyopathy. *Br Heart J* 1982;48:19–26.

CHAPTER 26
Pulmonary Heart Disease

William M. Girard
Richard W. Light

An important type of cardiac disease in the geriatric patient, and one which is easily overlooked, is pulmonary heart disease, or cor pulmonale. The World Health Organization has defined chronic cor pulmonale as some combination of right ventricular hypertrophy and dilatation due to hypertension of the pulmonary circulation, the cause of which lies within the pulmonary parenchyma or within the pulmonary vascular system between the origin of the main pulmonary artery and the entry of the pulmonary veins into the left atrium. Thus, pulmonary hypertension which is caused by left atrial hypertension (due to left heart disease or mitral valve disease) is not included as cor pulmonale. Furthermore, pulmonary hypertension secondary to increased pulmonary blood flow produced by an intracardiac shunt or patent ductus arteriosus is, by definition, not cor pulmonale. There are many different disorders of the respiratory system which can produce cor pulmonale and several different mechanisms by which they cause pulmonary hypertension. We will present a brief review of the normal anatomy and physiology of pulmonary hypertension before discussing the pathophysiology of pulmonary hypertension.

ANATOMY AND PHYSIOLOGY OF THE PULMONARY CIRCULATION

The anatomy and circulatory dynamics of the pulmonary vascular circuit differ from those of the systemic circulation. The pulmonary circulation is a low pressure, high compliance system and its anatomy and physiology are optimal for that type of function. The pulmonary artery pressure is one fifth to one sixth the systemic arterial pressure even though the right ventricular output is the same as the left. The right ventricle, in comparison with the left, is more thin-walled and compliant. Thus it is more efficient in handling volume loads, but less well able to work against pressure loads. Animal studies have demonstrated that an increase in right ventricular preload causes only a slight increase in right ventricular stroke work, but an increase in afterload significantly reduces right ventricular stroke volume.[1] The pulmonary arteries and arterioles are likewise more thin-walled and less muscular than the corresponding systemic vessels.

The distinctive feature of the pulmonary vascular system is its ability to handle increased volume or flow without a significant increase in pressure. This is due not to high compliance of the individual pulmonary vessels but to the phenomenon of recruitment. When pulmonary blood flow is increased, pulmonary arteriolar and capillary beds which were closed become open. Thus, as the flow increases, the opening of parallel circuits reduces the vascular resistance commensurate with the increased flow, resulting in very little change in pulmonary artery pressure. The right ventricle can thus increase its output without generating higher pressures.

Because the pulmonary vessels are surrounded by pulmonary parenchyma, their resistance to blood flow is influenced by lung volume. At very low and very high lung volumes the pulmonary vascular resistance is increased compared with that at midlung volumes. This is because at a high lung volume the distended alveoli partially compress the alveolar capillaries, and at a very low lung volume the larger, extraparenchymal vessels are partially compressed by the contracted lung tissues and high pleural pressure. Alveolar pressure may also become positive enough during a forced expiration to compress alveolar capillaries and increase their resistance to blood flow.

Alveolar gas tension and blood pH also influence pulmonary vascular resistance and pulmonary artery pressure. Hypoxia produces an increase in pulmonary artery pressure, generally observed in man when the systemic arterial oxygen saturation falls below 80%.[2] This is due primarily to active vasoconstriction, which increases vascular resistance. Hypoxia is the most potent pulmonary vasoconstrictor, but its exact mechanism of action is not known. Acidosis also causes vasoconstriction and acts synergistically with hypoxia; ie, a high pH blunts the response to hypoxia and a low pH increases the response. Hypercapnia does not appear to cause vasoconstriction itself but affects resistance only by its effect on hydrogen ion concentration.

The response of the pulmonary circulation to exercise is an increase in blood flow which is linearly related to the increase in oxygen consumption. At the start of exercise, pulmonary artery pressure increases by 3 to 5 mmHg and plateaus as exercise is continued. The calculated pulmonary vascular resistance usually decreases with light to moderate exercise because more pulmonary vessels are recruited. During heavy exercise accurate pulmonary artery pressure measurements are difficult because of the wide fluctuations in intrathoracic pressure, but it appears that, as pulmonary blood flow is more than tripled, pulmonary vascular resistance remains constant and pulmonary artery pressure rises. The higher the preexercise pressure, the higher the rise with exercise. Immediately after exercise the pulmonary artery pressure often falls below the control resting level because of the marked decrease in blood flow, while many of the recruited vessels remain patent.

PATHOPHYSIOLOGY OF COR PULMONALE

The basic mechanism by which disorders of the respiratory system produce cor pulmonale is through pulmonary hypertension. This increase in afterload of the right ventricle reduces its pumping efficiency, and stroke volume falls. The heart compensates for this in three ways: distention, hypertrophy, and increased catecholamine release. Distention, an increase in end-diastolic volume, increases stroke volume by the Frank-Starling mechanism, ie, increased muscle fiber length. Hypertrophy increases the myocardial contractility. Hypertrophy occurs gradually, whereas distention is the response to a more sudden increase in afterload.

Cardiac failure is defined as failure of the pumping function of the heart to provide enough cardiac output to meet the metabolic requirements of the tissues. Because metabolic demands are greatest during exercise, the earliest indication of cardiac impairment is a limitation of exercise capacity due to an inability to increase cardiac output, or a lower than normal cardiac output for the level of oxygen consumption. The latter response is observed in patients with pulmonary hypertension whose ventilation is not limited, ie, in patients with pulmonary hypertension due to recurrent thromboemboli or primary pulmonary hypertension.[3]

In the case of cor pulmonale, this failure of the pumping ability of the heart does not mean that the right ventricular myocardium itself is abnormal. The factor responsible for the decreased stroke volume is the increased afterload. Measurements of the contractile state of the right ventricle in patients with pulmonary hypertension with or without right ventricular failure have demonstrated that the contractile performance of the ventricle is not abnormal.[4] Thus, if the pulmonary hypertension is relieved, the myocardial pumping function may return to normal. Perhaps this explains the inability of digitalis to improve cor pulmonale in most patients. Of course, with time and continued hypertrophy and dilatation the right ventricular muscle may become intrinsically impaired.

Mechanisms of Pulmonary Hypertension

Pulmonary hypertension is considered to be present when the pulmonary artery systolic pressure exceeds 30 mmHg and the diastolic pressure exceeds 20 mmHg. Pulmonary hypertension may result from several different factors: (1) reduction in the extent and distensibility of the pulmonary vascular bed, (2) an increase in pulmonary blood flow, (3) an increase in pulmonary venous pressure, and (4) pulmonary vasoconstriction. In most cases, several of these factors are present.

The pulmonary hypertension produced by intrinsic disease of the lung is usually a result of both anatomic loss of vascular bed and hypoxia-induced vasoconstriction. In interstitial disease with pulmonary hypertension, both hypoxia and compromise of the vascular lumen by fibrosis or vasculitis are present. In chronic obstructive airway disease, hypoxia produces active vasoconstriction, and emphysematous destruction of pulmonary capillary beds eliminates much of the pulmonary vascular system. Prolonged vasoconstriction itself appears to initiate hypertrophy of the pulmonary arterial musculature which compromises the vascular lumen and may increase the degree of vasospasm which can be produced by hypoxia.

Pulmonary hypertension resulting from increased pulmonary blood flow or pulmonary venous hypertension is, by definition, not cor pulmonale. However, both may occur in a patient with vasoconstriction or obliteration of the pulmonary vascular bed and thus augment the elevated pulmonary artery pressure. Thus, during the exercise-induced increase in pulmonary blood flow, the pulmonary arterial pressure increases much more in a patient with a compromised vascular bed than in a normal subject. Also, pulmonary venous hypertension resulting from left ventricular failure augments preexisting pulmonary artery hypertension and worsens cor pulmonale.

DISEASES PRODUCING COR PULMONALE

Chronic Airflow Obstruction

The most common cause of cor pulmonale, particularly in the geriatric population, is chronic airflow obstruction. In a study of 61 patients with heart failure solely on the basis of cor pulmonale, chronic airflow obstructive disease (CAO) was responsible for 79% of the cases.[5] Cor pulmonale develops in those patients with CAO who have arterial hypoxemia. Since the PaO_2 normally decreases with aging, a geriatric individual with a given degree of airflow obstruction is more likely to be hypoxic and therefore have cor pulmonale. Although the reduction of pulmonary vascular bed which results from emphysematous destruction of the lung contributes to the pulmonary hypertension, especially during high blood flow conditions such as exercise, hypoxemia is the most important factor. Hypoxemia in CAO is due to hypoventilation or mismatching of ventilation and perfusion, with the result that blood flows through poorly ventilated areas of the lung and does not become fully oxygenated.

There have been a number of investigations which purport to demonstrate either a correlation or lack of correlation between the type of CAO and the presence or absence of hypoxemia and cor pulmonale. Burrows et al[6] studied hemodynamics in 50 patients with CAO. Patients with only mild obstructive dysfunction and without severe hypoxemia had normal pulmonary artery pressure and low normal cardiac output at rest, with slightly elevated pulmonary vascular resistance. During exercise pulmonary artery pressure rose abnormally in most patients. Pulmonary vascular resistance rose with exercise, as contrasted with the normal response of a fall or no change, indicating insufficient pulmonary vessels to allow for recruitment during exercise. With more severe obstructive disease, pulmonary vascular resistance was abnormally high even at rest. The hemodynamic response with this high pulmonary vascular resistance varied depending upon the arterial blood gases. In patients with relatively normal PaO_2, cardiac output was abnormally low, pulmonary artery pressure was slightly elevated at rest and became markedly so with exercise. In those patients with severe chronic hypoxemia, cardiac output was normal or increased and significant pulmonary hypertension was present even at rest. These hypoxemic patients often had clinical and ECG features of cor pulmonale. The authors felt that hypoxemia, pulmonary hypertension, and cor pulmonale occurred especially in patients with a bronchitic type of CAO, whereas patients with predominant emphysema had relatively normal oxygenation and near normal resting pulmonary artery pressures. Of the 50 patients studied, however, only 14 fell into one or the other of these categories. The majority of patients were considered to have a mixture of bronchitis and emphysema.

Thurlbeck et al[7] studied 61 patients with CAO and compared clinical, roentgenologic, and functional criteria with morphology of inflated lung specimens and concluded that the separation of patients into "bronchitis" and "emphysema" is an unwarranted oversimplification and that the majority of patients have features of both. They noted that cor pulmonale was more common in patients with severe emphysema, and was noted infrequently in patients with little emphysema. They agreed that abnormal blood gases and acidemia are the determinants of pulmonary hypertension in CAO, but noted that abnormal blood gases were more commonly found in patients with severe emphysema than in those with slight or no emphysema. They noted that chronic bronchitis did not produce pulmonary hypertension in patients with mild or no emphysema.

Recent studies of the chemical control of ventilation in patients with CAO suggest that central respiratory drive plays an important role in the degree of blood gas abnormality produced by obstruction to airflow in a particular patient.[8] When obstruction to airflow develops, it causes maldistribution of ventilation, thus reducing the efficiency of breathing. Because of this inefficiency the patient must increase his minute ventilation in order to maintain a normal $PaCO_2$ and PaO_2. But airway obstruction also increases the work of breathing. If a patient has a high sensitivity to hypoxia and hypercapnia, ie, a high respiratory drive, he increases his ventilation even though it requires an increase in work, and he maintains relatively normal blood gases. Thus he does not develop pulmonary hypertension until the obstruction becomes so severe that he is unable to adequately increase his ventilation in spite of great efforts. In contrast, a patient with a diminished sensitivity to hypoxia and hypercapnia does not increase his respiratory efforts in response to airflow obstruction, but allows his PaO_2 to fall and $PaCO_2$ to rise. And, consequent to the chronic hypoxemia, this patient develops pulmonary hypertension and cor pulmonale at an earlier stage in his disease. Since the geriatric individual on the average has a diminished ventilatory response to hypoxia and hypercapnia, he is more likely to develop cor pulmonale.

It appears that in patients with less severe disease, in whom some recruitment of closed pulmonary vessels can still occur, exercise results in improvement in ventilation-perfusion mismatching and a rise in PaO_2. Therefore, due to the fall in pulmonary vascular resistance, cardiac output is not as limited as it is in those patients who are unable to recruit vessels. In patients with more extensive disease, recruitment is not possible and metabolic demands exceed the ventilatory capacity, causing blood gases to deteriorate further. Pulmonary artery pressure increases abnormally during exercise in both groups, and because it was already elevated at rest in the more hypoxemic patients, it reaches higher levels in these patients during exercise. Administration of oxygen during exercise to patients with CAO lessens the rise in pulmonary artery pressure, either by reducing vasoconstriction or cardiac output at maximal exertion. Minute ventilation is also reduced and exercise capacity is often improved.[9,10] This occurs in patients who become hypoxemic during exercise as well as those who do not.

Sleep Disordered Breathing

Episodes of pulmonary hypertension may also occur during sleep. This occurs primarily in two groups of patients: those with CAO and those with sleep apnea. Many patients with CAO have frequent episodes of arterial oxygen desaturation during sleep. In 10 patients with awake resting hypoxemia and hypercapnia, decreases in saturation of 10% to 77% occurred during sleep which lasted from 2 to 100 minutes.[11] These episodes occurred most frequently during rapid eye movement (REM) sleep. This desaturation during sleep is associated with an increase in pulmonary artery pressure and may contribute significantly to the development of cor pulmonale. Episodic desaturation during sleep correlates with the patient's respiratory drive. Patients who desaturate during sleep are those who have decreased sensitivity to hypercapnia and hypoxemia. Administration of oxygen often prevents or ameliorates the desaturation and therefore also the episodic elevation in pulmonary artery pressure.

The oxygen desaturation which occurs during apnea in patients with sleep apnea is also associated with episodic increases in pulmonary artery pressure, and if the episodes are frequent or prolonged, the pulmonary hypertension may become persistent.[12] Because periodic breathing and sleep apnea occur more frequently in elderly subjects, it should be considered as a possible contributory factor to cor pulmonale in the geriatric patient.[13]

Interstitial Lung Disease

Pulmonary hypertension and cor pulmonale secondary to interstitial lung disease generally occur late in the course. When the vital capacity is greater than 80% of predicted, the pulmonary hemodynamics are normal. When the vital capacity lies between 50% and 80%, the pulmonary vascular resistance is increased but the resting pulmonary artery pressure lies at the upper limit of normal, although with exercise this group of patients develop pulmonary hypertension. When the vital capacity is less than 50%, pulmonary hypertension is present at rest.

With some diseases the pulmonary vasculature is affected disproportionately to the lung parenchyma. In many of these cases, the chest roentgenogram has been normal with the exception of changes in the pulmonary vasculature and secondary cardiomegaly. This has been noted in rheumatoid arthritis, systemic lupus erythematosis, and systemic sclerosis. The pulmonary hypertension is due to anatomic compromise of the small and medium-sized pulmonary arteries and pulmonary arterioles by intimal proliferation or thickening.

Thoracic Cage Abnormalities

Cor pulmonale in disorders of the thoracic cage occurs primarily in those with mechanical abnormalities (fibrothorax, scoliosis, obesity-hypoventilation, and thoracoplasty) and only infrequently in those with neuromuscular disease. Two possible explanations for this are: (1) the more severe decrease in lung volume and hence the decrease in caliber of pulmonary blood vessels, and (2) the more protracted course and hence the longer period of existence of those factors that lead to intimal hyperplasia and medial hypertrophy. Pulmonary hypertension in mechanical abnormalities of the chest wall is due to two factors: vasoconstriction and anatomical changes in the vessels, namely medial proliferation and compression of pulmonary blood vessels by the compressed or distorted lung. It is probable that episodic arterial desaturation contributes to the pulmonary hypertension in some of these patients.

Primary Pulmonary Hypertension

When pulmonary hypertension occurs with no apparent underlying pulmonary or cardiac disorder, it is called primary pulmonary hypertension. There is controversy as to whether this is a distinct entity or whether it is due to chronic recurrent clinically inapparent thromboemboli. The wide range in age of affected individuals as well as an increased incidence at certain ages suggests that several different unknown etiologic factors may result in pulmonary hypertension. The hemodynamic findings and clinical features of right ventricular failure are indistinguishable from pulmonary hypertension of other causes.[14] Primary pulmonary hypertension is distinctly uncommon in the geriatric population.

CLINICAL MANIFESTATIONS AND DIAGNOSIS

What are the clinical manifestations of pulmonary hypertension and cor pulmonale? Diminished exercise capacity and dyspnea on exertion are symptoms of most respiratory diseases. When pulmonary hypertension and cor pulmonale occur, these symptoms will be increased. Many patients with CAO also have a chronic productive cough. Often patients have had these symptoms for 10 to 20 years by the time they consult a physician. Right ventricular failure also causes fluid retention which presents as pedal edema and may progress to ascites and anasarca. Substernal chest pain is an occasional symptom of pulmonary hypertension.

Physical Signs

The physical signs of cor pulmonale are a systolic sternal lift, an increased pulmonic component of the second heart sound, persistent splitting of the second heart sound, jugular venous distention, hepatomegaly, and peripheral edema with or without ascites. A right-sided third or fourth heart sound may be heard along the left sternal border which is accentuated during inspiration. Tricuspid valvular insufficiency may develop, producing a holosystolic murmur along the sternal border which is accentuated during inspiration. Many of the cardiac findings may be obscured in patients with CAO by the hyperinflated lungs which dampen the heart sounds and by airway sounds which make them difficult to hear. In such patients the heart sounds are best heard in the epigastric area.

Chest Radiography

Chest radiography is also useful in evaluating a patient for pulmonary hypertension. The roentgenographic signs are related to enlargement of the proximal portion of the pulmonary arteries with or without evidence of right ventricular enlargement. In a report of 34 patients with CAO in which hemodynamic measurements were correlated with standard chest radiographs, the best test for pulmonary hypertension was a hilar thoracic index of 35 or greater.[15] The hilar thoracic index is determined by summing the horizontal distances from the midline to the first radiographically visualized upper lobe pulmonary arterial division on both sides, dividing this by the transverse diameter of the thorax, and multiplying by 100. Pulmonary hypertension is also indicated by a width of the descending branch of the right pulmonary artery greater than 20 mm or a hilar width greater than 11 cm. Patients with primary pulmonary hypertension have the same radiologic signs.[16]

Electrocardiography

Electrocardiography is useful in identifying some patients with right ventricular hypertrophy although it is a relatively insensitive test.[17] The characteristic features of cor pulmonale are right axis deviation, P pulmonale pattern (low P in lead 1 with tall, pointed P in leads 2, 3 and aV_F) and right ventricular hypertrophy (reversal of the precordial pattern with tall R waves over the right precordium and deep S waves over the left, and ST segment depression with upward convexity and inverted T waves in the right precordial leads and in whichever limb leads show tall R waves).

Acute changes in the ECG may occur during episodes of worsening hypoxemia associated with acute elevation of pulmonary artery pressure. These include: (1) a rightward shift of the mean QRS axis of 30 degrees or more from its previous position; (2) inverted, biphasic or flattened T waves in the right precordial leads; (3) depressed ST segments in leads 2, 3 and aV_F; and (4) incomplete or complete right bundle-branch block. These alterations revert with improvement in oxygenation but may become permanent if recurrences of desaturation are frequent.

Echocardiography

Because of the insensitivity of the ECG and physical examination in detecting cor pulmonale, other noninvasive technics have been utilized. In an evaluation of 43 patients suspected of having cor pulmonale, echocardiography demonstrated increased right ventricular internal dimension or hypertrophy of the right ventricular free wall in 37 (86%).[17] The ECG showed evidence of right ventricular hypertrophy in only 45% of the 37 patients. The echo confirmed that the ECG changes were specific for right ventricular hypertrophy but not sensitive. This study demonstrated that the echo was more sensitive than the ECG, but it did not determine the sensitivity of the echo in detecting less severe cor pulmonale.

Radionuclide Ejection Fractions

Measurement of right and left ventricular ejection fraction using noninvasive radionuclide technics has been utilized to assess cardiac function in patients with lung disease. In interpreting these studies it must be realized that ejection fraction is reduced by increased afterload. Thus, demonstration of a lower than normal ejection fraction does not necessarily imply abnormal myocardial contractility since patients with pulmonary hypertension have increased right ventricular afterload.

Two radionuclide technics have been utilized to measure the ejection fraction: first-pass angiography and equilibrium gated blood pool imaging. First-pass studies measure the radioactivity during the first transit of the tracer through the cardiac chambers following intravenous injection. A curve relating radioactivity counts to time is generated from the right ventricular blood pool by proper positioning of the probe. Activity during several beats is recorded and ejection fraction is calculated by comparing counts at end-diastole and end-systole. In equilibrium studies the radionuclide tracer is injected and allowed to achieve equilibrium. Counting is gated to a physiologic marker, usually the R wave of the ECG. This means that the counting device is given a signal to record the counts during a specific interval of time in relation to the ECG. Thus a greater number of beats can be monitored, increasing the resolution of the study. Ejection fraction is again calculated by comparing the counts during diastole and systole. These studies can be performed during exercise as well as at rest.

Right ventricular ejection fraction varies widely in patients with CAO.[18] It is usually low (<45%) in patients with clinical cor pulmonale and is also low in many patients with severe obstructive pulmonary disease without clinical evidence of cor pulmonale. Patients with worse hypoxemia or lower FEV_1 are more likely to have an abnormal ejection fraction. During exercise, the right ventricular ejection fraction in patients with severe CAO does not show the normal increase, and in some patients, it decreases. Thus, assessment of right ventricular ejection fraction may suggest cor pulmonale before it is detectable by other noninvasive means. Utilizing this technic, administration of oxygen has been shown to improve the ejection fraction response to exercise in some patients, possibly by decreasing the rise in pulmonary artery pressure during exercise. Long-term administration of oxygen has resulted in improvement in right ventricular ejection fraction as well as in pulmonary hypertension and pulmonary vascular resistance.[19]

It should be emphasized that assessment of right ventricular function via radionuclide ejection fraction is not without its problems. First, the ejection fraction is dependent upon the preload which determines the ventricular end-diastolic volume. The preload and the ventricular end-diastolic volume are not defined with the ejection fraction measurements. Accordingly, changes in ejection fractions may be due to changes in the preload rather than to changes in the right ventricular function or right ventricular afterload. Moreover, with multiple gated equilibrium right ventricular ejection fractions, a major problem arises from the underlying right atrial activity which can result in a fallacious right ventricular ejection fraction.[20] With the first-pass method, technical difficulties are encountered when there is marked pulmonary artery hypertension resulting in delayed radionuclide clearance from the right heart.

Thallium Scans

Another radionuclide technic which has been used to detect right ventricular hypertrophy is thallium 201 imaging. Thallium is concentrated in the myocardium, depending upon the adequacy of blood supply. It is primarily used to detect areas of myocardium with poor blood supply. Because the right ventricle normally constitutes only a small proportion of the total myocardium, it is not normally seen at rest on a thallium 201 scan. Right ventricular enlargement secondary to pressure or volume overload results in visualization of the right ventricle by thallium 201 scan. In 33 patients in whom the right ventricle was visualized clearly on thallium scan, 28 (85%) had pulmonary artery systolic pressure greater than or equal to 30 mmHg.[21] In 3 of the remaining 5 patients there was volume overload due to left-to-right shunt. Other tests detected right ventricular hypertrophy or pulmonary hypertension less often: chest radiograph (58%), echocardiogram (36%), and ECG (15%). In a second study of 71 patients with chronic obstructive pulmonary disease,[22] the right ventricle was visualized in 52 (73%). Patients with marked uptake had a significantly lower right ventricular ejection fraction, PaO_2, and FEV_1 than patients with normal scans. Of 23 patients with marked uptake, 20 had abnormal right ventricular ejection fractions but only 9 had right ventricular hypertrophy on ECG. Thus right ventricular uptake on thallium 201 scan was significantly more sensitive than ECG in detecting right ventricular hypertrophy.

TREATMENT

The central goal in the therapy of cor pulmonale is the alleviation of pulmonary hypertension. Relief of hypoxemia is of major importance in achieving this. Hypoxemia is relieved by measures which improve the patient's ventilation and by the administration of supplemental oxygen. Ventilation is improved by bronchodilator therapy, treatment of bronchopulmonary infection and pulmonary edema, and, if necessary, by mechanical ventilation. A detailed discussion of these therapeutic measures is beyond the scope of this chapter and may be found in standard textbooks of pulmonary medicine.

Oxygen

The acute effect of oxygen administration to patients with stable chronic airflow obstruction is a significant but variable fall in pulmonary pressure.[23] Oxygen lessens the abnormal rise in pulmonary artery pressure which occurs during exercise in these patients. This effect is more pronounced than the effect on the resting pulmonary artery pressure. Oxygen administration also improves the abnormal right ventricular ejection fraction response to exercise in some of these patients. These effects may be partly responsible for the increased exercise tolerance of some CAO patients when given oxygen.

The hemodynamic effect of oxygen when administered during an episode of acute decompensated CAO is controversial. Abraham et al[24] studied eight patients with acute respiratory failure secondary to chronic bronchitis. While the patients were breathing room air, the average pulmonary arterial mean pressure was 52.2 mmHg. This contrasted with a mean pressure of 36.5 mmHg upon the patients' discharge from the hospital after recovery. Administration of 28% oxygen resulted in a fall in mean pulmonary artery pressure by an average of 5 mmHg without a significant change in cardiac output. The authors concluded that hypoxia plays a major role in the reversible pulmonary hypertension of acute respiratory failure in chronic airflow obstruction.

Long-term administration of supplemental oxygen to patients with hypoxemia and pulmonary hypertension has been shown to reduce pulmonary vascular resistance, mortality, and hematocrit, and to increase right ventricular ejection fraction. The British oxygen therapy trial demonstrated that the administration of oxygen to hypoxemic (mean $PaO_2 = 51$ mmHg) CAO patients for at least 15 hours daily significantly reduces mortality.[25] The American trial[26] demonstrated that the administration of oxygen to markedly hypoxemic ($PaO_2 < 55$ mmHg) CAO patients for 24 hours a day was associated with a significantly lower mortality (11.9%) after 12 months than was the administration of oxygen for 12 hours a day (mortality 20.6%).

In view of the basic role that hypoxemia plays in the pathogenesis of cor pulmonale and in view of the decreased mortality of the hypoxemic CAO patient who is treated with oxygen, supplemental oxygen is recommended for all hypoxemic patients with cor pulmonale. The majority of patients who require oxygen for chronic hypoxemia are in the geriatric age range. Presently the mean age of the 72 patients that we have on home oxygen is 74 years. Sufficient oxygen should be administered to maintain the SaO_2 above 85% during rest, exercise, and sleep. The requirements for supplemental oxygen can be assessed noninvasively by monitoring the SaO_2 of the patient with an ear oximeter during various activities with different levels of supplemental oxygen. Supplemental oxygen at 2 L/min is also recommended during sleep for those patients with overt right ventricular failure even with an SaO_2 above 85% at rest while awake.

Supplemental oxygen on an outpatient basis is provided most economically by nasal prongs. Supplemental oxygen can be administered via gas cylinder, liquid containers, or oxygen concentrators. The interested reader is referred to a recent article for a discussion of the advantages and disadvantages of administering oxygen by each of these methods.[27] It should be noted that oxygen is expensive.

Digitalis

The use of digitalis glycosides in the treatment of cor pulmonale has been controversial for many years. Mathur et al[28] studied the effect of digoxin on the right and left ventricular ejection fractions in 15 patients with cor pulmonale secondary to CAO. The patients did not have clinical evidence of left ventricular disease. Radionuclide angiocardiography demonstrated reduced right ventricular ejection fraction in all patients and reduced left ventricular ejection fraction in four. After 8 weeks of digoxin treatment, the abnormal left ventricular ejection fractions were normal; right ventricular ejection fractions increased only in those patients who had abnormal left ventricular ejection fractions. These authors concluded that digoxin is only beneficial in cor pulmonale in those patients with abnormal left ventricular ejection fraction, and noted that the abnormal left ventricular function may not be clinically apparent.

In view of the fact that the geriatric patient is particularly susceptible to digitalis toxicity, digitalis preparations are recommended for geriatric patients with cor pulmonale only if there is coexisting left ventricular failure or if the patient has a supraventricular arrhythmia which is responsive to a digitalis preparation.

Diuretics

Diuretics are useful in patients with increased dyspnea due to right ventricular failure[29] since their administration leads to better gas exchange and improved pulmonary function and decreases the weight that the patient must carry to perform various activities. It is important to remember that oxygen is the best diuretic in patients with right ventricular failure who are hypoxemic.

Phlebotomy

Patients with cor pulmonale, particularly those with CAO and hypoxemia, may develop polycythemia with hematocrits of 60% or above. If such patients are subjected to phlebotomy, there is a significant decrease in the pulmonary artery pressure and the pulmonary vascular resistance.[30] It has recently been shown that the exercise capacity of patients with CAO and polycythemia is improved substantially (>25%) after therapeutic phlebotomy.[31] In view of these findings it is recommended that the hematocrit of the polycythemic COPD patient be maintained below 55%.[31] This is best accomplished by alleviating the hypoxemia with supplemental oxygen, but in certain patients periodic phlebotomies are necessary.

Bronchodilators

In addition to their bronchodilating effects, bronchodilators may improve the hemodynamics of patients with cor pulmonale. Parker et al[32] demonstrated that the intravenous administration of aminophylline to patients with cor pulmonale significantly reduces the mean pulmonary artery pressure and the pulmonary vascular resistance while increasing cardiac index. Intravenous aminophylline also increases right and left ventricular ejection fractions in patients with CAO as well as in control subjects.[33] Although FEV_1 improved in these patients, arterial oxygen tension did not; thus relief of hypoxemia was not responsible for the improvement. The improvement is probably secondary to increased myocardial contractility as well as reduction in pulmonary vascular resistance produced by dilatation of the pulmonary vasculature.

The beta-2-adrenergic stimulant terbutaline also has beneficial hemodynamic effects in addition to its bronchodilator action. In a group of patients with CAO, abnormal right ventricular performance, and elevated pulmonary vascular resistance, subcutaneous administration of terbutaline resulted in a decrease in pulmonary vascular resistance and increases in right and left ventricular ejection fractions and cardiac index.[34] Pulmonary artery pressure did not change significantly. Oxygen delivery was improved without a change in arterial oxygen tension. The hemodynamic effects of terbutaline in CAO patients at rest and during exercise were studied by Teule and Majid.[35] Terbutaline decreased pulmonary vascular resistance and pulmonary artery pressure both at rest and during exercise. Cardiac output and frequency were also increased both at rest and exercise. Therefore, a therapeutic level of a theophylline preparation and a beta-adrenergic stimulant is indicated for all patients with cor pulmonale. However, since geriatric patients have decreased theophylline clearances, a relatively low dose of theophylline (10 mg/kg/24 h) is recommended. Additionally, since elderly patients are likely to have difficulty from tremors with high-dose oral beta-adrenergic stimulants, only low doses of these compounds are recommended.

Vasodilators

In recent years several vasodilators including isoproterenol,[36] diazoxide,[37] nitroglycerine,[38] hydralazine, and nifedipine[39] have been given therapeutic trials in patients with pulmonary hypertension. In general the initial reports on each drug were very encouraging, but subsequent reports have been discouraging. At the present time, the rightful place of vasodilators in the treatment of pulmonary hypertension is unknown.

REFERENCES

1. McFadden ER Jr, Braunwald E: Cor pulmonale and pulmonary thromboembolism, in Braunwald E (ed): *Heart Disease, A Textbook of Cardiovascular Medicine.* Philadelphia, WB Saunders Co, 1980, pp 1643–1680.
2. Fishman AP, McClement J, Himmelstein A, et al: Effects of acute anoxia on the circulation and respiration in patients with chronic pulmonary disease studied during the steady state. *J Clin Invest* 1952; 31:770.
3. Gazetopoulos N, Salonikides N, Davies H: Cardiopulmonary function in patients with pulmonary hypertension. *Br Heart J* 1974;36:19–28.
4. Stein PD, Sabbah HN, Anbe DT, et al: Performance of the failing and non-failing right ventricle of patients with pulmonary hypertension. *Am J Cardiol* 1979;44:1050–1055.
5. Stevens PM, Terplan M, Knowles JH: Prognosis of cor pulmonale. *N Engl J Med* 1963;269:1289–1291.
6. Burrows B, Kettel LJ, Niden AH, et al: Patterns of cardiovascular dysfunction in chronic obstructive lung disease. *N Engl J Med* 1972;286:912–917.
7. Thurlbeck WM, Henderson JA, Fraser RG, et al: Chronic obstructive lung disease, A comparison between clinical, roentgenologic, functional and morphologic criteria in chronic bronchitis, emphysema, asthma and bronchiectasis. *Medicine* 1970;49:81–142.
8. Mountain R, Zwillich C, Weil J: Hypoventilation in obstructive lung disease: The role of familial factors. *N Engl J Med* 1978;298:521–525.
9. Cotes JE, Pisa Z, Thomas AJ: Effect of breathing oxygen upon cardiac output, heart rate, ventilation, systemic and pulmonary blood pressure in patients with chronic lung disease. *Clin Sci* 1963;25: 305–321.
10. Horsfield K, Segel N, Bishop JM: The pulmonary circulation in chronic bronchitis at rest and during exercise breathing air and 80% oxygen. *Clin Sci* 1968;43:473–483.
11. Douglas NJ, Calverley PM, Leggett RJ, et al: Transient hypoxemia during sleep in chronic bronchitis and emphysema. *Lancet* 1979;1:1–4.
12. Tilkian AG, Guilleminault C, Schroeder JS, et al: Hemodynamics in sleep induced apnea, studies during wakefulness and sleep. *Ann Intern Med* 1976; 85:714–719.
13. Webb P: Periodic breathing during sleep. *J Appl Physiol* 1974;37:899–903.
14. Fishman AP, Pietra GG: Primary pulmonary hypertension. *Ann Rev Med* 1980;31:421–431.
15. Chetty KG, Brown SE, Light RW: Identification of pulmonary hypertension in chronic obstructive pulmonary disease from routine chest radiographs. *Am Rev Respir Dis* 1982;126:338–341.
16. Lupi E, Dumont C, Tejada VM, et al: A radiologic index of pulmonary arterial hypertension. *Chest* 1975;68:28–31.
17. Lesser LM, Johnson M, Felner JM, et al: Echocardiography in patients with suspected cor pulmonale. *South Med J* 1982;75:388–391.
18. Berger HJ, Matthay RA, Loke J, et al: Assessment of cardiac performance with quantitative radionuclide angiocardiography: Right ventricular ejection fraction with reference to findings in chronic obstructive pulmonary disease. *Am J Cardiol* 1978;41: 897–905.
19. Ellis JH, Kirch D, Steele PP: Right ventricular ejection fraction in severe chronic airway obstruction. *Chest* 1977;71S:281–282.
20. Berger HJ, Zaret BL: Nuclear cardiology. *N Engl J Med* 1981;305:855–865.
21. Khaja F, Alam M, Goldstein S, et al: Diagnostic value of visualization of the right ventricle using thallium-201 myocardial imaging. *Circulation* 1979;59:182–188.
22. Berger H, Wackers F, Mahler D, et al: Right ventricle visualization on thallium-201 myocardial images in chronic obstructive pulmonary disease: Relationship to right ventricular function and hypertrophy. *Circulation* 1980;62(suppl 3):103.
23. Burrows B: Arterial oxygenation and pulmonary hemodynamics in patients with chronic airways obstruction. *Am Rev Respir Dis* 1974;110S:64–70.
24. Abraham AS, Cole RB, Green ID, et al: Factors contributing to the reversible pulmonary hypertension of patients with acute respiratory failure studied by serial observations during recovery. *Circ Res* 1969;24:51–60.
25. Medical Research Council Working Party: Long term domiciliary oxygen therapy in chronic cor pulmonale complicating chronic bronchitis and emphysema. *Lancet* 1981;1:681–685.
26. Nocturnal Oxygen Therapy Group: Continuous or nocturnal oxygen therapy in hypoxemic chronic obstructive lung disease. *Ann Intern Med* 1980;93: 391–398.
27. Petty TL: Home oxygen in advanced chronic obstructive lung disease. *Med Clin North Am* 1981; 65:615–627.
28. Mathur PH, Powles P, Pugsley S, et al: Effect of digoxin on right ventricular function in severe chronic airflow obstruction: A controlled clinical trial. *Ann Intern Med* 1981;95:283–288.
29. Turino GM, Goldring RM, Hememann HO: Water, electrolytes, and acid–base relationships in chronic cor pulmonale. *Prog Cardiovasc Dis* 1970; 12:467–483.
30. Weiss AB, Moschos CB, Frank MJ, et al: Hemodynamic effects of staged hematocrit reduction in patients with stable cor pulmonale and

severely elevated hematocrit levels. *Am J Med* 1975;58:92–98.
31. Chetty KG, Brown SE, Light RW: Improved exercise tolerance of the polycythemic lung patient following phlebotomy. *Am J Med* 1983;74:415–420.
32. Parker JO, Kelkar K, West RO: Hemodynamic effects of aminophylline in cor pulmonale. 1966;33:17–29.
33. Matthay RA, Berger HJ, Loke J, et al: Effects of aminophylline upon right and left ventricular performance in chronic obstructive pulmonary disease: Noninvasive assessment by radionuclide angiocardiography. *Am J Med* 1978;65:903–910.
34. Brent BN, Mahler D, Berger HJ, et al: Augmentation of right ventricular performance in chronic obstructive pulmonary disease by terbutaline: A combined radionuclide and hemodynamic study. *Am J Cardiol* 1982;50:313–319.
35. Teule GJJ, Majid PA: Haemodynamic effects of terbutaline in chronic obstructive airways disease. *Thorax* 1980;35:536–542.
36. Lupi-Herrera E, Bialostozky D, Sobrino A: The role of isoproterenol in pulmonary artery hypertension of unknown etiology (primary). *Chest* 1981;79:292–296.
37. Honey M, Cotter L, Davies H, et al: Clinical and haemodynamic effects of diazoxide in primary pulmonary hypertension. *Thorax* 1980;35:269–276.
38. Chick TW, Kochukoshy KN, Matsumoto S, et al: The effect of nitroglycerin on gas exchange, hemodynamics, and oxygen transport in patients with chronic obstructive pulmonary disease. *Am J Med Sci* 1978;276:105–111.
39. Wood BA, Tortoledo F, Luck JC, et al: Rapid attenuation of response to nifedipine in primary pulmonary hypertension. *Chest* 1982;82:793–794.

CHAPTER 27
Cardiomyopathy in the Elderly Patient

H. Malcolm Hodkinson

The term cardiomyopathy has been variously used, some authors such as Goodwin[1] restricting its use to those examples where there is no known cause for the heart muscle disease, while many others use cardiomyopathy to include heart muscle disorders of known cause and those occurring in association with known diseases.

In this account, cardiomyopathy will be used in this wider sense to refer to heart muscle pathology other than that resulting from hypertension, ischemic heart disease, or occurring in association with valvular disease or with other structural abnormalities of the heart or great vessels.

Cardiomyopathies may be subdivided into two principal types: hypertrophic obstructive cardiomyopathy (HOCM) and congestive cardiomyopathy (COCM). HOCM includes idiopathic hypertrophic subaortic stenosis as a subtype but obstruction, though a common finding, is not an essential feature of HOCM where the basic defect is impairment of ventricular filling in diastole. In contrast, COCM is characterized by failure of the ventricle to empty adequately during systole. HOCM and COCM appear to be quite distinct pathologic conditions which do not overlap with each other. Together, they account for almost all the cases of CM which are diagnosed in developed countries such as Britain.[2] However, though an occasional case of cardiomyopathy may be of the restrictive type, eg, that of secondary amyloidosis, the obliterative type of cardiomyopathy is very rarely seen outside the tropics.[3]

HOCM IN OLD AGE

HOCM is a relatively rare condition at any age but a substantial proportion of cases are diagnosed in the elderly.[3-6] The only difference from younger cases lies in the much lower proportion of the elderly who have a family history of the disease. Thus, whereas perhaps a third of younger patients have a positive family history, this was obtained in only one of the 15 patients over 60 in the series of Pomerance and Davies.[6] They also noted that only two patients had had the diagnosis of HOCM made in life while five were instances of sudden death and seven an unexpected postmortem finding. This suggests that HOCM is substantially underdiagnosed in elderly patients. However, even with allowance for this, the disease is uncommon in the elderly patient, no examples being found in two substantial postmortem series which were specifically directed toward cardiac pathology in old age.[7-8]

The pathology of HOCM consists of gross left ventricular hypertrophy with a small ventricular cavity. The etiology is unknown. The familial tendency suggests that an underlying genetic predisposition is important in its etiology but no evidence of a HLA antigen association has been demonstrated.[9] A variety of histologic and histochemical changes have been reported. Most characteristic of these are severe myofiber hypertrophy with whorling and an increase in glycogen while electron microscopy shows myofibrillar disarray.[10] Unfortunately, none of these changes appear to be entirely specific.

There is no effective medical treatment but surgical treatment can be beneficial where there is an appreciable obstructive element and recent reports indicate that good results can be obtained even when patients are elderly.[5,11]

COCM IN THE ELDERLY

COCM is characterized pathologically by gross dilatation of the heart which may often mask an accompanying moderate degree of left ventricular hypertrophy. There seems little doubt that COCM may represent a common end-stage of ventricular muscle damage from a wide range of different pathologic insults. These causes may or may not be clearly identifiable.

Infections

The dividing line between COCM and myocarditis is somewhat arbitrary and there seems little doubt that an infective myocarditis can progress to COCM even though such an evolution is not often clearly documented. A wide variety of infections can result in myocarditis and are thus at least possible causes of COCM. The range of such infective agents includes viruses, bacteria, rickettsiae, fungi, spirochetes, and protozoa. A full listing is provided by Hudson.[12] However, particular interest has attached to group B coxsackieviruses, for patients with apparently idiopathic COCM have a considerable excess of high antibody titers to B types 1 through 5 when their sera are compared with those of age- and sex-matched controls.[13] This is particularly seen where the disease is of more recent onset.

Autoimmune Damage

Immunofluorescent antibodies have been demonstrated in 40% of patients with idiopathic COCM, antibodies being detectable either in the serum or in the heart muscle obtained at biopsy.[14] This raises the possibility of some form of autoimmune damage though other etiologic factors, such as viral infection, for example, might well be responsible for triggering this.

Other Causes

There are many other occasional causes of COCM which have been recognized, and again Hudson[12] may be consulted for a reasonably comprehensive listing. These include such causes as hemochromatosis, siderosis, oxalosis and a wide variety of other inborn errors of metabolism. Cardiomyopathy may also occur in more generalized neuromuscular disorders such as Friedreich's ataxia, myotonia atrophica, and the myopathies. Toxic drugs and chemicals may also be responsible, cobalt as an additive in beers being a particularly well-documented example. However, though of considerable academic interest, none of these causes are of particular relevance to cardiomyopathy in old age where they would appear to account for only a tiny minority of cases.

SENILE CARDIAC AMYLOIDOSIS

Senile cardiac amyloidosis is probably the commonest form of cardiomyopathy in old age that can be recognized clearly. Many series have reported high postmortem prevalences, eg, our own study[8] showing it to be present in almost half of the hearts of geriatric patients. However, the extent of the amyloidosis was variable: in 22.5% of the series it amounted only to scanty atrial deposits while there were more extensive atrial deposits in 11%, and in 16% both the atria and ventricles were involved. We found a significant association with rising age and there was also a less striking female preponderance. In 31 patients over 90 years old, 84% had evidence of senile cardiac amyloidosis. A significant independent association between amyloidosis and cardiac failure was demonstrable at all grades of involvement excepting those with only scanty atrial deposits. Senile cardiac amyloidosis thus emerges as a clinically important type of heart muscle disease in old age and, with its association with heart failure, must rank as far and away the most frequent cause of COCM in old age. Indeed it may prove to be the commonest cause overall when all age groups are considered together.

The association with cardiac failure is a strong one. Indeed, senile cardiac amyloidosis, ischemic heart disease, and atrial fibrillation proved to be the main three independent factors predicting the presence of heart failure in the series.[15] However, more recent work suggests that there may be two quite separate types of senile cardiac amyloidosis.[16] Histochemical evidence suggests that there is a type confined to the atria with no associated deposits in other organs and which does not stain histochemically for tryptophan. The authors term this isolated atrial amyloidosis (IAA). In contrast, the second type, which they term generalized senile cardiac amyloidosis (SCA), occurs in both atria and ventricles and shows positive histochemical staining for tryptophan. Only in this second type where the ventricles are involved are there associated deposits in other organs. These consist of small deposits in the aorta, pulmonary vessels, and pulmonary alveolar septa and infrequently small scattered foci in small and medium-sized arteries elsewhere.[8,16] Clearly, if this distinction between two types is confirmed, the relationship of each type to cardiac failure and to atrial fibrillation will need to be re-examined. However, the earlier finding,[8] that scanty atrial deposits showed no association with either cardiac failure or atrial fibrillation while heavy atrial deposits or the combination of atrial and ventricular deposits did with both, would suggest that the IAA type may have no clinical significance while SCA does.

Amyloid of the SCA type has now been shown to contain a specific protein component, AScI[17] but this cannot be demonstrated in fibrils derived from deposits of the IAA type.[16] This protein has been partially characterized and has been shown to have peptic residues exhibiting sequence identity with prealbumin.[18] Interestingly, only one other form of amyloid has been found to have a relationship to prealbumin, the Portuguese familial Andrade type, but this latter can be immunostained with prealbumin antisera whereas the SCA type cannot. The SCA type of amyloid would thus appear to be unique and is quite distinct from that of senile plaques, pancreatic islet amyloid, myeloma-associated amyloid, amyloid of endocrine origin ("apudamyloid"), or classical secondary amyloidosis.[17] The amounts of amyloid deposited in the heart in SCA are modest so that there may be little or no hypertrophy. COCM results rather than the restrictive cardiomyopathy which is the consequence of the much heavier deposits in secondary amyloidosis which may occasionally be seen in elderly patients.

The underlying causes of either type of senile cardiac amyloidosis are as yet unknown. Nor at the present time is it possible to make the diagnosis in life given that cardiac biopsy could not be justified. Isotopic imaging might be possible but an extremely specific agent would be necessary in view of the generally small amounts of amyloid present.

ALCOHOLIC CARDIOMYOPATHY

Alcoholism is a common problem within the geriatric age group in many communities. Alcohol is now well recognized as an important cause of heart muscle disease and therefore needs to be actively considered as a cause of cardiomyopathy in old age. However, there have been no specific studies of alcoholic cardiomyopathy in the elderly and its prevalence is not properly known.

Typically, alcoholic cardiomyopathy develops against the background of many years of heavy drinking – generally in excess of 10 years. It is the amount of alcohol consumed rather than the form in which it is consumed which appears to be important, for the condition is seen in spirit, wine, beer, and cider drinkers alike. Onset of the cardiomyopathy may be insidious or sudden and is of the COCM type. Arrythmias are a common accompaniment and in particular many elderly patients develop atrial fibrillation.[19] Tachycardia is a very common feature.

Alcoholic cardiomyopathy is quite different from beriberi heart and from the cobalt cardiomyopathy described in beer drinkers, related to its addition to certain beers in the past as a frothing agent. It appears to represent a direct toxic effect of alcohol on the heart, though this may well be mediated through its first metabolite, acetaldehyde.[20] Acutely, alcohol gives rise to loss of intracellular constituents such as potassium, phosphate, magnesium, and enzymes. Free fatty acid levels are increased and the uptake of triglycerides by ventricular muscle is reduced. Mitochondrial damage and reduced myofibrillar adenosine triphosphatase (ATPase) activity are demonstrable.[20]

In the earlier stages of the disease the changes are reversible if alcohol intake ceases. Unfortunately, if drinking of alcohol continues the disease progresses and becomes irreversible, the prognosis then being quite as adverse as for other forms of COCM.[19] It is therefore of considerable practical importance that alcoholic cardiomyopathy should be recognized at the earliest possible time and that strenuous efforts are then made to persuade the patient to stop drinking.

SENILE CARDIOMYOPATHY

Are there other forms of cardiomyopathy related to the aging process itself? Burch[21] suggests that there may be a specific senile cardiomyopathy. However, he appears to be using the term to represent the general decline in cardiac reserve with age, comparable to the physiologic declines seen with age in other organ systems, rather than to any identifiable pathologic entity. He states that published studies of heart disease in old age have concentrated upon the demonstrable pathologic changes such as ischemic heart disease, valvular pathology, and the like, and have ignored the possibility of some more subtle yet perhaps widespread aging effect. This is a valid criticism, for while a great deal of recognizable pathology may be found in elderly hearts[7] and though cardiac failure may perhaps arise because of a summation of multiple pathologies which could individually be regarded as trivial in some patients, there remain other elderly patients in whom there is no demonstrable cardiac abnormality to account for heart failure.[15] Indeed, this series found no cardiac abnormalities in 14 of 71 hearts at autopsy from patients with cardiac failure and none of these 14 had atrial fibrillation nor other obvious extracardiac causes of heart failure such as thyrotoxicosis, chronic obstructive airways disease, or anemia. The possibility of there being hitherto unrecognized age-associated cardiomyopathies is thus a reasonably convincing one which is supported by their finding that age itself was an independent predictor of atrial fibrillation in combination with ischemic heart disease, senile cardiac amyloidosis, and mitral valve disease.[15] However, it did not make an independent contribution to the prediction of heart failure in combination with atrial fibrillation, senile cardiac amyloidosis, and ischemic heart disease in a multiple logistic analysis.

HOW IMPORTANT ARE THE CARDIOMYOPATHIES IN OLD AGE?

Senile cardiac amyloidosis is a form of cardiomyopathy which is extremely common in old age and which does appear to have serious consequences or at any rate associations. Such patients have a highly significant excess both of cardiac failure and of atrial fibrillation.[8] The prevalence of other cardiomyopathies in old age is far less certain. Certainly HOCM is something of a rarity but COCM is probably very much underdiagnosed. Alcoholic cardiomyopathy in particular is probably very often overlooked—an important error in view of its favorable prognosis if alcohol intake ceases. The possibility of other cardiomyopathies, perhaps including a specific senile cardiomyopathy, contributing to the development of cardiac failure in elderly patients must be seriously entertained. However, given our present inability to treat these, this is a somewhat academic matter though warranting further careful study.

REFERENCES

1. Goodwin GF: Hypertrophic cardiomyopathy: A disease in search of its own identity. *Am J Cardiol* 1980;45:177–180.
2. Goodwin GF, Oakley CM: The cardiomyopathies. *Br Heart J* 1972;34:545–552.
3. Pomerance A, Davies MJ: The pathology of the heart. Oxford, Blackwell Scientific Publications, 1975, pp 211–250.
4. Krasnow N, Stein RA: Hypertrophic cardiomyopathy in the aged. *Am Heart J* 1978;96:326–336.
5. Koch J-P, Maron BJ, Epstein SE, et al: Results of operation for obstructive hypertrophic cardiomyopathy in the elderly. *Am J Cardiol* 1980;46:963–966.
6. Pomerance A, Davies MJ: Pathological features of hypertrophic obstructive cardiomyopathy (HOCM) in the elderly. *Br Heart J* 1975;37:305–312.
7. Pomerance A: Pathology of the heart with and without cardiac failure in the elderly. *Br Heart J* 1965;27:697–710.
8. Hodkinson HM, Pomerance A: The clinical significance of senile cardiac amyloidosis: A prospective clinico-pathological study. *Q J Med* 1977;46:381–387.
9. Mourant AJ, Kafetz KM, Brigden WW, et al: HLA antigen associations in hypertrophic cardiomyopathy. *Tissue Antigens* 1982;20:389–393.
10. Olsen EGJ: The pathology of the cardiomyopathies: A critical analysis. *Am Heart J* 1979;98: 385–392.
11. Kafetz K: Surgical treatment of hypertrophic obstructive cardiomyopathy in the elderly. *Postgrad Med J* 1981;57:604–606.
12. Hudson REB: The cardiomyopathies: Order from chaos. *Am J Cardiol* 1970;25:70–77.
13. Waterson AP: Virological investigation of congestive cardiomyopathy. *Postgrad Med J* 1978;54:505–507.
14. Bolte H-D, Grothey K: Cardiomyopathies related to immunological processes, in Riecker G, Weber A, Goodwin J (eds): *Myocardial Failure*. Berlin, Springer-Verlag, 1977, pp 266–290.
15. Hodkinson HM, Pomerance A: The clinical pathology of heart failure and atrial fibrillation in old age. *Postgrad Med J* 1979;55:251–254.
16. Westermark P, Johansson B, Natvig JB: Senile cardiac amyloidosis: Evidence of two different amyloid substances in the aging heart. *Scand J Immunol* 1979;10:303–308.
17. Cornwell GG, Westermark P: Senile amyloidosis: A protean manifestation of the aging process. *J Clin Pathol* 1980;33:1146–1152.
18. Sletten K, Westermark P, Natvig JB: Senile cardiac amyloidosis is related to prealbumin. *Scand J Immunol* 1980;12:503–506.
19. Brigden W: Alcoholic cardiomyopathy. *Br J Hosp Med* 1977;12:122–125.
20. Goodwin JF: Alcohol and the heart: Alcoholic cardiomyopathy. *J Roy Coll Physicians Lond* 1977;12: 5–11.
21. Burch GE: Senile cardiomyopathy. *J Am Geriatr Soc* 1982;30:642–644.

CHAPTER 28
Mitral Annulus Calcification in the Elderly

Marcello Mellino

Calcific mitral annulus degeneration is frequently demonstrated with current echocardiographic technics, particularly in the elderly population.[1-4] This has enabled the clinician to study this interesting condition with a noninvasive and objective approach, thus rediscovering the important clinical implications of such a "disease".[5-7] Mitral annulus calcification (MAC) has been termed by D'Cruz et al[8] "subvalvular mitral annulus calcification" on the basis of their two-dimensional echocardiographic experience. In a recent study[9] we have suggested "perivalvular mitral valve degeneration" as a more descriptive and less limiting term. This term indicates that the calcific process is frequently *not* localized in the mitral annulus proper but more commonly below and around this structure as well as on the subvalvular endocardium. As the condition progresses the calcific deposition subsequently extends toward the true annulus creating a rigid and irregular structure. Such controversy is clinically not important. No significant differences in clinical presentation and its consequences have been reported between true annular and subvalvular calcification. MAC, although a misnomer, is a widely accepted term and it will be used throughout this paper, keeping in mind its spectrum of anatomical localizations.

PATHOLOGY

This calcific disease is a degenerative condition which begins at first in one of several mitral perivalvular locations. Initially this presents as a fibrosclerotic structure which subsequently becomes diffusely calcified. MAC has been reported in 8% to 13% of autopsies on elderly patients.[10-12] The prevalence of MAC is higher in females than in males. Pomerance[11] reported MAC in 11.5% of females and in 4.6% of males. Geill[12] found MAC in 9.4% and 2.7%, respectively. More frequent and greater amount of calcification is generally seen with increasing age with a predilection for females. Pomerance[11] demonstrated MAC in 8.5% of patients over 50 years of age. A marked correlation with age was found particularly in women who had a prevalence of MAC of 3.2% when under 70 years and of 43.5% when over 90 years. No valid explanations account for such sex predilection: infectious, hormonal, and trauma-mediated[13,14] mechanisms have been considered as well as derangements of calcium metabolism.[15]

Several authors[16] have described the distinctive pathologic features of MAC. Pathologic evidence of previous inflammation or of infectious processes is usually absent. The gross appearance is that of a ring or more commonly a U- or J-shaped rigid bar (Figure 28-1). This is usually localized below the posteromedial mitral leaflet, protruding toward the left ventricular cavity, often pushing the leaflet upward and stretching the chordae tendineae.[16,17] Because of their displacement, the involved leaflets may lose their mobility, although histologically they remain normal, differently from rheumatic valvulitis.[16] Small calcific spurs can at times project from the annulus toward the adjacent septal myocardium containing vital portions of the conduction system. The combination of displaced and less mobile leaflets with loss of the physiologic "sphincter" action of the mitral annulus due to calcification causes mitral regurgitation.[4,18]

PATHOPHYSIOLOGY

We have recently evaluated the angiographic presence of mitral regurgitation in patients with

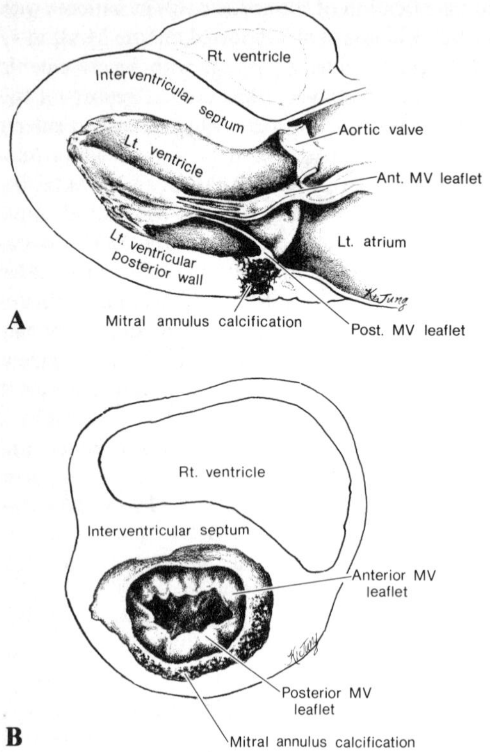

Figure 28-1 **A** Representation of mitral annulus calcification as seen along a long-axis view. **B** Same on a short-axis view. (Reproduced with permission from Mellino and Salcedo.[9])

echocardiographically demonstrated MAC[6] (Table 28-1). Previous observations[16] confirm the significant correlation between more severe degree of MAC and the presence of mitral regurgitation. Long-standing mitral insufficiency caused primarily by this process can lead to a hemodynamically severe disturbance with marked left ventricular dysfunction.

Heart failure is a common feature of patients with MAC. Clinically it is difficult to justify its onset simply on the basis of severe malfunction of the mitral annulus. Pomerance[19] demonstrated MAC in 45% of elderly patients with well-documented heart failure, second only to ischemic heart disease as a demonstrable etiology. In most patients, however, heart failure was multifactorial: in only 3% was MAC the only abnormality found.

In 60 patients[19a] the length of MAC was 12.5 ± 10.3 mm in males and 31.8 mm ± 23.5 mm in females with a highly positive correlation between its length and cross-sectional diameter, which was usually up to 10 mm. The location of MAC was typically posterior, as previously described by others.[10–12,16] Patients with thicker calcification demonstrated a significantly higher tendency toward anterior extension of this process.

A "circular" type of MAC has been occasionally reported,[16,20] usually in patients with massive degree of calcification and mostly in elderly females with congestive heart failure. These patients have hemodynamically significant mitral insufficiency and at times evidence of a diastolic mitral valve gradient as seen in rheumatic mitral stenosis. Contrary to what was initially believed, recent reports clearly suggest that heavy MAC can produce mitral stenosis, which may be severe enough to warrant mitral valve replacement.[21,22]

PATHOGENESIS

The average age of patients with MAC as reported in pathologic or clinico-echocardiographic studies (Table 28-2) does not clearly indicate when the process actually begins. This sclerocalcific, noninflammatory process might begin with scattered calcific foci within or below the posterior mitral annulus around the fourth decade of life. During the subsequent three to four decades a small group of patients develops progressively a higher degree of calcification. The asymptomatic patient with mild MAC might only be discovered at autopsy although by means of echocardiography we can now detect the earliest stages of this disorder before death. Patients with more severe MAC are more likely to develop clinical manifestations such as congestive heart failure, atrial fibrillation, and conduction problems, or to demonstrate associated aortic valve disease. They will likely come to the clinician's attention earlier, by means of radiographic or echocardiographic technics.[3,5–7] Certain "predisposing factors" have been suggested as favoring or leading to the development and progression of MAC. Some conditions cause increased and sustained "systolic stress" on the mitral valve apparatus such as systemic hyperten-

Table 28-1
Relationship of Mitral Annulus Calcification (MAC) and Left Atrial Dimensions (LA) to Mitral Regurgitation (MR)*

	No. of Patients	MAC	LA
MR	10	8.6 ± 2.3 mm	5.0 cm
No MR	14	6.1 ± 2.1 mm	4.2 cm
Total	24	$P < 0.02$	$P < 0.05$

Reproduced with permission from Mellino et al.[6]
*MR detected by angiography.

sion, hypertrophic cardiomyopathy, and valvular aortic stenosis.

Since most patients with MAC are in the age group with a significant incidence of hypertensive cardiovascular disease, it is difficult to prove an association between systemic hypertension and MAC. Fulkerson et al[5] found significant hypertension in 46% of their patients. Most other studies[1,4,6] have reported hypertension in 20% to 30% of patients with MAC. No conclusive studies have been done correlating controlled and uncontrolled hypertensive subjects with the development and progression of MAC. Hypertension and MAC appear to be coincidental occurrences rather than being causally related.

An interesting relation exists between aortic valvular stenosis and MAC. Several authors[1,3,5,6] have recognized an increased incidence of sclerosis or calcification of the aortic cusps in patients with MAC. Roberts et al[23] reported diffuse MAC in 17 of 21 (81%) elderly patients with severe calcific aortic valve stenosis. Most studies report on the incidence of calcific aortic valve disease in elderly patients with MAC. No data is available in relation to the prevalence of MAC in aortic valve disease patients of younger age. Mellino et al[6] have demonstrated significantly thicker MAC in patients with echographic evidence of aortic valve calcification. A recent study (Mellino et al, unpublished data) of 98 patients who underwent cardiac catheterization demonstrates more prominent MAC in older patients with angiographic evidence of aortic valve calcification. A group of patients with angiographically documented coronary atherosclerosis had significant correlations between MAC and coronary calcification (Table 28-3). It is

Table 28-2
Summary of Published Series of Patients with MAC

		No. of Patients	F/M	Mean Age (yr)
Gabor et al[1]	(E)	40	32/8	73
Schott et al[4]	(E)	41	30/11	63
Fulkerson et al[5]	(E)	80		73
Mellino et al[6]	(E)	123	85/38	70
Zoneraich et al[7]	(E)	65	43/22	75
D'Cruz et al[8]	(E)	84	67/17	74
Korn et al[16]	(P)	14	14/0	75
Rytand and Lipstich[18]	(P)	10	7/3	72
Nair et al[29]	(E)	68	41/27	68
Kronzon et al[33]	(E)	18	10/8	68
Curati et al[39]	(E)	21	17/4	70
Tanabe and Ibrahim[32a]	(E)	18	14/4	72
Nair et al[30a]	(E)	104	55/49	70
Simon and Liu[40]	(P)	59	36/23	69
Sugiura et al[19a]	(P)	60	40/20	82
		805		71.6

Abbreviations: E = echocardiographic study, P = pathologic study, F/M = female/male ratio.

Table 28-3
Severity of MAC Determined by M-mode Echocardiography Among 98 Patients Undergoing Cardiac Catheterization

A)	Age <60 yr	MAC	Age >60 yr	MAC
	F	6.1 ± 1.6 mm	F	6.6 ± 1.9 mm
	M	6.0 ± 1.8 mm	M	7.8 ± 2.5 mm
	F AS/AI	6.1 ± 1.6 mm	F AS/AI	6.6 ± 1.9 mm
	M AS/AI	6.0 ± 1.8 mm	M AS/AI	7.8 ± 2.5 mm
B)	− Ca	MAC	+ Ca	MAC
	− Ca AV	5.8 ± 1.7 mm	+ Ca AV	6.9 ± 2.0 mm
	CAD(F)	6.6 ± 2.0 mm	CAD(F)	6.9 ± 2.2 mm
	CAD(M)	5.2 ± 0.8 mm	CAD(M)	7.5 ± 2.4 mm

Abbreviations: Ca/AV = aortic valve calcification (+) present or (−) absent angiographically, AS/AI = aortic valve stenosis (AS) or aortic insufficiency (AI) determined angiographically, CAD/Ca = patients with presence of coronary atherosclerosis with (+ Ca) or without (− Ca) coronary calcification determined angiofluoroscopically.
Unpublished data from Mellino et al.

likely that MAC is part of a diffuse calcific process related to aging. This is at first localized at or below the mitral annular region. Subsequently, it gradually spreads across the fibrous skeleton of the heart to involve the aortic valve in those patients who have higher degree of annular calcification.

We found 6 patients with hypertrophic cardiomyopathy among 123 subjects with echocardiographic demonstration of MAC,[6] and 5 among 98 patients with MAC who underwent cardiac catheterization. Fulkerson et al[5] demonstrated this condition in approximately 6% of their patients with MAC. Kronzon et al[24] have reported 16 patients (24%) with MAC among 68 patients with hypertrophic cardiomyopathy. They observed that the patients with MAC were significantly older and they found a higher incidence of MAC among elderly patients with hypertrophic cardiomyopathy when compared with patients undergoing cardiac catheterization for other reasons. It is unlikely that patients with MAC have a higher incidence of hypertrophic cardiomyopathy as suggested by Kronzon et al,[24] but elderly subjects with hypertrophic cardiomyopathy might have a higher than normal incidence of MAC. Most studies on hypertrophic cardiomyopathy[25,26] have rarely mentioned the concomitant presence of MAC, perhaps because younger patients are commonly included. The long-standing elevation of left ventricular intracavitary pressure in patients with hypertrophic cardiomyopathy might account for increased lipid deposition in the mitral ring with subsequent calcification.

Mitral valve prolapse has been reported in patients with MAC.[5,27] Occasional reports of young patients with Marfan's syndrome and MAC have also appeared.[28] Fulkerson et al[5] noted that the group of patients with mitral valve prolapse and MAC were significantly younger than patients with MAC alone. They also had a higher incidence of significant mitral regurgitation and atrial fibrillation. Other studies of patients with MAC and associated rheumatic heart disease or chronic renal failure, have reported that these patients are also relatively younger than patients with MAC alone. Mitral valve prolapse, chronic renal failure, and rheumatic heart disease are likely true "predisposing factors" in the development of MAC, causing in different ways acceleration of this degenerative process and its earlier clinical manifestation.

SYMPTOMATOLOGY

No symptom is characteristic of MAC. The history is closely related to the onset of clinical complications due to MAC. Progressive heart failure will lead to dyspnea, orthopnea, and eventually symptoms of low cardiac output. The onset of atrial fibrillation or of high-degree conduction problems could aggravate heart failure. Presyncope and syncopal attacks are usually caused by the development of atrioventricular block. Retinal, cerebral, or systemic embolism is an uncommon complication of MAC. Infectious endocarditis can present with numerous and often misleading symptoms. Patients with MAC, often with associated calcific aortic valve, may develop infectious endocarditis. Whenever the symptoms are suggestive such patients should be carefully evaluated and multiple blood cultures obtained. Angina pectoris is usually due to associated coronary atherosclerosis and less commonly to aortic stenosis or insufficiency or to hypertrophic cardiomyopathy.

PHYSICAL EXAMINATION

The clinical manifestations of MAC are numerous. Most patients have apical systolic murmurs of variable quality and intensity, usually suggestive of mitral insufficiency or of aortic valve sclerosis or stenosis. A precise correlation between auscultatory characteristics of such murmurs and underlying mitral annular pathology is usually difficult because elderly patients often have similar murmurs due to ischemic papillary muscle or chordae dysfunction. A left lower parasternal or apical murmur is usually consistent with predominant posteromedial leaflet dysfunction with related mitral insufficiency, whereas an apical pansystolic murmur radiating to the left axillary region is more likely due to more extensive MAC with diffuse malfunction of both mitral leaflets.

Pomerance[11] and Sigiura et al[19a] mentioned systolic murmurs in 55% and 45% of their patients. We have found presence of systolic murmurs in 90% of our patients.[6] The higher prevalence is explained by the high incidence of severe MAC among our patients: 67% of 123 subjects had MAC of more than 5 mm in thickness, defined as "moderate to severe." Greater than 70% incidence of systolic murmurs has been reported by others[4,5,11] in severe MAC. The importance of MAC as a major cause of systolic murmurs in the elderly has been suggested by Pomerance.[13] In an autopsy study on subjects with known systolic murmurs, 48% showed MAC as the only or the predominant cardiac lesion. In contrast, calcification of the aortic valve was the predominant lesion in less than 20% of patients.

There appears to be a close correlation between increasing amount of calcium deposition on the mitral annulus and mitral insufficiency, even though only 50% to 60% of patients with MAC and systolic apical murmurs have angiographically demonstrable mitral insufficiency. Angiographic data in 24 patients with MAC (Table 28-1) revealed mitral insufficiency in 10 subjects with echocardiographically thicker MAC.

RADIOGRAPHIC EVALUATION

Prior to the availability of echocardiography, fluoroscopy was the only method for detection of MAC in vivo.[18] Chest films occasionally demonstrate MAC (Figure 28-2) as a J or U or inverted C calcific shape in the mitral region. The ability to detect MAC by chest roentgenography is minimal. We found that only 4% of 123 patients with echocardiographically demonstrated MAC showed MAC on chest film.[6] Others have reported similar results.[1,4]

Only a severe degree of MAC is recognized by routine chest film, while fluoroscopy is a more sensitive technic, although it does not provide the clinician with an objective, reproducible, or retrievable record. We found an excellent correlation between the amount of MAC measured by echocardiography and the amount seen on fluoroscopy.[9] The severity of MAC measured echocardiographically increased significantly among groups with fluoroscopically more severe MAC. If fluoroscopy is the most precise method for diagnosis of MAC, as suggested by Fulkerson et al,[5] our data demonstrate that the echocardiographic severity of this process is comparable to its fluoroscopic severity. In four patients with normal fluoroscopic examination and mild degree of MAC by M-mode echocardiography, two-dimensional echocardiography showed abnormal echoes in or below the mitral annular region as seen in the other patients with fluoroscopically demonstrated MAC, but of lesser degree.[9] These abnormal echoes could correspond to "precalcific lesions," perhaps an earlier stage in the development of more severe calcific annular lesions.

Normal fluoroscopy has not been reported in patients with severe MAC. We[6] and others[2-4] believe that M-mode echocardiography is extremely reliable in diagnosing MAC. There is no clear advantage in routinely examining such patients by fluoroscopy. If a false-positive echocardiographic diagnosis is made, this usually involves patients with a very limited amount of calcification of no clinical significance.

ECG FINDINGS

Most large clinical reports[4,5-7] have mentioned significant abnormalities of the conduction system in 25% to 50% of patients with MAC, often requiring a permanent pacemaker. High-degree atrioventricular (AV) block, often with syncopal or presyncopal episodes, is a frequent presentation.[18,29] Rytand[18] and others[30] have reported occasional cases of complete heart block

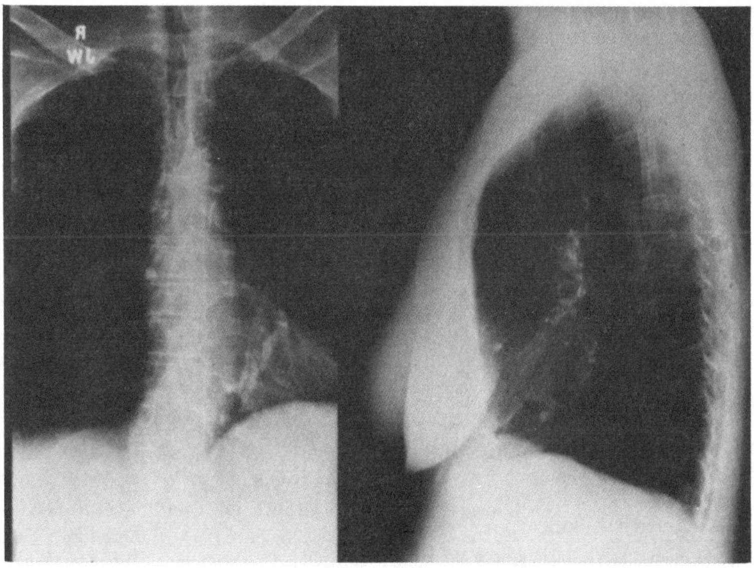

Figure 28-2 Chest film demonstrating mitral annulus calcification.

caused by calcification in the mitral annular region. This was usually extensive, encroaching the portion of the conduction system located medially to the calcified annulus within the interventricular septum. Calcific spurs have been noted to involve the interventricular septum, thereby increasing the chances of disruption of the conduction system. This could produce symptomatic bradyarrhythmias.

Of 123 patients studied by us[6] only 32 revealed a normal ECG (Table 28-4). Conduction problems were associated with significantly thicker MAC. Zoneraich et al[7] studied 65 patients with MAC and 65 matched controls, demonstrating in 23 with MAC the presence of conduction disturbances as compared to only 7 patients in the control group. Complete atrioventricular block necessitating a permanent pacemaker developed during hospitalization in 3 (4.6%) of the patients with MAC. Their study confirmed that focal disruption of the bundle of His with complete AV block can be caused by severe degree of MAC. Nair et al[30a] also demonstrated more frequent conduction disturbances in subjects with MAC than in controls. They did not find an increased incidence of conduction problems among patients with aortic valve calcification without MAC, nor in the group with "anterior" and "posterior" MAC, suggesting that a strategic localization of this process in the posteromedial aspect of the annulus is crucial for the development of heart block.

In a group of 68 patients with symptomatic bradyarrhythmias and with a permanent pacemaker,[29] of whom 59 (87%) had MAC, 23 (34%) had atrial fibrillation with slow ventricular response and 30 (44%) had intermittent sinus arrest. These are a common ECG presentation of patients with the sick sinus syndrome,[31] suggesting that patients with MAC frequently demonstrate a diffuse type of sclerodegenerative process which is not limited to or below the bundle of His. This concept is supported by the frequent demonstration of distal conduction disturbances in subjects with sick sinus syndrome.[32]

Atrial fibrillation has been reported in 25% to 40% of patients with MAC.[5-7] Multiple factors might be involved in the occurrence of atrial tachyarrhythmias in patients with MAC: (1) left atrial enlargement usually associated with mitral insufficiency; (2) diffuse sclerodegenerative abnormalities of the conduction system; (3) presence of heart failure and cardiac dilatation; (4) coronary atherosclerosis and myocardial ischemia; (5) systemic hypertension with left ventricular hypertrophy. Tanabe et al[32a] demonstrated significantly enlarged left atria in their patients with MAC, but this was not correlated with the presence of atrial arrhythmias. We[6] have demonstrated an echocardiographic correlation between significant degree of MAC, left atrial enlargement, and presence of atrial fibrillation. The 48 patients with atrial fibrillation revealed significantly thicker MAC and larger left atria than the patients in sinus rhythm (7.7 mm vs 6.3 mm and 5.0 cm vs 3.8 cm, respectively). In patients with heavy MAC, this correlation is probably mediated by the presence of mitral insufficiency and heart failure.

ECHOCARDIOGRAPHY

The M-mode echocardiographic appearance of MAC has been described in the recent literature.[1-4] MAC appears as a dense band of echoes of variable thickness localized behind the mitral

Table 28-4
Relation of MAC and Left Atrial Size to ECG Findings in 123 Patients

	No (%)	MAC (mean ± SD)	LA (mean ± SD)
Normal ECG	32 (26.0)	6.0 ± 2.1 mm	3.6 ± 0.7 cm
Abnormal ECG	91 (74.0)		
Atrial fibrillation	48 (39.0)	7.7 ± 2.4 mm	5.0 ± 1.0 cm
LVH	31 (25.2)	7.5 ± 2.4 mm	4.7 ± 0.9 cm
CLBBB	4 (3.2)	7.4 ± 2.4 mm (CLBBB through third-degree AV block)	4.7 ± 0.9 cm (CLBBB through third-degree AV block)
CRBBB	9 (7.3)		
LAHB	8 (6.5)		
CRBBB + LAHB	4 (3.2)		
First- and second-degree AV block	7 (5.6)		
Third-degree AV block	5 (4.0)		

Abbreviations: LVH = left ventricular hypertrophy, CLBBB = complete left bundle-branch block, CRBBB = complete right bundle-branch block, LAHB = left anterior hemiblock, LA = left atrial dimensions by M-mode echocardiography.

valve, at times obscuring the posterior leaflet. It is situated parallel and anterior to the endocardial surface of the left ventricular wall (Figure 28-3). A sweep from the left ventricular cavity to the aortic root and left atrial cavity will demonstrate sudden disappearance of the dense band of echoes at the AV junction. D'Cruz et al[3] and Zoneraich[7] had previously measured the severity of this calcific process by its echocardiographic thickness, but had not correlated the echocardiographic severity of MAC with its clinical or hemodynamic features. The echocardiographic quantification of the severity of MAC is of particular importance in relation to its clinical consequences. We have recently utilized M-mode echocardiography to study a large group of elderly patients with MAC.[6] Of 123 patients, 48% had evidence of congestive heart failure. Significant correlations were found between echographic severity of MAC and congestive heart failure. The mean MAC thickness for all patients was 6.9 mm and the mean left atrial size was 4.3 cm. In subjects with heart failure the MAC was 7.8 mm and the left atrium was 4.8 cm, whereas in patients without heart failure MAC was 6.1 mm and left atrial dimension 3.8 cm. MAC equal to or more than 5 mm (Table 28-5) was associated with the presence of heart failure, as well as with evidence of atrial fibrillation or diffuse conduction disease.

The echocardiographic quantification of MAC is valuable in relation to its possible complications. This could be also utilized as a prognostic indicator of onset of future complications. No

Table 28-5
Relation of MAC to Presence of Conduction Problems, Atrial Fibrillation, and Congestive Heart Failure

	MAC <5 mm	MAC >5 mm
Normal ECG	15	17
Conduction defects	4	21*
Sinus rhythm	33	42
Atrial fibrillation	8	40†
No congestive heart failure	31	33
Congestive heart failure	11	48‡

Chi-square test with Yates correction: $*P < 0.05$; $\dagger P < 0.01$; $\ddagger P < 0.001$.
Reproduced with permission from Mellino et al.[6]

prospective follow-up of patients with documented MAC is available to correlate the onset of conduction problems, heart failure, or significant valvular pathology with the severity of MAC. Also, further studies are needed to establish a direct comparison between the amount of MAC quantified echocardiographically and the amount measurable pathologically.

In the majority of patients the posterior calcification is not precisely in the annular region but "submitral" and localized in the angle between the posterior mitral leaflet and the left ventricular posterior wall. Kirk and Russell[10] had come to the

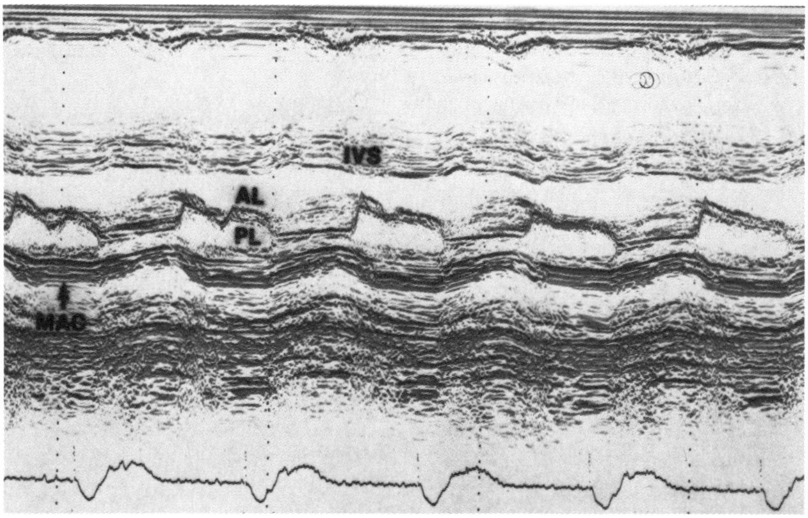

Figure 28-3 M-mode echocardiogram of patient with mitral annulus calcification (MAC). IVS = intraventricular septum, AL = anterior mitral leaflet, PL = posterior mitral leaflet. (Reproduced with permission from Mellino, M. et al.[6])

same conclusion, and more recent two-dimensional echocardiographic studies have further confirmed this.[9] Two-dimensional echocardiography offers a very precise and sensitive method for study of MAC (Figure 28-4). The advantages over M-mode echocardiography include better visualization of the contiguity of MAC with the conduction system, more precise definition of its extent, and better overall quantification of its severity.[33]

The mitral valve might exhibit several abnormalities related to the presence of MAC. Gabor et al[1] and others[2,3] demonstrated decreased diastolic anterior excursion of the anterior mitral leaflet. At times this is seen with decreased E-F slope of the anterior mitral leaflet but without thickening of the mitral leaflets, thus suggesting a nonrheumatic etiology for the mitral valve restriction. Few cases of MAC have been reported demonstrating a diastolic hemodynamic gradient across the mitral valve without documented rheumatic valvulitis.[21,22] All such cases had echocardiographically severe MAC which did not clearly involve the anterior region of the annulus. Roberts and Waller[20] studied two elderly females with "circular" MAC and found no evidence of diastolic gradient.

Anterior MAC usually is found only in patients with severe calcification. Utilizing M-mode echocardiography, anterior MAC can on occasion be differentiated with difficulty from echoes caused by a heavily calcified aortic root. The latter can create abnormal echoes anteriorly to the mitral leaflets and below the interventricular septum at the AV junction. Two-dimensional echocardiography more readily identifies anterior submitral calcification.[8] No clinical or hemodynamic consequences of anterior MAC have thus far been described. More detailed echocardiographic and angiographic observations of these patients might indicate a tendency toward mitral valve diastolic gradient. Abnormal anterior displacement of the mitral valve is also described with MAC.[3] Abnormal echoes originating from a heavily calcified aortic root can at times protrude toward the left ventricular cavity next to the interventricular septum, creating a confusing picture suggestive of hypertrophic cardiomyopathy.[3] Anterior displacement of the mitral valve with abnormal contiguity with the interventricular septum, decreased E-F slope of the anterior leaflet of the mitral valve, pseudoasymmetric septal hypertrophy and pseudosystolic anterior motion (SAM) of the mitral valve have also been described in patients with MAC.[3] However, few patients truly appear to have coexistent hypertrophic cardiomyopathy with indisputable echocardiographic criteria.

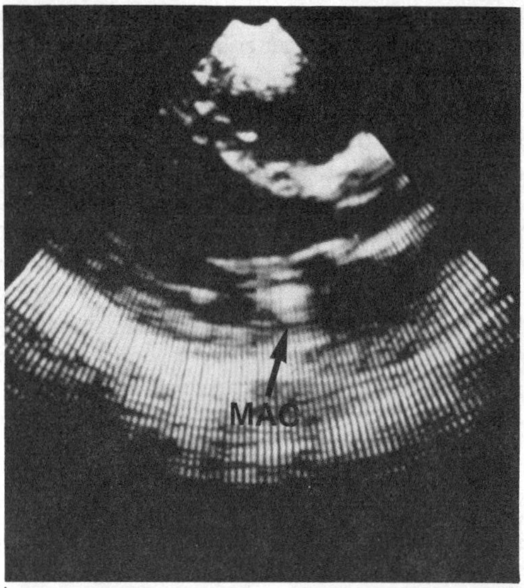

A

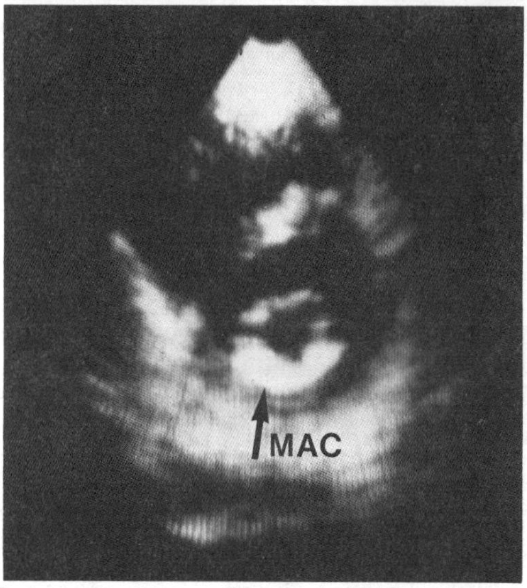

B

Figure 28-4 **A** Parasternal long-axis view of stop-frame photograph from a two-dimensional echocardiographic study of a patient with mitral annulus calcification (MAC). **B** Short-axis view.

Posterior pericardial effusion can be erroneously diagnosed if MAC is not correctly identified and its echoes felt to correspond to the posterior left ventricular wall. Consequently the clear space between MAC and the true posterior left ventricular wall could be erroneously interpreted as an "echo-free" space. Other echocardiographic findings in patients with MAC include left ventricular and left atrial enlargement and aortic valve sclerosis, stenosis, or evidence of aortic insufficiency (Figure 28-5).

ANGIOGRAPHY

There have been few angiographic reports on patients with MAC.[2,4] Most refer to unusual hemodynamic or clinical conditions associated with MAC. No large angiographic evaluation of patients with MAC is available, in spite of the potential value of such study in terms of quantification of mitral insufficiency as related to fluoroscopic and echocardiographic severity of MAC as well as evaluation of associated valvular, coronary, and myocardial function. The lack of such data is likely due to the advanced age of these patients.

MAC was not found among the etiologies of isolated, severe mitral insufficiency in a recently reported study of 97 patients undergoing mitral valve replacement.[34] Mitral valve prolapse was found in 60 (62%) of patients, who demonstrated a significantly increased mitral annular circumference (mean 13.4 cm) as compared with other patients. No mention was made of associated MAC in any of the groups reported.

We have evaluated 98 patients with MAC by angiography (Mellino et al, unpublished observations). Mitral insufficiency was found in 49 (50%) of patients, in whom MAC was significantly thicker when compared to patients without mitral insufficiency. These observations confirm a close relationship between severe MAC and mitral insufficiency as previously reported by clinicopathologic studies.[11]

The angiographic presence of calcific aortic stenosis in patients with MAC has been previously documented. Of 24 patients studied by Mellino et al, 37.5% had severe aortic valve gradient (mean 81 mmHg) and all required aortic valve replacement. Few reports of aortic valve replacement in elderly patients with MAC are available.[4,5] The presence of extensive calcification of the mitral and aortic annular regions is associated with conduction problems, endocarditis, and heart failure. This may increase the technical difficulties of implanting prosthetic valves in these patients.

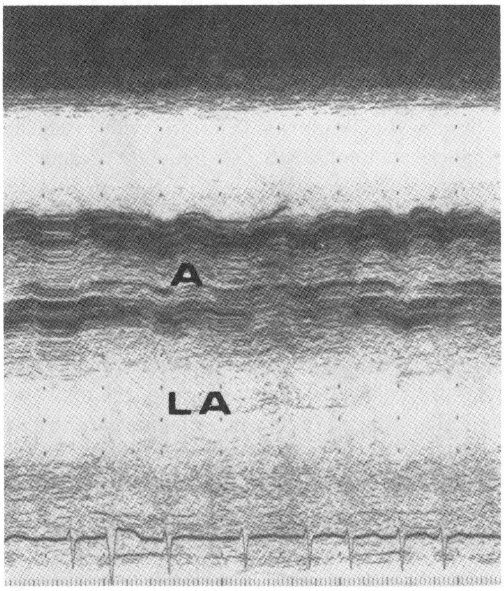

A

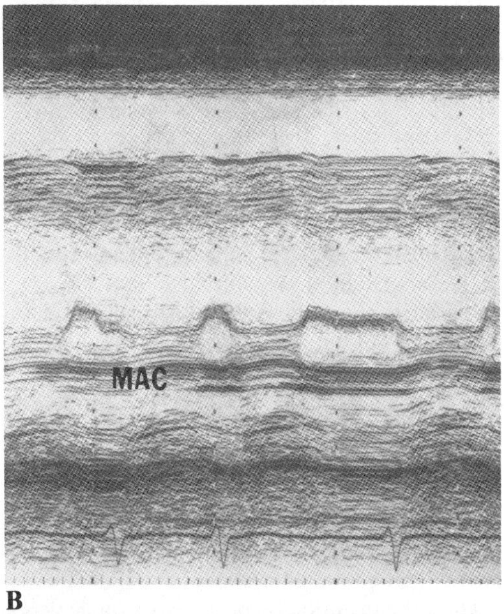

B

Figure 28-5 M-mode echocardiogram of a patient with calcific aortic stenosis, aortic insufficiency and mitral annulus calcification. A = aortic root, LA = left atrium, MAC = mitral annulus calcification.

ELECTROPHYSIOLOGY

Data available on a few patients with MAC who underwent electrophysiologic study[35] of the conduction system revealed a significant prolongation of the H-V interval among patients with complete heart block when compared with patients who had sick sinus syndrome. This observation, although limited, provides us with a better understanding of the mechanism of onset of symptomatic heart block in these patients. It suggests the need for close observation of elderly patients with MAC. A markedly prolonged H-V interval in subjects with chronic bifascicular or trifascicular block has been associated with a higher incidence of complete heart block and sudden death. Such events are strongly determined by the underlying presence of coronary or myocardial disease. Severe MAC with evidence of conduction problems in elderly patients presenting with intermittent dizzy spells or syncope could strongly suggest the possibility of intermittent high-degree AV block. The conduction impairment is probably related to disruption of the distal conduction system by the calcific process. Particularly when no neurologic or vascular process is demonstrable, electrophysiologic study of such patients revealing an H-V interval of more than 75 ms could justify the insertion of a permanent pacemaker.

CLINICAL IMPLICATIONS

Most large series[3,5,11,16] have reported a 50% to 60% prevalence of congestive heart failure among elderly patients with MAC. Multiple causes contribute to its development and rarely is MAC the only abnormality found.[28] The development of heart failure in patients with MAC is quite common; other concomitant factors are often involved, but MAC is usually extensive in these patients. Significant enlargement of the left ventricle and left atrium occurs more often in patients with MAC than among controls; many of such patients have heart failure.

Echocardiographic demonstration of more than 5-mm thickness significantly increases the possibility of presence of heart failure. Asymptomatic patients demonstrating MAC of more than 5-mm thickness, particularly if females and with ECG abnormalities related to the presence of MAC, should be followed closely since they might be at higher risk of developing heart failure or symptomatic conduction disturbances. This conclusion is supported by earlier clinicopathologic evidence of heart failure, most commonly in patients with "massive" MAC.[16,18]

Embolism caused by calcific debris detached from the mitral annulus most frequently causes retinal or cerebral ischemia[36] and rarely massive systemic emboli. This can also be caused by emboli from a calcific aortic valve. Septic embolism from infectious endocarditis involving a calcified mitral annulus is also a potential complication. In recent years several cases of bacterial endocarditis, often caused by *Staphylococcus aureus*, have been described.[37,38] The severity and complexity of infections involving the mitral annulus and at times extending with abscess formation toward the adjoining conduction system must be considered. Appropriate prophylactic antibiotics should be administered to elderly patients with documented MAC prior to any potentially bacteremic procedure.[37] The prognosis in such patients has been uniformly poor because of frequent perforation of mitral leaflets caused by the infectious process. Also, the unusual annular location makes surgical intervention difficult and frequently ineffective. No definite criteria are available to indicate the patients with MAC who are at high risk for bacterial endocarditis, but most reported cases had marked degree of calcification. Echocardiographic demonstration of MAC of significant degree (more than 5 mm) could be a valid criterion for selecting the patients at high risk.

Severe MAC with calcified aortic valve stenosis in elderly patients with nonrheumatic degenerative valve disease clearly suggests that a common pathogenesis leads to gradually more extensive cardiac calcification with eventual involvement of both contiguous valvular regions. Elderly patients with severe MAC and calcific aortic valve disease, particularly females with a small aortic orifice, should be carefully evaluated for the presence of hemodynamically significant aortic stenosis. The clinical findings of aortic stenosis are often difficult to elicit in elderly subjects, due to loss of compliance of their vessels and to inconspicuous cardiac murmurs caused by abnormalities of chest wall or lung parenchyma. Cardiac catheterization may be needed in order to define the severity of their valvular disease.

THERAPY

No specific therapy is indicated for MAC. Conventional medical therapy for congestive heart failure, atrial fibrillation, and mitral insufficiency include use of diuretics, digitalis, and other positive inotropic drugs, and the newer afterload and preload reducers for patients with severe congestive heart failure.

Some patients will need a permanent pacemaker if symptoms caused by conduction problems develop. In patients undergoing open-heart surgery, when significant conduction disturbances are present preoperatively, the need for a permanent pacemaker should be carefully evaluated. Intraoperative epicardial permanent pacing leads could be easily implanted in such high-risk subjects, facilitating the subsequent introduction of a pacing unit in selected cases.

Appropriate antibiotic prophylaxis for patients with MAC is indicated; patients with significant MAC by echocardiography (more than 5-mm thickness), with significant mitral insufficiency or associated aortic valve calcification or stenosis, or with mitral valve prolapse or associated hypertrophic cardiomyopathy, should be given prophylaxis. This might not be necessary in patients demonstrating only a mild degree of MAC (less than 5-mm thickness), particularly if no significant systolic murmur can be auscultated.

With improving surgical technics and increasing longevity, it is likely that patients with this type of valvular pathology will be seen more frequently. The clinician needs to become familiar with the precise anatomy and pathophysiology underlying this unusual valvular condition, as well as with its possible complications.

REFERENCES

1. Gabor GE, Mohr BD, Goel PC, et al: Echocardiographic and clinical spectrum of mitral annular calcification. *Am J Cardiol* 1976;38:836–842.
2. Dashkoff N, Karacuschansky M, Come PC, et al: Echocardiographic features of mitral annulus calcification. *Am Heart J* 1977;94:585–592.
3. D'Cruz IA, Cohen HC, Prabhu R, et al: Clinical manifestations of mitral annulus calcification, with emphasis on its echocardiographic features. *Am Heart J* 1977;94:367–377.
4. Schott R, Kotler MN, Parry WR, et al: Mitral annulus calcification—Clinical and echocardiographic correlations. *Arch Intern Med* 1977;137: 1143–1150.
5. Fulkerson PK, Beaver BM, Auseon JC, et al: Calcification of the mitral annulus—Etiology, clinical associations, complications and therapy. *Am J Med* 1979;66:967–977.
6. Mellino M, Salcedo EE, Lever HM, et al: Echographic-quantified severity of mitral annulus calcification: Prognostic correlation to related hemodynamic, valvular, rhythm and conduction abnormalities. *Am Heart J* 1982;103:222–225.
7. Zoneraich S, Zoneraich O, Patel M: Conduction disturbances in patients with calcified mitral annulus diagnosed by echocardiography. *J Electrocardiol* 1979;12:137–139.
8. D'Cruz I, Panetta F, Cohen H, et al: Submitral calcification or sclerosis in elderly patients: M-mode and two dimensional echocardiography in "mitral annulus calcification." *Am J Cardiol* 1979;44:31–38.
9. Mellino M, Salcedo EE: Fluoroscopy and echocardiography in patients with mitral annulus calcification, in Diethrich EB (ed): *Noninvasive assessment of the cardiovascular system.* John Wright-PSG Inc, 1982; pp. 159–163.
10. Kirk RS, Russell JGB: Subvalvular calcification of mitral valve. *Br Heart J* 1969;31:684–692.
11. Pomerance A: Pathological and clinical study of calcification of the mitral valve ring. *J Clin Pathol* 1970;23:354–361.
12. Geill T: Calcification of the left annulus fibrosus. *J Gerontol* 1951;6:327–333.
13. Pomerance A: Cardiac pathology and systolic murmurs in the elderly. *Br Heart J* 1968;30:687–689.
14. Bulkley BH, Morrow AG, Roberts WC: Calcification of the mitral annulus: A late complication of valve replacement with caged-ball prosthesis, abstracted. *Am J Cardiol* 1973;31:123.
15. Abrahams C, D'Cruz IA, Kathpalia S: Abnormalities in the mitral valve apparatus in patients undergoing long-term hemodialysis. *Arch Intern Med* 1982;142:1796–1800.
16. Korn D, Desanctis RW, Sell S: Massive calcification of the mitral annulus. A clinicopathological study of fourteen cases. *N Engl J Med* 1962;267: 900–909.
17. Roberts WC, Perloff JK: Mitral valve disease—A clinicopathologic survey of the conditions causing the mitral valve to function abnormally. *Ann Intern Med* 1972;77:939–975.
18. Rytand DA, Lipsitch LS: Clinical aspects of calcification of the mitral annulus fibrosus. *Arch Intern Med* 1946;78:544–564.
19. Pomerance A: Pathology of the heart with and without cardiac failure in the aged. *Br Heart J* 1965;27:697–710.
19a. Sugiura M, Uchiyama S, Kuwako K, et al: A clinicopathological study on mitral ring calcification. *Jpn Heart J* 1977;18:154–163.
20. Roberts WC, Waller BF: Mitral valve "annular" calcium forming a complete circle or "O" configuration: Clinical and necropsy observations. *Am Heart J* 1981;101:619–621.
21. Hammer WJ, Roberts WC, deLeon AC: "Mitral Stenosis" secondary to combined "massive" mitral annular calcific deposits and small, hypertrophied left ventricles. *Am J Med* 1978;64:371–376.
22. Ramirez J, Flowers NC: Severe mitral stenosis secondary to massive calcification of the mitral annulus with unusual echocardiographic manifestations. *Clin Cardiol* 1980;3:284–287.
23. Roberts WC, Perloff JK, Costantino T: Severe valvular aortic stenosis in patients over 65 years of age. *Am J Cardiol* 1971;27:497–506.
24. Kronzon I, Glassman E: Mitral ring calcification in idiopathic hypertrophic subaortic stenosis. *Am J Cardiol* 1978;42:60–66.
25. Tajik AJ, Giuliani ER, Weidman WH, et al: Idiopathic hypertrophic subaortic stenosis. Long-term surgical follow-up. *Am J Cardiol* 1974;34:815–822.
26. Nanda NC, Gramiak R, Shah PM, et al: Echocardiography in the diagnosis of idiopathic hypertrophic subaortic stenosis co-existing with aortic valve disease. *Circulation* 1974;50:752–757.
27. McLean J, Felner JM, Whipple R, et al: The echocardiographic association of mitral valve prolapse and mitral annulus calcification. *Clin Cardiol* 1979; 2:220–223.
28. Grossman M, Knott AP, Jacoby WJ: Calcified annulus fibrosus with mitral insufficiency in the Marfan syndrome. *Arch Intern Med* 1968;121:561–563.
29. Nair CK, Sketch MH, Desai R, et al: High prevalence of symptomatic bradyarrhythmias due to atrioventricular node-fascicular and sinus node-atrial disease in patients with mitral annular calcification. *Am Heart J* 1982;103:226–229.
30. Lewis T: Postmortem notes of Dr. J.H. Starling's care of heart block. *Heart* 1922;9:283–287.
30a. Nair CK, Runco V, Everson GI, et al: Conduction defects and mitral annulus calcification. *Br Heart J* 1980;44:162–167.

31. Scarpa WJ: The sick sinus syndrome. *Am Heart J* 1976;92:648-660.
32. Strauss HC, Bigger JT, Saroff AL, et al: Electrophysiologic evaluation of atrio-ventricular node function in patients with sinus node dysfunction. *Circulation* 1976;53:763-776.
32a. Tanabe J, Ibrahim F: Echocardiographic findings of mitral annulus calcification, in Diethrich EB (ed): *Noninvasive Cardiovascular Diagnosis—Current Concepts.* Baltimore, University Park Press, 1978; pp 383-392
33. Kronzon I, Mitchell J, Shapiro J, et al: Two dimensional echocardiography in mitral annulus calcification. *Am J Radiol* 1980;134:355-358.
34. Waller BF, Morrow AG, Maron BJ, et al: Etiology of clinically isolated, severe, chronic, pure mitral regurgitation: Analysis of 97 patients over 30 years of age having mitral valve replacement. *Am Heart J* 1982;104:276-288.
35. Mellino M, Salcedo EE: Mitral annulus calcification: Clinical implication. *Cleve Clin Q* 1983;50:6-11.
36. DeBono DP, Warlow CP: Mitral annulus calcification and cerebral or retinal ischemia. *Lancet* 1979; 25:383-385.
37. Burnside JW, Desanctis RW: Bacterial endocarditis on calcification of the mitral annulus fibrosus. *Ann Intern Med* 1972;76:615-618.
38. Mambo NC, Silver MD, Brunsdon DF: Bacterial endocarditis of the mitral valve associated with annular calcification. *Can Med Assoc J* 1978;119: 323-326.
39. Curati WL, Petitclerc R, Winsberg F: Ultrasonic features of mitral annulus calcification. *Radiology* 1977;122:215-217.
40. Simon MA, Liu SF: Calcification of the mitral valve annulus and its relation to functional valve disturbance. *Am Heart J* 1954;48:497-505.

CHAPTER 29
Valvular Heart Disease in the Elderly

Colin M. Bloor

Cardiovascular disease is a major cause of death in the elderly, accounting for 40% of deaths of individuals over 75 years old. Pomerance[1] has reviewed an autopsy series performed on 370 patients over 75 years old. One hundred sixty-two (44%) had congestive heart failure while the other 208 patients (56%) did not. She categorized the frequency of the different types of cardiovascular disease in this elderly population. In the 162 patients with congestive heart failure, ischemic heart disease was most common, occurring in 49%. In decreasing order of frequency were degenerative calcific changes of the atrioventricular valves, hypertension, senile cardiac amyloidosis, endocarditis, cor pulmonale, calcific aortic stenosis, rheumatic heart disease, mucoid degeneration of the mitral valve, and syphilis. In the 208 patients without congestive heart failure, degenerative calcific changes of the heart valves were most frequent, occurring in 29%. In decreasing order of frequency were ischemic heart disease, hypertension, cardiac amyloidosis, rheumatic heart disease, cor pulmonale, endocarditis, calcific aortic stenosis, and mucoid degeneration of the mitral valve.

In general, the incidence of these various cardiovascular diseases increased with age until the age of 90 years. Then hypertension and calcific degeneration of the semilunar valves decreased in patients older than 90 years who had congestive heart failure. Also, mucoid degeneration of the atrioventricular valves was less frequent in patients older than 90 years. The most striking feature of congestive heart failure in the elderly was the presence of multiple pathologic entities.

In another autopsy study comprising 805 patients ranging in age from 10 to 96 years, Pomerance[2] focused on the aging changes that occur in heart valves. Of particular interest are the changes that occur in the mitral valve. The anterior leaflet of the mitral valve has two types of changes that occur with increasing age: nodular thickening at the free edges and lipid deposition. The posterior leaflet has additional changes that occur with age: annular calcification, small puckered scars, diffuse opacification of the leaflet, and ballooning deformity. Changes that occur in the aortic valve with age include noduli Arantii, fenestrations, and calcification. Changes in the tricuspid valve with age include nodular thickening at the free margins of the leaflets while changes occurring in the pulmonary valve are minimal with increasing age.

Pomerance[2] discusses the possible etiologies of these lesions in elderly patients. The noduli Arantii of the aortic valve and the nodularity of the anterior leaflet of the mitral valve represent reactions to local injury. Lipid deposits in the anterior leaflet of the mitral valve are very frequent, occurring in 99% of patients older than 55 years. Otherwise, normal appearing valves in the elderly included the aforementioned changes.

Changes increasing in severity with age occurred only in the left heart. These changes included lipid deposits in the mitral valve, aortic valve calcification, and mitral valve annulus calcification. The first two entities increase in frequency with age and are not related to sex, but result from hemodynamic forces. The latter, mitral valve ring calcification, increases in frequency with age and is more common in women.

Changes occurring only during middle age which do not increase in frequency after 65 to 74 years of age include nodular sclerosis of the atrioventricular valves and mucoid degeneration of the mitral valve. Nodular sclerosis of the atrioventricular valves is frequently associated with chronic obstructive pulmonary disease.

VALVULAR LESIONS IN THE ELDERLY

Pathogenesis

In Western societies there is little doubt that changes occur in the heart valves as a person ages. In general it is believed that thickening of the valve substance occurs with aging, and calcification of the valve tissue is found in the aged population. Some of these changes are more pronounced in persons who have cardiac arrhythmias and may even account for the arrhythmias, since similar changes may also be found in the conduction tissue of the heart. In general, it is accepted that when these changes extend beyond a certain threshold, they may induce significant function abnormalities, eg, valve malfunction, arrhythmias, or even compromise of myocardial function.

Although such changes have been well described, several important issues have not been thoroughly explored. First, it is not clear to what extent these changes are related to the aging process itself or to what extent they are primarily related to other diseases that are common among the elderly. Valvular ring calcification, for example, may be related to other processes. The increased incidence in diabetics may be due to processes related to altered carbohydrate metabolism rather than to aging. Valvular ring calcification and mucoid degeneration of valve tissue are more prevalent in women than in men, for reasons that are not understood.

Aging Changes

From birth to maturity there is progressive thickening of the endocardium of the atrial aspect of the atrioventricular valves.[3] Similar changes occur in the atrial wall. The lines of closure of the valves become slightly thickened and nodular. Since these alterations are most marked in the anterior leaflet of the mitral valve and least marked in the septal leaflet of the tricuspid valve, it would seem that they are related to the degree of pressure to which the leaflet is subjected. In the elderly, the aortic valve cusps become palpably thickened at their bases and opaque ridges with central nodules (corpora Arantii) appear along their lines of closure. With increasing age, changes are normally found in the left heart valves only; they consist of increasing general opacity of the outflow surfaces and the appearance and growth of yellow lipid streaks on the ventricular surface of the anterior mitral leaflet. On microscopic examination, these plaques appear as fine sudanophilic droplets, have a foamy appearance, and are mainly in the fibrosa portion of the valve. The lipids are identical to those found in uncomplicated vascular atheroma (fatty streaks), but the thrombosis, calcification, and hemorrhage that complicate atheroma are not seen in these mitral valve lesions. The lesions are believed to result from the abrupt arrest of blood flow against the ventricular surface of the anterior leaflet of the mitral valve during the cardiac cycle. Increasing quantities of lipid also appear in the fibrosa of the aortic valve cusps in the elderly, but this is not usually apparent macroscopically.[4,5] With aging, changes also occur in the collagen fibers and metachromasia is well marked. In the elderly, the collagen becomes denser, its staining becomes variable, the parallel orientation is lost, and the nuclei are less numerous. Acid mucopolysaccharide content decreases.[6] Lipid begins to appear in the third decade and increases in amount with the age of the subject. Microscopic calcification is common in persons older than 40 years and in those cardiac règions where calcification of the valve leaflets subsequently develops.

The incidence of minor adhesions of the aortic commissures and agglutination of mitral chordae tendineae increase with the subject's age, but these changes are found in only a small number of elderly patients. They are extreme forms of the irritational hyperplasia of the endocardium that occurs with aging and they are of no clinical significance. Certainly, they are not indicative of healed rheumatic valvulitis. These changes alone do not cause significant functional disturbances. Of more clinical importance in the elderly are the "degenerative" changes.

Degenerative Changes

In the elderly, degenerative changes affecting the heart valves involve the fibrosa and take either of two forms: calcification or mucoid degeneration. Both processes are uncommon in right-sided heart valves. In the left-sided heart valves, degenerative calcification is a common finding in elderly patients, even exceeding the incidence of ischemic myocardial disease. Examples of degenerative calcification of the left-sided heart valves that reach clinical significance are calcific aortic stenosis and calcified mitral annulus. Examples of mucoid degeneration of the left-sided heart valves reaching clinical significance are mitral valve prolapse and ruptured chordae tendineae.

Calcific aortic stenosis In a series of autopsies on patients over 75 years of age, degenerative calcification of aortic or mitral valves was identifiable microscopically in about one third.[7] Twenty-one percent of unstenosed aortic valves showed that calcification first appears in the fibrosa at the base of the aortic cusps.[8] The development is probably related to the repeated mechanical stresses of normal valve action. With increasing severity of calcification, the deposits extend toward the free margin of the cusps, but very rarely do they involve the free edges. Large masses of calcium may project into the sinuses of Valsalva. On microscopic examination there are solid zones of calcification expanding and occasionally breaking through the fibrosa. Thin-walled vascular channels and scanty chronic inflammatory cell infiltrates may be present adjacent to the calcified regions. This condition is easily distinguished grossly from calcification due to endocarditis by the absence of commissural adhesions or distortion of the free edges of the cusp, and macroscopically by the absence of thick-walled vessels, fibrous disorganization of valve architecture, or involvement of the ventricular endocardium.

Pomerance reviewed 111 cases of isolated aortic stenosis.[7] Calcified congenitally bicuspid valves were most common, occurring in 43%. These were characterized by a transverse slitlike or crescentic orifice and occurred most often in men. Senile degenerative calcification was responsible for aortic stenosis in 31% of the patients. It was characterized by a triradiate orifice without adhesions of the commissures and was most frequent in women. Postinflammatory aortic stenosis, usually secondary to rheumatic heart disease, resulted in fixed central circular or triangular orifices (Figure 29-1) and occurred in 24% of the series. Inflammatory fusion of a congenital bicuspid valve occurred in 7%. The relative frequencies, presented in Table 29-1, can be summarized as follows: (1) Stenosis due to previous inflammation occurs in patients younger than 60 years; (2) calcification in congenitally bicuspid valves occurs most frequently in patients 60 to 75 years old; (3) degenerative calcification is not seen in patients younger than 75 years, is the predominant lesion in patients older than 75 years and is responsible for all cases of aortic stenosis in patients older than 85 years.

Clinical features In most cases aortic valve calcification is of no clinical significance other than as a source of aortic systolic murmurs. However, in a small proportion of patients, calcification may become extensive enough to restrict valve opening, resulting in aortic stenosis. The frequency of the aortic stenosis increases with age; it is 15 times more common in patients of the 60 to 80-year age group than in those under 30 years. Its incidence in patients over the age of 65 years is about 4% to 6% in various autopsy series. Isolated aortic valvular stenosis is more common in men than in women in a ratio of about 4:1. However, in older age brackets, eg, over 80 years of age, women predominate with respect to isolated aortic stenosis.

In older patients with aortic stenosis caused by calcific deposits on the surfaces of otherwise normal tricuspid aortic valves, the murmur in the sec-

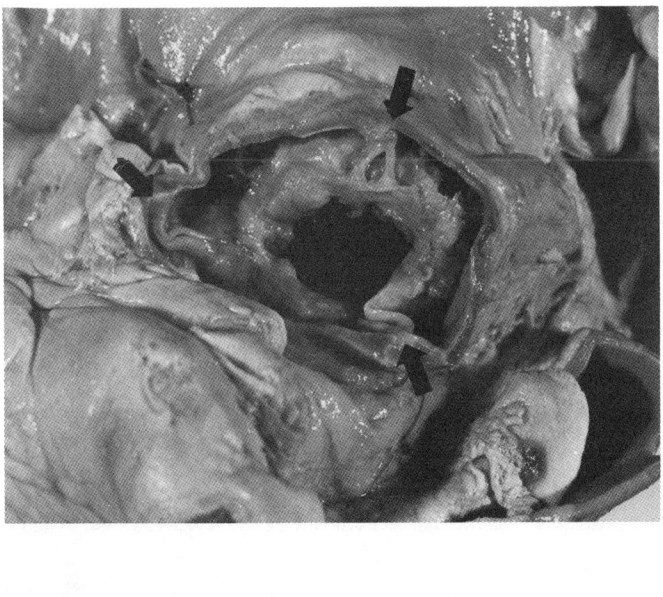

Figure 29-1 Postinflammatory aortic stenosis due to rheumatic heart disease. The valve cusps are markedly thickened due to extensive scarring and calcification. The commissures are fused (arrows). These changes result in a fixed circular valve orifice.

Table 29-1
Frequencies of Aortic Stenosis Etiologies

Age	Inflammatory	Inflammatory on Congenital	Congenital	Senile
85	1 (M)			6 (M) 11 (F)
75–84	3 (F)		10 (M) 7 (F)	9 (M) 8 (F)
60–74	4 (M) 10(F)	1 (M) 1 (F)	16 (M)	
50–59	7 (M) 1 (F)	5 (M)		

Adapted from Pomerance.[7]

ond right interspace tends to be harsh and noisy, whereas the murmur at the apex may be pure and musical. The noisy murmur originates at the aortic root because of the disturbance caused by the high-velocity jet. The musical murmur has been ascribed to periodic vibrations of the stenotic valve itself and may be well recorded within the cavity of the left ventricle.[8]

Pathologic features Large masses of calcification distort a three-cusped aortic valve without evidence of previous inflammation (Figure 29-2). It appears to be an extreme form of the moderate calcification that is common in otherwise normal aortic valves in the elderly. The process starts at the base of the cusps and rarely involves the free edges, although large masses of calcium may fill the sinuses of Valsalva.

Calcified mitral annulus With increasing longevity, mitral ring calcification is one of the commonest cardiac abnormalities seen by general pathologists.[9,10] It has been reported in up to 10% of autopsies on patients over 50 years of age. Mitral ring calcification is essentially a disease of the elderly. Most cases are in patients over 70 and the frequency increases with age.[11,12] Women are affected much more often than men, the relative incidence being about 4:1.[11]

Clinical features Until recently, mitral annular calcification was dismissed as having no clinical importance, but it is now apparent that this lesion often results in mitral insufficiency or conduction abnormalities and, less often, in mitral stenosis. In many cases it is an important contributing factor to congestive heart failure in the elderly and is one of the conditions predisposing to the development of endocarditis. Restriction of the normal systolic contraction of the atrioventricular orifice results when a sufficiently large part of the annulus is made rigid by calcification and distortion, and atrial displacement of the posterior mitral valve leaflet prevents coaptation of the valve margins. Mitral stenosis results when subvalvular or intravalvular extensions are sufficient to form a rigid shelf. The degree of stenosis is usually minor, although it has been a prominent feature in some instances. Conduction disturbances are expected because of the anatomical relationship of the atrioventricular node and the bundle of His to the mitral annulus. Massive mitral calcification alone may be respon-

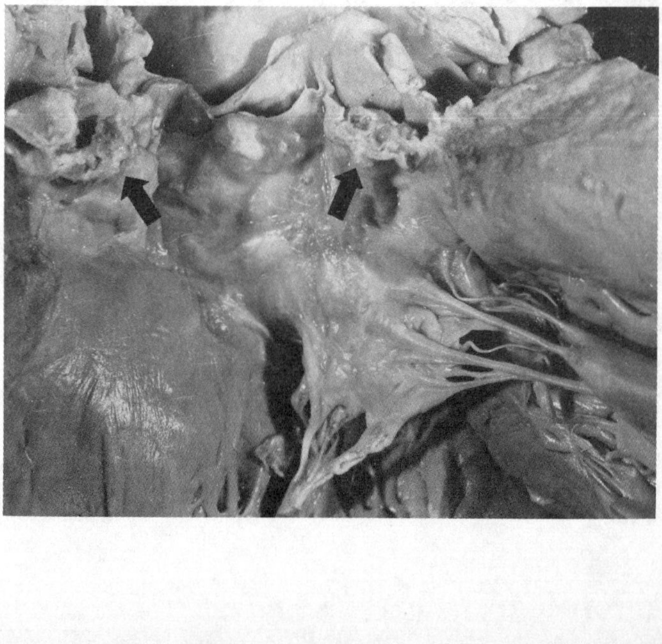

Figure 29-2 Calcific aortic stenosis. The aortic valve cusps are thickened due to diffuse calcification (arrows). Since the calcium deposits first appear in the base of the valve cusps, the commissures are not yet fused.

sible for cardiac failure. Lesser degrees of calcification are present in a high proportion of elderly patients in whom multiple cardiac lesions are associated with heart failure.

Mitral annulus calcification is the most common cardiac abnormality in elderly patients with apical systolic murmurs.[12,13] Systolic murmurs and clinical diagnoses of mitral insufficiency have been reported in a high percentage of cases. Not unexpectedly, murmurs are heard far more frequently when distortion of the leaflets is present. In some series, systolic murmurs have been reported three times as often as in patients in whom calcification has not been sufficiently advanced to have produced distortion.

Mitral annular calcification is unrelated to rheumatic heart disease, rheumatoid disease, or any known form of cardiac inflammation. An increased incidence has been reported in patients with diabetes mellitus or osteitis deformans.[14,15] The mitral annulus is one of the sites affected in patients with metastatic calcification. However, no abnormality of calcium metabolism has been demonstrated in the majority of cases. The condition is considered to be an exaggerated form of the normal aging changes already described, but it is not clear why they should occur in only a portion of even the most elderly patients and why women should be predominantly affected in contrast to the reverse sex incidence in aortic valve calcification. Mitral annular calcification is sometimes regarded as a wear-and-tear change due to the pull of the left ventricular myocardium and aortic and mitral valves on their attachments to the cardiac skeleton.[16] The probable importance of hemodynamic factors is emphasized by the rarity of calcification in the tricuspid ring, except in association with pulmonary hypertension or the increased incidence of systemic hypertension in cases of mitral annular calcification. A possible explanation for the different incidence of mitral annular calcification between the sexes has been suggested. Since senile osteoporosis is more common in women, perhaps a factor exists that affects calcium distribution between bone and soft tissue and this factor is more active in elderly women.[9] It is also possible that the mitral valve region is more prone to an exaggerated response to injury in women. This hypothesis is supported by observations that inflammatory changes in mitral annular calcification are more common in women and by the well-known preponderance of rheumatic mitral stenosis in women, although rheumatic carditis is equally common in both sexes.

Pathologic features The gross appearances vary from small localized palpable nodules or spicules of calcium to transformation of the entire mitral annulus into a rigid C-shaped or J-shaped bar up to 2 cm in thickness (Figure 29-3). The early lesions are usually located in the midportion of the posterior leaflet attachment or at the junction of the medial commissure with the ventricular wall. Calcification frequently extends into the subvalvular angle, sometimes forming a prominent ridge over which the posterior cusp is stretched. Distortion and upward displacement of the valve leaflet by irregular calcified spurs is also common. The calcified masses may erode through the atrial surface of the leaflets, but this is surprisingly infrequent. When erosion through the leaflet does occur, thrombotic or infective endocarditis is likely to develop. The thrombus may reach a large size, and fatal aortic embolism may occur from tumorlike masses. Sometimes the calcified annulus shows extensive central softening resembling a caseous abscess. Often this is mistaken for an infective process, possibly a tuberculoma. However, this finding does not seem to be associated with any particular coexisting disease such as rheumatoid arthritis; thus, its only practical importance

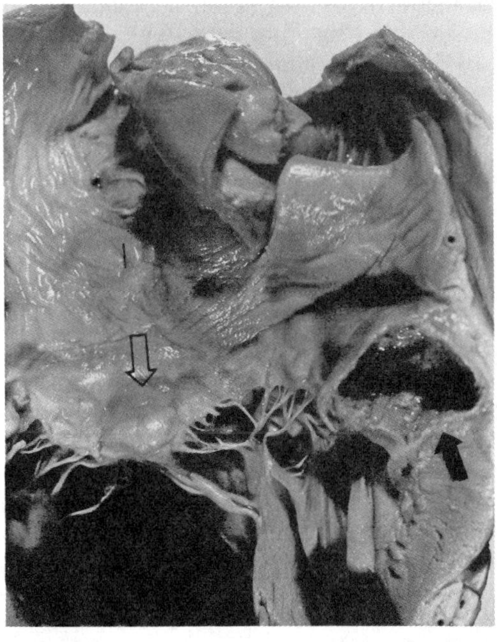

Figure 29-3 Calcified mitral annulus. A large mass of calcification (solid arrow) lies beneath the posterior leaflet of the mitral valve. The leaflet is intact and is free of similar deposits. Degenerative change in the mitral valve leaflet is evidenced by mild ballooning deformity (open arrow) near the free margin.

lies in the possibility of confusion with tuberculoma or gumma. Mitral annular calcification may be extensive enough to erode through adjacent portions of the conduction bundle. In one case the author observed, such extensive calcification caused third-degree heart block in a woman 88 years old. She lived for 4 more years, to the age of 92 years, at which time the calcifications eroded through the posterior left ventricular wall, resulting in a sterile abscess and cardiac tamponade.

Microscopically, the calcification appears as large masses of amorphous eosinophilic material, often with basophilic granular zones. The calcification is first apparent in the fibrosa of the annulus. When more advanced, it extends into the myocardium. Thin-walled vascular channels and focal inflammatory cell infiltrates are common at the margins of the calcification. Occasionally seen are hemorrhage, marked inflammatory changes with myocardial or valvular necrosis, foreign body–type giant cells, palisading fibroblast proliferation of the rheumatoid type, and cartilage. On rare occasions bone may be present.

Mitral valve prolapse Mucoid degeneration mainly affects the mitral valve and is characterized by transformation of normally dense valve fibrosa into a loose metachromatically staining connective tissue.[17,18] This softening of the fibrosa permits stretching of the mitral leaflet under normal intracardiac pressure. When this change is sufficiently extensive, a large ectatic "floppy" leaflet prolapses into the left atrium during systole. A variety of names has been attached to this condition, describing the characteristic microscopic features; floppy valve, describing its appearance at operation; and ballooning, billowing prolapse or aneurysmal protrusion of the posterior mitral leaflet, describing the valve's appearance on angiography. This change also accounts for the late systolic murmur or nonejection click murmur syndrome.

Severe mucoid degeneration of the mitral valve has been found in about 1% of autopsies on patients over 50 years of age.[18] Probably it is more common in men than in women, but some clinical series have shown a preponderance of women. Of the 35 cases reported by Pomerance[18] 19 patients had congestive heart failure and systolic murmurs were present in 67%. The complications that were observed included bacterial endocarditis (2 of 35), ruptured chordae tendineae (2 of 35), and mitral regurgitation which was present in most patients.

Clinical features There seems to be no doubt that mucoid degeneration of the mitral valve is associated with mitral insufficiency. Obvious left atrial dilatation and regurgitant murmurs are common. Almost all cases show mitral systolic murmurs varying from late apical to pansystolic with thrills. Whenever regurgitant flow is directed against the anterior mitral leaflet, a basal murmur suggesting aortic valve disease may predominate. Ballooning of the mitral valve without a murmur may occur, but it is uncommon. A critical factor may be the degree of elongation of the chordae tendineae of the mitral valve. Mitral insufficiency associated with ballooning deformity appears to be well tolerated. In one series 57% of the patients were known to have had murmurs for more than 25 years. The number of cases in which mitral insufficiency becomes severe enough to require surgery is small. Several patients with this clinical syndrome have abnormal ECGs and chest pain suggestive of ischemic heart disease, and sudden death has been reported. No pathologic correlates have been shown. Arrhythmias may be provoked by exercise. In one autopsy series, the valve abnormality was an incidental finding in about one half of the patients, although almost all had mitral systolic murmurs during life. Death was directly due to the valve disease in only 20% of cases, mainly because of ruptured chordae tendineae. The remainder had mitral insufficiency as one of two or more cardiac abnormalities contributing to heart failure. It appears that mitral insufficiency due to mucoid degeneration has a long natural history and that death will therefore often be due to unrelated conditions. The main clinical significance of mucoid degeneration lies in the predisposition to infective endocarditis and to spontaneous rupture of the chordae tendineae.

Pathologic features The abnormal characteristics are usually limited to the mitral valve. The posterior leaflet is more often and more severely affected than the anterior leaflet (Figure 29-4). The striking change is marked increase in the surface area of the affected leaflet. It may be twice the depth of the anterior leaflet instead of the normal one third or one half. Sometimes only one or two of the normal three "scallops" are involved. The affected leaflets are voluminous, opaque, and white, resembling a partly collapsed parachute. The mucoid consistency of the core of the leaflet is often grossly apparent when the valve leaflet is cut. Small regions of ulceration and thrombus formation are common on the atrial surface of the affected leaflet and, occasionally, on the apposing surface of the anterior leaflet. Superficial vascularity of the leaflets, commonly observed in

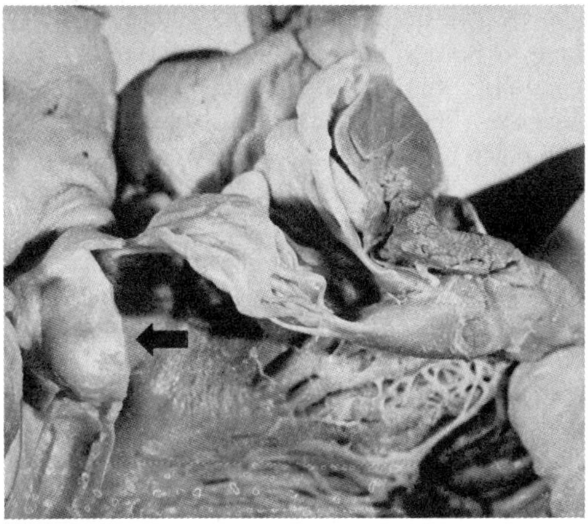

Figure 29-4 Mitral valve prolapse. The posterior leaflet of the mitral valve shows severe ballooning deformity (arrow). A section has been removed from the leaflet for histologic examination.

rheumatic valvular disease, is absent in mucoid degeneration. The chordae tendineae are usually thin, often to an abnormal degree. Some localized thickening may be seen at their insertions into the valve leaflet. Friction lesions are often present on the chordae of the affected leaflet, and when these lesions are well developed, the chordae tendineae themselves may become fused to the regions of mural endocardial fibrosis. Jet lesions are not uncommon, either on the posterior wall of the left atrium or, more often, on the septal wall or at the base of the anterior mitral leaflet. In about 25% of cases, the tricuspid valve will show similar ballooning changes, usually to a lesser degree.

Microscopically, regions of loose spongy tissue replace the normal dense homogeneous collagen of the fibrosa of the leaflet. This abnormal tissue stains metachromatically with toluidine blue and may contain stellate cells. Histochemical studies show it is a complex mucoprotein or acid mucopolysaccharide. Metachromasia is not usually present in the normal adult mitral valve, although small zones of mucoid degeneration are not uncommon near the free edge. The atrial side of the leaflet shows a variable degree of fibroelastic proliferation, which is presumably a nonspecific response to stretching. Superficial ulceration and noninfective thrombotic endocarditis are common. The anatomical layers of the mitral leaflet remain indistinct. There is no vascularization or other evidence of previous inflammation. The collagen of the chordae tendineae show degenerative changes similar to those of the fibrosa. Ultrastructural studies show loss of the normal orderly arrangement and cross-banding of collagen fibers and increased translucency of extrafibrillary ground substance.

Ruptured chordae tendineae

Clinical features Rupture of the chordae tendineae is the most common complication of mucoid degeneration of the mitral valve.[19,20] It is responsible for death in about 16% to 20% of cases in which it occurs. Indeed, mucoid degeneration appears to be associated with most cases of "isolated" rupture of the chordae tendineae, particularly those of the posterior mitral leaflet. The exact mechanism of rupture is variable; there is no doubt that the chordae attached to the ballooned portion of the leaflet are subject to excessive tension, because the main stress on a competent valve is taken by the apposing leaflet margins. This support is no longer present in the prolapsed leaflet. The mechanical stress alone may cause attenuation and finally, rupture of the chordae. Alternatively, the collagen of the chordae tendineae may show the same mucoid degeneration as the leaflet fibrosa, and these changes could increase the chances of rupture.

Pathologic features Mucoid degeneration is not related to rheumatic fever or any specific previous illness. The pathologic features resemble those of Marfan's syndrome. It has been suggested that this isolated mucoid degeneration of the mitral valve is a forme fruste of Marfan's syndrome, a concept that should be discouraged. This condition is a localized bioatrophy, whereas the syndrome described by Marfan consists of widespread abnormalities of the connective tissue and skeleton. Genetic factors are present in some cases, particularly in younger patients. Several familial cases have been described, the inheritance following an autosomal dominant pattern. Mucoid degeneration of the chordae tendineae is also more common in hearts with congenital abnormalities, particularly atrial septal defects. Some skeletal abnormalities of the chest have been noted in many patients. This observation also supports a congenital pathogenesis. A high incidence of the lesion has been observed in Ugandan Africans (15% of patients over 60 years of age) who showed severe mucoid degeneration of the mitral valves. It is of interest that a similar disease occurs in dogs of certain breeds. However, most human cases have been isolated examples with no relevant family history. Emphysema is often associated with mucoid degeneration of the chordae tendineae, and this suggests a common weakness of pulmonary and valvular connective tissue. In dogs, the lesion is related to age. Some observers have claimed that aging is a significant factor in human cases. Certainly, most reported autopsy cases have been in the elderly, the highest incidence in one series being in the ninth decade. Experimental observations show that mucoid accumulation in heart valves occurs after interruption of cardiac lymphatic drainage. This raises the possibility that the lymphatic system may play a role in the etiology. However, no studies on human subjects have been published.

The pathogenesis in most cases of mucoid degeneration of the mitral valve is still obscure. The most likely explanation is that the mucoid degeneration is a nonspecific change and may result from a number of factors that include genetic and possibly aging changes.

INFECTIVE ENDOCARDITIS

Before the use of antibiotics, infective endocarditis occurred predominantly in young adults. About 67% of patients with acute endocarditis were between 20 and 40 years of age. However, since the introduction of antibiotics and cardiovascular surgery and the rise in age range of patients with the disease, a significantly greater proportion of patients is now older than 50 years. In one series, the ages ranged from 8 months to 85 years. In another series, 40% of the patients were over 50 years of age. The author observed a case of acute infective endocarditis in a 64-year-old woman who had been a heroin addict for more than 40 years (Figure 29-5). Thus, infective endocarditis may occur at any age, and the clinician's index of suspicion should always be high when the clinical features are suggestive.

SUMMARY AND CONCLUSIONS

Examination of the heart valves of an elderly patient requires that a distinction be made between changes that simply represent the accumulated injuries of one or more disease processes and changes that are an inevitable part of aging. Aging changes alone do not cause significant clinical disease. Although all types of valvular heart disease have been reported in the elderly, certain entities are of particular interest. The clinically significant lesions are due to either extensive calcification or mucoid degeneration of the valves and their annuli. The most important valvular lesions occurring in the elderly include calcific aortic stenosis, calcified mitral annulus, mitral valve prolapse due to mucoid degeneration, and ruptured chordae tendineae. Even though these entities have been thoroughly described, further study is needed to explain which pathogenetic mechanisms are related to the aging process itself as contrasted to those secondary to other concurrent diseases.

It should be emphasized that with the current advances in clinical practice, we are observing an increased frequency of infective endocarditis in the elderly. When diagnosed early it can often be successfully treated.

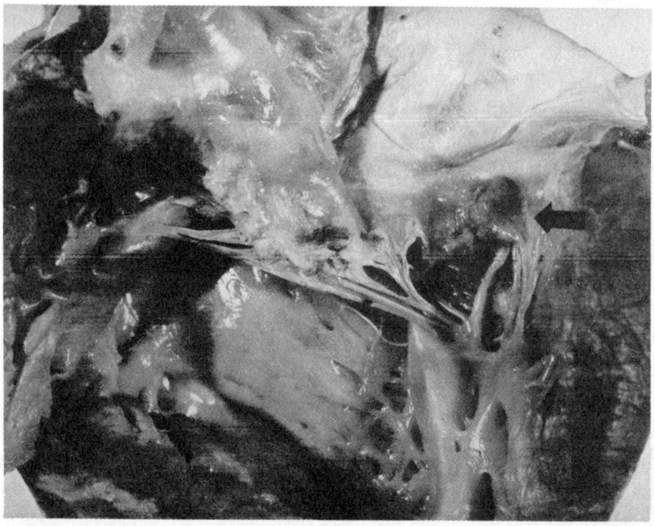

Figure 29-5 Acute infective endocarditis. A large friable vegetation (arrow) is present on the mitral valve of a 64-year-old woman. Cultures of the vegetation grew *Serratia marascens*.

REFERENCES

1. Pomerance A: Pathology of the heart with and without cardiac failure in the aged. *Br Heart J* 1965;27:697–702.
2. Pomerance A: Aging changes in human heart valves. *Br Heart J* 1967;29:222–226.
3. McMillan JB, Lev M: The aging heart. I. Endocardium. *J Gerontol* 1959;14:268–273.
4. Kim KM, Valigorsky JM, Mergner WJ, et al: Aging changes in the human aortic valve in relation to dystrophic calcification. *Hum Pathol* 1976;7:47–52.
5. Sell S, Scully RE: Aging changes in the aortic and mitral valves: Histologic and histochemical studies, with observations on the pathogenesis of calcific aortic stenosis and calcification of the mitral annulus. *Am J Pathol* 1965;46:345–349.
6. Torii S, Bashey RI, Nakao K: Acid mucopolysaccharide composition of human heart valve. *Biochim Biophys Acta* 1965;101:285–290.
7. Pomerance A: The pathogenesis of aortic stenosis and its relation to age. *Br Heart J* 1972;34:569–574.
8. Roberts WC: The structure of the aortic valve in clinically isolated aortic stenosis. *Circulation* 1970; 42:91–94.
9. Korn D, DeSanctis RW, Sell S: Massive calcification of the mitral annulus: A clinicopathological study of 14 cases. *N Engl J Med* 1962;367:900–905.
10. Pomerance A: Pathological and clinical study of calcification of the mitral ring. *J Clin Pathol* 1970; 23:354–359.
11. Pomerance A, Darby AJ, Hodkinson HM: Valvular calcification in the elderly: Possible pathogenic factors. *J Gerontol* 1978;33:672–676.
12. Sugiura M, Uchiyama S, Kuwako K, et al: A clinicopathological study on mitral ring calcification. *Japan Heart J* 1977;18:154–159.
13. Simon MA, Liu SF: Calcification of mitral annulus and its relationship to functional valvular disturbance. *Am Heart J* 1954;48:497–501.
14. Harrison CV, Lennox B: Heart block in osteitis deformans. *Br Heart J* 1948;10:167–171.
15. Kirk RS, Russel JGB: Subvalvular calcification of mitral valve. *Br Heart J* 1969;31:684–689.
16. Lev M: Anatomic basis for atrioventricular block. *Am J Med* 1964;37:742–746.
17. Crawford MH, O'Rourke RA: Mitral valve prolapse syndrome, in Braunwald E, et al (eds): *Principals of Internal Medicine*, ed 9, New York, McGraw-Hill, 1981, p 91.
18. Pomerance A: Ballooning deformity (mucoid degeneration) of the atrioventricular valves. *Br Heart J* 1969;31:343–348.
19. Caulfield JB, Page DL, Kastor JA, et al: Connective tissue abnormalities in spontaneous rupture of chordae tendinae. *Arch Pathol* 1971;91:537–542.
20. Osmunsdon PJ, Callahan JA, Edwards JE: Ruptured mitral chordae tendineae. *Circulation* 1961;24:42–47.

CHAPTER 30
Venous Thromboembolism in the Elderly

J. Leclerc
R. D. Hull
J. Hirsh

Venous thromboembolism is a very important clinical problem in the elderly population primarily because of its high prevalence but also because of certain inherent problems related to the diagnosis, prevention, morbidity, and treatment of this disease in older patients. The high prevalence of venous thromboembolism in elderly patients is explained by the fact that age itself[1] is an important risk factor and also because elderly patients are prone to develop illnesses such as congestive cardiac failure, malignant disease, and hip fracture, which are additional risk factors for venous thromboembolism. In addition, elderly patients frequently have associated cardiorespiratory disease which renders them more vulnerable to the effects of even small or moderate-sized pulmonary embolism.

The clinical diagnosis of venous thromboembolism may be particularly difficult in elderly patients if they are confused or if they have an associated disorder such as chronic obstructive lung disease, congestive cardiac failure, paralytic stroke with leg swelling, or hip fracture, which may mask some of the manifestations of venous thrombosis.

Prophylaxis of venous thromboembolism presents a particular problem in the elderly patient with hip fracture since there is no proven efficacious and safe method of prevention in this patient group. Finally, there is evidence that the risk of hemorrhage is increased in elderly patients on long-term oral anticoagulant therapy and in elderly females treated with intravenous heparin.[2]

Despite these difficulties, there have been marked improvements in the clinical management of venous thromboembolism in both young and old patients over the last decade. Important advances have been in the areas of diagnosis and clinical trial methodology[3] which have produced reliable information, and which now provide the clinician with a rational approach to the diagnosis, prevention, and treatment of venous thromboembolism.

In this chapter, we will discuss the diagnosis, prevention and treatment of the complete clinical spectrum of venous thromboembolism, which includes acute deep vein thrombosis, acute recurrent deep vein thrombosis, the postphlebitic syndrome, and pulmonary embolism.

CLINICAL DIAGNOSIS OF VENOUS THROMBOSIS

It is now generally accepted that the clinical diagnosis of venous thrombosis is inaccurate, both because of low sensitivity and low specificity.[4,5] Clinical diagnosis is nonspecific because none of the symptoms and signs of venous thrombosis (Table 30-1) is unique to this condition and all can be caused by nonthrombotic disorders. Most patients who present with clinically suspected venous thrombosis do not have this diagnosis confirmed when they are investigated with accurate objective tests.[4] Clinical diagnosis has a low sensitivity because many potentially dangerous venous thrombi are nonobstructive and not associated with inflammation of the vessel wall or surrounding perivascular tissues and therefore have no detectable clinical manifestations. Consequently, patients with relatively

Table 30-1
Clinical Manifestations of Venous Thrombosis

Clinical Feature	Mechanism
Pain and tenderness	Vascular and perivascular inflammation and venous distention
Swelling	Venous obstruction and inflammation
Venous distention	Raised venous pressure
Discoloration	
Pallor	Arterial spasm
Cyanosis	Stagnant anoxia due to impaired venous return
Redness	Vascular and perivascular inflammation
Palpable cord	Thrombosed vein or thickened vein wall

minor symptoms and signs may have large and extensive venous thrombi. Because of this, management of venous thrombosis based on clinical diagnosis alone is no longer acceptable.[4]

DIAGNOSIS OF VENOUS THROMBOSIS USING OBJECTIVE TESTS

In recent years, objective tests have superseded clinical evaluation as the diagnostic standard for deep vein thrombosis.[5] The available objective diagnostic tests which have been adequately evaluated are venography,[6,7] impedance plethysmography (IPG),[6] Doppler ultrasound[8,9] and fibrinogen I 125 leg scanning.[6,10] The choice of the objective test to be used depends on whether it is required for the detection of subclinical thrombosis in high-risk patients or whether it is required to confirm the diagnosis of clinically suspected venous thrombosis.

Venography

Ascending venography is the standard reference method for the diagnosis of venous thrombosis.[6,7] The aim of venography is to inject radiopaque contrast medium into a dorsal foot vein to outline the deep venous system of the leg.[11] The most reliable criterion for the diagnosis of acute deep vein thrombosis is a constant intraluminal defect seen in two or more projections.[6,7] Other criteria, such as failure to fill a deep vein segment, are less reliable and may be due to technical factors. In expert hands, this method yields very accurate results. Special care must be taken to obtain adequate visualization of the entire deep venous system of the leg including the external (Figure 30-1) and common iliac veins and also to minimize the frequency of artifacts such as nonfilling of venous segments.

Venography has the disadvantage of being invasive. It may produce pain in the foot while the dye is being injected and may cause transient pain in the calf, one to two days after.[11] It may induce clinically significant phlebitis in a small percentage of patients (2%).[7] Fluid overload from the hyperosmotic dye may occur in elderly patients who have impaired cardiac function. Extravasation of dye at the site of injection may cause local skin and tissue necrosis[11] and this may lead to serious consequences in elderly patients with peripheral arterial insufficiency. Finally, venography cannot be used for the screening of high-risk patients and cannot be conveniently used for follow-up. For these reasons, noninvasive technics have been developed to replace ascending venography for the diagnosis of deep vein thrombosis.[5]

Impedance Plethysmography

Occlusive cuff impedance plethysmography (IPG) is a noninvasive technic based on the

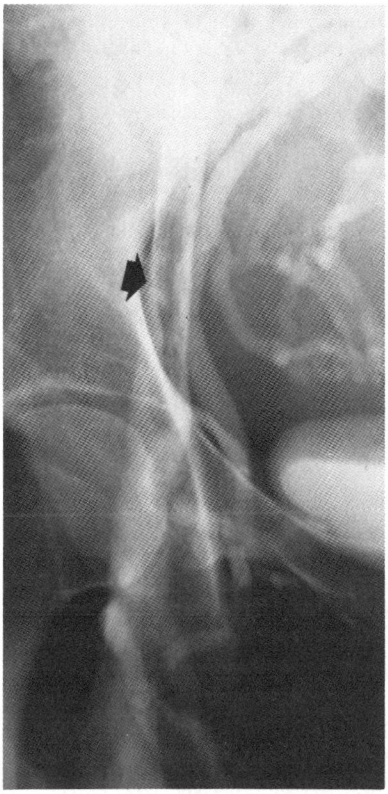

Figure 30-1 Acute venous thrombosis of the external iliac vein, showing a large filling defect in the distal external iliac vein. Note collaterals in the pelvis.

principle that blood volume changes in the calf produced by inflation or deflation of a pneumatic thigh cuff results in changes in electrical resistance (impedance) detected by skin electrodes placed around the calf.[5,6] The change in impedance is recorded on an ECG paper strip and both the total rise during cuff inflation and the fall occurring during the first 3 seconds of deflation are plotted on a two-way type IPG graph.[5] The graph includes a discriminant line separating normal and abnormal results.[5] With this method, plethysmography is 95% sensitive and specific to thrombosis of the popliteal, femoral, or iliac veins,[6] but it is relatively insensitive to calf vein thrombosis.

Impedance plethysmography does not distinguish between thrombotic and nonthrombotic obstruction to venous outflow. It may be falsely positive[5] (1) if the patient is positioned incorrectly or is inadequately relaxed (the vein is constricted by contracting muscles), (2) if the vein is compressed by an extrinsic mass (eg, pelvic tumor), or (3) if the venous outflow is impaired by raised central venous pressure (congestive heart failure, constrictive pericarditis). Reduced arterial inflow to the limb due to severe obstructive arterial disease can also lead to reduced venous outflow and consequently produce a false-positive result.[5] Finally, this test cannot be performed in patients with a leg in traction or wearing a plaster cast.

Fibrinogen I 125 Leg Scanning

The diagnosis of venous thrombosis by radioiodine-labeled fibrinogen scanning depends upon incorporation of circulating labeled fibrinogen into the thrombus which is detected by measuring the increase in overlying surface radioactivity with an isotope detector.[5,12] The measured surface radioactivity is expressed as a percentage of the surface radioactivity measured over the heart. Readings are taken over both legs. Venous thrombosis is *suspected*[5] if there is an increase in the radioactive reading of more than 20% (1) at any point compared with readings over adjacent points of the same leg, (2) over the same points on the previous day, or (3) over the corresponding point on the opposite leg. Venous thrombosis is *diagnosed*[5] if the scan remains abnormal at repeated examination 24 hours later. This test is very sensitive (95%) for detection of calf vein thrombosis in patients who have had symptoms for less than 8 days.[6] It is less sensitive for detection of proximal vein thrombosis[6] and is unreliable in the upper thigh because of the close proximity of the bladder (containing radioactive urine) and the presence of large veins and arteries which produce an increase in the background count.[5] It is insensitive to pelvic vein thrombosis because these veins are situated posteriorly and the relatively weak gamma rays which are emitted by the ^{125}I are not detected on the anterior abdominal surface.

Fibrinogen I 125 leg scanning should never be used alone for the diagnosis of symptomatic deep vein thrombosis because it is insensitive to high femoral and iliac vein thrombi and because there may be a 24- to 48-hour delay before sufficient radioactivity is incorporated into the symptomatic thrombus.[5] Falsely positive results are obtained when scanning is performed over hematoma or cellulitis. Patients with superficial varicosities may have a positive leg scan result and when this occurs, the test should be repeated after the leg has been wrapped in a compression bandage and elevated in order to decrease venous pooling. Because of the lack of specificity of fibrinogen I 125 leg scanning, a positive result with this test requires confirmation by venography.

The major use of fibrinogen I 125 leg scanning is for screening high-risk patients and for the diagnosis of acute recurrent deep vein thrombosis. These will be discussed later in the chapter.

Doppler Ultrasound

Doppler ultrasound is a noninvasive method for qualitative evaluation of venous blood flow.[8,9] The Doppler ultrasound flowmeter detects changes in the velocity of blood flow in the veins which are induced by normal respiratory excursions and by compressing and releasing the vein being examined. The ultrasound detector is placed over the vein and the 5-MHz ultrasound beam which is transmitted percutaneously is reflected from blood cells in the underlying vein. If the blood cells are stationary, the frequency of the reflected beam is identical to the frequency of the incident beam and no sound is recorded. If the blood cells are moving, the beam is reflected at an altered frequency (the Doppler shift) that is proportional to the velocity of blood flow. The difference in frequency between the incident and the reflected beam is translated into an audible signal. Venous blood flow produces a characteristic low-pitched sound that is phasic and changes in intensity with respiration, producing a "windstorm" effect. The sound is abolished by venous occlusion and when compression is released, an augmented sound is heard as blood flow in the vein suddenly increases. An augmented sound is also obtained by compression of the vein being examined distal to the ultrasound probe.

For a Doppler ultrasound study, the following veins are examined individually: common femoral, superficial femoral, popliteal, and posterior tibial. If the probe is placed over a thrombus, no Doppler shift or sound will be heard because the blood is stationary. If the probe is placed proximal to the thrombus and the vein is compressed distal to the thrombus, no augmented sound will be heard because of the obstructing thrombus.

Venous Doppler ultrasound is highly sensitive to proximal vein thrombosis but less sensitive to calf thrombi.[5] The major pitfall of this technic is that it requires an experienced examiner and the interpretation is subjective. This technic is useful for the diagnosis of venous thrombosis in patients in whom IPG is not possible (eg, leg in traction, leg amputation). It is also a useful method for demonstrating deep venous incompetence in patients with the postphlebitic syndrome.

A PRACTICAL APPROACH FOR THE DIAGNOSIS OF DEEP VEIN THROMBOSIS

Background

Over the last decade, we have performed a number of studies evaluating noninvasive tests for the diagnosis of venous thrombosis. In the first of these studies, the combined use of impedance plethysmography and fibrinogen I 125 leg scanning was evaluated for the diagnosis of deep vein thrombosis. In this study, all patients referred with clinically suspected deep vein thrombosis had an IPG on the day of referral and then daily for three days concurrently with leg scanning. All patients underwent bilateral venography either on the third day or earlier if either noninvasive test was positive. This combined approach was highly sensitive (sensitivity 94%) and specific (specificity 91%) for the diagnosis of deep vein thrombosis. In the subsequent study, we demonstrated the safety of not treating patients with anticoagulants if the results of both the IPG and leg scan were negative.[10]

Based on the foregoing, the following approach for the diagnosis of a first episode of deep venous thrombosis in symptomatic patients is recommended:

1. IPG should be performed on the day of referral and if positive, in the absence of conditions known to produce a false-positive result, a diagnosis of venous thrombosis can be made. In patients with a condition known to produce a falsely positive IPG result (eg, congestive heart failure), ascending venography is required to confirm the diagnosis of deep vein thrombosis.

2. If the IPG is negative on the day of referral, the clinician is faced with two alternatives. These are: (*a*) to repeat the test at intervals to detect extending calf vein thrombosis; or (*b*) perform 72-hour fibrinogen I 125 leg scanning. Serial IPG with repeated examination on day 5 to 7 is being used with apparent safety in many centers but requires formal evaluation in a prospective study. The addition of fibrinogen I 125 leg scanning when impedance plethysmography is negative is currently the most thoroughly evaluated approach. Patients do not need to be hospitalized or receive anticoagulants while undergoing serial IPG testing or leg scanning. For practical purposes, a negative IPG and leg scan result excludes the diagnosis of deep vein thrombosis in symptomatic patients and there is no need for further investigation or treatment.

3. Patients with deep vein thrombosis should have their IPGs repeated at 1 month, 3 months and then three times a month until it returns to normal. This provides a valuable base line which can be used for the diagnosis of acute recurrent deep vein thrombosis. In our experience, 30% of patients with deep vein thrombosis have a normal IPG after 3 weeks, 50% after 3 months, and 70% after 6 months.[13]

4. If impedance plethysmography is not available, then all patients with clinically suspected venous thrombosis should be tested by venography or by Doppler ultrasound.

5. In the hands of an expert, Doppler ultrasound can probably be used interchangeably with impedance plethysmography and a diagnostic algorithm similar to that described for impedance plethysmography should be followed.

ACUTE RECURRENT DEEP VENOUS THROMBOSIS

When patients present with pain or swelling in the leg that has been the previous site of proven venous thrombosis, it is difficult to establish a diagnosis of acute recurrent thrombosis on clinical grounds alone. Venography is also of limited value because the diagnostic hallmark of recurrent thrombosis, a constant intraluminal defect, may be masked due to obliteration and recanalization of the involved veins. We have recently demonstrated the value of the combination of impedance plethysmography and fibrinogen I 125 leg scanning in ruling in or ruling out acute recurrent deep vein thrombosis.[14] In this prospective study, we evaluated impedance plethysmography and fibrinogen I 125 leg scanning plus venography for the diagnosis of recurrent deep vein thrombosis in 270 patients considered by their physician to be experiencing symptoms and signs of acute recurrent deep vein thrombosis. The results demonstrated that symptomatic patients can be separated into two groups: (1) a negative cohort (patients in whom both noninvasive tests are negative and in whom it is safe to withhold anticoagulant therapy), and (2) a positive cohort (patients in whom either noninvasive test is positive and who require anticoagulant therapy).

Of 270 patients, 182 (67%) had negative impedance plethysmograph and leg scanning results; only 3 of these 181 patients (1.7%) returned with recurrent venous thromboembolism during long-term follow-up and no patient died from pulmonary embolism. In contrast, patients with positive impedance plethysmograph or leg scan results had a high frequency of acute recurrent deep venous thrombosis on long-term follow-up; 18 of 89 (20.8%) developed new episodes of documented venous thromboembolism including 4 deaths from pulmonary embolism, a highly statistically significant difference. In the majority of positive patients, recurrent venous thromboembolism occurred after anticoagulant therapy had been terminated either inadvertently or following three months of therapy.

On the basis of our studies, we recommend the following diagnostic approach (Figure 30-2), in patients with clinically suspected acute recurrent venous thrombosis:

1. IPG should be performed first and if positive in the absence of conditions known to produce a false-positive result, a diagnosis of recurrent venous thrombosis can be made.

2. If the IPG is negative, a leg scan should be done and both the leg scan and the IPG repeated 24 and 72 hours later. If either of these tests is positive in the absence of conditions known to produce a false-positive result, a diagnosis of recurrent venous thrombosis can be made.

3. If both tests are negative, then a diagnosis of recurrent venous thrombosis can be excluded. Using this approach, a small percentage of patients with suspected recurrent venous thrombosis who have a positive IPG as a result of their previous thrombotic episode may be treated unnecessarily, but at present there is no alternative approach which is as safe and effective.

This diagnostic approach has a high clinical utility since it allows the clinician to establish a definitive management in most patients with clinically suspected recurrent deep vein thrombosis. It is also highly cost-effective since patients with negative noninvasive tests are spared the need for in-hospital care and long-term anticoagulant therapy.

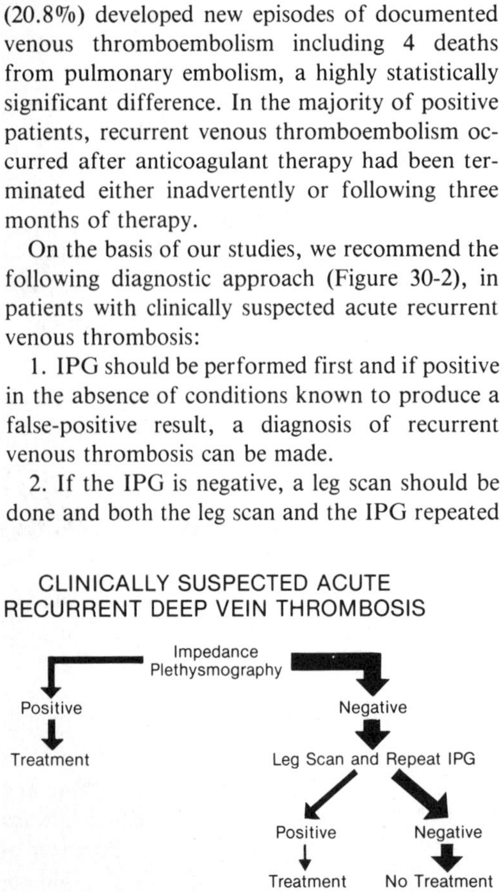

Figure 30-2 Recommended approach for patients with clinically suspected acute recurrent deep vein thrombosis.

THE POSTPHLEBITIC SYNDROME

The postphlebitic syndrome refers to a disorder caused by deep venous incompetence and/or persistent obstruction following deep vein thrombosis.[15] The postphlebitic syndrome occurs as a consequence of the generation of abnormally high pressure in the deep veins of the leg (Figure 30-3).[16,17] Chronic venous hypertension is secondary to deep valve incompetence with or without outflow obstruction. Incompetence of the valves may be caused by their direct involvement by the thrombotic process or by dilatation of the distal veins as a consequence of proximal obstruction. It has been suggested that the competence of the popliteal valves is an important factor in determining the ambulatory venous pressure in post-thrombotic limbs. In more advanced cases, perforator valves became incompetent and cause direct transmission of ambulatory venous hypertension to the superficial veins and dermal vessels. The development of perforator incompetence is thought to be an important mechanism for the development of venous ulcers.

The clinical manifestations of the postphlebitic syndrome are caused by chronic venous hypertension, perforator incompetence, and incompetence of the superficial veins. The initial symptoms are caused by *venous hypertension* and include swelling and edema of the ankle and the calf which are most marked after the patient has been standing or walking.[18] The swelling may be intermittent and is usually relieved by rest and leg elevation. Marked swelling of the thigh may also occur after

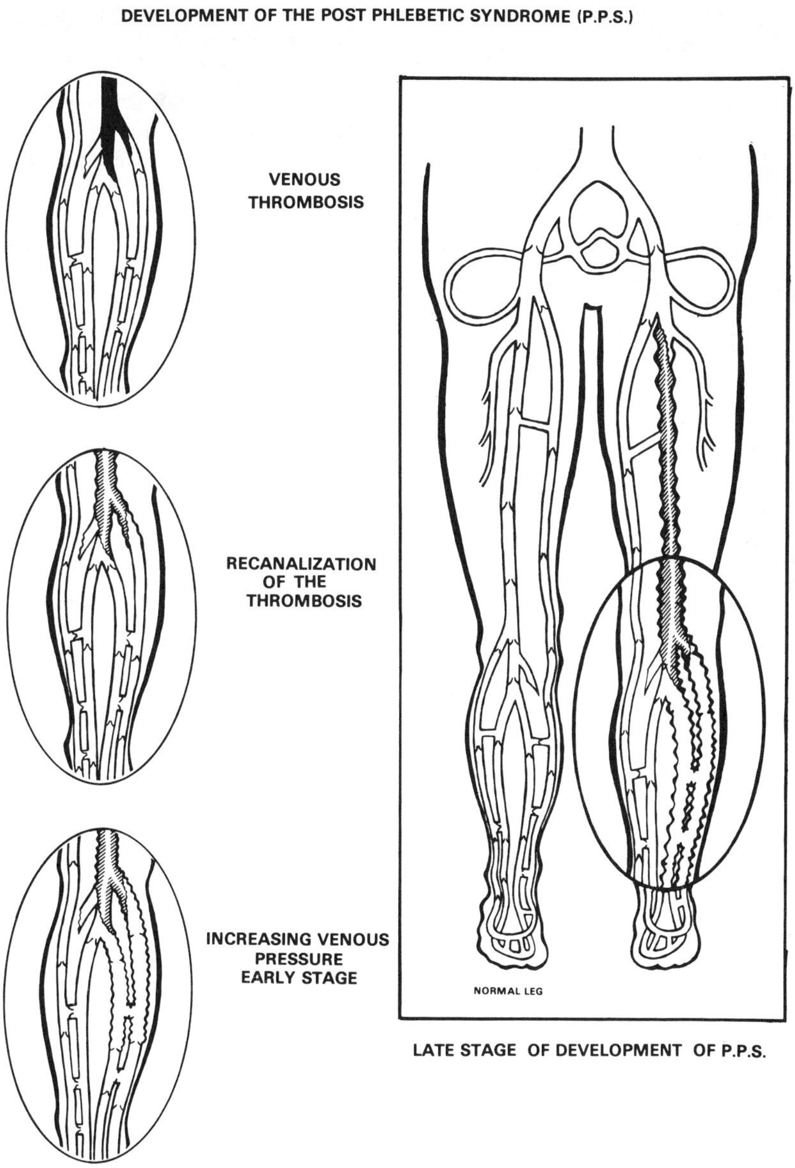

Figure 30-3 Development of postphlebitic syndrome (PPS). Following acute venous thrombosis (upper left) the thrombus recanalizes (middle left) leading to valvular destruction and an increase in venous pressure; this in turn results in distention of veins distal to the recanalized segment (lower left). The resulting venous distention produces further venous dilatation which in turn leads to more extensive valvular incompetence and the development of the postphlebitic syndrome with pain, swelling, pigmentation and, in its most severe form, ulceration (right).

proximal vein thrombosis. Heavy, aching pain in the calf and proximal leg is typically present and is exacerbated by standing and relieved by rest and leg elevation. Venous claudication may occur after iliofemoral thrombosis. Patients with this disorder complain of a "bursting" pain in the thigh or calf which is produced by walking and particularly by climbing. It can mimic arterial claudication. With time and the development of *incompetent perforators*, pigmentation, induration, and prominent venules develop around the ankle and the lower third of the leg.[19] The skin pigmentation is caused by repeated bleeding from dermal capillaries which results in the deposition of hemosiderin. There is also a thickening of the skin and subcutaneous tissue called lipodermatosclerosis. Venous ulceration occurs as a late manifestation. The ulcers usually develop in the region of the medial malleolus. Venous ulceration is the most serious manifestation of the postphlebitic syndrome and is responsible for marked disability. Venous ulcers respond to conservative management but have a tendency to recur.[19] *Superficial varicosities* may occur and they are caused by secondary destruction of the valves of the superficial veins.

There is no definitive diagnostic test for the postphlebitic syndrome, but objective evidence of a prior episode of deep vein thrombosis, or the demonstration of deep valve incompetence in a patient with appropriate symptoms, constitute sufficient evidence to make the diagnosis. Qualitative evaluation with Doppler ultrasound is the most simple and rapid method to detect venous reflux. The presence of reflux is elicited by compressing the area proximal to the valve being examined and placing the probe distally. A positive test for venous reflux in the presence of the appropriate signs and symptoms supports a diagnosis. If venous Doppler ultrasound is not available, ascending venography can be performed to confirm the previous episode of venous thrombosis and to demonstrate the persistent abnormalities (recanalized postphlebitic veins, collateral channels, varicose superficial veins) which frequently accompany the postphlebitic syndrome.

SUBCLINICAL THROMBOSIS IN HIGH RISK PATIENTS

The majority of venous thrombi that lead to fatal pulmonary embolism are asymptomatic.[20] Therefore, prevention of fatal pulmonary embolism can only be achieved by detecting subclinical thrombi and treating them before they become dangerous or by using primary prophylaxis.[21,22] Of the two methods, primary prophylaxis is by far the most cost-effective[23] and is the method of choice in most clinical circumstances. Fatal pulmonary embolism is an important complication in the elderly because these patients frequently have morbid conditions which predispose to venous thrombosis such as congestive cardiac failure, immobility, fractured hip, malignant disease, stroke.

PROPHYLAXIS OF VENOUS THROMBOEMBOLISM

A number of prophylactic methods are effective in preventing venous thrombosis and pulmonary embolism. The most extensively tested methods are low-dose heparin,[22] intermittent pneumatic compression of the leg,[23,24] dextran,[25] and oral anticoagulants.[26] Low-dose heparin is usually given in a dose of 5000 units 2 hours preoperatively and then either at 12 or 8 hours postsurgery. This form of prophylaxis is effective in preventing symptomatic calf vein thrombi, proximal vein thrombi, and major pulmonary emboli. It is the most convenient prophylactic method in high-risk medical and surgical patients. External pneumatic compression is a highly effective form of prophylaxis which can be used as an alternative to low-dose heparin in patients in whom low-dose heparin is either contraindicated or ineffective. Dextran is a useful method with demonstrated efficacy in orthopedic patients[25] with hip fracture, but its use may be complicated by volume overload in elderly patients who have impaired cardiac function.

CHOICE OF PROPHYLAXIS IN THE VARIOUS HIGH-RISK GROUPS

Elective Abdominal and Thoracic Surgery

The risk of venous thromboembolism in patients undergoing abdominal or thoracic surgery is influenced by the patient's age, the nature and extent of the operative procedure, and on whether or not there is a history of previous venous thromboembolism. Without prophylaxis, patients over the age of 40 and more so over the age of 60, who have abdominal or thoracic surgical procedures performed under general anesthesia which last at least 30 minutes, have a risk of developing calf vein thrombosis that varies between 20% and 40%,[27] a risk of proximal vein thrombosis of between 4% and 8%,[27] and a risk of fatal pulmonary embolism of between 0.2% and 0.7%. These patients should be given prophylaxis either with low-dose heparin or external pneumatic compression. Patients with a history of recent venous thromboembolism, or who have extensive pelvic or abdominal surgery, or advanced *malignancy*[28] are even at higher risk. Without prophylaxis, these patients have a 30% to 60% risk of developing fibrinogen I 125 leg scan–detected calf vein thrombosis, a 6% to 12% risk of developing proximal vein thrombi, and a 1% to 2% risk of fatal pulmonary embolism.

The best prophylaxis for this very high risk category has not been established but it is reasonable to suggest that an effective method of primary prophylaxis such as low-dose heparin or external pneumatic compression be combined with fibrinogen I 125 leg scanning to detect patients who break through primary prophylaxis.

Hip Surgery

Without prophylaxis, over 50% of patients who have elective hip surgery or who have a fractured hip develop venous thrombosis[29]; 20% develop proximal vein thrombosis, and between 1% to 5% have a fatal pulmonary embolism. Two forms of prophylaxis, oral anticoagulants[26] and dextran,[25] are effective in preventing venous thromboembolism in these patients. Oral anticoagulants are most effective when treatment is initiated before surgery or at the time of surgery, but this is associated with an increased risk of bleeding which is considered unacceptable by most orthopedic surgeons. Bleeding is reduced if oral anticoagulants are started 48 hours after completing surgery in a dose which is aimed to prolong the prothrombin time to approximately 1.2 to 1.5 times control (rabbit brain thromboplastin) on the fourth or fifth postoperative day. Although this approach needs to be evaluated further in properly designed studies, we use this method in fractured hip patients with a previous history of deep venous thrombosis. Dextran commenced preoperatively is effective but because of the risk of volume overload, it is not recommended in elderly patients. At the present time, the combination of screening tests (IPG and fibrinogen I 125 leg scanning), although expensive, is the most appropriate preventive measure in these patients until a safe and effective prophylactic method becomes available.

Major Knee Surgery

Without protection between 60% to 70% of patients undergoing major knee surgery develop calf vein thrombosis and 20% develop proximal vein thrombosis.[23] External pneumatic compression is highly effective in these patients and is the prophylactic method of choice.[23] In these patients, external pneumatic compression is continued postoperatively until patients are ambulatory. In patients with a plaster cast, prophylaxis with oral anticoagulants or subcutaneous heparin started postoperatively is the method of choice and should be continued until the plaster cast is removed.

Genitourinary Surgery

Trans-urethral resection of the prostate carries a 7% to 10% risk of developing ^{125}I leg scan-detected calf vein thrombosis.[24,30] The risk is even higher in patients having retropubic prostatectomy or an equivalent operation: 25% to 50% of these patients develop leg scan-detected calf vein thrombosis. The results of low-dose heparin have been inconsistent in this group. On the other hand, external pneumatic compression is effective and is the method of choice to prevent calf vein thrombosis.[24]

High Risk Medical Patients

Myocardial infarction Between 20% to 40% of patients who sustain an acute myocardial infarction develop calf vein thrombosis and the risk is higher in patients who also develop congestive heart failure. Low-dose heparin is effective in reducing the frequency of leg scan-detected venous thrombosis in these patients.[31]

Cerebrovascular accidents Approximately 60% of all patients who sustain a paralytic stroke develop leg scan-detected venous thrombosis. Although not definitively established, it is likely that either external pneumatic compression or low-dose heparin would be effective in preventing serious venous thromboembolism in this patient group. External pneumatic compression is the prophylactic method of choice in patients with intracerebral hemorrhage.

DIAGNOSIS OF PULMONARY EMBOLISM

The clinical diagnosis of pulmonary embolism is unreliable because all symptoms and signs are nonspecific.[32] Although dyspnea, tachypnea, and pleuritic chest pain occur in a majority of patients with angiographically demonstrated emboli, these clinical features do not reliably differentiate pulmonary embolism from other cardiopulmonary disorders.

Historically, a number of laboratory investigations have been used either as screening tests or as definitive diagnostic tests in patients with clinically suspected pulmonary embolism.[33] These investigations, which include serum enzymes and bilirubin, levels of fibrin split products, arterial blood gas analysis, chest films, and ECG findings, have all been shown to lack sensitivity and specificity. The chest film and ECG are important to rule out other disorders which may simulate pulmonary embolism but cannot be used to diagnose pulmonary embolism.

The diagnostic approach to pulmonary embolism is not as clear-cut as the diagnostic approach to venous thrombosis because the diagnostic standard, pulmonary angiography, cannot be performed in all centers and the noninvasive tests, particularly lung scanning, which are used as a substitute for pulmonary angiography, have not been as carefully evaluated as the noninvasive tests for venous thrombosis.[5]

Lung Scanning

Perfusion scintigraphy with technetium-Tc 99m is widely used as a screening test in patients with clinically suspected pulmonary embolism. This technic detects occluded vessels more than 3 mm in diameter and is virtually 100% sensitive in its ability to detect clinically significant pulmonary emboli.[32] When this test was first introduced in the late 1960s, it became rapidly accepted as a valid test for the diagnosis of pulmonary embolism and it was believed that most patients with clinically suspected pulmonary embolism who had an abnormal perfusion lung scan and a normal chest film, had pulmonary embolism. However, it was soon realized that the perfusion lung scan was nonspecific, since it could not distinguish pulmonary embolism from a number of nonembolic pathologic processes which also affect pulmonary blood flow.[32]

With the advent of ventilation scanning in the late 1970s, a new diagnostic concept was developed to improve the specificity of the perfusion lung scan. This concept was based on the premise that patients with pulmonary emboli have an abnormal perfusion scan and a normal ventilation scan (a so-called ventilation/perfusion mismatch), whereas patients with a primary ventilation defect have a matching abnormality on the perfusion and ventilation scan. When studies comparing the results of pulmonary angiography with ventilation and perfusion scans were performed in patients with clinically suspected pulmonary embolism, it became evident that the mismatch concept was an oversimplification. These studies demonstrated that the probability of pulmonary embolism is 80% or greater when the perfusion scan shows a large defect (segmental or larger) with a normal ventilation scan (Figure 30-4).[34] On the other hand, patients with smaller perfusion defects (subsegmental or smaller) often do not have pulmonary embolism even though they have a normal ventilation scan. Patients with abnormal perfusion and ventilation lung scans sometimes have pulmonary embolism demonstrated by pulmonary angiography.

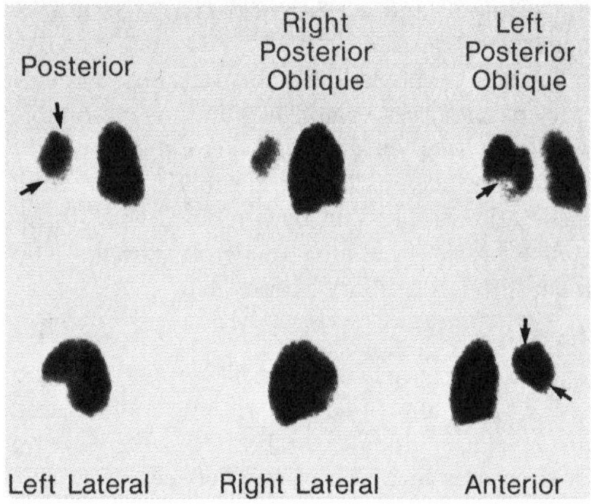

Figure 30-4 A segmental ventilation-perfusion mismatch characteristic of pulmonary embolism. Perfusion scan (posterior view) reveals a segmental filling defect involving the apical segment of the left upper lobe, while the xenon 127 ventilation scan is normal.

In summary, therefore, it can be concluded (1) that perfusion scintigraphy is a sensitive screening test for patients with clinically suspected pulmonary embolism, (2) that the ventilation scan is a useful addition to the diagnostic process in patients with large (segmental or larger) perfusion defects if the ventilation scan is normal since 80% or more of these patients have pulmonary embolism documented by pulmonary angiography, and (3) that ventilation-perfusion scanning is not useful for making management decisions in patients with small defects (subsegmental or smaller) or in patients with large matched defects since it is not possible to rule in or rule out pulmonary embolism in patients with these patterns of perfusion-ventilation scan abnormalities.

Pulmonary Angiography

Pulmonary angiography is the most definitive means of making the diagnosis of pulmonary embolism and it is the reference method. Technical improvements in recent years have made this method more accurate and safer to perform even in elderly patients. Selective pulmonary angiography is performed by passing a catheter through the right heart and then injecting dye selectively in each of the main pulmonary artery branches. With selective filling of the artery, accuracy is markedly improved and much less dye needs to be injected. The most reliable criterion for the diagnosis of pulmonary embolism is the presence of an intraluminal filling defect (Figure 30-5). A sharp vessel cut-off is an indirect sign and is not diagnostic of pulmonary embolism. When indicated, pulmonary angiography should be performed as soon as possible after a provisional diagnosis of pulmonary embolism has been made by lung scan because thrombi fragment after a few days and a false-negative result may occur.[32]

A SUGGESTED APPROACH TO THE DIAGNOSIS OF PULMONARY EMBOLISM

On the basis of our studies and other reports in the literature,[34-36] we have evolved an approach to the diagnosis of pulmonary embolism which is summarized in Figure 30-6. Three investigations are the key to this diagnostic algorithm: ventilation-perfusion lung scanning, pulmonary angiography, and objective tests for deep vein thrombosis. There are four major components to this algorithm: First, all patients should have a chest film and ECG to rule out other conditions which may mimic pulmonary embolism (eg, pneumothorax, myocardial infarction, pneumonia, etc). Second, a perfusion lung scan should be performed, and if normal, clinically significant pulmonary embolism can be excluded and no further investigation is required. If the perfusion lung scan is abnormal and the defect is segmental or greater in size, then a ventilation scan should be performed, and if the perfusion-ventilation scan pattern shows one or more segmental or greater defect(s) which ventilate normally, a diagnosis of pulmonary embolism can be made. Pulmonary angiography is the most definitive means to diagnose pulmonary embolism in patients who have an abnormal perfusion scan that does not fall into the category of high probability (see above), since none of the patterns have sufficiently high or low predictive power to rule in or rule out pulmonary embolism. Objective tests for venous thrombosis are extremely useful since a positive IPG or venogram increases the likelihood of pulmonary embolism and in patients with an abnormal perfusion scan, a decision to treat with anticoagulants can be made without performing a pulmonary angiogram. Pulmonary angiography should be performed in patients with clinically suspected pulmonary embolism and an abnormal lung scan who have normal venograms or in patients where the nature of the underlying pulmonary abnormality needs to be clarified (eg investigation of a pulmonary infiltrate, pleural effusion).

TREATMENT OF VENOUS THROMBOEMBOLISM

Proximal Deep Vein Thrombosis and/or Pulmonary Embolism

The main objectives of the treatment of venous thromboembolism are (1) to prevent death from

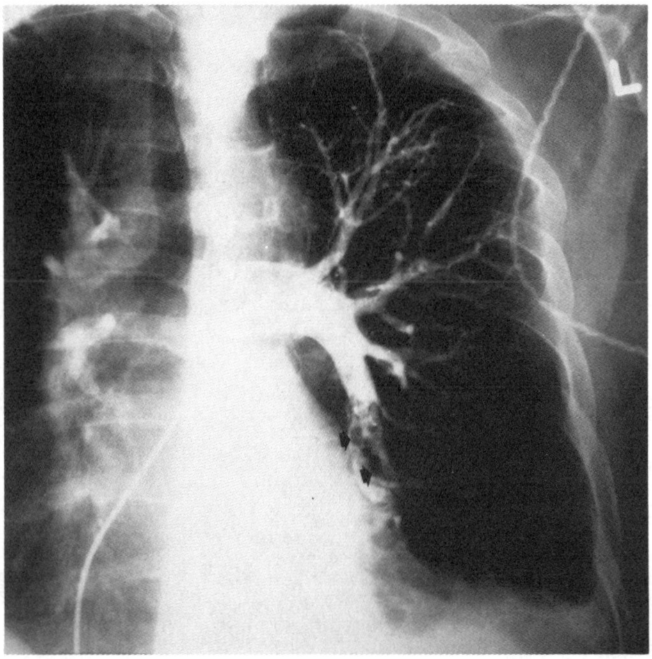

Figure 30-5 Selective left pulmonary angiogram: an intraluminal filling defect at the first bifurcation of the left lower lobe main pulmonary artery establishes a definitive diagnosis of pulmonary embolism.

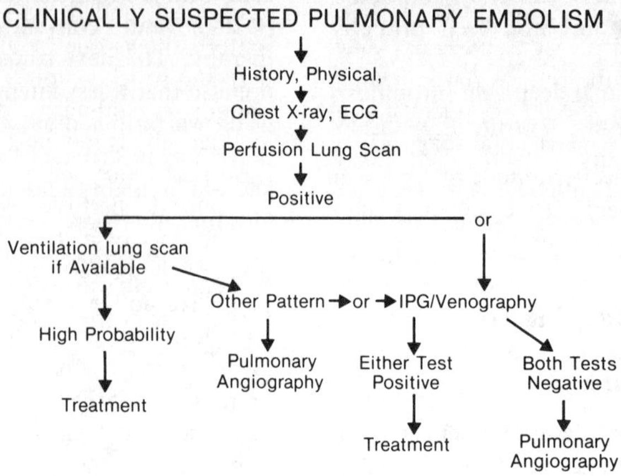

Figure 30-6 Recommended approach for patients with clinically suspected pulmonary embolism.

pulmonary embolism, (2) to reduce morbidity from the acute event, and (3) to achieve these objectives with a minimum of side-effects. In most patients, these objectives can be achieved with anticoagulants but because they are not free from side-effects, it is important to ensure that the diagnosis of venous thromboembolism is confirmed by objective tests before initiating treatment.[5]

Heparin is the treatment of choice in patients with proximal deep vein thrombosis and/or pulmonary embolism because it is effective in both preventing extension of venous thrombi and fatal pulmonary embolism. The standard approach is to administer an initial bolus of heparin sodium followed by either a continuous infusion or by 4-hourly intermittent injections.[37] For most patients, an initial loading dose of 5000 units is sufficient, but patients with extensive proximal vein thrombosis or pulmonary embolism usually require a higher dose (7000 to 10,000 units) and old and frail patients a lower dose (approximately 3000 units). The continuous infusion of heparin is administered in a dosage of 24,000 units/24 h and the dose adjusted according to results of the monitoring test.

The activated partial thromboplastin time (APTT) is one of the most commonly used methods to monitor the anticoagulant effect of heparin in North America. When the continuous infusion method is used, the aim is to maintain the test result at approximately 1.5 times control. When intermittent intravenous (IV) heparin is used, the aim is to maintain the APTT at approximately 1.5 times control before the next injection is due. It may be useful to obtain a heparin level in patients who fail to demonstrate adequate prolongation of the APTT despite treatment with what appears to be adequate doses of heparin. In these patients, failure to prolong APTT may be associated with either low "therapeutic" levels of circulating heparin (0.3 to 0.5 units/ml). If the heparin level is low, the dose of heparin should be increased. If, however, the heparin level is within the therapeutic range,[37] it is recommended that the dose not be increased further. The reason why the APTT remains relatively short in the presence of adequate heparin level is not always clear, but in many cases it is due to very high levels of coagulation factors (particularly factor VIII) which artificially shorten the APTT.

Intermittent IV injection of heparin can be used as an alternative to full-dose continuous IV heparin infusion. This approach has been reported to produce a greater frequency of bleeding in patients at high risk of hemorrhage.[38] It should be noted, however, that in these studies, higher doses of heparin were used in the group given IV heparin, so that the increased rate of bleeding could have been related to the dose rather than the method of administration.[38] Intermittent injection should be administered every 4 hours in a dose of between 4000 to 7000 units per injection. Although it is recommended that the dose be adjusted to produce an APTT of approximately 1.5 times control immediately before the next injection is due, in practice careful laboratory monitoring with intermittent heparin is difficult. Subcutaneous heparin given in full therapeutic doses has been reported to be another effective method of heparin administration and preliminary studies suggest that it may cause less bleeding. However, this method has not been properly evaluated.

In patients with proximal deep vein thrombosis or pulmonary embolism, treatment with IV heparin is followed by oral anticoagulants for a period of 12 weeks. Oral anticoagulants are given to prevent the late recurrence of venous thromboembolism. In patients with an underlying risk factor (eg, lower limb fracture, paralytic stroke), it is sensible to continue therapy until the risk factor is reversed. Oral anticoagulants should be started 4 to 5 days before heparin is stopped since the full antithrombotic effect of oral anticoagulants is delayed.

The administration of vitamin K antagonists monitored by conventional level of anticoagulant control is associated with an appreciable risk of bleeding (5% major bleeding episodes). Recently we have conducted a series of clinical trials designed to answer the question of whether protection against late recurrence of venous thromboembolism can be achieved without exposing patients to a substantial risk of hemorrhage. In these studies, three anticoagulant regimens for long-term treatment of proximal deep vein thrombosis were successfully explored. These are:

1. Adjusted intermediate dose of subcutaneous heparin
2. Conventional oral anticoagulant therapy using sodium warfarin[39] with prothrombin time (using Simplastin) maintained at 1.5 to 2 times the control
3. A less intense anticoagulant approach using sodium warfarin with prothrombin time (using Simplastin) maintained at approximately 1.25 times the control[39]

In the first of these studies, conventional warfarin sodium therapy was compared with an adjusted dose of subcutaneous heparin which we predicted might be associated with a lesser risk of hemorrhage without loss of effectiveness in preventing recurrent venous thromboembolism. The dose in the subcutaneous heparin group was adjusted to maintain the mid-interval APTT (determined 6 hours after injection) at 1.5 times the control value. The dose was then fixed after the initial 3 days and no further anticoagulant monitoring was performed over the 3 months of long-term therapy. Adjusted dose subcutaneous heparin regimen proved effective in preventing recurrent venous thromboembolism and its use was associated with a significantly lower risk of bleeding (<2%) than conventional warfarin sodium therapy. The next study was designed with the premise that a less intense anticoagulant regimen using warfarin sodium might also be effective in preventing recurrence of venous thromboembolism and that it might be associated with a lower risk of bleeding; therefore, conventional oral anticoagulant therapy was compared with a less intense regimen using warfarin sodium. The patients randomized into the less intense oral anticoagulant group had their warfarin therapy monitored to maintain the prothrombin time using human brain thromboplastin (Manchester Comparative Reagent) at twice the control values. This is comparable to a prothrombin time using Simplastin of approximately 15 seconds (or 1.25 times the control). This study demonstrated that warfarin sodium administered to provide a less intense anticoagulant effect retained its effectiveness against recurrent venous thromboembolism (the frequency of recurrence was less than 2%) with a greatly reduced frequency of bleeding (less than 5% compared to 20% in the conventional warfarin sodium group).

The findings of these randomized trials indicate that the hemorrhagic risk of long-term therapy for venous thrombosis can be substantially reduced by either a regimen using an adjusted dose of subcutaneous heparin or a less intense oral warfarin sodium regimen. The adjusted-dose regimen can be used in patients who cannot take oral medication but it should be used with caution in elderly patients in view of the risk of osteoporosis associated with long-term administration of heparin. A less intense oral anticoagulant regimen can be achieved either by maintaining prothrombin time using Simplastin at approximately 1.25 times control, or by using a more sensitive human brain thromboplastin (eg, Manchester Comparative Reagent, which is widely available in Europe) maintained between 24 to 28 seconds (control of 12–13 seconds).

Calf Deep Vein Thrombosis

Patients with isolated calf vein thrombosis are usually treated in hospital with heparin for 7 days, followed by either oral anticoagulants or by subcutaneous heparin at the dose of 5000 units every 12 hours for 6 weeks.[40]

Major Pulmonary Embolism

In some patients the clinical manifestations of pulmonary embolism are accompanied by hemodynamic impairment as manifested by hypotension and/or acute cor pulmonale. These very ill patients are at risk of dying over the next 12 to 24 hours as a result of pulmonary vascular obstruction, severe hypoxemia, arrhythmia, acidemia, or even a small recurrent embolism. This clinical picture is seen in patients with massive embolism or with pre-existing cardiac or pulmonary disease. The first step in the management of this condition is to confirm pulmonary embolism by objective testing. The differential diagnosis includes other conditions which may simulate massive pulmonary embolism such as acute myocardial infarction, dissecting aneurysm of ascending aorta, pericardial tamponade, tension pneumothorax, hemorrhage, and septic shock. Although the indications for thrombolytic therapy in patients with acute pulmonary embolism have not been definitely established, rapid lysis of emboli in these critically ill patients is desirable.[41] In this situation, pulmonary embolism should be confirmed by pulmonary angiography and thrombolytic therapy started as soon as possible and continued for 12 to 24 hours, followed by heparin and oral anticoagulants.

Recurrent Venous Thromboembolism

The first step in the management of acute recurrent deep vein thrombosis is to confirm the diagnosis by using objective tests. Patients are treated with IV heparin for a period of 7 to 10 days followed by oral anticoagulants for at least a year, in view of the high recurrence rate (20% in the following year) in patients who received only three months of oral anticoagulants.[23] In addition, life-long anticoagulation should be considered (1) in patients with more than two episodes of well-documented venous thromboembolism, and (2) after a first episode of pulmonary embolism in patients who have a severe underlying cardiopulmonary condition in whom a small or moderate-sized pulmonary embolism could be fatal.

Postphlebitic Syndrome

Treatment of patients with postphlebitic syndrome is conservative and aimed at increasing venous return to the heart and preventing stasis.[42] Symptoms of pain and dependent edema are best relieved by periodic leg elevation. Pressure-gradient elastic stockings compress the superficial veins, force blood flow into the deep veins, and prevent venous stasis.[43] Although graduate pressure stockings do not completely correct the abnormal venous hemodynamics, most patients experience subjective relief and they may be useful in preventing venous ulcers. Patients should be instructed to wear the stockings continuously. Patients should also be instructed to protect the lower ankle area against trauma, which is often an initiating factor in the development of venous ulcers. The treatment of venous ulceration is also conservative[42] and consists of rest, leg elevation, control of infection, and topical applications of proteolytic enzymes. Venous ulcers rarely require ablative surgery.

REFERENCES

1. Hirsh J, Genton E, Hull R: Risk factors in thrombosis, in Hirsh J, Genton E, Hull R (eds): *Venous Thromboembolism.* New York, Grune and Stratton, 1981, pp 19–41.
2. Vieweg WVR, Piscatelli RL, House JJ, et al: Complications of intravenous administration of heparin in elderly women. *JAMA* 1970;213:1303–1306.
3. Hull R: Venous thromboembolism: Applying epidemiology to controversies. *Vascular Diagnosis and Therapy* April/May, 1981.
4. Hirsh J, Genton E, Hull R: Venous thrombosis, in Hirsh J, Genton E, Hull R (eds): *Venous Thromboembolism.* New York, Grune and Stratton, 1981, pp 42–52.
5. Hirsh J: Noninvasive tests for thromboembolic disease. *Hospital Practice* 1982;17:77–93.
6. Hull R, Hirsh J, Sackett DL, et al: Combined use of leg scanning and impedance plethysmography in suspected venous thrombosis, an alternative to venography. *N Engl J Med* 1977;296:1497–1500.
7. Hull R, Hirsh J, Sackett DL, et al: Clinical validity of a negative venogram in patients with clinically suspected venous thrombosis. *Circulation* 1981;64: 622–625.
8. Evans DS: The early diagnosis of thromboembolism by ultrasound. *Ann R Coll Surg Engl* 1971; 49:225–249.
9. Strandness DE, Sumner DS: Ultrasonic velocity detector in the diagnosis of thrombophlebitis. *Arch Surg* 1972;104:180–183.
10. Hull R, Hirsh J, Sackett DL, et al: Replacement of venography in suspected venous thombosis by impedance plethysmography and ^{125}I-fibrinogen leg scanning. *Ann Intern Med* 1981;94:12–15.
11. Hirsh J, Hull R: Comparative value of tests for the diagnosis of venous thrombosis. *World J Surg* 1978;2:27–28.
12. Kakkar VV, Nicholaides AN, Renney JTG, et al: ^{125}I-labelled fibrinogen test adapted for routine screening for deep-vein thrombosis. *Lancet* 1972;1: 540–542.
13. Jay R, Hull R, Carter C, et al: Outcome of abnormal impedance plethysmography results in patients with proximal-vein thrombosis: Frequency of return to normal. In Press.
14. Hull RD, Carter C, Jay R, et al: The diagnosis of acute recurrent deep vein thrombosis: A diagnostic challenge. *Circulation* 1983;67:901–906.
15. Hirsh J, Genton E, Hull R: The post-phlebitic syndrome, in Hirsh J, Genton E, Hull R (eds): *Venous*

Thromboembolism. New York, Grune and Stratton, 1981, pp 63–66.

16. DeCamp PT, Ward JA, Ochsner A: Ambulatory venous pressure studies in post-phlebitic and other disease states. *Surgery* 1951;29:42–52.
17. Hojemsgard IC, Sturp H: Venous pressure in primary and post-thrombotic varicose veins. *Acta Chir Scand* 1950;99:133–153.
18. Negus D: Calf pain in the post-thrombotic syndrome. *Br Med J* 1968;2:156–158.
19. Browse NL: Venous insufficiency: Nonoperative management, in Bang N, Glover J, Holden R, et al (eds): *Thrombosis and Atherosclerosis.* Chicago, Year Book Medical Publishers, 1982, pp 275–281.
20. Bell WR, Simon TL: Current status of pulmonary thromboembolic disease: Pathophysiology, diagnosis, prevention and treatment. *Am Heart J* 1982; 103:239–262.
21. Clagett GP, Salzman EW: Prevention of venous thromboembolism. *Prog Cardiovasc Dis* 1975;17: 345–366.
22. Kakkar VV, Stamatakis JD, Bentley PG, et al: Prophylaxis for postoperative deep-vein thrombosis. *JAMA* 1979;241:39–42.
23. Hull R, Delmore TJ, Hirsh J, et al: Effectiveness of intermittent pulsatile elastic stockings for the prevention of calf and thigh vein thrombosis in patients undergoing elective knee surgery. *Thromb Res* 1979;16:37–45.
24. Salzman EW, Ploetz J, Bettman M, et al: Intraoperative external pneumatic calf compression to afford long-term prophylaxis against deep vein thrombosis in urological patients. *Surgery* 1980;87: 239–242.
25. Gruber UF, Saldeen T, Brokop T, et al: Incidence of fatal postoperative pulmonary embolism after prophylaxis with dextran 70 and low-dose heparin. An international multicentre study. *Br Med J* 1980;280:69–72.
26. Coventry MB, Nolan DR, Beckenbaugh RD: "Delayed" prophylactic anticoagulation. A study of results and complications in 2,012 total hip arthroplasties. *J Bone Joint Surg* 1973;55A,1487.
27. Rosenberg L, Evans M, Pollock AV: Prophylaxis of postoperative leg vein thrombosis by low dose subcutaneous heparin or preoperative calf muscle stimulation: A controlled clinical trial. *Br Med J* 1975;1:649–651.
28. Roberts VC, Cotton LT: Prevention of postoperative deep vein thrombosis in patients with malignant disease. *Br Med J* 1974;1:358–360.
29. Hull R, Hirsh J, Sackett DL, et al: The value of adding impedance plethysmography to ^{125}I-fibrinogen leg scanning for the detection of deep vein thrombosis in high risk surgical patients: A comparative study between patients undergoing general surgery and hip surgery. *Thromb Res* 1979;15: 227–234.
30. Coe NP, Collins RE, Klein LA, et al: Prevention of deep vein thrombosis in urological patients: A controlled randomized trial of low-dose heparin and external pneumatic compression boots. *Surgery* 1978;83:230–234.
31. Handley AJ, Emerson PA, Fleming PR: Heparin in the prevention of deep vein thrombosis after myocardial infarction. *Br Med J* 1972;2:436–438.
32. McNeil BJ, Bettmann MA: The diagnosis of pulmonary embolism, in Colman RW, Hirsh J, Marder VJ, et al (eds): *Hemostasis and Thrombosis.* Philadelphia, Lippincott, 1982, pp 844–856.
33. Hirsh J, Genton E, Hull R: Diagnosis of pulmonary embolism, in Hirsh J, Genton E, Hull R (eds): *Venous Thromboembolism.* New York, Grune and Stratton, 1981, pp 94–107.
34. McNeil BJ: A diagnostic strategy using ventilation-perfusion studies in patients suspect for pulmonary embolism. *J Nucl Med* 1976;17:613–616.
35. Moses DC, Silver TM, Bookstein JJ, et al: The complementary roles of chest radiography, lung scanning and selective pulmonary angiography in the diagnosis of pulmonary embolism. *Circulation* 1974;49:179–188.
36. Biello DR, Mattar AG, McKnight RC, et al: Ventilation-perfusion studies in suspected pulmonary embolism. *Am J Roentgenol* 1979;133:1033–1037.
37. Chiu HM, Hirsh J, Yung WL, et al: Relationship between the anticoagulant and antithrombotic effects of heparin in experimental venous thrombosis. *Blood* 1977;49:171–184.
38. Hirsh J, Genton E, Hull R: Heparin, in Hirsh J, Genton E, Hull R (eds): *Venous Thromboembolism.* New York, Grune and Stratton, 1981, pp 155–183.
39. Hull R, Hirsh J, Carter C, et al: Different intensities of oral anticoagulant therapy in the treatment of proximal-vein thrombosis. *N Engl J Med* 1982; 307:1676–1681.
40. Hull R, Delmore T, Genton E, et al: Warfarin-sodium versus low-dose heparin in the long-term treatment of venous thrombosis. *N Engl J Med* 1979;301:855–858.
41. Verstraete M: Biochemical and clinical aspects of thrombolysis. *Semin Hematol* 1978;15:35–54.
42. Browse NL: Venous insufficiency: Nonoperative management, in Bang N, Glover J, Holden R, et al (eds): *Thrombosis and Atherosclerosis.* Chicago, Year Book Medical Publishers, 1982, pp 275–281.
43. Jones MAG, Webb R, Ree I, et al: A physiological study of elastic compression stockings in venous disorders of the leg. *Br J Surg* 1980;67:569–572.

CHAPTER 31
Bundle-Branch Block in the Elderly

John H. McAnulty
Shahbudin H. Rahimtoola

Unexplained dizzy spells, syncope, and even sudden death are common in the elderly and cardiovascular abnormalities are frequent causes. Still, it is often difficult to make the connection between recognized cardiovascular abnormalities and the symptoms and to know how to direct treatment.

There are concerns about bundle-branch block as well. It, on occasion, is associated with heart block, syncope, and with sudden death. Again the association between the ECG findings and the events is frequently difficult to demonstrate. Because so many symptoms in the elderly are difficult to explain and because bundle-branch block is frequently recognized in these individuals, it is appropriate to ask whether the two are related. This chapter will review the significance of bundle-branch block in the elderly and will discuss management of this conduction abnormality.

It is recognized, particularly by these authors, that there is no clear definition of "elderly." Still, for the purposes of this chapter, the elderly will be defined as being 60 years of age or older. "Younger" individuals will be assumed to be less than 60 years of age. Although this is clearly arbitrary, one reason why this age division is selected is that some of the studies that have looked at the significance of bundle-branch block as it relates to age have used these age ranges.[1,2]

GENERAL CONCERNS

Unrelated to age, there are a number of reasons why bundle-branch block is of general clinical significance. First, it is not an unusual finding. Occurring in 1% to 2% of the adult population,[2-4] it is encountered frequently in clinical practice.

Second, it is an indication of heart disease.[1-5] Coronary artery disease is recognized in almost half of those with bundle-branch block and hypertension and systemic arterial hypertension is found in up to two thirds of bundle-branch block patients. Others have valve disease, myocardial disease, or congenital heart disease, and in only 20% to 25% does the conduction system abnormality appear to be a primary process.

Third, whether a primary process or secondary to associated cardiovascular disease, bundle-branch block is an indication of disease of the conduction system. Since this can predispose individuals to both tachycardias and bradycardias, and since these arrhythmias are potential explanations for both symptoms and sudden death, the bundle-branch block is worthy of consideration when establishing diagnostic and therapeutic plans.

Fourth, an understanding of the anatomy of the distal conduction system has increased the concern that bundle-branch block patients are at risk of heart block (Figure 31-1).[6] There are at least three distal pathways (fascicles) connecting the atrium and the atrioventricular (AV) node to the ventricle, the right bundle, the anterior fascicle of the left bundle, and the posterior fascicle of the left bundle. This allows access of the electrical impulse to the ventricle from multiple approaches. If an individual has unifascicular block (Table 31-1) or block of one of the pathways, there may be little concern as there are at least two others to allow conduction to the ventricle. However, evidence of block in two fascicles—bifascicular block—raises theoretical concern of an increased risk of heart block. Now, only one pathway is available for conduction from the atrium to the

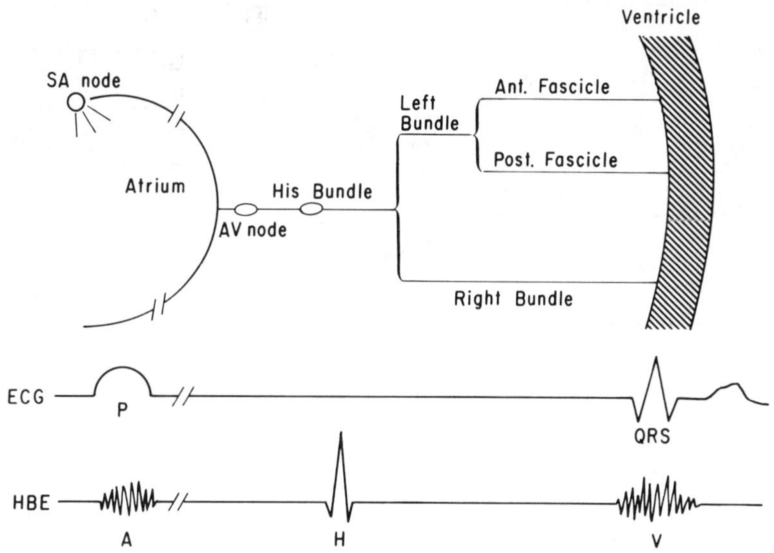

Figure 31-1 Below this schematic representation of the cardiac conduction system are the ECG and the intracardiac His bundle electrogram (HBE) tracings. Atrial depolarization is represented by the P complex on the ECG and by the A deflection on the HBE. AV node depolarization is not seen on either tracing. His bundle depolarization is not seen on the surface ECG but produced the recognizable H deflection on the HBE. Ventricular depolarization is represented by the QRS complex on the ECG and by the V deflection on the HBE.

ventricle and it is appropriate to be concerned that the disease process causing block of the other two pathways could be affecting the third, possibly increasing the risk of transient complete heart block.

Finally, bundle-branch block has been documented in some cases to progress to complete heart block (Figure 31-2). Although this is an uncommon progression, it is worthy of consideration in patients with symptoms compatible with that arrhythmia.

Table 31-1
Types of Fascicular Disease

Unifascicular disease*
Surface ECG evidence of isolated RBBB, LAFB, *or* LPFB
Bifascicular disease*
Surface ECG evidence of
LBBB
RBBB and LAFB
RBBB and LPFB
Alternating LAFB and LPFB
Trifascicular disease
Surface ECG evidence of
Alternating RBBB and LBBB
RBBB with alternating LAFB and LPFB

*Trifascicular disease cannot be excluded in these patients without measurement of an HV interval. If the HV interval is normal, trifascicular disease as manifest by conduction delay is excluded, and if the HV interval is prolonged, trifascicular disease is likely to be present. The PR interval does not differentiate bifascicular from trifascicular disease. RBBB = right bundle-branch block; LAFB = left anterior fascicular block; LPFB = left posterior fascicular block; LBBB = left bundle-branch block.

BUNDLE-BRANCH BLOCK IN THE ELDERLY

Although the concerns listed are not restricted to the elderly, it is this group of individuals in whom an understanding is most important as they are more likely to have symptoms suggestive of bradyarrhythmias and are more likely to have bundle-branch block. Just enough complete heart block and sudden death has been observed in patients with bundle-branch block to wonder if the conduction abnormality is a predictable cause. Recently, this association of AV block with bundle-branch block has been looked at from the other side. That is, in an elderly patient population with bundle-branch block, but without documented bradyarrhythmias, prospective follow-up studies have been carried out to determine the incidence of progression to complete heart block, to sudden death, and to sudden death likely or possibly due to the bundle-branch block.[1,2] These have helped clarify the significance of the conduction abnormalities in the elderly.

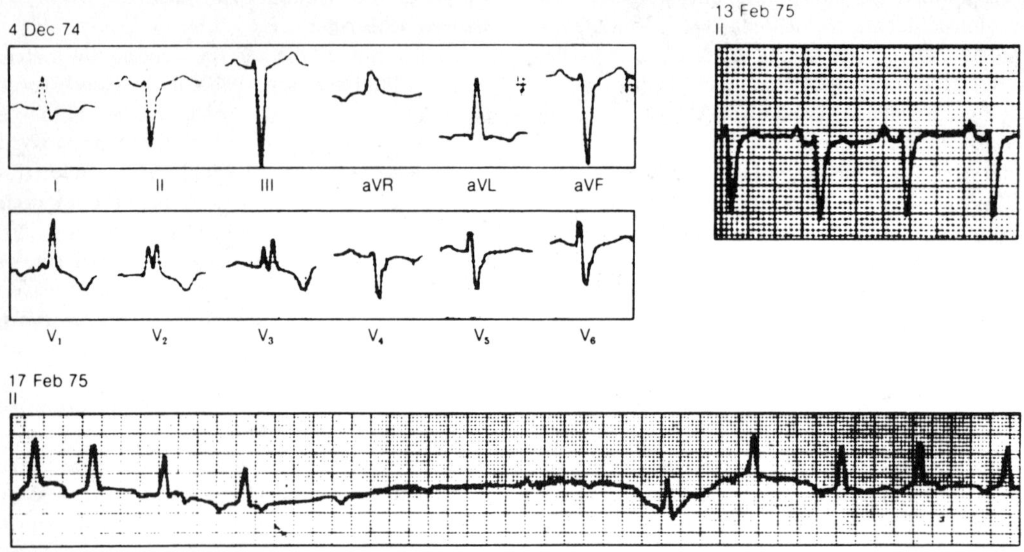

Figure 31-2 A woman with right bundle-branch block and left anterior fascicular block (bifascicular block) was asymptomatic (upper left). Because of a syncopal episode, monitoring was begun two months later with the initial tracing showing sinus rhythm (upper right). With a repeat syncopal episode, monitoring documented transient complete heart block as the cause.

Incidence

The incidence of bundle-branch block increases with age. In younger individuals, as represented by a large group of US government personnel averaging under 40 years of age, bundle-branch block was found in only 0.2%.[7] It was found on the ECG in 0.6% of those entered into the Framingham study with the affected individuals averaging 48 and 49 years of age for right[3] and left bundle-branch block[4] respectively. During the course of follow-up in that study, the conduction abnormality developed in another 2.4% at an average age of 61 years. When large groups of hospital-based patients have been evaluated, bundle-branch block has been recognized on almost 1% of ECGs, with the average age of those involved being in the mid 60s.[1,2,5]

Etiology

In patients 60 years and older, bundle-branch block is usually associated with recognizable organic heart disease (Table 31-2).[1,2] Up to one half have clinically recognizable coronary artery disease. This is a significantly ($P < .10$) greater incidence than the 20% to 27% found in individuals with bundle-branch block who are less than 60 years of age. In the elderly, 28% to 46% will have other recognized forms of heart disease (hypertensive heart disease, primary myocardial disease, valve disease, or congenital disease). In 19% to 20% of those 60 years and over, there will be no recognized associated heart disease. It is likely that many of these have primary disease of their conduction system, possibly the direct result of increased fibrosis and sclerodegenerative changes occurring with age.[8,9] However, in some, associated disease may not be recognized. This was observed in the Framingham study.[3,4] Individuals, who first presented with bundle-branch block and no apparent associated heart disease, when followed, had a significantly increased chance of developing recognized clinical coronary artery disease (at least a twofold increase) and up to a sevenfold increase in the subsequent development of congestive heart failure. In the elderly, as in younger individuals, associated heart disease is so common with bundle-branch block that the conduction abnormality can be considered, if nothing else, a marker for this process.

Events

Progression to complete heart block In a large group of patients 60 years of age or older (mean age 73 ± 0.1 years), followed for three years at the University of Illinois,[1] clinically recognized spontaneous AV block was documented to occur in just over 1% per year. In the University of

Oregon study,[2] patients in the same age group had an almost identical incidence of spontaneous complete heart block (unpublished data from this study). The incidence of complete heart block is not significantly different from that observed in younger individuals with bundle-branch block. In both series the patients presented for clinical care and were treated with pacemakers. In the Oregon study, patients with bundle-branch block and unexplained syncope had a higher chance of eventually being shown to have complete heart block (17%) within four years as compared to those without syncope (2%) ($P < .05$).

Death Overall mortality in the elderly with bundle-branch block approaches 9% per year.[1,2] It is not surprising that this is higher than that in individuals under 60 years of age with bundle-branch block considering the progression of associated disease with increasing age.

The concern about bundle-branch block as it relates to death focuses around bradyarrhythmias. It would seem that if the bundle-branch block is the direct cause of death, it would be by progression to AV block, with no adequate escape rhythm. Such a death is likely to be sudden. For that reason, studies have focused on the incidence of sudden death in this population. It does occur, and at a rate of 3% to 4% per year in the elderly. This incidence is similar to that observed in younger patients with this conduction abnormality.[1,2]

Deaths documented to be, or possibly, due to complete heart block Although sudden death could be caused by complete heart block in patients with bundle-branch block, it is probably unusual. Serious tachyarrhythmias and acute myocardial infarctions have been the demonstrated cause in most cases.[1,2,10] However, some patients have died from the bradyarrhythmia itself; others have unexplained sudden death that possibly could have been due to bradyarrhythmias. In the Oregon study, such deaths have been labeled "special events." These special events occurred in the elderly at a rate of 1% to 2% per year. This would seem to be the maximum incidence as it is likely (based on the experience with observed sudden deaths) that many of the unexplained sudden deaths were due to something else other than complete heart block. Still, it is possible that some of these special events could have been prevented had a permanent pacemaker been inserted when the bundle-branch block was first detected. The incidence of special events in the elderly was not significantly different from that observed in younger individuals.[2]

Progression of Conduction System Disease with Age

To determine whether the conduction system abnormalities are more severe in the elderly (even though the progression to complete heart block is no more frequent) intracardiac electrophysiologic data has been reviewed (Table 31-2). With this testing, the conduction time through the AV node can be evaluated by measuring the interval between the atrial depolarization potential (the A wave) and the His bundle potential (the H wave). The AH interval in the elderly with bundle-branch block does not differ significantly from that recorded in younger individuals.[1,2]

Conduction through the unblocked portion of the bundle branches is measured by the HV interval, the time from the His bundle potential to the ventricular activation (the V wave). In the elderly with bundle-branch block, up to 46% have a prolonged HV interval (56 to 75 ms) and an additional 12% have a greatly prolonged HV interval (> 75 ms). It was hoped that the HV interval could be used as a way of defining those bundle-branch block patients at high risk of proceeding to AV block. Its predictive value has been disappointing, however, and the rate of progression to heart block is so low that pacemaker insertion based on HV interval measurements alone (without documented AV block) is, at very best, controversial.[1,2,5]

MANAGEMENT OF BUNDLE-BRANCH BLOCK

There is more to be learned about management of bundle-branch block but the information already available makes it possible to make some recommendations. In the elderly, management should not differ from that of younger individuals. In individuals with bundle-branch block in whom there are no symptoms suggesting a bradyarrhythmia, no evaluation of the conduction system or treatment is required. The associated heart disease may require treatment in some cases, but therapy directed at the conduction system is not appropriate.

In the patient with bundle-branch block documented to develop complete heart block or high-degree AV block, the approach is also noncontroversial. The reversible causes of heart block (hyperkalemia, antiarrhythmia drugs, acute ischemic events) should be treated if recognized and, if the rhythm normalizes, pacemaker therapy is not indicated.[11] In most, however, a reversible

Table 31-2
Clinical Characteristics of the Study Population

	Age (yr)	
	< 60	≥ 60
No. of Patients	106	229
Male/Female	66/40	166/63
Age (mean ± SD)	47 ± 13	70 ± 8
Range	10–59	60–94
Associated heart disease		
Coronary artery disease	27%	52%*
Primary conduction system disease	25%	20%
Other‡	48%	28%*
ECG abnormality		
Left bundle-branch block (LBBB)	41%	35%
Left bundle-branch block, left axis deviation	6%	11%
Right bundle-branch block (RBBB), left axis deviation	25%	34%†
Right bundle-branch block, right axis deviation	23%	13%
Other§	5%	7%
Symptoms		
Syncope	25%	33%
Electrophysiologic data (mean ± SE, ms)		
AH interval, ms	90 ± 3.4	97 ± 2.3
SNRT at heart rate 130/bpm	1024 ± 24	1050 ± 21
HV interval, ms	58 ± 1.3	59 ± 1.0
HV ≤ 55 ms (normal)	48%	46%
HV 56–75 ms	44%	42%
HV > 75 ms	8%	12%

*$P < 0.01$.
†$P > 0.05$.
‡Includes valvular, primary myocardial, hypertensive, and congenital heart disease.
§Includes RBBB with indeterminate axis, RBBB with alternating axis, alternating RBBB and LBBB.
Unpublished data from prospective evaluation of bundle-branch block performed at the University of Oregon. See McAnulty et al.[2]

cause cannot be recognized and permanent pacemaker insertion is required.

Much more difficult is the management of patients with bundle-branch block who have symptoms suggestive of transient complete heart block (dizziness, syncope, episodic fatigue, and chest pain) but in whom a bradyarrhythmia cannot be demonstrated. The concern that they may be having complete heart block makes them particularly difficult to manage. If no other recognizable explanation is immediately defined, a diligent search for bradyarrhythmias is appropriate. Ambulatory monitoring for at least 72 to 96 hours is indicated and should be repeated with recurrence of symptoms. Although the yield is low, because of the episodic nature of the arrhythmias, this will reveal heart block as a cause on some occasions (Figure 31-2). It is this interruption of AV conduction which is suspected to be the most likely arrhythmia in bundle-branch block patients. Monitoring, however, may reveal bradyarrhythmias due to another cause entirely (sinus node disorders) or tachyarrhythmias as the cause of symptoms.[2,10–12] Additionally, the monitoring may be useful by showing a normal rhythm at the time of symptoms, excluding arrhythmias as a cause. In those with symptoms related to exercise, an exercise stress test may occasionally demonstrate the cause.

If rhythm monitoring and observation do not explain the symptoms, and particularly if symptoms are recurrent, additional studies are indicated. Based on the description of symptoms, evaluation for noncardiac causes such as inner ear disease, seizure disorders, metabolic abnormalities, or cerebrovascular abnormalities may be appropriate.

If the workup is unremarkable, rhythm provocation studies may on occasion reveal a likely cause of symptoms. This is done during an intracardiac electrophysiologic study. Although perhaps not appropriate in all, in patients with at least a marker suggesting heart disease and possible rhythm abnormalities, its application is a consideration. During this study, intravenous wires are advanced into the heart. Intracardiac conduction intervals are evaluated and using pacing provocation technics, the susceptibility to bradyarrhythmias and tachyarrhythmias is evaluated. A high incidence of either inducible arrhythmias or of prolonged intracardiac conduction times is likely to be demonstrated.[2,13-16] It is not always clear what to do with the information but some have elected to treat prolonged conduction intervals as the explanation for the syncope and to insert pacemakers (without documenting AV block). Symptoms have persisted in some (despite a pacemaker) and there has been no demonstrated beneficial effect on survival.[5,14,15] If a tachyarrhythmia is induced during the study, treatment directed toward its inducibility may also be beneficial. Expense is a consideration and there is some risk (although it is trivial and a study death has never been reported) but this approach may be of value in selected patients with recurrent symptoms.

It has not been demonstrated that the presence of symptoms in patients with bundle-branch block is an indication that they are at high risk of sudden death. Because of this it seems appropriate to make the general recommendation that *permanent pacemaker insertion should be reserved for those with documented bradyarrhythmias.* On occasion, recurrent syncope is such a significant problem that a pacemaker is inserted on the presumption that a bradyarrhythmia is the cause. Pacemaker implantation is not without its own risks and expense but if these are recognized by both the patient and the physician, this approach may be warranted. An inappropriate pacing unit may cause symptoms that outweigh potential protective effects of the unit.

SELECTED CLINICAL SITUATIONS

Acute Myocardial Infarction

Patients with an acute myocardial infarction have an increased chance of developing arrhythmias. This includes bradyarrhythmias as well as tachyarrhythmias. Complete heart block occurs in up to 6% of those admitted to the coronary care unit. Although this is a remarkedly high incidence, insertion of a prophylactic temporary pacemaker wire in each case is not general practice. This approach should be considered, however, in many patients who have or develop bundle-branch block. Complete heart block will develop in 20% to 46% of patients and the in-hospital mortality rate exceeds 40%.[17-20] Most of the deaths are due to associated severe myocardial damage or to ventricular tachyarrhythmias but some can survive both of these if protected against bradyarrhythmias. Based on information from a large retrospective collaborative study,[18,19] some patients with infarctions and bundle-branch block appear to be at high enough risk of developing heart block that temporary pacemaker placement is recommended. These include patients with new bundle-branch block involving a portion of both the right and the left bundles or that occurs in association with first-degree AV block.

If patients with a myocardial infarction and bundle-branch block develop transient complete heart block and survive the infarction, some have recommended insertion of a permanent pacemaker before hospital discharge.[19] The value of this approach is still unclear.

General Surgical Procedures

There has been concern that individuals with bundle-branch block undergoing general surgical procedures are at increased risk of developing complete heart block at the time of surgery. Occurring in less than 2% of patients,[21] however, the risk is low and a temporary pacemaker wire before surgery is not appropriate in all bundle-branch block patients. Continuous cardiac monitoring in the perioperative period (prior to premedication, during the surgery, and for at least 24 hours after surgery) is required and it is prudent to have a large central venous line in place during surgery for pacemaker insertion, should it be necessary.

Cardiac Catheterization

When a catheter is positioned in the right ventricle, transient right bundle-branch block can occur in up to 10% of patients, probably from the trauma of the catheter. This is of no clinical significance in patients without bundle-branch block. In the patient with left bundle-branch block, however, the addition of right bundle-branch block results in complete heart block. Although quick withdrawal of the catheter usually results in normalization of conduction, this is not invariable. Thus, in a patient with left bundle-branch block undergoing a right heart catheterization, careful observation of the possibility of complete heart block is necessary. The same is true for a patient with right bundle-branch block undergoing left ventricular catheterization. It is not recommended that all these patients receive temporary pacemakers, but each should be monitored carefully and the pacing wire and access site should be immediately available.

Medication Use

Any drug should be used cautiously in a patient with heart disease but selected drugs, particularly cardiac drugs, can interrupt conduction. Digitalis can be used as safely in elderly patients with chronic bundle-branch block, as at other times, because it has little effect on the distal conduction system.[22] All of the available group I antiarrhythmic agents (quinidine, procainamide, and disopyramide) prolong the AV conduction time and should be used cautiously in patients with chronic bundle-branch block.[6] They have been documented in some cases to cause complete heart block. If a patient has symptoms of possible transient complete heart block and if the drug is considered necessary, it is best started during monitoring in the hospital. Although the group II antiarrhythmic agents (lidocaine and phenytoin) are less likely to interfere with distal conduction they also should be used at the time of rhythm monitoring in bundle-branch block patients. The beta-blocking agents and calcium channel blockers are unlikely to affect distal conduction. However, because many patients with bundle-branch block also have associated AV node and sino-atrial disease,[12] the toxic manifestations of these drugs, particularly in the elderly with bundle-branch block, should be watched for carefully.

ACKNOWLEDGMENT

The skills of Ms. Barbara Lewis were essential in preparation of this chapter and are gratefully acknowledged.

REFERENCES

1. Dhingra RC, Wyndham C, Deedwania PC, et al: Effect of age on atrioventricular conduction in patients with chronic bifascicular block. *Am J Cardiol* 1980;45:749–756.
2. McAnulty JH, Rahimtoola SH, Murphy E, et al: Natural history of "high-risk" bundle branch block. *N Engl J Med* 1982;307:137–143.
3. Schneider JF, Thomas HE Jr, Kreger BE, et al: Newly acquired left bundle branch block: The Framingham study. *Ann Intern Med* 1979;90:303–310.
4. Schneider JF, Thomas HE Jr, Kreger BE, et al: Newly acquired right bundle branch block: The Framingham study. *Ann Intern Med* 1980;92:37–44.
5. Scheinman MM, Peters RW, Sauve MJ, et al: Value of the H-Q interval in patients with bundle branch block and the role of prophylactic permanent pacing. *Am J Cardiol* 1982;50:1316–1322.
6. McAnulty JH, Rahimtoola SH: The etiology, prognosis, and treatment of bilateral bundle branch block, in Hurst JW (ed): *The Heart Update IV.* New York, McGraw-Hill Book Company, 1981, pp 173–191.
7. Rotman M, Triebwasser JH: A clinical and followup study of right and left bundle branch block. *Circulation* 1975;51:477–484.
8. Lev M: The pathology of complete atrioventricular block. *Prog Cardiovasc Dis* 1964;6:317–326.
9. Lenegre J: Etiology and pathology of bilateral bundle branch block in relation to heart block. *Prog Cardiovasc Dis* 1964;6:409–444.
10. Denes P, Dhingra RC, Wu D, et al: Sudden death in patients with chronic bifascicular block. *Arch Intern Med* 1977;137:1005–1010.
11. Dhingra RC, Wyndham C, Amat-y-Leon F, et al: Incidence and site of atrioventricular block in patients with chronic bifascicular block. *Circulation* 1979;59:238–246.
12. Wyse DG, McAnulty JH, Rahimtoola SH, et al: Electrophysiologic abnormalities of sinus node and atrium in patients with bundle branch block. *Circulation* 1979;60:413–420.
13. Dhingra RC, Wyndham C, Bauernfeind R, et al: Significance of block distal to the His bundle induced by atrial pacing in patients with chronic bifascicular block. *Circulation* 1979;60:1455–1464.
14. DiMarco JP, Garan H, Harthorne JW, et al: Intracardiac electrophysiologic techniques in recurrent syncope of unknown cause. *Ann Intern Med* 1981;95:542–548.
15. Hess DS, Morady F, Scheinman MM: Electrophysiologic testing in the evaluation of patients with syncope of undetermined origin. *Am J Cardiol* 1982;50:1309–1315.
16. Li CK, McAnulty JH, Morton M: Are electrophysiologic studies in patients with syncope without heart disease of diagnostic value?, abstracted. *Am J Cardiol* 1983;1(2):607.
17. Mullins CB, Atkins JM: Prognosis and management of ventricular conduction blocks in acute myocardial infarction. *Mod Concepts Cardiovasc Dis* 1976;45:129–134.
18. Hindman MC, Wagner GS, JaRo M, et al: The clinical significance of bundle branch block complicating acute myocardial infarction. 1. Clinical characteristics, hospital mortality and one year followup. *Circulation* 1978;58:679–699.
19. Hindman MC, Wagner GS, JaRo M, et al: The clinical significance of bundle branch block complicating acute myocardial infarction. 2. Indications for temporary and permanent pacemaker insertion. *Circulation* 1978;58:689–699.
20. DeGuzman M, Rahimtoola SH: What is the role of pacemakers in patients with coronary artery disease and conduction abnormalities?, in Rahimtoola SH (ed): *Current Controversies in Coronary Heart Disease.* Philadelphia, FA Davis, 1983, 191.
21. Pastore JO, Yurchak PM, Janis KM, et al: The risk of advanced heart block in surgical patients with right bundle branch block and left axis deviation. *Circulation* 1978;57:677–680.
22. Kauffman S, McAnulty JH, DeMots H, et al: Digitalis in bifascicular and trifascicular conduction disease: Its effect on the H-V interval, abstracted. *Clin Res* 1976;24:224A.

CHAPTER 32
Sick Sinus Syndrome in the Elderly

Edgar Lichstein

Sick sinus syndrome describes a clinical syndrome characterized by abnormalities of the sinus node associated with various and sometimes vague symptoms.[1-6] The term was first used by Lown to describe arrhythmias noted after cardioversion. Most early reports emphasized sinus bradycardia or arrest as the main feature of this syndrome. The association of sinus bradycardia with periods of paroxysmal supraventricular tachycardia was noted by Short and is now referred to as the bradycardia-tachycardia syndrome.[7] The various abnormalities of sinus and atrioventricular (AV) nodal function that constitute the sick sinus syndrome are listed in Table 32-1.

Many of the ECG abnormalities listed in Table 32-1 are very common, especially in the elderly. There is a question whether an abnormality such as sinus bradycardia actually represents disease or is merely an expected or normal finding in a particular age group. The symptoms of sick sinus syndrome include various manifestations of cerebral dysfunction. These symptoms may be difficult to interpret in the elderly, since they may be vague and nonspecific and also because they are produced by many other diseases common to the elderly.

ANATOMY AND ELECTROPHYSIOLOGY

The ultrastructure of the sinus node, which comprises P cells and transitional cells, has been described by James et al.[8] The sinus node has a unique blood supply which is primarily from a single vessel. This vessel arises from the right coronary artery in 55% of the cases and the left circumflex artery in 45%. This large vessel passes directly through the center of the sinus node, suggesting the possibility that there is a relationship between pulsation of this artery and sinus node function.

Sinus node dysfunction is thought to be a disorder of both impulse generation and impulse conduction.[1] In addition to abnormal impulse generation in the sinus node, there is also an abnormality of impulse formation in the AV node. This explains the failure of the AV node to escape promptly when the sinus slows or arrests. Abnormal autonomic tone may influence both of these pacemakers.[9] Patients with this syndrome may have enhanced parasympathetic tone and decreased sympathetic tone. Dighton[10] suggests that atrial cholinesterase activity is reduced in sino-atrial (SA) disease, thus leading to a build-up of acetylcholine in atrial tissues. Vagal stimulation by acetylcholine may slow automaticity of the sinus node by reducing the slope of phase 4 depolarization.[11] The response or lack of response to atropine may differentiate patients with actual sinus node disease from those with increased vagal tone.

CAUSES OF SICK SINUS SYNDROME

Coronary heart disease, and particularly myocardial infarction, is reported to be the most common underlying disease.[12] This is important in a discussion of the elderly, since coronary disease becomes more prevalent with increasing age. The effects of coronary disease may be due to either acute myocardial infarction, or chronic disease producing fibrosis and scarring of the sinus node.

Sinus node dysfunction occurs in approximately 5% of acute myocardial infarctions.[13] Occlusion of the right coronary artery or left circumflex artery

Table 32-1
ECG Manifestations of Sick Sinus Syndrome

1. Severe sinus bradycardia with no significant response to exercise or atropine
2. Sinus arrest or SA block
3. Chronic or recurrent atrial fibrillation with slow ventricular response
4. Periods of sinus arrest or marked sinus bradycardia following atrial tachycardia
5. Greater than 3-second sinus pause with carotid massage
6. Failure to resume sinus rhythm following DC cardioversion

produces the ECG picture of inferior myocardial infarction and infarction of the sinus node and atria. Sinus node disease has been found in over 50% of patients with acute myocardial infarction.[14]

Sinus node dysfunction usually occurs within the first few days after myocardial infarction. Occasionally this dysfunction is not permanent and is due to reversible ischemia. Ischemia to cholinergic terminals near the sinus node may cause sinus bradycardia, which is easily reversed with atropine.[1] Some of these patients who have reversible ischemia will eventually develop fibrosis of the sinus node and develop symptoms months to years after the myocardial infarction.

A sclerotic, degenerative process is thought to be responsible for most cases of sick sinus syndrome not due to coronary heart disease.[15] A large group of miscellaneous conditions may also produce sick sinus syndrome. These include myocarditis, pericarditis, cardiomyopathy, rheumatic heart disease, collagen vascular disease, metastatic disease, Friedreich's ataxia, diphtheria, hemochromatosis, and amyloidosis. Amyloidosis is of particular interest, since this disease is present in many elderly patients. Kaplan et al[16] described one patient with sick sinus syndrome with amyloid deposits in the atrium. Allensworth et al[17] reported amyloid deposits in the myocardium in two patients with persistent atrial standstill.

Sick sinus syndrome may rarely occur as a congenital defect.[18,19]

EFFECT OF AGE ON HEART RATE

Sinus bradycardia and atrial fibrillation are common arrhythmias in sick sinus syndrome. These arrhythmias are also found in the apparently healthy elderly population. This raises the question of which rhythm abnormalities represent disease and which represent the normal change with age.

Mihalick and Fish[20] reviewed ECGs of 671 patients aged 65 to 96. They found only two patients with sinus bradycardia and 34 with atrial fibrillation. Camm et al[21] used Holter monitoring to study patients, all above 75 years of age. The heart rate fell below 50 in only 11 cases (10%). In 70 of these cases the bradycardia occurred only during sleep. Gavey[22] reported only a 2.5% incidence of sinus bradycardia and Kirk and Kvorning[23] noted a 5.8% incidence in patients over age 65. In this latter study the incidence of sinus bradycardia in patients less than 40 years of age was 9.3%. Other studies of younger populations have found a higher incidence of sinus bradycardia. Brodsky et al[24] noted a 24% incidence of severe sinus bradycardia (less than 40 bpm) and frequent sinus pause (less than 1.5 seconds) in 50 young, healthy medical students.

Since some elderly patients may have sinus bradycardia, the next question is whether it actually represents disease. Agrus et al[25] studied seven elderly asymptomatic patients with sinus bradycardia and compared them with four age-matched controls. Autonomic function, stroke volume, and cardiac output were evaluated. Although both groups achieved similar levels of cardiac output during exercise, the bradyarrhythmia group did so by means of a higher stroke output and lower heart rate. Following atropine, the bradycardia subjects had a much greater percentage increase in heart rate, suggesting the importance of vagal tone in this group. They conclude that significant sinus bradycardia may be associated with aging. Increased vagal tone may be a significant contributing factor and, more importantly, normal cardiac performance may still be present. The complications and management of sinus bradycardia depend on whether or not the heart can increase its rate when needed, and also whether or not the cardiac output remains normal.

Kostis et al[26] noted that a problem in studying the effect of age on the heart is the difficulty in separating the true effects of aging from those due to deconditioning or unrecognized disease. They performed 24-hour Holter monitoring and maximum exercise stress tests in 101 subjects with normal hearts. They found a decrease in maximum heart rate with increasing age. They found that the resting heart rate was not affected by age. They speculate that there may be a decline in the capacity of the sinus node to increase the heart rate. Aging changes pacemaker tissue and leads to a decrease in the responsiveness of autonomic cardiovascular reflexes and decreased adrenergic receptor sensitivity. Decreased responsiveness of the sinus node to catecholamines may also explain the lower nighttime maximum heart rate in older patients, despite increased plasma norepinephrine at night.[27]

Since some of the sinus bradycardia noted in the elderly may be changes in autonomic tone, it must be determined whether or not the intrinsic heart rate decreases with age. Jose and Collison[28] studied intrinsic heart rate by taking a group of normal volunteers and giving them intravenous (IV) propranolol and atropine. They found a negative relationship to age, which was described by the regression equation: Intrinsic heart rate = 118.1 − (0.57 × age).

It thus appears that intrinsic heart rate does decrease with age. The actual observed resting heart rate may be decreased in the elderly, but this is actually less common in the elderly than in younger populations. The decrease in heart rate observed in the elderly is mostly due to a decrease in the intrinsic rate, in addition to decreased responsiveness of the sinus node to catecholamines. The sinus bradycardia observed in the young is mostly due to increased vagal tone, which becomes less of a factor with increasing age.

SYMPTOMS

The majority of symptoms of sick sinus syndrome result from decreased perfusion of the brain. A small decrease in cerebral flow may produce subtle changes, such as fatigue, memory loss, and irritability. Many of these symptoms are ascribed to senility.

A sudden or more significant decrease in cerebral perfusion may cause dizziness or syncope. Moss and Davis[7] report syncope or near syncope in 41% of their patients and note a 69% incidence in a review of the literature. Syncope was noted in 25/56 of Rubinstein et al's[4] patients and was recurrent in 16. Both of these studies noted a significant incidence of cerebral embolism, particularly in patients with the bradycardia-tachycardia syndrome as a cause of cerebral symptoms. Fairfax et al[29] found evidence of embolus in 16/100 patients with chronic SA nodal disease. Fifteen of these patients had bradycardia-tachycardia syndrome. They claim that the risk of embolism persists, even if chronic atrial fibrillation is present and is due to impaired atrial function.

A decreased rate or a sudden tachycardia may produce cardiac symptoms. The most common cardiac symptom is palpitation and is usually noted with sudden change in heart rate. The irregular beating of atrial fibrillation is also commonly described as palpitation. Sinus node disease may increase symptoms of congestive heart failure and may even precipitate acute pulmonary edema. Angina may also occur due to decreased coronary artery perfusion and increased myocardial oxygen demands which may occur during periods of tachycardia.

Burch[30] has emphasized the difficulty in interpreting symptoms in the elderly population. He points out that elderly people frequently have disease of multiple organ systems. For instance, it may be difficult to make a definite diagnosis of heart failure if the patient also has evidence of chronic pulmonary disease. Many of the symptoms that are seen are actually due to an additive effect of symptoms due to more than one disease process. For example, a patient with minimal sinus node disease is more likely to manifest definite cerebral symptoms if he has concomitant disease of the cerebrovascular system.

The drugs used to treat other diseases may also cause symptoms. Common examples of this are digitalis used for congestive heart failure and beta-blockers used for angina. Many elderly patients may have borderline sinus node function which decreases to the point of symptoms because of one of these medications. Patients with heart failure receiving digitalis may complain of dizziness or syncope. It may be difficult to determine if this is due to the heart failure or sinus node disease precipitated by the digitalis. The diagnosis is usually clarified by discontinuing digitalis and attempting to treat the heart failure with other medications.

ESTABLISHING A DIAGNOSIS

The history is important, as in all other disease, in making a diagnosis of sick sinus syndrome. As I have already indicated, questions must be asked to rule out other causes of cerebral and cardiac symptoms. The physical examination may serve to document a slow heart rate and to document the presence of congestive heart failure. The physical examination should also rule out other causes of cerebral symptoms, such as aortic stenosis and carotid artery disease.

The ECG abnormalities, which are the hallmark of sinus node disease, are documented either by the standard ECG or, more commonly, by 24-hour Holter recording. The most certain way of establishing a diagnosis is to note the presence of a symptom such as dizziness or syncope coinciding with an observed significant arrhythmia, such as sinus arrest on the Holter recording. Documenting the presence of disease by this technic will make certain that there will be a response to therapy such as pacemaker insertion. Unfortunately, we do not always see the clear relationship between symptoms and ECG abnormalities. We are, therefore, faced with interpreting the presence of symptoms without ECG abnormalities, and the presence of ECG abnormalities without symptoms.

Symptoms that occur without ECG abnormalities may be simply due to other types of disease. Since these arrhythmias are frequently transient, it is possible that the technic being used fails to record the arrhythmia at the appropriate time. The technic used to document the presence of arrhythmia in most instances is the 24-hour Holter recording. It is important that the patient keep a symptom diary so that the physician may see if an arrhythmia was present at the time the patient experienced symptoms. If a symptom was described and no arrhythmia is found, then the physician may conclude that the symptom was produced by other disease. Frequently the patient does not have any symptoms on the day the recording is taken, so no definite conclusions can be made. The technic of transtelephonic monitoring can be used after Holter monitoring has failed to document sinus node disease. Figure 32-1 illustrates the transtelephonic transmission of a 70-year-old female who frequently complained of palpitations. Two Holter recordings had failed to document any significant arrhythmia, but were not conclusive, since the patient did not have symptoms on those days. This rhythm strip, which clearly shows an episode of atrial fibrillation, was transmitted transtelephonically when symptoms were present.

ECG abnormalities may be present without symptoms. This requires that we establish rigid criteria as to what abnormalities constitute disease even in the absence of symptoms. For example, is a resting heart rate of 45 bpm abnormal in an 85-year-old asymptomatic male? What about a resting heart rate of 40 or of 35? When the resting heart rate is consistently lower than 40 we usually think sinus node disease is definitely present. It also must be remembered that symptoms are subjective and their elucidation depends in part on the skill of the examiner. Elderly patients may be less active and, therefore, not experience symptoms that a younger and more active person might

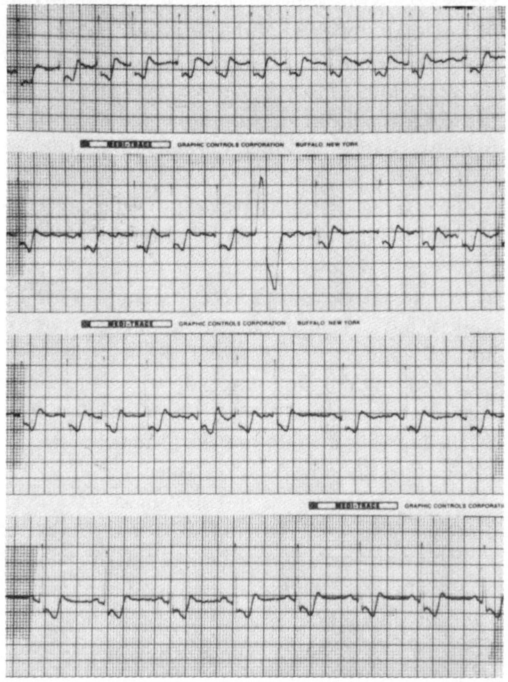

Figure 32-1 Transtelephonic ECG transmission showing an episode of atrial fibrillation with one ventricular premature beat. The bottom strip taken 1 hour after the episode of palpitation shows a return to normal sinus rhythm.

notice. Symptoms may occasionally be present and be misinterpreted by both the patient and his family. An interesting example is shown in the following case history:

> A 76-year-old male was evaluated because of questionable cerebral symptoms and sick sinus syndrome. A 24-hour Holter recording was performed and showed a 21-second period of asystole (Figure 32-2). The patient claimed that he felt well and had absolutely no symptoms during the recording. This was initially substantiated by his wife. On careful questioning it was learned that at the time the patient had his asystole he was sitting and watching television. His wife heard him make some unusual noises which she thought represented snoring. It is clear that the patient actually lost consciousness and was actually convulsing at that time.

Provocative tests are occasionally used to either bring out or prove the absence of significant sinus node disease. Carotid massage may be done to document a hyperactive carotid sinus reflex which may be leading to sinus arrest and syncope. In performing this test, especially in the elderly, it is important to plapate both carotid arteries before

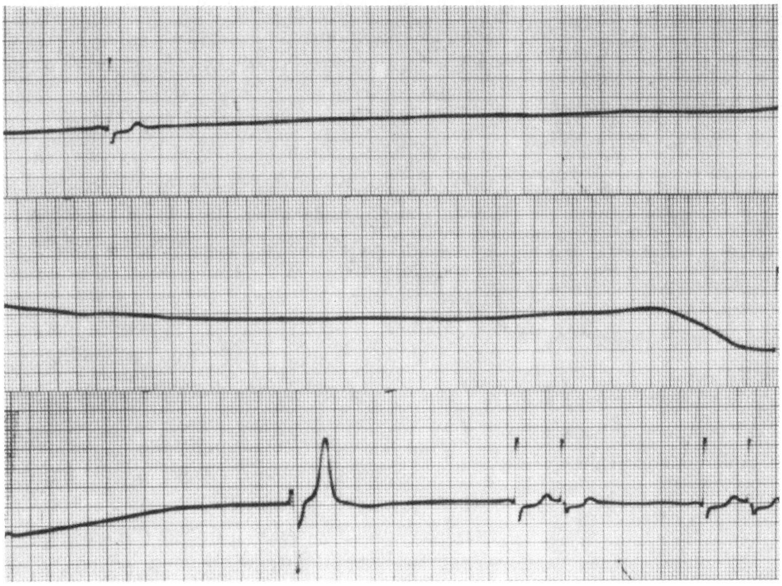

Figure 32-2 Holter recording showing a 21-second period of sinus arrest.

compressing one. If a patient has an absent carotid impulse on one side due to previous occlusion, a stroke may result from compressing the remaining side. This test must be done with ECG monitoring and with the immediate availability of IV atropine.

As previously mentioned, significant sinus bradycardia may be seen in asymptomatic patients. It is more important to note the response of the heart to exercise than to note the resting rate. If the patient is able to walk on the treadmill, a very limited stress test may be done just to see if the heart rate does accelerate with exercise and to make certain that no symptoms occur with exercise. Since many elderly patients are not able to walk, or walk with difficulty, IV atropine may be given to determine the heart rate response. It must be remembered, especially in the elderly, that atropine may precipitate urinary retention and glaucoma.

Atrial pacing is used to document sinus node disease and is, in effect, an attempt to reproduce the bradycardia-tachycardia syndrome in the laboratory. With this technique the right atrium is paced at rates of 90 to 150 bpm for periods of 2 to 5 minutes at each rate, with a rest of 1 to 2 minutes between each advance in rate. Atrial pacing is abruptly stopped and the time measured for the next sinus impulse to reappear. Sinus node recovery time is determined by measuring from the last atrial paced beat to the following sinus escape beat. The corrected sinus node recovery time is obtained by subtracting the average P-P interval from the sinus node recovery time. Mandel et al[31] and Narula et al[32] found these tests to be clinically useful in the diagnosis of sick sinus syndrome. Gupta et al[33] did not find the tests as useful and noted that only a limited number of patients with sick sinus syndrome have an abnormal corrected sinus node recovery time. In addition to the limitations of the study, one must be careful when accelerating the heart rate of elderly patients. Angina pectoris may occur when the heart rate approaches 140 to 150 bpm.

Figures 32-3 through 32-8 show other examples of ECG manifestations of sick sinus syndrome.

THERAPY

Treatment of sick sinus syndrome is recommended for the following three conditions: (1) presence of definite symptoms, (2) arrhythmia thought to be so abnormal that therapy is recommended even without documented symptoms, (3) the need to use medication which will further suppress sinus function.

The first consideration in therapy is to attempt to discontinue any medications that may be suppressing the sinus node. The most common examples are digitalis, which may be used for heart failure, and beta-blockers, which may be used for hypertension or angina pectoris. Whenever possible, other types of medication should be considered.

The administration of drugs for sick sinus syndrome is limited entirely to suppressing tachycardias

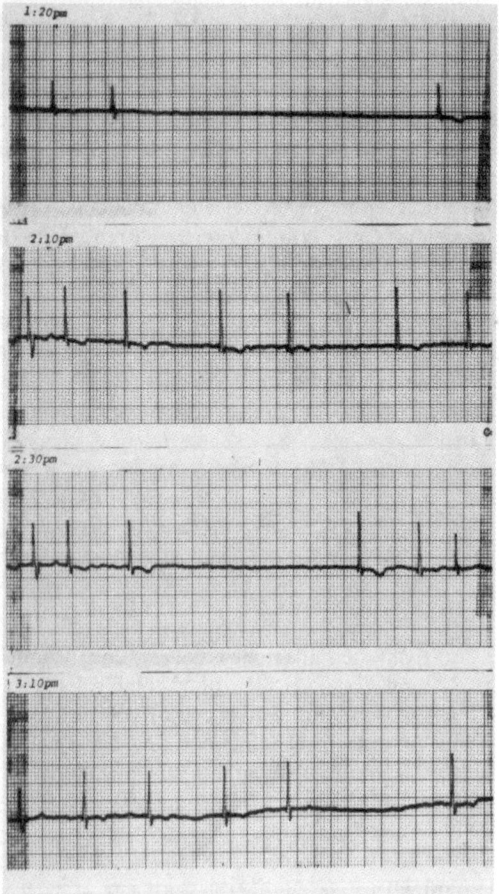

Figure 32-3 Holter recording showing atrial fibrillation with several periods of extremely slow ventricular response.

or controlling the ventricular response of atrial fibrillation. Vagolytic or sympathomimetic drugs which might increase sinus rate are theoretically possible but not practical to use. If a patient has episodes of atrial tachycardia, quinidine is frequently used with frequent Holter recordings to make certain that the sinus rhythm that occurs after the tachycardia does not become further suppressed by the quinidine. Small doses of digoxin may be used to control the ventricular response to atrial fibrillation. Frequently, no drug is necessary, since these patients commonly have concomitant AV nodal disease, and therefore, a slow ventricular response.

Although anticoagulants are not actual therapy for sick sinus syndrome, they are occasionally given to these patients.[34] This is because of the risk of systemic embolus when patients are in chronic atrial fibrillation. Coumadin should be considered in patients with chronic atrial fibrillation and an enlarged left atrium.

The most common therapy is insertion of a permanent pacemaker. This type of invasive therapy was once avoided in the elderly population, but is now more acceptable because of the ease of insertion and the low morbidity of this procedure. Endocardial pacemakers are inserted transvenously using only local anesthetic. Even in the elderly, chronically ill patient, the risks are minimal. There are three choices for type of permanent pacemaker: (1) atrial pacing, (2) ventricular pacing, and (3) AV sequential or physiologic pacing. Atrial pacing has the advantage that it is physiologic and maintains the patient's atrial contribution. However, it is usually not advised, since 25% of the patients with sick sinus syndrome either have AV nodal disease at the time of diagnosis or will develop it during the next several years. If an atrial pacemaker is considered, a His bundle electrogram should be first recorded to make certain that AV nodal conduction is completely normal. A ventricular demand pacemaker is probably the most commonly used and the simplest. It deprives the patient of a normal atrial

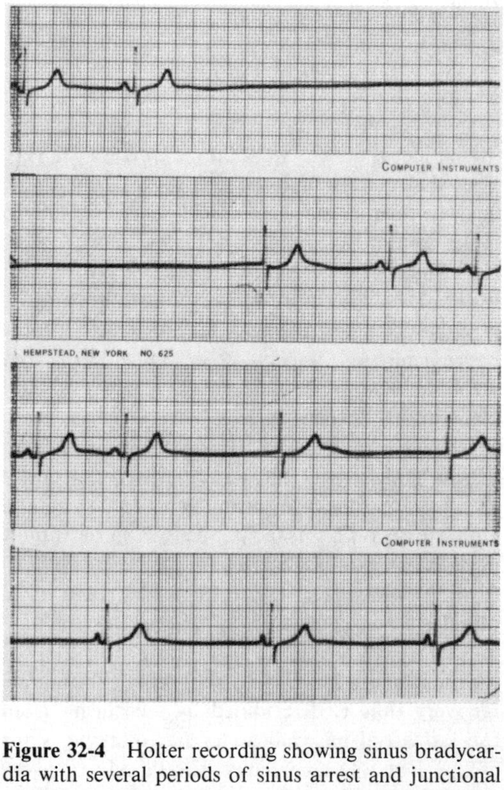

Figure 32-4 Holter recording showing sinus bradycardia with several periods of sinus arrest and junctional escape.

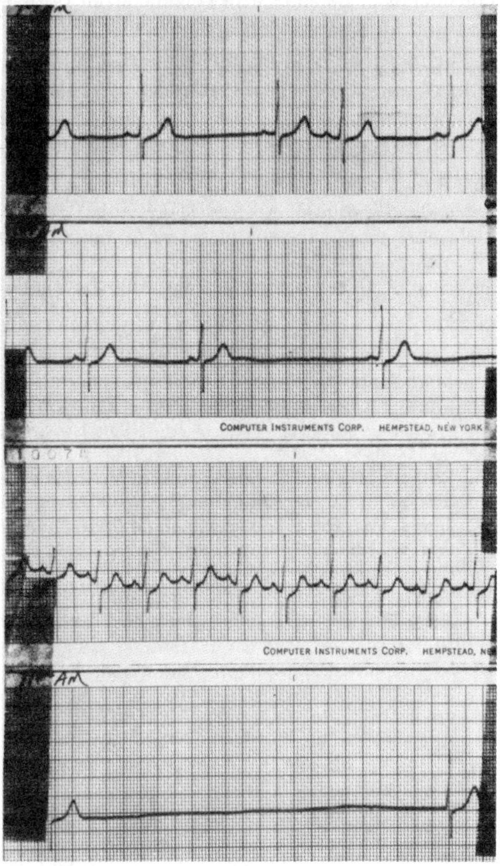

Figure 32-5 Holter recording showing both periods of sinus bradycardia and sinus tachycardia. There is a period of sinus arrest with a junctional escape rhythm.

contraction, but this may not be a problem if the patient has no evidence of heart failure. The most physiologic pacemaker and the one being more commonly used is the AV sequential pacemaker. Pacing wires must be inserted in both the atrium and ventricle and result in normal atrial synchrony, even in the presence of AV block. These pacemakers are now quite reliable and have a generator life expectancy of approximately 10 years.

It should be noted that permanent pacing will abolish the symptoms of sick sinus syndrome, if the patients have been chosen correctly.[35,36] However, this procedure does not alter the frequently severe underlying heart disease present in many of these patients. Wohl et al[37] and Lichstein et al[38] have shown that long-term survival is frequently not altered by permanent pacemaker insertion.

ACKNOWLEDGMENT

Mrs. Carol Scott and Mrs. Shaye Komitau assisted in the preparation of this manuscript.

REFERENCES

1. Ferrer MI: The sick sinus syndrome. *Circulation* 1973;47:635–641.
2. Lien WP, Lee YS, Chang FZ, et al: The sick sinus syndrome. Natural history of dysfunction of the sinoatrial node. *Chest* 1977;72:628–634.
3. Reiffel JA, Bigger JT, Cramer M, et al: Ability of Holter electrocardiographic recording and atrial stimulation to detect sinus nodal dysfunction in symptomatic and asymptomatic patients with sinus bradycardia. *Am J Cardiol* 1977;40:189–194.
4. Rubenstein JJ, Schulman CL, Yurchak PM, et al: Clinical spectrum of the sick sinus syndrome. *Circulation* 1972;46:5–11.
5. Easley RM, Goldstein S: Sino-atrial syncope. *Am J Med* 1971;50:166–177.

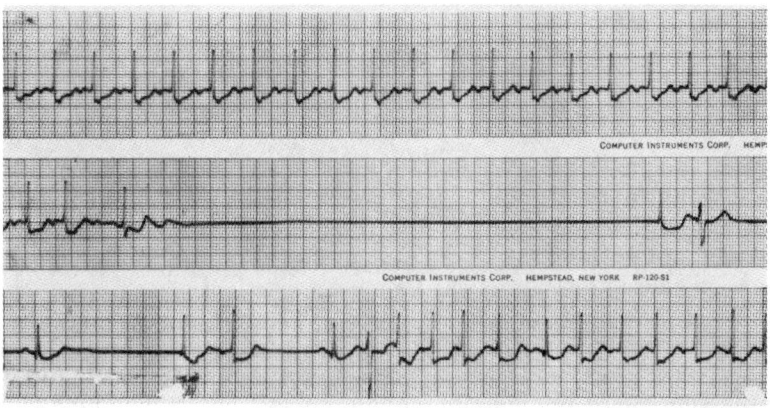

Figure 32-6 Supraventricular tachycardia with a long period of sinus arrest following spontaneous cessation of this arrhythmia. The episode of sinus arrest is terminated by a junctional escape beat.

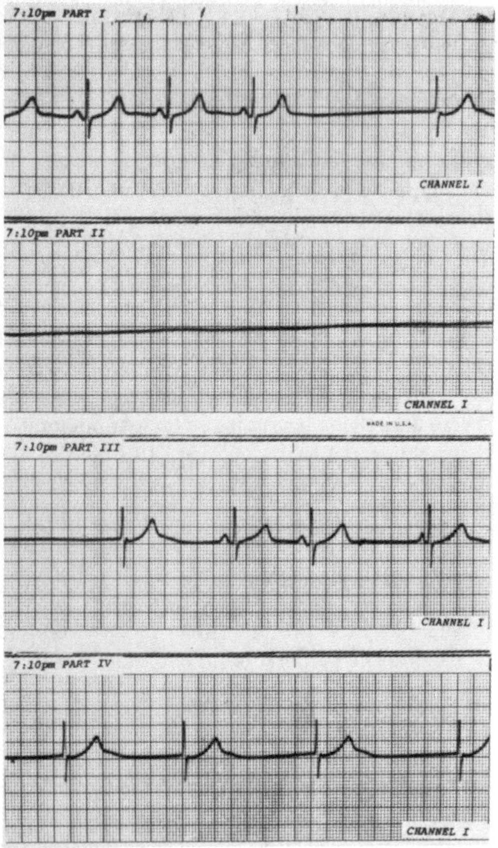

Figure 32-7 Holter recording showing sinus rhythm with sudden onset of sinus arrest. At 7:10, part IV, there is sinus arrest with a slow junctional escape rhythm.

6. Scarpa WJ: The sick sinus syndrome. *Am Heart J* 1976;92:648–660.
7. Moss AJ, Davis RJ: Brady-tachy syndrome. *Prog Cardiovasc Dis* 1974;16:439–454.
8. James TN, Sherf L, Fine G, et al: Comparative ultrastructure of the sinus node in man and dog. *Circulation* 1966;34:139–163.
9. Talano JV, Euler D, Randall, WC, et al: Sinus node dysfunction. An overview with emphasis on autonomic and pharmacologic consideration. *Am J Med* 1978;64:773–781.
10. Dighton DH: Sinus bradycardia. Autonomic influences and clinical assessment. *Br Heart J* 1974;36: 791–797.
11. Chung EK: Sick sinus syndrome: Current views. *Mod Concepts Cardiovasc Dis* 1980;49:61–66.
12. Chung EK: *Artificial Cardiac Pacing: Practical Approach.* Baltimore, Williams & Wilkins Co, 1979, pp 119–149.
13. Rokseth R, Hatle L: Sinus arrest in acute myocardial infarction. *Br Heart J* 1971;33:639.
14. James TN: The coronary circulation and conduction system in acute myocardial infarction. *Prog Cardiovasc Dis* 1968;10:410.
15. Evans R, Shaw DB: Pathological studies in sinoatrial disorder (sick sinus syndrome). *Br Heart J* 1977;39:778.
16. Kaplan BM, Langendorf R, Lev M, et al: Tachycardia-bradycardia syndrome (so-called "sick sinus syndrome"). *Am J Cardiol* 1973;31:497–507.
17. Allensworth DC, Rice GJ, Lower GW: Persistent atrial standstill in a family with myocardial disease. *Am J Med* 1969;47:775.
18. Yabek SM, Swensson RE, Jarmakani JM: Electrocardiographic recognition of sinus node dysfunction in children and young adults. *Circulation* 1977; 56:235–239.
19. Goyal SL, Lichstein E, Gupta PK, et al: Sick sinus syndrome requiring permanent pacemaker implantation in a patient with mirror-image dextrocardia. *Chest* 1976;69:558–561.

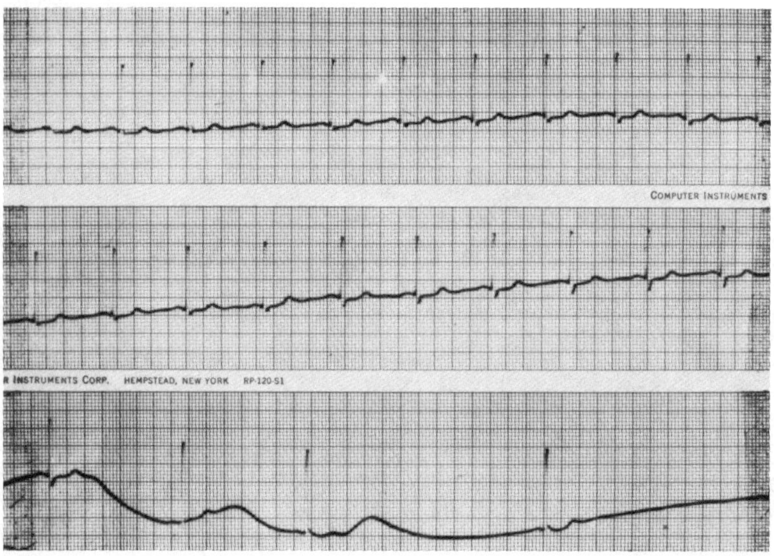

Figure 32-8 Holter recording showing sinus rhythm with sudden onset of sinus arrest and a junctional escape rhythm.

20. Mihalick MJ, Fisch C: Electrocardiographic findings in the aged. *Am Heart J* 1974;87:117–128.
21. Camm AJ, Evans KE, Ward DE, et al: The rhythm of the heart in active elderly subjects. *Am Heart J* 1980;99:598–603.
22. Gavey CJ: The cardiology of old age. *Lancet* 1949;2:725.
23. Kirk JE, Kvorning SA: Sinus bradycardia. A clinical study of 515 consecutive cases. *Acta Med Scand* 1952;266:625.
24. Brodsky M, Wu D, Denes P, et al: Arrhythmias documented by 24 hour continuous electrocardiographic monitoring in 50 male medical students without apparent heart disease. *Am J Cardiol* 1977;39:390–395.
25. Agruss NS, Rosin EY, Adolph RJ, et al: Significance of chronic sinus bradycardia in elderly people. *Circulation* 1972;46:924–930.
26. Kostis JB, Moreyra AE, Amendo MT, et al: The effect of age on heart rate in subjects free of heart disease. Studies by ambulatory electrocardiography and maximal exercise stress test. *Circulation* 1982; 65:141–145.
27. Bixler EO, Kales A, Soldatos CR, et al: Prevalence of sleep disorders in the Los Angeles metropolitan area. *Am J Psychiatry* 1979;136:1251.
28. Jose AD, Collison D: The normal range and determinants of the intrinsic heart rate in man. *Cardiovasc Res* 1970;4:160–167.
29. Fairfax AJ, Lambert CD, Leatham A: Systemic embolism in chronic sinoatrial disorder. *N Engl J Med* 1976;295:190–192.
30. Burch GE: Interesting aspects of geriatric cardiology. *Am Heart J* 1975;89:99–114.
31. Mandel WJ, Hayakawa H, Allen HN, et al: Assessment of sinus node function in patients with the sick sinus syndrome. *Circulation* 1972;46:761–769.
32. Narula OS, Samet P, Javier RP: Significance of sinus-node recovery time. *Circulation* 1972;45: 140–158.
33. Gupta PK, Lichstein E, Chadda KD, et al: Appraisal of sinus nodal recovery time in patients with sick sinus syndrome. *Am J Cardiol* 1974;34:265–270.
34. Radford DJ, Julian DG: Sick sinus syndrome: Experience of a cardiac pacemaker clinic. *Br Med J* 1974;3:504–507.
35. Rokseth R, Hatle L: Prospective study on the occurrence and management of chronic sinoatrial disease, with follow-up. *Br Heart J* 1974;36:582–587.
36. Shokshi DS, Mascarenhas PS, Center S: Treatment of sinoatrial rhythm disturbances with permanent cardiac pacing. *Am J Cardiol* 1973;32:215–219.
37. Wohl AJ, Laborde J, Atkins JM, et al: Prognosis of patients permanently paced for sick sinus syndrome. *Arch Intern Med* 1976;136:406–408.
38. Lichstein E, Aithal H, Jonas S, et al: Natural history of severe sinus bradycardia discovered by 24 hour Holter monitoring. *PACE* 1982;5:185–189.

CHAPTER 33
Characteristics of Myocardial Infarction in the Elderly

Eugene L. Coodley
Diane Zebari

It is well recognized that coronary heart disease constitutes a major problem in mortality and morbidity in the US population. Moreover, although the number of patients over the age of 65 is approximately 11% at the present time, it is projected that 20% of the population will be above this age limit before the end of this century. It is clear that there are a number of significant differences between the appearance and behavior of coronary heart disease in the younger and older patient and it is important that physicians be aware of the many subtle and gross differences in enabling them to make an accurate diagnosis, take appropriate therapeutic steps, and have some basis for a prognostic index. While coronary heart disease reaches its maximum incidence in the fifth, sixth, and seventh decades of life, there is comparatively little information available on the precise differences in presentation and course between the younger and older patient. It is well known that coronary artery disease is four to six times more frequent in men than in women, but differences between the sexes in terms of presentation are not as well recognized. There is a later incidence in women than men, a relatively higher mortality in women than in men in the lower age groups, and a considerably smaller rise in mortality with increasing age in women.

METHODS

The present study is a retrospective review of the charts of patients above and below the age of 60 with proven myocardial infarction (MI). Sixty-eight consecutive patients with MI above age 60 were studied with particular reference to mode of presentation, symptomatology, physical findings, specific laboratory parameters, course and prognosis, role of more sophisticated technology in diagnosis and prognosis, and therapeutic approaches. Fifty-one patients below the age of 60 were selected for comparison.

Myocardial infarction was felt to be present when a combination of the following criteria were met: (1) typical ECG evidence of either transmural or subendocardial infarction, (2) significant total creatine phosphokinase (CPK) elevation together with a positive MB fraction, (3) clinical features compatible with MI. In some instances the use of a pyrophosphate isotope scan was also included in the diagnostic workup. For each of these patients, tabular data was secured. The background data are shown in Table 33-1.

The literature was reviewed for other experience with patients in the elderly age group with MI as well as for comparative data on MI in patients in other defined age groups. Immediate mortality in short-term prognosis (up to 3 weeks) has been assessed in relation to episodes of MI and associated factors.

RESULTS

The demographic features of the two groups of patients are illustrated in Table 33-1. The mean age of the nonsurvivors in group 1 was consistently higher and this approached statistical significance. Initial symptoms including chest pain did not differ in the two groups while precipitating factors were more frequently identified in the older age group.

Table 33-1
Background Data on 119 MI Patients—A Comparative Study

	Patients >60 yr		Patients <60 yr	
	Surviving (52)	*Dead in Hospital (16)*	*Surviving (44)*	*Dead in Hospital (7)*
Age (mean)	66.6	72.3	53.6	54.6
Symptoms				
Chest pain	45	11	37	6
Shortness of breath	3	0	2	0
Abdominal pain	0	2	1	1
Miscellaneous	4	3	4	0
Precipitating factor				
At rest	29	14	13	6
With exertion	8	0	8	0
Unknown	15	2	23	1
Diagnosis				
Anterior MI	13	3	8	1
Lateral MI	1	3	3	0
Inferior MI	9	3	16	2
Diffuse MI	10	3	8	1
Subendocardial MI	17	3	9	2
Unknown	0	1	0	1
Associated disease				
Hypertension	23	5	22	3
Chronic obstructive pulmonary disease	2	3	2	0
Heart failure	13	8	2	2
Diabetes mellitus	13	4	6	2
None	15	4	19	2
Smokers				
Yes	36	10	32	4
No	14	4	8	3
Unknown				
Alcohol use				
None	19	8	11	2
Mild	17	5	10	4
Heavy	5	1	16	1
Heart size pre-MI				
Normal	17	5	17	1
Enlarged	8	5	3	2
Preceding angina				
Yes	25	11	24	6
No	22	2	15	0
Preceding MI				
Yes	22	12	17	4
No	25	3	25	2
Family history				
Positive	17	2	17	3
Negative	13	11	15	4

Mortality was higher in the older group, 23.5% compared to 13.7%, though this did not reach statistical significance ($P = .10$). While anterior infarction was also more common in this group, this was unrelated to such mortality since the latter was equally divided between anterior, lateral, inferior, and subendocardial infarctions. Inferior MI occurred in 12/68 (17.6%) of the older group; it was present in 18/51 (35.3%) of the younger group ($P = .05$).

Transmural MIs were more frequently associated with mortality but did not reach statistical significance ($P > .10$) because of small sample size in the total group.

Both diabetes and heart failure were more commonly associated diseases in the older patient group and mortality was particularly striking in those patients with associated heart failure.

Smoking incidence was similar in the two groups and more frequently associated with mortality but was not statistically significant ($P > .10$).

History of preceding MI was far more frequent in the older group and especially in nonsurvivors (12/34 [35%] compared to 4/21 [19%]).

Table 33-2 gives data obtained following infarction. Complications were statistically more frequent in the older group (46/68 compared to 22/51) $P < .01$. Mortality after complication was similar in the two groups. Shock and significant ventricular arrhythmias were seen in a high percentage of nonsurvivors in both groups. Abnormal isotope scans were infrequent in both groups while heart size was abnormal in a higher percentage of older patients and more so in nonsurvivors in the older group. Ejection fraction was less than 50% in the majority of patients tested in both groups and was unrelated to subsequent mortality in these patients. Posthospital cardiac events were confined to the older group. Heart failure in the older group after MI proved to have a poor prognosis ($P = .05$). Catheterization studies showed predominantly two- and three-vessel disease in both age groups. The longer hospital stay for older patients was probably related to more frequent complications and more associated diseases.

The laboratory data was essentially similar in the two groups except for higher mean potassium levels in the nonsurvivors of the older group. There was no difference in mean CPK values between the two groups of patients, suggesting that the normals used in younger patients were probably applicable in older patients.

DISCUSSION

In a study reported by Peel[1] the ratio of males with MI compared to females was approximately 4:1 in patients between the ages of 60 and 69 while from 70 onward it was somewhat less than 2:1. He indicated that in females episodes of cardiac ischemia with or without infarction were almost equal in number in all ages with half of the coronary episodes in women being associated with infarction. On the other hand, in males the same ratio occurred up to the age of 50 but at a later age infarction became more frequent. He postulated that the difference late in life was related to the development of the collateral circulation which was sufficiently well developed to prevent infarction in many instances of coronary ischemia and that males seem to lose this advantage once the age of 50 has been passed. With regard to mortality, Peel indicated that there is a steady rise in mortality in males up to the age of 65, whereas the rise in mortality with increasing age in females is minimal.

In that study, it appeared that the age of onset was the most important factor in determining the probable expectation of life; it was best in patients with an early onset of MI. In males on the other hand, the optimum ages from the point of view of life expectancy were from 50 to 54 and the worst prognosis was at ages 60 to 64.

Rodstein[2] reviewed the records of 700 ambulatory residents of a home for the aged for evidence of MI in early 1950. He described 51 patients who were considered to have had an acute nonfatal MI during that time. In 16 of these 51 patients, no history was attainable of any symptoms referable to heart disease, and they were thought to be cases of silent infarction. In 21 patients classical chest or neck pain was absent, but substitute symptoms such as dyspnea, syncope, vertigo, or abdominal pain were predominant. There were 16 patients with classical symptoms and these were hypertensive males under the age of 71 with normal hearts on x-ray film and ECG. The infarctions were accompanied by the expected changes in WBC counts and ESR and there was a high incidence of significant Q waves and reciprocal ST segment changes. Of the patients with atypical presentations, most had no Q waves and few had the expected fall in blood pressure. Silent infarcts were found in 16 patients between the ages of 70 and 90, half were hypertensive, and typical changes in ESR and WBC count were found infrequently. He concluded that the appreciation of pain in the typical group could be explained on the basis of their being younger with better mental function and the ability to verbalize a sensation of pain more clearly. He postulated that the absence of stimuli of preceding cardiac damage, ie, coronary disease by ECG, might be correlated with a less well-developed collateral circulation. He felt that the lack of pain and presence of atypical symptoms in the middle group were related to the following: (1) early mental deterioration with a loss in the ability to interpret pain sensation; and (2) a reduction in arterial elasticity and degenerative vascular changes in the cerebral vessels with aging, which sensitizes the cerebrum to reductions in blood flow resulting in cerebral anoxia, which in turn would result in less pain sensation. Infarction without pain frequently occurs in the presence of an acute exacerbation of heart failure with characteristic symptoms of dyspnea.

With regard to the large proportion of cases of silent infarction, it was suggested that these may be the result of a better collateral circulation, be related to gradual progressive coronary artery narrowing resulting in an area anesthetized by destruction of nerves and vessels, or result from destruction of only a few fibers at a time resulting

Table 33-2
Postinfarction Data on 119 MI Patients—A Comparative Study

	Patients >60 yr		Patients <60 yr	
	Surviving (52)	*Dead in Hospital (16)*	*Surviving (44)*	*Dead in Hospital (7)*
Age (mean)	66.6	72.3	53.6	54.6
Isotope scan				
Normal	3	2	3	1
Abnormal	24	2	10	2
Not performed	25	12	31	4
Complications				
Shock	2	7	0	4
Heart failure	7	7	7	0
Atrial arrhythmias	6	1	7	0
Ventricular arrhythmias	7	6	5	3
Conduction defect	6	1	1	0
Other	9	1	6	2
None	20	0	29	0
Predischarge stress test				
Not performed	22	14	19	6
Normal	14	2	17	0
Abnormal	11	0	5	1
Heart size post-MI				
Normal	18	0	27	2
Enlarged	22	8	10	2
Left ventricular function				
Ejection fraction <50%	18	1	12	2
Ejection fraction >50%	8	1	7	0
Posthospital cardiac event				
MI	4	2	0	0
Unstable angina	1	0		
Cardiac deaths (non-MI) within 18 months			0	1
None	36	0	36	0
Bypass surgery				
Prior to MI	3	1	0	0
Following MI	3	0	4	0
Catheterization				
One-vessel	0		1	1
Two-vessel	14	2	9	0
Three-vessel	4		5	1
Hospital stay (days)	25.2	12.4	15.1	16.2
Laboratory data				
K	4.25	4.55	4.24	4.29
WBC	10.3	13.2	9.7	8.8
Hematocrit	41.6	40.7	44.5	38.6
Glucose	171	173	149	146
CPK	1262 ± 552	1038 ± 385	1245 ± 1019	621 ± 572

in insufficient sensory awareness. It is well recognized that there is associated with age a relative increase in insensitivity to pain as well as to other sensations.

Rodstein emphasized the importance of suspecting acute MI in aged patients who show unexplained behavior changes, acute signs of cerebral insufficiency, present with unexplained abdominal complaints, or who present with an acute fall in blood pressure of unknown origin.

Latting and Silverman[3] have analyzed the age, sex, hospital mortality rate, and factors influencing prognosis in a group of patients aged 70 or older with acute myocardial infarction. They combined this study with a comparison of a similar group of patients under the age of 70. This data was obtained retrospectively from a comprehensive data base similar to the study described by us. Their comparison group included 772 patients below the age of 70 while the study group comprised 175 patients having criteria of an acute MI. They reported a mortality rate for the elderly group of 32% with no significant difference between those patients between 70 and 79 years and those between 80 and 89 years. There was no statistical difference in the mortality rate for elderly females as compared to males, although there was a slightly increased percentage. Looking at patients below the age of 70, they confirmed that there was an increase in mortality which was progressive for each decade of life and this was true for both men and women. In addition, they described a slightly higher mortality rate for each decade after age 49 in women. In the group of patients under age 70, the mortality rate was 8.2%. Looking at prognostic factors in the elderly group, they described a history of angina in 54.3%, a history of prior MI in 33.1%, a history of hypertension in 44%, a history of heart failure in 20%, and a history of diabetes mellitus in 21.7%; no single prognostic factor was associated with a significant increase in mortality rate during the hospital course. In comparing the mortality rate of patients with none of the above prognostic factors with patients having adverse prognostic factors, there did not appear to be any associated increase in mortality rate with an increase in the number of prognostic factors per patient, although there was an increase in mortality with some prognostic factors as compared to none.

In looking for factors associated with an increased hospital mortality rate they found no significant difference related to the type or location of MI, but the development of either complete heart block or new bundle-branch block was associated with a higher mortality rate. The mortality rate of all patients with old or new bundle-branch block was 42.9%.

The presence of cardiogenic shock, pulmonary edema on chest film, heart failure on physical examination, and occurrence of complete heart block during admission or while in hospital were all associated with a significant mortality rate.

In their analysis of the elderly group who died in hospital, the major cause of death was found to be shock, which accounted for approximately one third of the deaths. These were predominantly present in patients with anterior MIs. The second major cause of death was external cardiac rupture, which was noted in almost 18% of the deaths. The major cause of death in the patients with anterior MI was extensive muscle damage with associated shock or severe heart failure. Of the ten patients with autopsy-documented external cardiac rupture, the majority were females. Virtually none of the patients had a history of prior MI, the cardiac rupture generally occurred during the first 48 hours of hospitalization, and most of the ruptures involved the anterior wall. The location of the rupture was always in the site of the acute MI as determined by ECG.

In analyzing the differences of MI in the group aged 70 and older as compared to patients younger than 70, the major findings included a lower male to female ratio in the older patients, ie, 0.9:1.0 compared to 2.77:1. Patients under the age of 60 had a male/female ratio of 3.85:1. They commented on the prevalence of certain prognostic factors in the older age group and indicated that the prevalence was much higher than the incidence of similar factors reported in younger age groups. Other studies of younger patients have indicated an incidence of angina pectoris of 17%, hypertension of 25%, heart failure of 4%, and diabetes mellitus of 11%, whereas this study demonstrated two to three times the incidence of the same prognostic factors. As indicated above, hospital mortality rate was not influenced by the number of prognostic factors present in individual patients nor by the overall prevalence of prognostic factors in this study group. Factors that significantly influenced hospital mortality rate from acute MI included: shock, pulmonary edema, heart failure, and development of complete heart block or new bundle-branch block. The incidence of cardiac rupture in the elderly group of 28.6% is two to three times the incidence of cardiac rupture reported in other series and indicates that the elderly dying of acute MI have a higher incidence of such complications. Most series have reported an incidence of about 10%.[4-6]

With regard to the hospital mortality rate from acute MI in the over 70 age group, the 32% incidence was almost four times greater than the mortality rate of 8.2% in the group under age 70; the mortality rate reported in studies in the literature for younger hospitalized patients with MI ranges between 8% and 20%, with an average of 15%.[7-9]

This study clearly indicated that age was a significant independent prognostic factor even when good risk older patients were compared with younger patients. This increased mortality was felt to be possibly related to the high incidence of existing pathologic processes which could contribute to pump failure.

Tinker[10] reported on a one-year study of elderly in-patients with MI in England and suggested that atypical presentation may be less common than previously thought. He described a total of 87 patients studied over a one-year period with the average age being 73.8 years. Of these, 51 patients had classical symptoms, 19 patients presented with symptoms of heart failure, and the remaining patients presented with stroke, syncope, or weakness. Only one patient presented with a silent infarction. Of the patients who presented with more classical symptoms, 21.6% had a history of prior angina, a much higher incidence than in the other presentations. Mortality rate was 37.9% and did not appear to be correlated with age, sex, or mode of onset. This author cited Williams et al[11] as showing a relationship between mortality with MI and age, but was unable to demonstrate that phenomenon in this group.

Berman[12] described the incidence of MI in 55 of 130 elderly patients. He found that the overall incidence of arrhythmias was similar to that for younger patients and that the period of stay in the coronary care unit (CCU) and the CCU mortality was similar in both elderly and younger patients. Of those patients surviving hospitalization, 76% were living 18 months after MI and his conclusion was that the elderly patient was as likely as the younger one to benefit from admission to the CCU. He indicated that prior studies of mortality in MI have stressed an increased mortality among older patients but this may reflect the selection process in regard to admission of the elderly. The study, which was conducted in 1976, indicated no difference in the rate of MI between patients below and above age 70. He emphasized that treatment was essentially the same, that resuscitation was as successful in the elderly as in the younger patient, and that the mortality in the elderly group was similar to the current average mortality for CCU care of acute MI in general. He also cited the report of Williams[11] who indicated that mortality of elderly patients with infarction was at least double that of younger patients and that serious complications were more common in the elderly. In addition, no difference in mortality was noted over a period of 3 successive years. The strong conclusion of this author was that the elderly patient was as likely to survive hospitalization following MI in the coronary care unit as the younger patient.

Sugura et al[13] performed extensive clinical pathologic correlation studies in a total of 203 elderly patients with myocardial infarction, the average age being 78.5 years. They noted 117 cases of massive MI. With aging, there tended to be a decreased proportion of large MIs and an increased number of moderate-sized MIs. When coronary stenosis of more than 75% was considered significant, there were 97 cases with three-vessel disease, 51 patients with two-vessel disease, and 30 patients with one-vessel disease. There were 25 patients with MI with no significant coronary stenosis. The largest MIs were associated with marked coronary stenosis.

The ECG diagnosis was correct in 65% of new large MIs. The incidence of chest pain was reported to be 48% with large MIs and only 27.8% in smaller infarctions, but complications including shock, heart failure, and arrhythmias were found in the majority of patients. They described 15 patients with cardiac rupture, all of which occurred within 5 days of the onset of the acute MI. Again the majority of ruptures were anterior. Twenty-one patients were found to have papillary muscle dysfunction, the majority being due to old MI. They described an incidence of 29% of conduction disturbances.

Sugura et al indicated that almost half the patients had painless infarction as described above by one of the other studies. The average age in painless infarction was not dissimilar from that of painful infarction. In general, painless infarction was thought to have a good prognosis. But this was not true in this study and most cases of painless infarction showed more severe symptoms and major complications such as cardiac rupture, heart failure, shock, and arrhythmias.

Roberts and Jones[14] also reported on pathologic findings in patients with acute MI with particular reference to quantification of coronary arterial narrowing. They studied 27 necropsy patients with transmural anterior MI. In 26 of the 27 patients, the ECG was either diagnostic or strongly suggested anterior infarction and in all patients anterior infarction was diagnosed on a clinical basis. Death resulted from cardiogenic shock, uncontrolled arrhythmias, rupture of the ventricular free wall or septum, acute pulmonary edema, and in two patients from intracerebral hemorrhage while on heparin therapy. These patients averaged 60 years in age. Results of the study indicated that severe narrowing was present in virtually every 5-mm segment of coronary artery. The degree of narrowing in the distal portions of the arteries was as great as in the proximal halves of the artery indicating that coronary atherosclerosis among patients with fatal transmural anterior infarction is a diffuse process. In patients over the age of 65 the extent of narrowing was somewhat greater than that in younger patients.

Chaturvedi et al[15] reviewed 105 patients aged 71 or over with MI in a coronary care unit in Belfast. They commented on frequent arrhythmias during the first 24 hours and indicated that the mortality in hospital at the end of three months appeared to be influenced by the interval between the onset of the attack and entry into the CCU. Hospital mortality was described as 27% and was lower (18%) in patients seen within four hours of onset of the MI. The mortality in late admissions ran as high as 53%. Other studies[16,17] have shown that in patients over the age of 70 not treated in a CCU the mortality was 43% compared to a mortality of 33% in a small group of patients treated in a CCU.

Pathy[18] has emphasized that clinical features of MI in the elderly may be extremely variable and the diagnosis easily overlooked. He reported on the clinical presentation of infarction in a series of 387 patients aged 65 and over, of whom 121 patients were aged 80 years or older, and 17 patients were aged 90 years or older. Among the clinical features of MI in those over 80, he indicated that the most common were either acute dyspnea, exacerbation of heart failure, or classical symptoms; many patients were admitted with acute confusion, syncope, stroke, vertigo, peripheral gangrene, palpitation, and acute renal failure, among other symptoms. This large series was diagnosed as MI primarily by ECG patterns since the majority of patients were seen in the 1960s. Of the patients who presented with more classical symptoms, a prior history of angina was noted in approximately one fourth and this was higher than in any other group of presentation. Acute hemiplegia was the presenting clinical problem in approximately 8% of the patients and was associated with atrial fibrillation in a small number of these patients. Of the patients presenting with an acute occlusive arterial episode, this involved the axillary artery, brachial artery, popliteal artery, and femoral artery. Patients having ischemic involvement of the upper limbs were predominantly women. Only a small percentage of such patients had preceding or accompanying atrial fibrillation. A small number of patients presented with clinical features of pulmonary embolization and at autopsy these patients had evidence of both pulmonary emboli and recent cardiac infarction.

Pathy indicated that in his experience an unequivocal diagnosis of an old cardiac infarction by ECG evidence alone is difficult to make in the elderly patient. He emphasized that the incidence of painless infarction (60%) was higher in his study than in any study previously described.

Pathy and Peach[19] reviewed the prevalence of psychological impairment and disability among elderly patients three years after MI. In reviewing 100 patients their results confirmed that elderly patients who were disabled at three months after their MI will, if they survive, make little or no progress toward their preinfarction way of life. The prevalence of symptoms and drug usage also did not change over a three-year period. Similar results have been described among middle-aged patients. The data from a questionnaire they used in their study indicated that the pattern of psychological impairment and disability appeared to be fixed at a three-month interval following MI and did not change during the subsequent three years, and they felt that such a survey might be helpful in planning the future care for such patients.

Yamour et al[20] followed 23 elderly patients, aged 75 years or older, with prior MI for an average of two years after cardiac catheterization in order to characterize elderly patients and their response to therapy. The mortality rate for medically treated patients was 13% and for the surgically treated patients was 28%. All of the surgically surviving patients were symptomatically improved while the medically treated patients remained relatively unchanged in their functional activity level. Burch[21] had indicated that the prognosis for elderly patients who had a MI and had continued to have angina was uniformly poor. In this study, of the patients with angina pectoris at catheterization, 83% had coronary occlusive disease in addition to the vessels supplying the area of prior infarct. They demonstrated that three-vessel coronary occlusive disease had approximately the same incidence with prior myocardial infarction of the anterior wall as that involving the inferior wall. They cited several studies, previously reported, describing the natural history of coronary artery disease in the elderly without surgical intervention. In the study by Peterson et al[22] which involved almost 7000 patients, it was observed that age was the only factor that significantly influenced subsequent hospital mortality and that the average mortality in patients aged less than 60 years was 12% and exceeded 50% in patients over the age of 80. On the other hand, Norris et al[23] found that the mortality rate from 0 to 6 years postinfarction was 67% for patients 70 to 79 years old and 74% for those over 80. Alternatively Kitchin and Milne[24] found the five-year cardiac mortality in survivors of MI in patients over 70 to be 40%. In the study of Yamour et al,[20] the overall prognosis in elderly patients with ischemic heart disease was felt to be not as limited as previously thought and they indicated that coronary bypass surgery may substantially improve the functional activity level in selected elderly patients without prohibitive risk. He also indicated that the mortality of the group was less than in previously described studies and that the mortality of the surgical and medical groups was comparable.

Boucek et al[25] reviewed the sex differences in obstructive coronary artery disease in patients 65 years of age or older with angina pectoris. They indicated that coronary atherosclerosis begins in early life and advances more rapidly in men than in women and that sex differences are maximal in the fifth decade and diminish after the seventh decade. This study indicated that there were no sex differences in the quality or duration of angina pectoris. They also indicated that rest or nocturnal angina pectoris alone was somewhat less common in geriatric than in younger adult patients with coronary artery disease. They demonstrated a greater incidence of significant stenosis of the left coronary artery in male geriatric patients with angina pectoris and more extensive disease of the circumflex and right coronary arteries in males than in females. There was a high incidence of one-vessel disease with predominant involvement of the proximal segments of any one of the three major arteries and predominance of incidence of left anterior descending artery disease.

White et al[26] have reviewed the relationship of the degree of coronary atherosclerosis with age in male patients by examining 100 consecutive males from each of the decades between age 30 and age 90. Of 600 hearts studied for the extent of coronary sclerosis it was shown that the degree of coronary sclerosis and necropsy material is not linearly related to age but increases rapidly in the 30- to 49-year-old age group, and reaches a maximum in the 50- to 59-year age group. From that point on no marked changes occur. Beyond the age of 49, the average male at the time of death had severe degree of atherosclerosis in both the left and right coronary arteries. Hypertension was not found to be a primary factor in the production of coronary atherosclerosis. The proximal segment of the anterior descending branch of the left coronary artery had the highest average grade of atherosclerosis of any of the 16 segments studied, but the pattern of development of sclerosis was similar in the right coronary artery as compared to the left coronary artery.

Ueda et al[27] studied the incidence of cardiac lesions in 184 autopsied aged patients with disseminated intravascular coagulation. They found coronary thrombosis in 16.8%, acute myocardial necrosis in 32.6%, and massive myocardial hemorrhage in 26.6% of the patients. A fresh MI was present in 8.7% of the patients. Only 3 of 16 patients with disseminated coagulation and acute MI had typical cardiac symptoms and in most patients the ECG changes were equivocal or not diagnostic for MI. They emphasized the importance of recognizing the frequency of cardiac involvement in aged patients who have underlying disseminated intravascular coagulation. The average age in this group of patients was 76.5 years. With regard to the etiology of the underlying coagulation defect, the majority of patients had neoplastic tumors and a significant percentage had sepsis.

In studying the effect of coronary artery disease in the aging heart, Bove et al[28] showed that normal aging effects are both peripheral, involving systemic and pulmonary pressures, and combined, involving cardiac output and A-VO_2 difference. Coronary disease was found to exaggerate age-related cardiac abnormalities but had no effect on peripheral circulatory changes due to age. In separating the changes in cardiac function related to age as compared to coexisting coronary disease, it was shown that there was a reduction of cardiac output with age as well as a rise in systemic blood pressure. There was no change in left ventricular systolic volume with age, but there was an increase in the presence of coronary disease. Left ventricular ejection fraction fell significantly with age and this was exaggerated by coexisting coronary artery disease. Pulmonary artery pressure rose with age alone. Systemic A-VO_2 difference rose with age and this was unaffected by coexisting coronary artery disease. Oxygen consumption declined with age but was unrelated to coexisting coronary artery disease. The one measurement affected by coronary disease and not by age was left ventricular end-diastolic volume, which increased in coronary disease but not with age.

Blaustein[29] indicated that an enzymatic pattern involving high myocardial isoenzyme levels when total creatine kinase activity is normal tends to occur more frequently in the elderly. He felt that this represented definite myocardial damage and should be considered as part of the spectrum of nontransmural myocardial infarction. He reported that approximately 20% of patients with MI had elevated myocardial isoenzymes with normal total creatine kinase activity and that these patients had clinical and laboratory characteristics of myocardial infarction. The majority of such patients tended to be older than other patients and age was suggested as an explanation for the atypical presentation. Fewer criteria of classical infarction were present in patients with this particular enzyme pattern.

Adair and Kasahara[30] studied the adrenal cortical response to acute MI in aged patients and demonstrated that the mean serum cortisol level in nine patients over 80 years old was similar to that in five patients less than 60 years old. However, in all patients who died or in whom shock developed, the serum cortisol concentration was significantly elevated. This study was related to the phenomena of increased mortality in aged myocardial patients as compared to younger patients[31,32]; the study was based on the possibility that relative adrenal cortical insufficiency might contribute to the excess mortality and incidence of shock observed in patients with acute MI. It was concluded that most aging patients have a normal adrenal cortical response to severe stress as judged by serum cortisol concentrations at the time of hospital admission for acute MI.

Warnowicz et al[33] studied the prognosis of patients with acute pulmonary edema and normal ejection fraction following acute MI. They studied 39 survivors of acute MI with an average age of 64.9 years. They found that the predischarge ejection fraction did not predict prognosis for this group of patients. However, patients with acute pulmonary edema in the course of MI formed a high-risk group despite good resting left ventricular function at discharge and had a significant incidence of recurrent MI and death. Since they had good residual left ventricular function, it was suggested that they might be good candidates for surgical intervention.

Goldberg and Kennedy[34] examined the influence of race on prognosis after acute MI. They found that accrued in-hospital case fatality rates were not significantly different between whites and blacks but that a significantly greater proportion of white men had transmural MIs as compared to black men. There was a significantly greater in-hospital case fatality rate among white women as compared to white men but no such differences were noted between black men and black women. These conclusions appear to be valid without relationship to age since approximately the same percentage of patients were over the age of 60 in both the male and female studies.

Ueda et al[35] studied the influence of vasodilator therapy on the prognosis of acute MI complicated by left ventricular failure in aged patients; the mean age was 75.7 years. The study demonstrated the beneficial influence of vasodilator therapy in the early prognosis in aged patients but failed to show a prolonged influence or lower mortality.

Two significant studies on the role of anticoagulants in elderly patients after MI have been reported. The first study was a double-blind trial to assess the efficacy of long-term oral anticoagulant therapy.[36] In this study of selected elderly patients over the age of 60, intensive oral anticoagulant therapy substantially reduced the risk of recurrent MI and cardiac deaths. The two-year total mortality was 13.4% in the placebo group and 7.6% in the treated group while the two-year incidence of recurrent MI was 15.9% in the placebo group and 5.7% in the anticoagulant-treated group.

A second study on oral anticoagulants in elderly patients after MI reviewed the risks involved in such therapy. Ross[37] described 12 intracranial events occurring in the anticoagulant group and 20 in the placebo group. The accumulated periods of neurologic disability amounted to 120 days in the anticoagulant group and 1204 days in the placebo group. Of the 106 extracranial bleeding episodes observed in the anticoagulant group, 28 were felt to be major, but none of the patients with major bleeding died. Minor episodes were noted 78 times in 56 anticoagulant patients and 6 times in 5 placebo patients. Over 75% of the bleeding episodes occurred when the prothrombin time was prolonged 2.5 to 4.5 times the desired level. No relationships could be demonstrated between the incidence of bleeding with sex, age, or duration of therapy.

Gundersen et al[38] reviewed the role of beta-blockers in reducing mortality in patients between the ages of 65 and 75 who survived an acute MI, and described sufficient benefit.

Long-term beta-receptor blockade after acute MI has been associated with a reduction in overall mortality.[39-43] Only a few studies, however, have evaluated the use of such blockers in elderly patients. Anderson et al[44] found that treatment with alprenolol in patients with acute MI increased mortality in those older than 65 years.

In the study described by Gundersen et al,[38] long-term treatment with timolol maleate in patients between the ages of 65 and 75 who survived MI was related to a significant reduction in overall mortality, total cardiac deaths, sudden deaths, and reinfarction. The study included 732 patients who were followed for 12 to 33 months (mean 17 months). Medication was timolol maleate in a dosage of 10 mg twice daily. There was a reduction of 35.5% in mortality and a reduction of 39.2% in the reinfarction rate. There was no difference in the reduction in mortality or reinfarction between patients 65 to 75 years of age and patients less than 65 years of age, thus implying that age should not be a decision factor in timolol maleate therapy in postinfarction patients.

In contrast to the material cited above and reported in our study, several studies have emphasized the features of MI in younger age groups. Uhl and Farrell[45] reviewed the natural history and risk factors of MI in several groups of young adults. They compared 165 patients under age 40 with a mean age of 35 to a second group of 100 patients over age 40 with a mean age of 50. They analyzed six risk factors: smoking, elevated lipids, hypertension, family history, diabetes mellitus, and obesity. Of the patients under age 40, 18% were without risk factors, whereas 41% in the group over age 40 were without risk factors. The younger group had hyperlipidemia, obesity, and positive family history more commonly than did the group over age 40 while hypertension was more frequent in the older patients. Physical exertion just prior to MI was more common in the younger age group. Death at the time of MI was more frequent in the older age group, but heart failure occurred in 17% of both groups. On follow-up, approximately half of both groups had no complications and the rates of subsequent MI and angina pectoris were similar in both groups. Late death was less frequent in the younger age group and patients under 40 with MI were found to have more risk factors than older patients.

In a study by Rubin et al[46] the extent of coronary vessel involvement after MI was analyzed in patients 60 years of age and younger. They studied 229 hospital survivors of acute MI who were age 60 or younger and followed for a period of 2 years. There was a 96% survival at 1 year and 95% survival at 2 years; this was partially the result of the high prevalence of one-vessel disease in these patients. In the cohort of younger patients with a mean age of 51 years, they indicated that prophylactic therapy, ie, bypass surgery, may not be justified because of the low mortality and should be reserved for identifiable high-risk groups. The mean age of the patients described above was 51 years with a range of 27 to 60 years. They demonstrated that none of the patients younger than age 40 had three-vessel disease and only 18% had two-vessel disease, whereas 40% of the patients aged 40 years or older had either two- or three-vessel disease. In this study extent of coronary vessel involvement correctly predicted survival.

A study by Taylor et al[47] indicated that in patients 70 years or younger the prevalence of one-vessel disease was only 26%, whereas the prevalence of multivessel disease was around 70%. It was emphasized that age was an important prognostic variable and that mortality increased exponentially beginning at age 65. They also emphasized that ejection fraction was felt to be an independent prognostic factor after MI and that a low ejection fraction enhances mortality in association with two- or three-vessel disease but not necessarily with one-vessel disease.

SUMMARY

Compared to several of the studies previously cited, we also showed a higher mortality associated with age and a higher mortality associated with heart failure, cardiomegaly, and preceding MI. We confirmed the occurrence of MI to be more frequent in older patients while at rest.

Our review did not show marked difference in the incidence of chest pain in the older patient as compared to the younger patient as was described in several other studies. We were unable to confirm the discrepancy in the relationship of total CPK and MB fraction of CPK that was noted in several other studies in older patients. We were also unable to demonstrate a difference in survival based on ejection fraction, but the number studied may have been too few to demonstrate this.

Our study did demonstrate a significant difference in the length of hospital stay in older patients vs younger patients ($P < .05$). There was also a significant difference in hospital stay between survivors and nonsurvivors of MI ($P < .025$).

Factors associated with a higher mortality included the presence of shock and an enlarged heart after infarction as well as a history of preceding

MI. A history of preinfarction heart failure and/or a preceding history of angina were significant predictors of mortality in the older age group.

ACKNOWLEDGMENT

The statistical analysis was prepared by Mark Ofstein, MD, Section of Gerontology, Medical Service, Long Beach VA Medical Center, California.

REFERENCES

1. Peel AAF: Age and sex factors in coronary artery disease. *Br Heart J* 1955;17:319–320.
2. Rodstein M: The characteristics of nonfatal myocardial infarction in the aged. *Arch Intern Med* 1956;98:84–90.
3. Latting CA, Silverman ME: Acute myocardial infarction in hospitalized patients over age 70. *Am Heart J* 1980;100:311–318.
4. Bates RJ, Beutler S, Resnekov L, et al: Cardiac rupture—Challenge in diagnosis and management. *Am J Cardiol* 1977;40:429–435.
5. Mundth ED: Rupture of the heart complicating myocardial infarction. *Circulation* 1972;46:427–431.
6. Biorck G, Mogensen L, Myquist O, et al: Studies of myocardial rupture with cardiac tamponade in acute myocardial infarction. I. Clinical features. *Chest* 1972;61:4–8.
7. Madias JE, Chahine RA, Gorlin R, et al: A comparison of transmural and nontransmural acute myocardial infarction. *Circulation* 1974;49:498–503.
8. Armstrong A, Duncan B, Oliver MF, et al: Natural history of acute coronary attacks. A Community Study. *Br Heart J* 1972;34:67–72.
9. Gross H, Vaid AK, Levine HS, et al: Anticoagulant therapy in myocardial infarction. An overview of methodology. *Am J Med* 1972;52:421–427.
10. Tinker GM: Clinical presentation of myocardial infarction in the elderly. *Age Ageing* 1981;10: 237–240.
11. Williams BO, Begg TB, Semple T, et al: The elderly in a coronary unit. *Br Med J* 1976;2:451–455.
12. Berman ND: The elderly patient in the coronary care unit. I. Acute myocardial infarction. *J Am Geriatr Soc* 1979;27:145–151.
13. Sugura M, Ohkawa S, Hiroaka K, et al: Clinicopathologic aspects of ischemic heart disease in the elderly. *Japan Heart J* 1981;22:15–30.
14. Roberts WC, Jones AA: Quantification of coronary arterial narrowing at necropsy in acute transmural myocardial infarction. *Circulation* 1980;61:786–790.
15. Chaturvedi NC, Walsh MJ, Shivalingappa G, et al: Myocardial infarction in the elderly. *Lancet* 1972; 49:280–282.
16. Norris RM, Brandt PWT, Caughey DE, et al: Myocardial infarction in the elderly. *Lancet* 1969; 1:274–279.
17. Pentecost BL, Mayne MMC: CCU care after MI for elderly patients. *Br Med J* 1968;1:830–835.
18. Pathy MS: Clinical presentation of myocardial infarction in the elderly. *Br Heart J* 1967;29:190–199.
19. Pathy MS, Peach H: Disability among the elderly after myocardial infarction: A 3-year follow-up. *J R Coll Physicians Lond* 1980;14:221–223.
20. Yamour B, McMartin D, Masden R, et al: Patient profile and follow-up in medically and surgically treated elderly adults with myocardial infarction. *Clin Cardiol* 1982;5:584–589.
21. Burch PRJ: Coronary heart disease risk factors and aging. *Gerontology* 1978;24:123–127.
22. Peterson DR, Thompson DJ, Chinn N: Ischemic heart disease prognosis. A community-wide assessment (1966–1969). *JAMA* 1972;219:1423–1427.
23. Norris RM, Caughey DE, Mercer CJ, et al: Prognosis after myocardial infarction. Six year follow-up. *Br Heart J* 1974;36:786–792.
24. Kitchin AH, Milne JS: Longitudinal survey of ischemic heart disease in randomly selected sample of older population. *Br Heart J* 1977;39:889–895.
25. Boucek RJ, Romanelli R, Willis WH, et al: Sex differences in obstructive coronary artery disease in patients 65 years of age or older with angina pectoris. *Circulation* 1982;66:926–929.
26. White NK, Edwards JE, Dry TJ: The relationship of the degree of coronary atherosclerosis with age. *Circulation* 1983;67:330–334.
27. Ueda K, Sugura M, Shinichiro O, et al: Disseminated intravascular coagulation in the aged complicated by acute myocardial infarction. *Japan J Med* 1981;20:202–210.
28. Bove AA, Bodurian EN, Santamore WP: Prognostic induction in patients with coronary artery disease, abstracted. *J Am Coll Cardiol* 1983;1(2): 718–725.
29. Blaustein AS: Elevated myocardial isoenzymes with normal creatine kinase. *Pract Cardiol* 1983;9: 21–26.
30. Adair R, Kasahara M: Serum cortisol response to acute myocardial infarction in the aged. *J Am Geriatr Soc* 1980;28:472–476.
31. Harris R, Piracha A: Acute myocardial infarction in the aged: Prognosis and management. *J Am Geriatr Soc* 1970;18:893–898.
32. Konu V: Myocardial infarction in the elderly. *Acta Med Scand* (suppl) 1977;604:3–68.
33. Warnowicz MA, Parker H, Cheitlin M: Prognosis of patients with acute pulmonary edema and normal ejection fraction after acute myocardial infarction. *Circulation* 1983;67:330–334.
34. Goldberg RJ, Kennedy HL: The influence of race on prognosis after acute myocardial infarction: A community-wide perspective. *J Cardiac Rehab* 1983;3:195–201.
35. Ueda K, Mifune J, Hiroshi I, et al: Influence of vasodilator therapy on prognosis of acute myocardial infarction in the aged patient. *Japan Heart J* 1980;41:35–45.
36. Ross J: A double blind trial to assess long-term oral anticoagulant therapy in elderly patients after myocardial infarction. *Lancet* 1980;2:989–994.
37. Ross J: Risks of long-term oral anticoagulant therapy in elderly patients after myocardial infarction. *Lancet* 1980;1:64–68.
38. Gundersen T, Abrahamsen AM, Kjekshus J, et al: Timolol-related reduction in mortality and reinfarction in patients ages 65–75 years surviving acute

myocardial infarction. *Circulation* 1982;66:1179-1184.
39. The Norwegian Multicentre Study Group: Timolol-induced reduction in mortality and reinfarction in patients surviving acute myocardial infarction. *N Engl J Med* 1981;304:801-807.
40. Wilhelmsson C, Vedin JA, Wilhelmsen L, et al: Reduction of sudden deaths after myocardial infarction by treatment with alprenolol: Preliminary results. *Lancet* 1974;2:1157-1161.
41. Multicentre International Study: Improvement in prognosis of myocardial infarction by long-term beta-adrenoreceptor blockage using practolol: A multicentre international study. *Br Med J* 1975; 3:35-41.
42. Hjalmarson A, Elmfeldt D, Herlitz J, et al: Effect on mortality of metoprolol in acute myocardial infarction. *Lancet* 1981;2:823-827.
43. Beta-blocker Heart Attack Study Group: The beta-blocker heart attack trial. Preliminary report. *JAMA* 1981;247:2073-2079.
44. Andersen MP, Bechsgaard P, Frederiken J, et al: Effect of alprenolol on mortality among patients with definite or suspected acute myocardial infarction. Preliminary results. *Lancet* 1979;2:865-871.
45. Uhl GS, Farrell PW: Myocardial infarction in young adults: Risk factors and natural history. *Am Heart J* 1983;105:548-553.
46. Rubin GS, Harris PJ, Bernstein L, et al: Coronary anatomy and prognosis after myocardial infarction in patients 60 years of age and younger. *Circulation* 1983;67:743-749.
47. Taylor GJ, Humphries JO, Mellitus ED, et al: Predictors of clinical course, coronary anatomy and left ventricular function after recovery from acute myocardial infarction. *Circulation* 1980; 62:960-967.

CHAPTER 34
Infective Endocarditis in the Elderly

David W. Webb
Frederic A. Wyle

Although infective endocarditis occurs in all age groups, there are important differences in infective endocarditis occurring in the elderly. In recent years there has been an increase in the average age of the patient with endocarditis due to an increased incidence of endocarditis in older patients.[1] Underlying cardiac diseases in the older patient with infective endocarditis differ significantly from those in younger endocarditis patients. Instead of rheumatic or congenital heart disease, these patients often have degenerative heart disease such as calcification of the aortic valve or mitral annulus.[2] Additionally, older patients more frequently have foreign bodies such as pacemakers or prosthetic valves that may predispose them to infective endocarditis.

The organisms responsible for infective endocarditis in the elderly differ only slightly. Enterococci have an increased incidence in the older age groups while viridans streptococci are less commonly seen than in younger patients.[1] These differences in causative organisms may reflect the increased risk of the elderly of undergoing invasive procedures such as catheterization of the urinary bladder or the insertion of intravenous lines, thus predisposing them to bacteremia from opportunistic organisms.

The clinical presentation of infective endocarditis may also differ in the elderly. The disease more often presents insidiously with symptoms such as weakness, fatigue, and weight loss predominating. Occasionally patients may present with no fever or murmur, leading to delays in diagnosis. Complications such as congestive heart failure occur more commonly in the elderly. Unfortunately, the frequent finding of murmurs and congestive heart failure in the elderly may be responsible for the diagnosis of endocarditis being overlooked in such patients.

The frequent delay in diagnosis, the higher incidence of certain complications, and the underlying debilitated state of elderly patients may explain the increased mortality that has been reported in infective endocarditis of the elderly.[3] Despite the foregoing, infective endocarditis in the elderly can be successfully treated, providing the diagnosis is considered and confirmed early and appropriate antimicrobial therapy is rapidly instituted.

DEFINITIONS

Infective endocarditis refers to an infectious process involving the endocardium. Most commonly the endocardial surface of a heart valve is involved. However, the infection can involve the mural endocardium or a septal defect of the heart.

Endocarditis has traditionally been divided into acute and subacute, based on the course of the untreated disease. Although some authors have contended that the terms acute and subacute endocarditis are mainly of historical interest,[4] they serve a useful purpose in separating two groups of patients that must be approached differently. Patients with acute endocarditis usually present with severe symptoms and rapid progression of valvular destruction. Institution of immediate antibiotic therapy prior to the results of cultures may be indicated in such situations. Subactue endocarditis usually presents insidiously and severe toxicity it unusual. Because valve destruction does not progress rapidly, short delays in antibiotic therapy pending culture results do not usually jeopardize a good outcome. Acute and subacute endocarditis, while useful in terms of describing the clinical features of the disease, do not discriminate among the organisms or the valves involved.

EPIDEMIOLOGY

Although it has been stated that the incidence of infective endocarditis has fallen in recent years due to increased use of antibiotics,[5] there is no conclusive evidence that this is true.[6] Chemoprophylaxis of high-risk patients and a lessening incidence of rheumatic heart disease may have led to some decline in infective endocarditis, but this has probably been more than offset by an increase in the number of individuals with prosthetic heart valves and degenerative heart disease who are at risk of developing infective endocarditis.

The average age of patients with infective endocarditis has gradually increased over the past 30 years. Data from Columbia-Presbyterian Hospital show the mean age of patients with infective endocarditis was 34.8 from 1932 to 1942, 47.4 from 1963 to 1967, and 55 from 1968 to 1973.[1] A significant proportion of patients with infective endocarditis are now over age 60, and patients over age 70 are not rare. Between 1970 and 1977, at Montefiore Hospital, 35% of patients with infective endocarditis were over age 65 and the average age of these patients was 71.7.[6a] This shift of patients with infective endocarditis to an older age group is most pronounced in males. At the University of Iowa, between 1940 and 1971, the male to female ratio of all patients with infective endocarditis was 2:1; whereas among patients over age 60 with infective endocarditis, the ratio was 4:1.[6b]

Reasons for this dramatic increase in the age of patients with infective endocarditis probably relate not only to the increasing life span of patients with predisposing cardiac lesions but also to a change in the nature of the cardiac lesions underlying endocarditis.

UNDERLYING HEART DISEASE

The underlying heart diseases that are responsible for predisposing patients to infective endocarditis differ in elderly patients. Congenital heart disease is a common predisposing condition in younger patients, but is an uncommon cause of infective endocarditis in older patients. In elderly patients with infective endocarditis, congenital heart disease is found in less than 12%. As the incidence of rheumatic fever has fallen, the relative importance of rheumatic heart disease as a predisposing cause of infective endocarditis has decreased, being associated with 28% of elderly patients with infective endocarditis at Montefiore Hospital (New York) from 1931 to 1938, but only 11% from 1970 to 1977.[6a]

Proportionally, elderly patients with infective endocarditis are more likely than the young to have underlying degenerative or atherosclerotic heart disease. Degenerative diseases of the heart include calcified mitral annulus and calcified aortic valve.[2] Both of these diseases occur principally in older age groups; the mean age of one group of 80 patients with calcified mitral annulus was 73 years.[7] Calcified mitral annulus occurs more commonly in female patients (2.5:1), while calcification of the aortic valve most commonly occurs in males.

Calcification of the aortic valve may occur in either a congenitally bicuspid or a normal tricuspid valve. Calcification of a normal valve usually occurs at a later age than calcification of a bicuspid valve. Although the cause of this abnormal calcification is unknown, it is thought to be due to degeneration of the fibrous skeleton of the heart. Hypertension, hypertrophic cardiomyopathy, aortic stenosis, and mitral valve prolapse all predispose the patient to development of calcification of the mitral annulus.[7] In most cases the valvular abnormality produced by the calcification is minor and significant stenosis or regurgitation is not produced. However, such valves are prone to the development of infective endocarditis. Aortic valvular calcification has been associated with 5% to 14% of cases of infective endocarditis in the elderly. Calcified mitral annulus was reported to be associated with 26% of patients with staphylococcal endocarditis in one series of patients over age 60.[7a] In a report from Massachusetts General Hospital, of seven patients with calcification of the mitral annulus and infective endocarditis, five were female and all were infected by virulent organisms such as *Staphylococcus aureus*, *Escherichia coli* and *Streptococcus pneumoniae*.[8] Calcified aortic valvular and mitral annular disease may be associated with infective endocarditis to a greater extent than is appreciated clinically, as such calcification may not always be apparent on roentgenography of the chest. Diagnosis may require fluoroscopy or echocardiography.[7]

Atherosclerotic heart disease is frequently reported in elderly patients with infective endocarditis; whether this is a coincidental finding or a predisposing condition to endocarditis is somewhat controversial. Although it has been postulated that atherosclerosis may cause subtle functional valvular changes which predispose to infective endocarditis, this remains unproven. Infective endocarditis may rarely follow myocardial infarction with infection of a mural thrombus and resultant structural damage to the valves, papillary muscles, or heart wall.[9]

Other cardiac abnormalities associated with an increased risk of infective endocarditis include idiopathic hypertrophic subaortic stenosis (IHSS) and prolapse of the mitral valve.[10] These entities are not common predisposing conditions in elderly patients. Increasingly important predisposing conditions are prosthetic valves and pacemakers. As patients who have had prosthetic valves inserted at a young age grow older, the elderly susceptible population increases. Furthermore, in recent years more elderly patients have undergone valve replacement. In one review of 320 elderly patients who underwent valve replacement, and were followed for a mean of 30.2 months, eight developed infective endocarditis.[11] Patients with prosthetic valves have accounted for about 5% of cases of infective endocarditis in elderly patients.

Many elderly patients have no known underlying cardiac disease. Infective endocarditis may occur on normal cardiac valves; this is particularly likely to occur when virulent organisms such as *S aureus* are involved.

CAUSATIVE ORGANISMS

There are minor differences in the frequency of different organisms causing infective endocarditis in elderly and younger patients.

Streptococci are the most frequent cause of infective endocarditis in all age groups. *S aureus* causes 21% to 29% of cases of infective endocarditis in the elderly. These percentages are not significantly different from those in younger patients. *S epidermidis* is an unusual cause of native valve endocarditis but is one of the most frequent causes of both early and late prosthetic valve endocarditis (causing from 20% to 25% of cases).[12]

Enteric gram-negative bacilli, *Pseudomonas* species and *Acinetobacter* organisms more commonly cause infective endocarditis in younger patients; they are unusual causes in elderly patients.[13]

Anaerobic bacteria, *Haemophilus* species, *Cardiobacterium hominus*, *Brucella* species, *Streptobacillus moniliformis*, and *Erysipelothrix* and *Listeria* organisms are rare causes of infective endocarditis. Corynebacteria (diphtheroids) are not uncommon causes of prosthetic valve endocarditis.[14] *Coxiella burnetti* (the cause of Q fever) may cause infective endocarditis but this is rare in the United States. The disease is more commonly seen in Britain, Ireland, and Australia. Patients as old as 67 have been reported.[15]

Candida and *Aspergillus* fungi, while rare causes of native valve endocarditis, are more frequently found as etiologic agents in prosthetic valve endocarditis.[16] *Candida* endocarditis may also occur as a complication of transient fungemia in patients receiving intravenous therapy, particularly parenteral hyperalimentation.

PATHOGENESIS

Infective endocarditis occurs when bacteria which are present in the bloodstream invade and proliferate on a heart valve. Many bacteremias due to relatively avirulent organisms are transient and of no consequence to the host. However, infective endocarditis can occur if the bacteria are able to invade the endothelial surface of the heart valves. This is most likely to occur in previously damaged valves but may occur on normal valves. Because of their inherent virulence, pathogenic bacteria such as *S aureus* are more likely to infect normal valves. Abnormal valves are more likely to be infected if the abnormality causes a venturi effect such that blood flows from a high pressure source through a narrow orifice into a low pressure area. In such situations, the site of infection characteristically occurs in the low pressure area.[17] Infective endocarditis therefore occurs more commonly in valvular insufficiency than stenosis. It has been stated that congestive heart failure and atrial fibrillation reduce the risk of infective endocarditis by attenuating these pressure changes and reducing blood turbulence. However, others have felt this reduced incidence in such patients may be due to their higher early mortality and consequent less risk of exposure to bacteremia.[18]

PORTAL OF ENTRY

Transient bacteremias are relatively common and can occur from a variety of sources:

Dental procedures are frequently associated with transient bacteremia. The risk is higher for those procedures that cause local trauma to the gingiva such as tooth extraction. The risk is also higher for those with gingival disease. The usual organisms causing transient bacteremia in such cases are the viridans streptococci, which also are the most common causes of infective endocarditis in the elderly. In view of the fact that elderly patients frequently have dental disease and may require dental procedures such as extractions, it has been felt that the oral cavity is the most common source of the initial bacteremia causing infective endocarditis in this age group. Dental procedures are an important precipitating event but account for only 5% to 25% of cases in the elderly despite the fact viridans streptococci account for from 17% to 40% of cases in these patients.

Skin infections may be responsible for transient bacteremias. Skin infections such as carbuncles may produce a bacteremia due to *S aureus* or *S epidermidis*. The debilitated aged patient may also develop bacteremia from infected decubitus ulcers.[19]

Urologic infections such as urinary tract infection may be associated with a bacteremia which can lead to infective endocarditis. In such a setting, the enterococcus is most frequently involved. Even though gram-negative bacteria are more common causes of urinary tract infection, a gram-negative bacteremia is less likely to lead to infective endocarditis, perhaps because of their lower inherent virulence. Urologic infections or procedures are associated with 4% to 7% of cases of infective endocarditis in the elderly.

The bowel can also be a source of bacteremia. *Streptococcus bovis* may colonize the bowel, and infective endocarditis may follow spontaneous bacteremia from this organism. Patients with *S bovis* colonization have a high rate of colon carcinoma and adenomatous polyps. These patients are typically elderly; the average age in one series was 70. Enterococci are a common component of bowel flora; endocarditis from this organism may follow surgery or instrumentation of the gastrointestinal (GI) tract.

Because of an increased incidence of hospitalization for associated diseases, elderly patients are subject to the risk of hospital-acquired infections. Bacteremias from such infections may lead to infective endocarditis.

VALVE INVOLVEMENT

Left-sided cardiac involvement is more commonly seen than right-sided in elderly patients with infective endocarditis. Both mitral and aortic valves are involved in approximately 10% to 20% of cases. Mitral valve endocarditis may occur as a complication of aortic valve endocarditis; in aortic insufficiency a jet stream may be created resulting in implantation of bacteria on the mitral valve.[17]

CLINICAL FEATURES

The classical clinical features of infective endocarditis are well known: fever, murmur, splenomegaly, and peripheral manifestations such as petechiae, Roth's spots, splinter hemorrhages, Osler's nodes, and Janeway's spots are often described but seldom seen together in a single patient. There has been a well-documented decrease in the peripheral manifestations of infective endocarditis over the past 30 years, eliminating many of the clues that clinicians have used to make the diagnosis. In addition, fever and murmurs are not invariably present. The situation is even more problematic in the elderly patient; the diagnosis is often not suspected in the older age group for a variety of reasons. Classic findings such as fever and murmur may be absent. Fever, when present, is often attributed to other causes coincidentally present in the elderly such as urinary infection. Murmur, when present, is often felt to be due to atherosclerotic heart disease. Patients often present with complaints relating to other organ systems, and because of the high incidence of chronic disease in this age group, infective endocarditis is often not considered. Patients presenting with musculoskeletal complaints may be thought to have degenerative arthritis. Those presenting with neurologic abnormalities may be thought to have cerebrovascular disease. Those presenting primarily with cardiac manifestations such as congestive heart failure or myocardial infarction may be thought to have atherosclerotic heart disease. Those presenting with weight loss, anorexia, and anemia may be thought to have malignancy. Indeed, in one recent series of patients over age 60 with infective endocarditis, the diagnosis was not made until death in 60%.

CLINICAL PRESENTATION

Nonspecific but common symptoms such as malaise, fatigue, anorexia, weakness, and weight loss may be the presenting complaints in elderly patients with infective endocarditis. The incidence of fever in several large series of elderly patients with infective endocarditis has been 55% to 95%.

Musculoskeletal symptoms may be the predominant presenting feature of patients with infective endocarditis. At the Mayo Clinic 44% of patients with infective endocarditis exhibited some form of musculoskeletal complaint, primarily arthralgias, arthritis, low back pain, and localized or diffuse myalgias.[20]

Patients with infective endocarditis may present with abdominal pain due to emboli and microinfarcts of the spleen or other organs. Elderly endocarditis patients may present primarily with abdominal pain.

A variety of neurologic abnormalities may occur in patients with infective endocarditis, including cerebral embolism and toxic encephalopathy. The overall rate of neurologic complications among 218 patients at Massachusetts General Hospital with infective endocarditis was 39%; there were no apparent age-related differences.[21]

Elderly patients with infective endocarditis may present with congestive heart failure; the true diagnosis may not be suspected as readily because patients in this age group have a high incidence of hypertension and atherosclerotic heart disease which may cause congestive heart failure.

Although not common in the elderly, patients with tricuspid endocarditis may present with septic pulmonary emboli masquerading as pneumonitis or pulmonary embolism.

Elderly patients often present with a prolonged illness ranging from two to six months. Acute infective endocarditis presents more abruptly; among patients with *S aureus* endocarditis who are over the age of 60, the duration of symptoms may range from one to seven days. Such patients usually appear very ill and toxic and the disease often has a fulminant course.

PHYSICAL FINDINGS

With regard to the incidence of abnormal findings in elderly patients with infective endocarditis, from 66% to 100% of patients have some type of murmur. The absence of a murmur does, therefore, not mitigate against the diagnosis of endocarditis. A changing pre-existent murmur is uncommon, although in acute endocarditis with rapid valvular destruction, new murmurs may develop. Some patients will develop murmurs during or after completion of successful therapy.

Splenomegaly is present in from 16% to 43% of elderly patients with infective endocarditis. Splenomegaly is more frequently found in patients with a more prolonged course of illness. Signs such as Osler's nodes, Janeway's spots, petechiae, splinter hemorrhages, and clubbing are helpful when present but are found only in a minority of patients. Splinter hemorrhages may be due to trauma and as such are not a highly reliable sign of endocarditis.

LABORATORY FEATURES

Anemia is a frequent manifestation of infective endocarditis in the elderly. Leukocytosis is more likely to be present in acute than in subacute infective endocarditis. Microscopic hematuria is often considered a classical finding in infective endocarditis, being present in approximately 50% of patients. The cause of microscopic hematuria, which is often accompanied by proteinuria, is thought to be immune complex focal glomerulonephritis or microemboli to the kidneys. Renal function remains normal in these entities. Rarely a diffuse glomerulonephritis will cause renal insufficiency.

An elevated erythrocyte sedimentation rate (ESR) is usually present in all patients with infective endocarditis. Rheumatoid factor has been reported to be positive in 47% of patients with infective endocarditis, most often in those with disease of over six weeks' duration.[22]

A majority of patients with infective endocarditis will have circulating immune complexes. The incidence has been found to be higher in subacute endocarditis (89%) than in acute endocarditis (66%).[23] Immune complexes are not usually present in patients with bacteremias without infective endocarditis. These immune complexes may be important in the pathogenesis of the peripheral lesions and the glomerulonephritis seen in this disease; their titer usually drops with effective therapy.[24] The diagnostic usefulness of this test remains to be determined, but it has been suggested that the test may be helpful in establishing the diagnosis of infective endocarditis in patients who have received prior antimicrobial therapy and therefore have negative blood cultures.

The electrocardiogram (ECG) is normal in most patients with infective endocarditis. Abnormalities on the ECG often indicate extension of the infection from the heart valve into the myocardium.

The chest roentgenogram is usually normal in patients with infective endocarditis except with certain complications. Signs of congestive heart failure may indicate valve dysfunction in acute infective endocarditis. Tricuspid endocarditis may present with septic pulmonary emboli and "pneumonia."

Studies in patients with infective endocarditis have shown vegetations detected in about 50% by M-mode and 80% by two-dimensional echocardiography.[25] Two-dimensional echocardiography is more sensitive than M-mode echocardiography, particularly in demonstrating vegetations of the aortic and tricuspid valves.

Blood cultures remain the single most useful test in the diagnosis of infective endocarditis. Blood cultures are positive in up to 97% of patients with infective endocarditis when optimal microbiologic technics are employed. Blood should be cultured both aerobically and anaerobically. As most patients with infective endocarditis have a continuous bacteremia, the timing of blood cultures is not crucial. Although two blood cultures will yield the etiologic agent over 90% of the time,[26] it is recommended that from three to six sets be obtained from separate venipuncture sites. The larger number should be employed in patients who have previously received antibiotics. Arterial blood offers no advantage over venous blood.

Blood cultures should be obtained in all elderly patients with fever; they are helpful not only in making the diagnosis of infective endocarditis but also in establishing the etiology of other infections such as pneumonias. Blood cultures should also be obtained in all elderly patients with undiagnosed illnesses in which infective endocarditis cannot be ruled out, whether or not a fever or murmur is present. This may entail taking cultures from many patients but will ensure that the diagnosis is not missed. A high index of suspicion is a most valuable attribute in making the diagnosis of infective endocarditis in the elderly patient.

PRINCIPLES OF THERAPY

Cure of infective endocarditis can best be achieved if a bactericidal antibiotic is given parenterally for a prolonged period of time. Bacteriostatic antibiotics or short courses of therapy are too frequently followed by relapses. Although there has been some success with oral therapy in some forms of infective endocarditis, this form of therapy cannot be recommended at present until further experience is available.

Selection of the proper antibiotic depends on isolation and identification of the organism from blood cultures. In most instances when infective endocarditis is suspected, blood cultures can be obtained and therapy may be withheld until the organism has been identified. However, in the patient with rapid onset of illness and a fulminant course consistent with acute endocarditis, therapy should be instituted immediately to prevent valvular destruction. Therapy should be directed at those organisms commonly associated with acute endocarditis, such as *S aureus*, gram-negative bacteria, and enterococci. A combination of nafcillin, penicillin, and gentamicin would be an appropriate combination. Patients with a presumptive diagnosis of prosthetic valve endocarditis (PVE) should also be treated immediately to prevent loss of valve function. Because *S epidermidis* is one of the most common causes of both early and late PVE, therapy must be directed at this organism as well as *S aureus*, streptococci, and gram-negative bacteria. In this setting, a combination of vancomycin, gentamicin, and rifampin is recommended. Vancomycin is preferable to nafcillin in this situation due to the frequent occurrence of nafcillin resistance in *S epidermidis.*[27] Vancomycin and rifampin are usually highly active in vitro against such strains. Presumptive therapy should always be modified based on the results of cultures and sensitivities as they become available.

Antibiotic selection and dosing should be based on the results of in vitro antibiotic susceptibility testing. Quantitative susceptibility testing of the organism should be done with determination of the minimal inhibitory concentration (MIC) and minimal bactericidal concentration (MBC) for all antibiotics which are potentially useful for the involved pathogen. Antibiotic selection should be made from among those agents which best kill the organism at clinically achievable levels.

Occasionally *S aureus* will demonstrate a phenomenon known as tolerance in which the organism will be inhibited but not killed by achievable levels of vancomycin or a beta-lactam antibiotic. Tolerance is defined as an MBC more than 32 times greater than the MIC. Clinical failures have been associated with the use of beta-lactam antibiotics to which *S aureus* is tolerant. However, in other instances the antibiotic has been effective despite in vitro tolerance. The clinical relevance of in vitro tolerance is still controversial. Patients who fail to respond to an antibiotic to which the organism is tolerant should either be given an alternative agent or have a second antibiotic, such as an aminoglycoside or rifampin, added to the beta-lactam antibiotic.

Once therapy has been selected based on initial in vitro susceptibility studies, the adequacy of therapy must be monitored carefully. Repeat blood cultures should be obtained every 48 hours until negative and then weekly until therapy has been completed (and monthly for 2 months after termination of therapy). Persistently positive blood cultures may indicate an inadequate antibiotic regimen or a myocardial or metastatic abscess.

The adequacy of the antibiotic regimen may be determined by measurement of the serum bactericidal titer. This is the highest dilution of the patient's serum that will kill 99.9% of a standard inoculum of the patient's organism. It is commonly accepted that a peak serum bactericidal titer equal to or greater than 1:8 is desirable.[28] However, there has been considerable controversy over the significance of this test; methodologies have often differed and some authors have recommended achieving a trough level of equal to or greater than 1:8.[29] None of 17 studies showed any correlation between serum bactericidal titers of equal to or greater than 1:8 and clinical outcome.[30] However, all studies were too small to exclude false-negative results. Until a definitive study has been carried out, it is prudent to attempt to achieve a peak titer of equal to or greater than 1:8 by adjustment of the antibiotic dose as long as this can be accomplished with nontoxic doses of the antibiotic. Even more controversial is whether the dose of an antibiotic can be safely lowered in the presence of a high serum bactericidal titer. Some authors have suggested that when the serum bactericidal titer is equal to or greater than 1:16, the dose of antibiotic used can be decreased.[31]

In general, the therapy of infective endocarditis in elderly patients does not differ significantly from that in younger patients. The reduced renal function that occurs with aging[32] often necessitates modification of the dosage of antibiotics as well as careful monitoring of their blood levels and close observation for drug toxicity.

Viridans streptococci are usually exquisitely susceptible to penicillin (MIC < 0.2 μg/ml). The optimal therapy of endocarditis due to this organism remains controversial; three separate regimens have been found to be efficacious and each has its own advocates[33] (Table 34-1).

Streptococcus faecalis is not as susceptible to penicillin as are viridans streptococci and needs combination therapy.[34] Penicillin plus streptomycin should be given for four to six weeks when the organism is susceptible to streptomycin (Table 34-1). Recently, 10% to 40% of enterococci have been reported to show high level resistance to streptomycin.[29] Most such strains are susceptible to gentamicin and therefore the combination of penicillin and gentamicin should be employed for four to six weeks if the isolated organism is resistant to streptomycin.[29]

A semisynthetic penicillinase-resistant penicillin should be given for six weeks to patients with *S aureus* endocarditis (Table 34-1). Nafcillin offers advantages over methicillin or oxacillin; the incidence of complications is higher with the latter two drugs (interstitial nephritis from methicillin,[34,35] hepatitis with oxacillin[36]). Furthermore, the dose of nafcillin does not have to be altered in renal failure.[37] In the penicillin-allergic patient, a cephalosporin may be used if the reaction was not of the immediate type; otherwise, vancomycin should be used.

Because of the relative resistance of gram-negative bacteria to antimicrobial agents, gram-negative bacterial endocarditis is often difficult to cure with antibiotic therapy alone. Many patients require valve replacement due to antimicrobial failure. A combination of antibiotics should always be used. One of the broad spectrum penicillins or cephalosporins plus an aminoglycoside should be selected based on in vitro susceptibility testing. In vitro antibiotic synergism studies may be helpful in determining which combination to employ.[29]

Most anaerobic bacteria except *Bacteroides fragilis* are susceptible to penicillin. *B fragilis* endocarditis has been successfully treated with metronidazole[38] which presently is the only agent bactericidal for this organism.

Ampicillin alone has been shown to be effective therapy for *Hemophilus* endocarditis. Although some authors have advocated concomitant treatment with an aminoglycoside, this should be avoided in elderly patients.

Combination therapy should be employed for *S epidermidis* endocarditis of a prosthetic valve. Most isolates are resistant to the penicillins and cephalosporins.[27] Vancomycin should be employed initially until susceptibility studies have been done. If the organism is susceptible, nafcillin may be substituted for the vancomycin. In nafcillin resistance, rifampin should be added to the vancomycin as this drug further increases bactericidal activity. Concomitant use of an aminoglycoside as a third drug is frequently employed; the necessity of its use is currently being evaluated by a multicenter trial.

Corynebacteria (diptheroids) are frequent causes of prosthetic valve endocarditis. The combination of penicillin and gentamicin may be used if the isolate is susceptible to gentamicin. Vancomycin, either alone or with an aminoglycoside, may be used for those isolates resistant to gentamicin and penicillin.[12]

Fungal endocarditis usually occurs in the setting of a prosthetic valve. Anti-infective therapy alone is inadequate and valve replacement should be carried out in all patients.[39,40] Antifungal agents should be used before and after surgery. Ampho-

Table 34-1
Specific Therapy for Infective Endocarditis

Organism	Antibiotic	Duration	Alternative if Penicillin-Allergic
Streptococci			
Viridans streptococci (MIC to Penicillin ≤0.2 μg/ml)	Penicillin G 16 million U/day IV*	4 weeks	Cephalothin 9 g/day *or* vancomycin 1.5 g/day
S pyogenes or *S bovis* or *S pneumoniae*	Penicillin G 16 million U/day IV	4 weeks	Cephalothin 9 g/day *or* vancomycin 1.5 g/day
S faecalis (enterococcus) or other relatively penicillin-resistant *Streptococcus*	Penicillin G 20 million U/day IV + streptomycin† 1 g q 12h IM then 0.5 g q 12h IM	4–6 weeks 2 weeks 2–4 weeks	Desensitize to penicillin or vancomycin 2 g/day + streptomycin† 0.5 q 12h
Staphylococci			
S aureus	Nafcillin 12 g/day IV‡	6 weeks	Vancomycin 2 g/day
S epidermidis	Nafcillin 12 g/day IV *or* vancomycin 2 g/day§ IV + rifampin 900 mg/day‖ PO		Vancomycin 2 g/day + rifampin 900 mg/day
Corynebacteria sp (diptheroids)	Penicillin G 20 million U/day IV + gentamicin sulfate¶ 3 g/kg/day IV or IM	4–6 weeks 4–6 weeks	Vancomycin 2 g/day
Haemophilus sp	Ampicillin 12 g/day IV	4 weeks	Cefamandole 12 g/day
Enterobacteriaceae	Ampicillin (or other broad-spectrum penicillin) or cephalosporin# IV + aminoglycoside**	6 weeks	Cephalosporin# IV + aminoglycoside**
Pseudomonas aeruginosa	Carbenicillin 36 g/day IV (or other anti-pseudomonal penicillin) + aminoglycoside**	6 weeks	Aminoglycoside** alone or desensitize to penicillin
Anaerobic bacteria			
B fragilis	Metronidazole 1 g q 8h IV	4 weeks	—
Others	Penicillin 20 million U/day IV	4 weeks	Cefoxitin or clindamycin

*Streptomycin may be added for the first two weeks if risk of relapse is high (eg, illness greater than three months duration or prosthetic valve).
†Gentamicin 3 mg/kg/day should be substituted if organism is resistant to streptomycin.
‡Penicillin G may be used if organism is susceptible to penicillin. Vancomycin should be used if organism is methicillin-resistant.
§Vancomycin should be used until organism is shown to be susceptible to methicillin as many strains are now methicillin-resistant.
‖Many authorities would add gentamicin 3 mg/kg/day if serum bactericidal level ≤1:8 or if patient does not respond promptly.
¶If organism is resistant to gentamicin, vancomycin should be given alone.
#Choice of broad-spectrum penicillin or cephalosporin to be based on in vitro susceptibility results.
**Choice of aminoglycoside to be based on in vitro susceptibility results. Dose should be maximum recommended dose.
MIC = minimal inhibitory concentration.

tericin B may be given for aspergillus endocarditis; a combination of amphotericin B and 5-fluoro-cytosine should be employed for *Candida* endocarditis.

COMPLICATIONS

Patients with infective endocarditis may develop a number of complications, even while on effective chemotherapy. The most common complications seen in elderly patients are cardiac in nature, ie, congestive heart failure and acute myocardial infarction. Other complications include a high incidence of neurologic complications (cerebral embolic phenomena, toxic encephalopathy, seizures). Renal insufficiency occurs in 10% to 20% of these patients.

Cardiac Complications

Congestive heart failure is the leading cause of death in patients with infective endocarditis. Infective endocarditis of the aortic valve is particularly likely to result in congestive heart failure. Whenever congestive heart failure associated with aortic insufficiency occurs in patients with infective endocarditis, consideration of early valvular replacement must be made. If the congestive heart failure is mild, the patient may be treated medically with digitalis and diuretics and observed carefully. Patients who develop moderate to severe congestive heart failure and do not immediately improve with digitalis and diuretics should have emergency aortic valve replacement.[41] The valvular surgery is crucial; surgery should not be delayed to complete a course of antibiotic therapy but rather should be based solely on the hemodynamic status of the heart. Delaying surgery in patients with severe congestive heart failure due to aortic insufficiency results in a fatal outcome, whereas the success of surgical replacement of an actively infected heart valve has been well demonstrated. Surgery should be followed by a complete course of antibiotics.

Valve ring or myocardial abscess may occur as a result of direct extension of infection from the valve. Most cases are due to virulent organisms such as *S aureus*. This most commonly occurs in infective endocarditis of the aortic valve.

CNS Complications

Major cerebral embolic events have been reported to occur in 17% of all patients with infective endocarditis; no relationship to age has been found.[21] When embolization occurs in an elderly patient, it can be difficult to determine the etiology. Coincidental cerebrovascular disease may be present and cloud the issue. Echocardiography is helpful in detecting large mobile vegetations which are prone to embolize. If cardiac echocardiography demonstrates large mobile valve vegetations following a major embolic event, cardiac surgery with valve replacement must be considered. Anticoagulation is contraindicated in such patients because of the risk of producing a hemorrhagic infarct in the brain.

Mycotic aneurysms of cerebral vessels may occur when septic emboli lodge in the vessels and weaken the arterial wall. This is an uncommon complication of infective endocarditis. When such an aneurysm ruptures, death may occur. Recent experience indicates that such aneurysms may be diagnosed before they rupture. The diagnosis should be suspected in patients with unilateral headache or focal neurologic symptoms. CT scanning may reveal evidence of leakage from a mycotic aneurysm. Arteriography remains the definitive test and should be performed if the CT scan is abnormal or if the patient undergoes unexplained neurologic deterioration.[21]

Embolization from infective endocarditis may produce one of two syndromes. Bland infarcts may occur if the embolus is sterile or if the organism is relatively avirulent. Septic emboli with metastatic infection may result if the organism is highly virulent (such as *S aureus*).

Patients with infective endocarditis due to highly virulent organisms, such as *S aureus*, may develop one or more metastatic abscesses as a result of their bacteremia.

RELAPSE

Relapse of infective endocarditis usually occurs within two months following cessation of antibiotic therapy. When infective endocarditis relapses, the organism should be fully identified and antibiotic susceptibility tests should be carried out to ensure that the episode is truly a relapse and not a reinfection with a different organism.

The first approach to relapsed infective endocarditis should be a thorough search for a metastatic abscess or extension of the infection to the myocardium. Should no suppurative focus of infection be found, the patient may be treated with a repeat full course of antibiotics. Surgery should be considered following the first relapse in instances where the organism is only marginally susceptible to antibiotics (eg, gram-negative bacteria).

MORTALITY

Death in patients with infective endocarditis is usually due to congestive heart failure or complications of embolization. The mortality in elderly patients with infective endocarditis is considerable, ranging from 45% to 70%. The mortality of patients with infective endocarditis has been shown to increase with advancing age.[3]

PROSTHETIC VALVE ENDOCARDITIS

In recent years the safety of valvular replacement in elderly patients has been demonstrated and such surgery is now often carried out in elderly patients. Unfortunately, patients with prosthetic valves are at increased risk of developing infective endocarditis. One study of elderly patients who underwent valve replacement showed that 8 of 320 developed infective endocarditis after a mean follow-up of 30 months.[11] Prosthetic valve endocarditis (PVE) is traditionally divided into early (occurrence within two months of surgery) and late (occurrence more than two months after surgery).[4] Early PVE is often related to intraoperative implantation of organisms or postoperative wound, urinary, pulmonary, or intravenous site infection. The most common causative organisms are *S aureus* and *S epidermidis* which together account for about 50% of cases.[12] Gram-negative bacteria are responsible for about 20% of cases and streptococci, fungi, and diptheroids about 10% each. Late PVE is most commonly caused by streptococci (40%), *S epidermidis* causes about 20%, and gram-negative bacteria about 15% of cases.[12]

The mortality of PVE is considerable; early PVE mortality has been 60% to 80%, late PVE 35% to 60%.[12] The mortality may be higher still in elderly patients. Survival in late PVE is related to the causative organism. Streptococcal PVE carries the best prognosis. New regurgitant murmurs and onset of moderate to severe congestive heart failure are associated with mortality rates of 65% to 85%.

Antibiotic treatment of PVE should be started empirically when the diagnosis is strongly suspected after blood cultures are obtained (as discussed under therapy). Antibiotics should be adjusted when culture and sensitivity studies have been completed. Surgery is often necessary to cure patients with PVE. It has been suggested that valve replacement should be carried out if two out of the following three risk factors are present: nonstreptococcal etiology, moderate to severe congestive heart failure, or presence of a new regurgitant murmur.[41a]

CULTURE-NEGATIVE ENDOCARDITIS

Although positive blood cultures are often considered the sine qua non of infective endocarditis, occasional patients will have negative blood cultures. Fastidious organisms such as *Brucella*, fungi, rickettsiae, *Chlamydia*, pyridoxal requiring streptococci,[42] or cell wall–deficient L-forms[43] may cause infective endocarditis. Prior antibiotic treatment may sterilize the blood. Blood cultures are more often negative in right-sided endocarditis and in uremic patients. With improved bacteriologic technics, culture-negative endocarditis has become less common.

PREVENTION

It is widely accepted that antibiotic prophylaxis may prevent infective endocarditis. Patients with known or suspected cardiac lesions that may predispose them to infective endocarditis should receive prophylaxis whenever they undergo a procedure that may result in bacteremia. The American Heart Association has published guidelines for such antibiotic prophylaxis.[44]

Patients with predisposing cardiac lesions undergoing dental procedures such as cleaning, extractions, or any other procedure that may lead to gingival bleeding should receive prophylaxis directed at viridans streptococci (Table 34-2).

Patients undergoing surgery or instrumentation of the lower GI or genitourinary tract should have prophylaxis directed against enterococcus (Table 34-2). Penicillin plus streptomycin is appropriate. Vancomycin plus streptomycin may be used if the patient is allergic to penicillin. Procedures likely to produce bacteremia include insertion or removal of an indwelling bladder catheter, prostatic surgery, colonic or rectal surgery, and colonoscopy or sigmoidoscopy with biopsy. Barium enemas and sigmoidoscopies without biopsy present a low risk of bacteremia; however, it may be prudent to provide prophylaxis for patients with prosthetic valves undergoing these procedures.

Hospitalized elderly patients with valvular disease are at particular risk of developing infective endocarditis. This risk should be minimized by avoiding indwelling intravascular or bladder catheters if at all possible. Such patients should be treated promptly for any infection they develop

Table 34-2
Prophylaxis for Infective Endocarditis

	Initial Dose	Follow-up
(Patient Undergoing Dental, Oral or Respiratory Procedure)		
	1 h before procedure	
Penicillin G	1 million U IM	
+		
Procaine penicillin G	0.6 million U IM	500 mg q 6h × 8 doses
or		
Penicillin V	2 g PO	
Penicillin allergy		
Erythromycin	1 g PO	500 mg q 6h × 8 doses
or		
Vancomycin	1 g IV	
Patients with prosthetic valves should also receive streptomycin 1 g IM as part of initial regimen 1h before procedure.		
(Patient Undergoing GI or GU Procedure)		
	1 h before procedure	
Penicillin G	2 million U IV or IM	2 million U q 8–12h × 2 doses
or		
Ampicillin	1 g IV or IM	1 g q 8–12h × 2 doses
+		
Streptomycin	1 g IM	1 g q 12h × 2 doses
or		
Gentamicin	1.5 mg/kg IV or IM (but no more than 80 mg)	1.5 mg/kg q 8h × 2 doses
Penicillin allergy		
Vancomycin	1 g IV	1 g IV q 12h × 1 dose
+		
Streptomycin	1 g IM	1 g IM q 12h × 1 dose

which may be associated with bacteremia, such as pneumonia, pyelonephritis, cholecystitis, etc. Patients with infected ulcers due to pressure, ischemia, or diabetes should be given antibiotics prior to débridement of the lesions. The importance of antimicrobial prophylaxis for elderly patients with degenerative heart disease such as a calcified aortic valve or calcified mitral annulus cannot be overemphasized. Physicians caring for elderly patients should thoroughly familiarize themselves with guidelines for prophylaxis. It remains the physician's responsibility to ensure that such prophylaxis is always carried out.

REFERENCES

1. Cherubin CC, Neu HC: Infective endocarditis at the Presbyterian Hospital in New York City from 1938-1967. *Am J Med* 1971;51:83–96.
2. Pomerance A: Cardiac pathology in the elderly. *Cardiovasc Clin* 1981;12:9–54.
3. Pearce ML, Guze LB: Some factors affecting prognosis in bacterial endocarditis. *Ann Intern Med* 1961;55:270–282.
4. Kaye D: Definitions and demographic characteristics, in Kaye D (ed): *Infective Endocarditis.* Baltimore, University Park Press, 1976, pp 1–10.
5. Wilson LM: Etiology of bacterial endocarditis. *Ann Intern Med* 1963;58:946–952.
6. Durack OT, Petersdorf RG: Changes in the epidemiology of endocarditis, in Raplam EL, Taronta AV (eds): *Infective Endocarditis—An American Heart Association Symposium.* Dallas, American Heart Association, 1977, pp 3–8.

6a. Robbins N, Demaria A, Miller MH: Infective endocarditis in the elderly. *South Med J* 1980;73: 1335–1338.

6b. Mabte-Gabr E, January LE, Smith IM: Bacterial endocarditis: The need for early diagnosis. *Geriatrics* 1973;28:164–170.

7. Fulkerson PR, Beaver BM, Aueseun JC, Graber HL: Calcification of the mitral annulus. *Am J Med* 1979;66:967–976.

7a. Watunakunakorn C, Tan JS: Diagnostic difficulties of staphylococcal endocarditis in geriatric patients. *Geriatrics* 1973;28:168–173.

8. Burnside JW, Desanctis RW: Bacterial endocarditis on calcification of the mitral annulus fibrosus. *Ann Intern Med* 1972;76:615–618.
9. McCallum OG, Grow J: Mural thrombus endocarditis complicating an acute myocardial infarction: Report of a case. *Arch Intern Med* 1981;141:527–528.
10. Clemens JD, Horwitz RI, Jaffe CC, et al: A controlled evaluation of the risk of endocarditis in persons with mitral valve prolapse. *N Engl J Med* 1982;307:776–782.
11. Jamieson WRE, Dooner J, Numro AI, et al: Cardiac valve replacement in the elderly in a review of 320 consecutive cases. *Circulation* 1981;64:177–183.
12. Wilson WR, Danielson GR, Giuliani ER, et al: Prosthetic valve endocarditis. *Mayo Clin Proc* 1982; 57:155–161.
13. Cohen PS, Maguire JH, Weinstein L: Infective endocarditis caused by gram negative bacteria: A review of the literature 1945–1977. *Prog Cardiovasc Dis* 1980;22:205–242.
14. Murray BE, Karchmer AW, Moellering RC: Diptheroid prosthetic valve endocarditis. A study of clinical features and infecting organisms. *Am J Med* 1980;69:838–848.
15. Varma MSS, Adgey AAJ, Connolly JH: Chronic Q fever endocarditis. *Br Heart J* 1980;43:695–699.
16. Rubinstein E, Noriega ER, Simberkoff MS, et al: Fungal endocarditis: An analysis of 24 cases and review of the literature. *Medicine* 1975;54:331–344.
17. Weinstein L, Schlesinger JJ: Pathoanatomic, pathophysiologic and clinical correlation in endocarditis. *N Engl J Med* 1974;291:832–837;1122–1126.
18. Durack OT, Beeson PB: Pathogenesis of infective endocarditis, in Rahimtoola SH (ed): *Infective Endocarditis.* New York, Grune & Stratton, 1978, pp 1–53.
19. Musher DM, McKenzie SD: Infections due to *Staphylococcus aureus. Medicine* 1977;56:383–409.
20. Churchill MA, Geraci JE, Hunder GG: Musculoskeletal manifestations of bacterial endocarditis. *Ann Intern Med* 1977;87:754–759.
21. Pruitt AA, Rubin RH, Karchmer AW, et al: Neurologic complications of bacterial endocarditis. *Medicine* 1978;57:329–343.
22. Messner RP, Laxdal T, Quie PG, et al: Rheumatoid factors in subacute bacterial endocarditis—Bacteremia, duration of disease or genetic predisposition. *Ann Intern Med* 1968;68:746–754.
23. Cabane J, Godeau P, Herreman G, et al: Fate of circulating immune complexes in infective endocarditis. *Am J Med* 1979;66:277–282.
24. Bayer AS, Therfilopoulos AN, Eisenberg R, et al: Circulating immune complexes in infective endocarditis. *N Engl J Med* 1976;295:1500–1505.
25. Melvin ET, Berger M, Lutzker LG, et al: Noninvasive methods for detection of valve vegetations in infective endocarditis. *Am J Cardiol* 1981;47:271–278.
26. Werner AS, Cobbs CG, Kaye D, et al: Studies on the bacteremia of bacterial endocarditis. *JAMA* 1967;202:199–203.
27. Karchmer AW, Dismukes WE, Johnson WD, et al: *Staphylococcus epidermidis* prosthetic valve endocarditis, in Nelson JD, Brassi C (eds): *Current Chemotherapy and Infectious Disease.* Washington, DC, American Society for Microbiology, 1980 vol 2, pp 904–906.
28. Mandell GL, Sande MA: Some newer aspects of infective endocarditis. *Geriatrics* 1975;30:97–102.
29. Sande MA, Scheld M: Combination antibiotic therapy of bacterial endocarditis. *Ann Intern Med* 1980; 92:390–395.
30. Coleman DL, Horwitz RI, Andriole VT: Association between serum inhibitory and bactericidal concentrations and therapeutic outcome in bacterial endocarditis. *Am J Med* 1982;73:260–267.
31. Scheld WM, Sande MA: Endocarditis and intravascular infections, in Mandell GL, Douglas RG, Bennett JE (eds): *Principles and Practice of Infectious Disease.* New York, John Wiley and Sons Inc, 1979, pp 653–690.
32. Ouslander JG: Drug therapy in the elderly. *Ann Intern Med* 1981;95:711–722.
33. Bisno AL, Dismukes WE, Durack DT, et al: Treatment of infective endocarditis due to viridans streptococci: AHA Committee Report. *Circulation* 1981;63:730A–733A.
34. Sande MA: Antimicrobial therapy for two serious bacterial infections: Enterococcal endocarditis and nosocomial pneumonia. *Arch Intern Med* 1982; 142:2033–2034.
35. Galpin JE, Shinaberger JH, Stanley TM, et al: Acute interstitial nephritis due to methicillin. *Am J Med* 1978;65:756–765.
36. Onorato IM, Axelrod JL: Hepatitis from intravenous high dose oxicillin therapy—Findings in an adult inpatient population. *Ann Intern Med* 1978;89:497–500.
37. Diaz CR, Kane JG, Parker RH, et al: Pharmacokinetics of nafcillin in patients with renal failure. *Antimicrob Agents Chemother* 1977;12:98–101.
38. Galgiani JN, Busch DF, Brass C, et al: *Bacteroides fragilis* endocarditis, bacteremia and other infections treated with oral or intravenous metronidazole. *Am J Med* 1978;65:284–289.
39. McLeod R, Remington JS: Fungal endocarditis, in Rahimtoola SH (ed): *Infective Endocarditis.* New York, Grune & Stratton, 1978, pp 211–290.
40. Kammer RB, Utz JP: Aspergillus species endocarditis—The new face of a not so rare disease. *Am J Med* 1974;56:506–521.
41. Griffin FM, Jones G, Cobbs CG: Aortic insufficiency in bacterial endocarditis. *Ann Intern Med* 1972;76:23–28.
41a. Karchmer AW, Dismukes WE, Buckley M, et al: Late prosthetic valve endocarditis: Clinical features influencing therapy. *Am J Med* 1978;64:199–206.
42. Roberts RB, Krieger AG, Schiller NL, Gross KC: Viridans streptococcal endocarditis: The role of various species, including pyridoxal-dependent streptococci. *Rev Infect Dis* 1979;1:955–966.
43. Neu HC, Goldreyer B: Isolation of protoplasts in a case of enterococcal endocarditis. *Am J Med* 1968; 45:784–788.
44. Kaplan EL, Anthony, BF, Bisno A, et al: Prevention of bacterial endocarditis: American Heart Association Committee Report. *Circulation* 1977; 56:139A–143A.

CHAPTER 35

Prognosis of Coronary Heart Disease in the Elderly Patient: The CASS Experience

Michael B. Mock
Lloyd D. Fisher
Bernard J. Gersh
Richard A. Kronmal
Robert L. Frye
David Fray
Thomas Killip III
and participants in the Coronary Artery Surgery Study (CASS)

Cardiovascular disease, coronary artery disease in particular, is the most common cause of death in persons 65 years of age or older in the United States.[1] The older patient with ischemic heart disease may present with angina or myocardial infarction or, less frequently, with congestive heart failure.

The clinician has available many diagnostic technics for confirming the clinical diagnosis of coronary artery disease. Today, the older patient is more commonly considered for a bypass operation, with a resultant increase in use of coronary arteriography.[2]

The Coronary Artery Surgery Study (CASS) (see Appendix) registry contains 24,959 patients who were admitted to one of the 15 cooperating centers because of suspected or proven coronary artery disease.[3] From August 1975 through May 1979, 20,088 registry patients who had not undergone previous cardiac operation were enrolled.

Coronary angiography was performed on all of the patients by either the brachial or the femoral technic. Ventriculography was performed in at least one view. The criterion for determining the extent of clinically significant one-, two-, or three-vessel coronary artery disease was based on reduction of 70% or more in the internal diameter of the major coronary arteries. For the left main coronary artery, reduction of 50% or more was considered significant. The ejection fraction was calculated from the left ventricular angiogram.

The survival of the medically treated patients in the CASS registry has been reported.[4] This chapter compares the natural history of the older patients in the CASS registry with that of the patients in the registry younger than age 65. The registry included 2186 patients who were 65 years of age or older and had been treated medically. The age distribution of the medically treated patients at the time of angiography is shown in Figure 35-1.

For the individual patients in the CASS registry, the decision for surgical or medical therapy was made by the responsible treating physicians. Eighty-five percent of the older patients in the study had at least one operable vessel. Patients who were chosen for surgical therapy were regarded as initially being medically treated. Many patients who were initially treated medically subsequently underwent coronary artery bypass graft operation for increasing severity of symptoms. These patients were withdrawn from further analysis at the time of operation. The survival curves were calculated by the life-table method

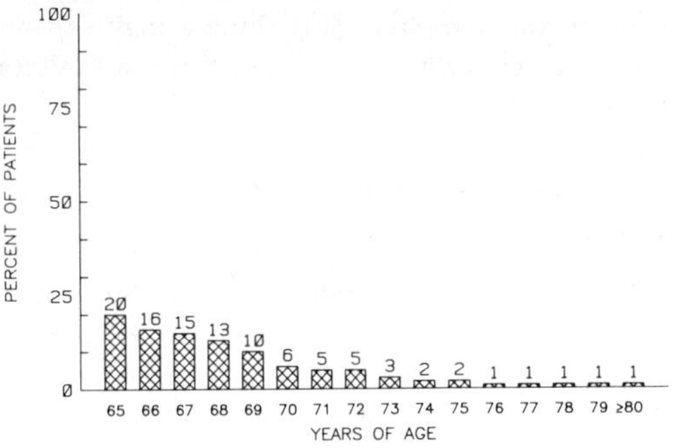

Figure 35-1 Age distributions of the 2186 patients from age 65 to 80 or more years. Each bar represents a yearly increment, except for bar representing patients aged 80 years or more.

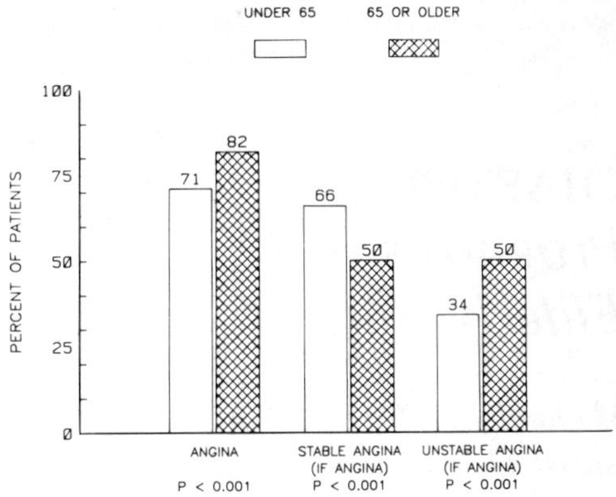

Figure 35-2 Percentage of patients in each age group who presented with angina. These patients were subdivided into those who had stable or unstable angina.

and were compared by log-rank statistics. Long-term follow-up of patients in the CASS registry is excellent—the vital status of 99% of the patients is known.

This chapter compares the symptoms, the anatomic extent of obstructive coronary artery disease, the left ventricular function, and the survival of medically treated patients aged 65 years or older with those of patients younger than age 65.

CLINICAL PRESENTATION AND BASELINE CHARACTERISTICS

Angina was the presenting symptom in more of the older patients (82% of patients 65 or older vs 71% of patients younger than 65). Half of the patients aged 65 years or older and about one third of patients younger than age 65 presented with unstable angina (Figure 35-2).

The elderly patients infrequently presented with atypical chest pain (only 8% of patients aged 65 years or older vs 16% of patients younger than age 65, $P < 0.001$).

The incidences of prior myocardial infarction were similar in older and younger patients. Figure 35-3 shows the incidences of prior myocardial infarction established by history and by ECG evidence (as determined by the Central Electrocardiographic Laboratory) for all patients.

Fewer of the older patients were current smokers, and more of the older patients had never been smokers (Figure 35-4). More of the older patients had hypertension and diabetes, but significant elevation of cholesterol was comparable in both groups (Figure 35-5).

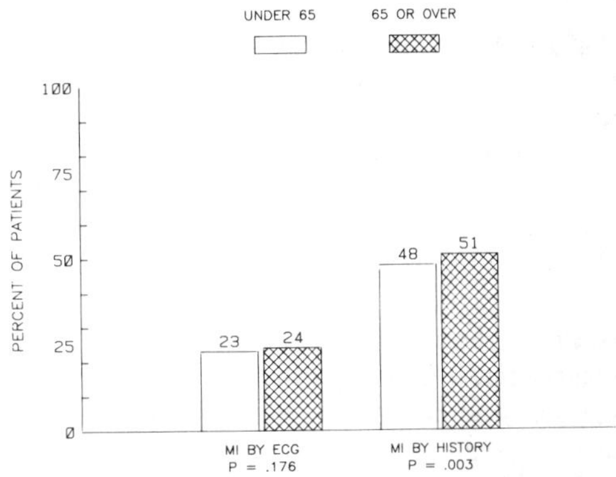

Figure 35-3 Percentage of patients in each age group with prior myocardial infarction, determined by ECG criteria (measured at Central Electrocardiographic Laboratory) and by medical history. MI = myocardial infarction.

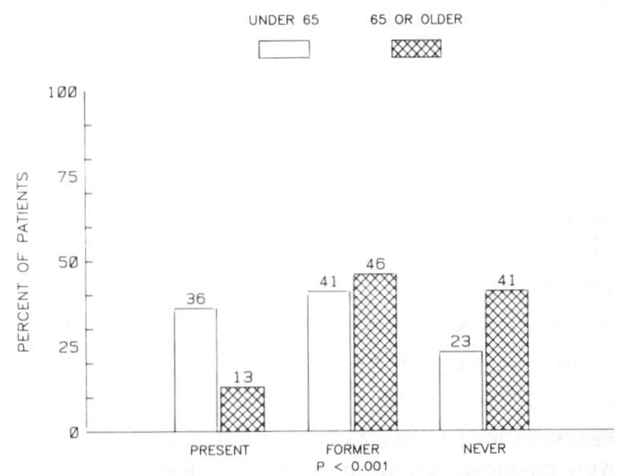

Figure 35-4 Percentage of patients in each age group who were present smokers, former smokers, or had never smoked.

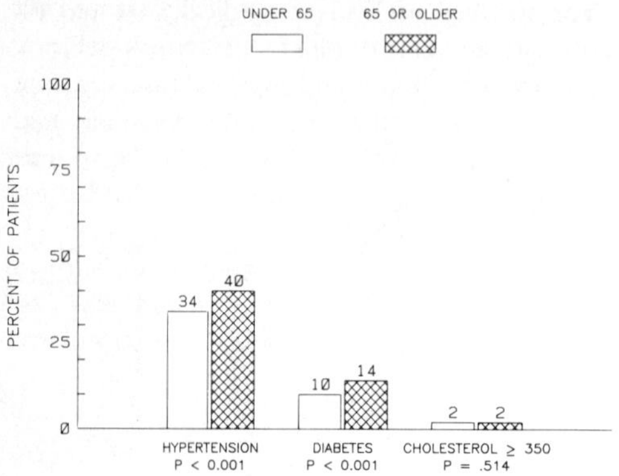

Figure 35-5 Percentage of patients in each age group who presented with hypertension, diabetes, and hypercholesterolemia.

ANGIOGRAPHIC FINDINGS

The older patients had evidence of more extensive disease on coronary angiography than did patients younger than age 65. Left main coronary artery disease occurred more frequently in the older patients (14% vs 7%, $P < 0.001$), and they had a statistically significant excess of three-vessel disease. Figure 35-6 shows the extent of coronary occlusive disease based on at least 70% luminal occlusion.

Figure 35-7 compares the ejection fraction in patients younger than age 65 with that of patients aged 65 years or older in the categories 0% to 35%, 36% to 49%, and 50% to 100%. The older patients had more impairment of left ventricular function more frequently (determined by left ventricular angiography). This finding may explain the increased frequency of congestive heart failure (Figure 35-8).

SURVIVAL OF MEDICALLY TREATED PATIENTS

In both groups, mortality of medically treated patients increased as the extent of obstructive disease increased. The comparative survival of patients younger than age 65 and aged 65 years or older is shown in Figure 35-9. As would be expected, there was a higher risk of death in the older patients. Although there was an increased risk of death in both groups with more extensive coronary disease, the gradient between the two groups also increased when coronary obstructive disease affected three vessels.

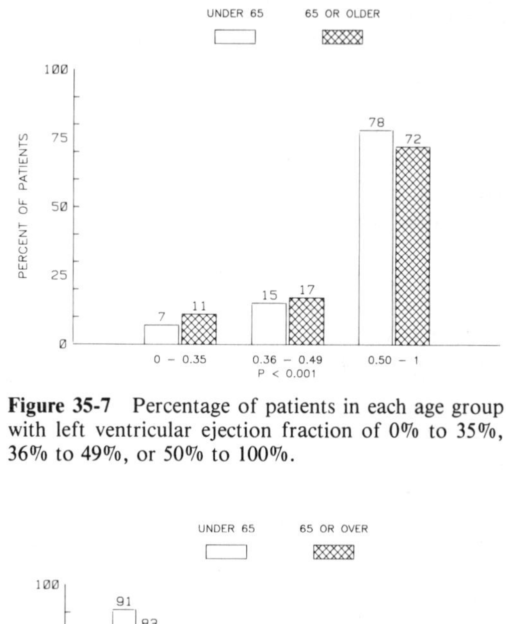

Figure 35-7 Percentage of patients in each age group with left ventricular ejection fraction of 0% to 35%, 36% to 49%, or 50% to 100%.

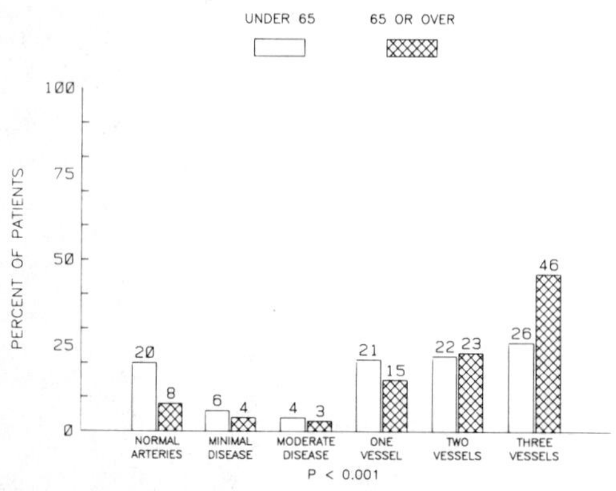

Figure 35-6 Percentage of patients in each age group with angiographic determination of normal coronary arteries, minimally diseased coronary arteries (≤30% obstruction), moderate coronary obstructive disease (>30% to 50% obstruction), and one-, two-, or three-vessel disease based on ≥70% obstruction.

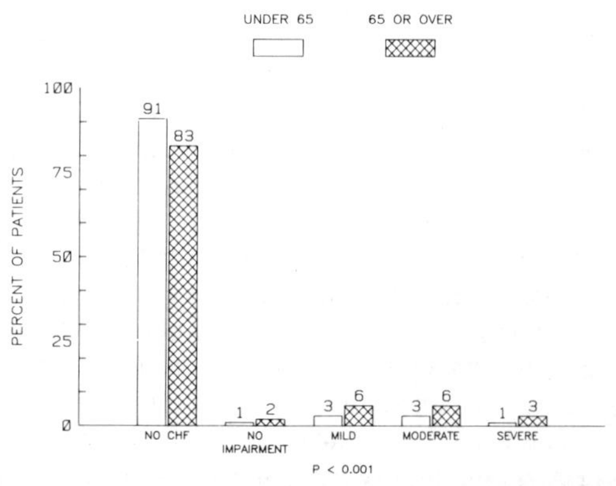

Figure 35-8 Percentage of patients in each age group who presented without symptoms of congestive heart failure. Percentages of patients who presented with clinical history of congestive heart failure and had no impairment or mild, moderate, or severe impairment are also presented.

The six-year survival of medically treated patients aged 65 years or older with zero-vessel (normal coronary arteries and minimal disease), one-vessel, or two-vessel disease was surprisingly high (86%, 76%, and 69%, respectively). The six-year survival of patients with three-vessel disease was considerably less (40%).

The correlation between cumulative survival and left ventricular ejection fraction was also significant. Figure 35-10 compares the cumulative

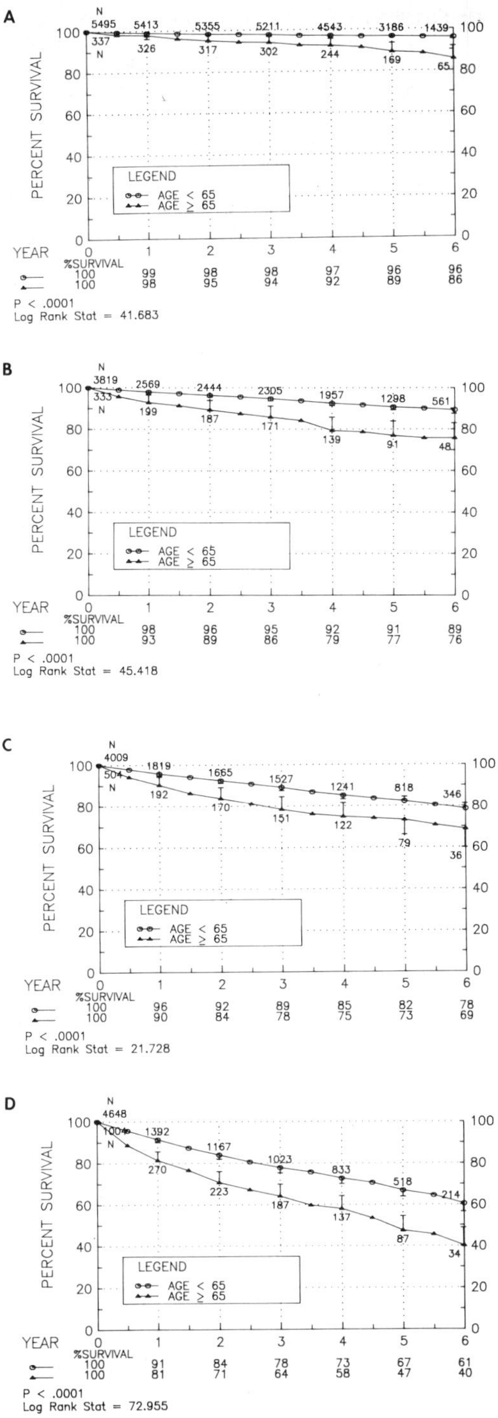

Figure 35-9 Six-year survival data for patients in each age group with zero-, one-, two-, or three-vessel coronary obstructive disease. **A**, Zero-vessel disease (normal coronary arteries and <70% obstruction). **B**, One-vessel disease (≥70% obstruction). **C**, Two-vessel disease (≥70% obstruction). **D**, Three-vessel disease (≥70 obstruction).

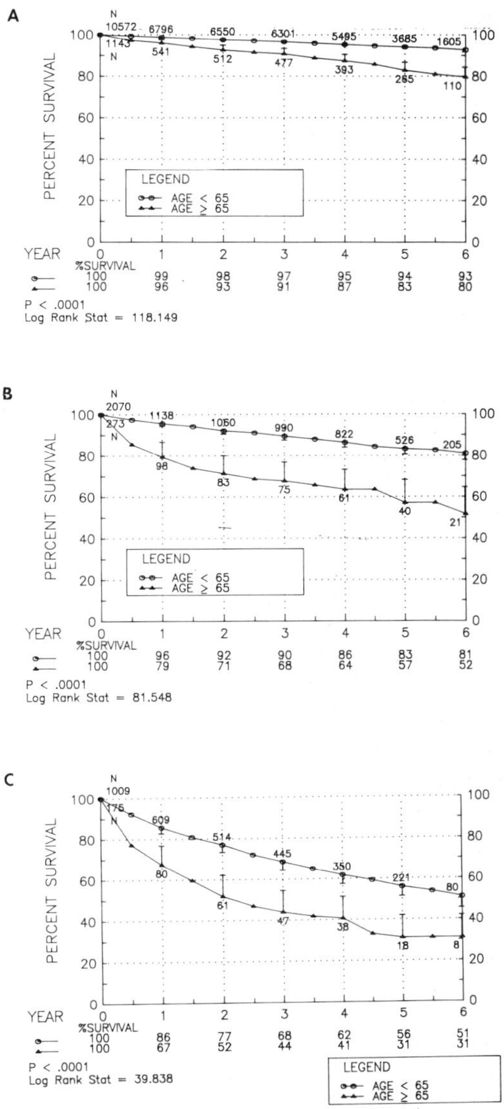

Figure 35-10 Six-year survival data for patients in each age group based on ejection fraction. **A**, Left ventricular ejection fraction of ≥50%. **B**, Left ventricular ejection of 36% to 49%. **C**, Left ventricular ejection fraction of ≤35%.

survival of patients younger than age 65 with that of patients 65 years of age or older; the patients were divided into three groups based on the global left ventricular ejection fraction (≥50%, 36% to 49%, and ≤35%).

SUMMARY

The older patients with coronary artery disease presented less frequently with atypical chest pain and more frequently with angina. The older patient with acute myocardial infarction often has atypical chest pain or no chest pain.[5]

The older patients in the CASS registry presented with a higher incidence of more severe and unstable angina than the group of patients younger than age 65; they also had a higher incidence of associated medical diseases such as hypertension and diabetes, which increase the risk of ischemic heart disease. Surprisingly, significant elevation of serum cholesterol was comparable in the two groups. Fewer of the older patients were current smokers, and more of the older patients had never smoked. These risk factors have been chiefly associated with premature atherosclerosis in younger patients, but relationships to coronary artery disease in the elderly are less well established.[6,7]

On coronary angiography, the older patients had more extensive obstructive coronary disease—statistically higher levels of both left main coronary artery disease and three-vessel disease—than those patients younger than age 65. The older patients also had poorer left ventricular function and were more likely to present with symptoms of congestive heart failure than the younger patients. Although both anatomical extent of disease and ventricular function have an important impact on subsequent survival, ventricular function is the principal determinant of long-term survival.

The large number of patients in the registry 65 years of age or older with arteriographically documented coronary anatomy is an excellent group in which to evaluate the "natural history" of medically treated older patients. The long-term survival of the subgroups within this study provides useful information for the physician who is pondering therapeutic options for the older patient. Coronary artery bypass graft operation in the elderly patient is considered elsewhere in this monograph. The alternative, a less invasive revascularization procedure (percutaneous transluminal coronary angioplasty), is also considered in a separate chapter.

REFERENCES

1. US President's Commission on Heart Disease, Cancer and Stroke: Report to the President; A national program to conquer heart disease, cancer and stroke. Washington, DC, 1964.
2. Gersh BJ, Kronmal RA, Frye RL, et al: Coronary arteriography and coronary artery bypass surgery: Morbidity and mortality in patients ages 65 years or older; A report from the Coronary Artery Surgery Study. *Circulation* 1983;67:483–491.
3. The Principal Investigators of CASS and their Associates: The National Heart, Lung, and Blood Institute Coronary Artery Surgery Study (CASS). *Circulation* 1981;63(suppl 1):1–81.
4. Mock MB, Ringqvist I, Fisher LD, et al: Survival of medically treated patients in the Coronary Artery Surgery Study (CASS) registry. *Circulation* 1982; 66:562–568.
5. Williams BO, Begg TB, Semple T, et al: The elderly in a coronary unit. *Br Med J* 1976;2:451–453.
6. Kannel WB, Gordon T: Evaluation of cardiovascular risk in the elderly: The Framingham Study. *Bull NY Acad Med* 1978;54:573–591.
7. Vlietstra RE, Kronmal RA, Seth AK, et al: Correlation of risk factors for coronary artery disease with coronary angiographic findings. *Kardiologiia* 1982;22:67–72.

APPENDIX

Participants in the Coronary Artery Surgery Study

1. University of Alabama in Birmingham: William J. Rogers, MD,* Richard O. Russell, Jr, MD, Albert Oberman, MD, and Nicholas T. Kouchoukos, MD

2. Albany Medical College: Eric D. Foster, MD,* Julio A. Sosa, MD,* Joseph T. Doyle, MD, Martin F. McKneally, MD, Joseph B. McIlduff, MD, Harry Odabashian, MD, and Thomas M. Older, MD

3. Boston University: Thomas Ryan, MD,* David Faxon, MD, Laura Wexler, MD, Robert L. Berger, MD, Donald Weiner, MD, and Carolyn H. McCabe, BS

4. Loma Linda University: Melvin P. Judkins, MD,* and Joan Coggin, MD*

5. Marshfield Medical Foundation, Inc, and Marshfield Clinic: William Myers, MD,* Richard D. Sautter, MD,* John N. Browell, MD, Dieter M. Voss, MD, and Robert D. Carlson, MD

6. Massachusetts General Hospital: J. Warren Harthorne, MD,* W. Gerald Austen, MD,* Robert Dinsmore, MD, Frederick Levine, MD, and John McDermott, MD

*Denotes principal investigator.

7. Mayo Clinic and Mayo Foundation: Robert L. Frye, MD,* Bernard Gersh, MD, David R. Holmes, MD, Michael B. Mock, MD, Hartzell Schaff, MD, and Ronald E. Vlietstra, MD

8. Miami Heart Institute: Arthur J. Gosselin, MD,* Parry B. Larsen, MD, and Paul Swaye, MD

9. Montreal Heart Institute: Martial G. Bourassa, MD,* Bernard R. Chaitman, MD, Claude Goulet, MD, and Jacques Lesperance, MD

10. New York University: Ephraim Glassman, MD,* and Michael Schloss, MD

11. St. Louis University: George Kaiser, MD,* J. Gerard Mudd, MD,* Robert D. Wiens, MD, Hendrick B. Barner, MD, John E. Codd, MD, Denis H. Tyras, MD, and Vallee L. Willman, MD

12. St. Luke's Hospital Center: Harvey G. Kemp, Jr, MD,* and Airlie Cameron, MD

13. Stanford University: Edwin Alderman, MD,* Francis H. Koch, MD, Paul R. Cipriano, MD, James F. Silverman, MD, and Edward B. Stinson, MD

14. Medical College of Wisconsin: Felix Tristani, MD,* Harold L. Brooks, MD,* and Robert J. Flemma, MD

15. Yale University: Lawrence S. Cohen, MD,* Rene Langou, MD, Alexander S. Geha, MD, Graeme L. Hammond, MD, and Richard K. Shaw, MD

Central Electrocardiographic Laboratory, University of Alabama: L. Thomas Sheffield, MD,* David Roitman, MD, and Carol Troxell, BS

Coordinating Center, University of Washington: Lloyd Fisher, PhD,* Mary Jo Gillespie, MS, Kathryn Davis, PhD, J. Ward Kennedy, MD, and Richard Kronmal, PhD

National Heart, Lung, and Blood Institute: Eugene R. Passamani, MD, Peter L. Frommer, MD, Suzanne Mullin, RN, MPH, Kent Bailey, PhD, and David DeMets, PhD

Chairman of Steering Committee: Thomas Killip, MD, Henry Ford Hospital

*Denotes principal investigator.

CHAPTER 36
Resting Electrocardiograms and Subsequent Mortality

Kevin Cullen
N. S. Stenhouse

The use of the electrocardiogram (ECG) as a routine screening measure has long been common practice in hospitals and private consulting rooms. Many abnormalities occur in people who are symptom-free and have no other clinical evidence of heart disease. It has been apparent that the prognosis of individual or isolated ECG changes are best measured prospectively in unbiased population samples. By this, we compare the risk of death for a given abnormality with a matched sample that is free of the abnormality. As there have been relatively few longitudinal population studies, a good deal of useful inferences have been made from observations in selected populations. These include hospitals, younger age groups of civil servants, defense forces, or company employees. For this chapter, the selection of the literature has reflected a preference for studies on samples containing diseased and control groups, particularly from the general population. In many instances, the number of cases has been quoted to indicate the scarcity of the accumulated evidence. The larger numbers in many hospital-based series have been omitted in view of the known bias involved in such patients. Comment will be mainly concerned with the evidence on ECG changes found in the resting ECGs of people over 40 years of age. Preference has been given to studies making correction for the effect of age by stating age-specific mortality ratios. Mortality ratios represent the mortality from cardiovascular disease (CVD) associated with the specific ECG divided by the mortality from a population with normal ECGs.

ABNORMALITIES IN RESTING ECGs COEXISTING WITH ADDITIONAL ECG ABNORMALITIES

The prognosis of any ECG abnormality depends on whether or not there are coexisting ECG abnormalities or other clinical evidence of heart disease. ECG abnormalities have a better prognosis occurring in isolation, than when observed in conjunction with one or more additional ECG changes. It is a frequent clinical situation for an abnormality to occur in conjunction with one or more ECG codes. For example, Table 36-1 outlines the risk ratios of significance for the ECG abnormalities in the Busselton study. These were found by Cullen et al[1] to have an increased 13-year mortality compared with the remainder of an age-adjusted population without the ECG abnormality. These included Q and QS patterns, left axis deviation, ST depression, T wave depression, flat or biphasic T waves, atrial fibrillation or flutter, and ventricular extrasystoles. Elsewhere in this chapter, left and right bundle-branch block and intraventricular conduction defects coexisting with other ECG abnormalities in the heart, have also been reported to have significant increased risk of death. The remainder of this chapter will be concerned with assessing the prognosis of ECG abnormalities found.

ISOLATED ABNORMALITIES OF THE ECG AND MORTALITY

Q-QS Waves

Large abnormal Q waves occurring as an isolated finding in symptom-free men have been

Table 36-1
Risk Ratios of Significance for ECG Abnormalities in Busselton Study

	All Subjects				
	No. of Age Contributing Groups	*Total No. of Subjects*	*No. of Deaths*	*Mortality Ratio*	*Statistical Significance*
Q and QS patterns	7	58	29	3.82	7.60†
Left axis deviation > −30°	8	119	32	1.64	2.46*
ST segment depression 1 mm or more	3	20	15	3.82	5.53†
ST 0.5 to 1 mm horizontal or downward	5	37	18	2.81	4.69†
ST downward by 0.5 mm	6	51	26	2.81	5.14†
T wave negative 1-5 mm	6	79	53	4.5	11.07†
T wave flat or biphasic < 1 mm	7	69	31	3.3	6.64†
Ventricular extrasystoles > 10%	2	10	4	2.8	2.29†
Atrial fibrillation or flutter	1	5	4	2.4	2.04*
Ventricular extrasystoles infrequent	8	84	25	2.2	3.93†
All ventricular extrasystoles	8	106	35	2.6	5.62†

*$P < 0.05$, †$P < 0.001$.
Thirteen-year cardiovascular mortality in 2119 subjects for specific ECG codes were compared with a population with normal ECGs each standardized in five-year age groups for the Busselton population aged 40 to 79 years.

reported by Rose et al,[2] in 18,403 British male civil servants of 40 to 64 years of age to have had a five-year age-adjusted mortality ratio of 27.9:1. They found a risk ratio of 4.1:1 for medium-sized Q waves and a ratio of 2.1:1 for small Q waves. By comparison, Caird et al[3] studied, during a three-year period, 2254 people aged 65 years and over living at home, and found a mortality risk ratio of 1.8:1 for all types of Q waves. Blackburn et al[4] reported a slight (but nonsignificant) increase in coronary heart disease (CHD) events in those with minor Q waves, among 12,770 men aged 40 to 59 years over a five-year period. In summary, the literature on isolated Q waves indicates that risk ratios were raised for large and moderate-sized Q waves, but were not significantly increased for small Q waves.

Left Ventricular Hypertrophy

In Framingham study subjects, Kannel et al[5] have described increased cardiovascular disease (CVD) mortality in those with left ventricular hypertrophy (LVH), compared with the population at large. In the 13-year Busselton results, 29 symptom-free persons with isolated LVH were observed, of whom 3 (10.3%) died of CVD causes—a mortality ratio of 0.67 (ie, below 1.0). Where LVH was combined with one or more ECG codes, the CVD mortality ratio rose to 2.0:1 (21 deaths in 68 subjects, 31%, compared with a death rate of 15.3% in subjects without LVH). The CVD mortality ratio for all types of Busselton's LVH was 1.6 (ns). During this 13-year period of 1967–1979, blood pressures in 68% of the Busselton study's hypertensives had their average diastolic pressures lowered by treatment to below 95 mmHg.[6] As the early period of the Framingham study occurred before many subsequent advances in antihypertensive drugs, the current therapies for hypertensives could be improving the previous prognosis of LVH. No other reports have recently been available on the prognosis of LVH.

ST Segment Depression

ST depression in symptom-free subjects showed no significant increase in risk in the study by Rose et al,[2] but the risks were markedly increased in the presence of a history of angina/myocardial infarction where they found a ratio of 9.0:1. Medalie et al[7] showed no increase in risk ratio over five years in 963 affected subjects with ST depression. In the elderly subjects of Caird et al,[3] the mortality ratio for isolated major ST patterns was 1.4:1, and for minor ST changes the ratio was 2.2:1. In unselected Busselton subjects[1] the risk ratios for major ST depression found with other ECG codes was 3.8:1, but the risk ratios became insignificant in those with isolated ST depression, without previous angina, or myocardial infarction. Despite the lack of risk in these reports, it should be borne in mind that Froelicher et al[8] revealed significant coronary heart disease in 60% of airmen with abnormal ST depression in their resting ECGs.

T Wave Changes

In the subjects of Rose et al[3] with isolated T wave inversion, the mortality ratios were 2.7:1 for intermediate T wave inversion, and 2.5:1 for minor inversion/flattened T waves. For all cases with T wave inversion (ie, not found in isolation), the mortality ratios were 7.4:1 for intermediate T wave inversion and 3.0:1 for minor inversion. Blackburn et al[4] reported no increase in risk for negative T waves independent of ST depression. In unselected Busselton subjects,[1] T wave inversion showed a risk ratio of 4.5:1, flat or biphasic T waves had a ratio of 3.3:1, but isolated T wave changes in symptom-free people showed no significant increase in risk. Higgins et al[9] reported from the Framingham study that there were no significant risks for isolated minor T wave inversion or flattened T waves.

AV CONDUCTION DEFECTS

Sino-Atrial Block

Concerning severe bradycardia, there has been no information published on the prognosis of this disturbance.

First-Degree AV Block

Blackburn et al[4] showed that there was a significant increase in the 5-year incidence of new CHD events in 12,770 male workers with first-degree AV block compared with carefully matched controls (risk ratio of 1.8:1). There were no significant increases in mortality. In the remaining literature, neither Packard et al,[10] Rose et al,[2] nor Cullen et al[1] reported on a sufficient number of cases to draw any conclusions about first-degree AV block. At present, it is fair to assume that first degree AV block in otherwise normal people appears to involve no increase in mortality ratios.

Second-Degree AV Block

There have been some follow-up studies on Mobitz type 1 AV block (Wenckebach block). Amat-Y-Leon et al[11] noted no cardiac deaths over three years in 15 people with Mobitz 1 block who were otherwise clinically normal. Zepilli et al[12] found a benign prognosis in top-ranking athletes, provided the AV block improved with sympathetic maneuvers and disappeared after cessation of training. In two cases reported by Cullen and Collin,[13] the Mobitz 1 AV block disappeared in a few weeks with cessation of exercise. Both subjects are alive 20 years later, the AV block reappearing and persisting with the resumption of exercise in one of the subjects. The prognosis of second-degree AV nodal block type 1 (proximal to the band of His) in 56 patients was studied by Strasberg et al[14] over a mean period of 3.82 years. In the prospective observation of 19 of these subjects who had no other evidence of organic heart disease, one patient required pacing because of a brady arrhythmia, and a further two died—neither suddenly. In the remaining 37 patients with other evidence of organic heart disease the prognosis was good although 12 died of CVD causes and four died from noncardiac causes. All 56 patients had type 1 second-degree block and five of them had additional episodes of 2:1 heart block.

Mobitz type 11 AV block is a rare phenomenon in normal subjects. Although it has not been the subject of long-term follow-up, experienced cardiologists (particularly A.R. Gilchrist of Edinburgh) would probably agree with the conclusion that Mobitz 11 AV block should be viewed as having similar prognosis to that of either bifascicular block or third-degree AV block.

Third-Degree AV Block

AV block associated with coronary heart disease (CHD) requires careful assessment of the need for a pacemaker. In the absence of overt CHD, the available literature on third-degree AV block in otherwise normal people contains relatively few subjects. Hatle et al[15] followed 10 people for five years and no deaths were observed. Reid et al[16] reported on 35 people aged 12 days to 35 years with congenital complete AV block. Permanent pacing was eventually required in 21 of the patients. In their views, most congenital AV blocks will require pacing before their 50th birthday, thus necessitating long-term supervision. Other contemporary data on third-degree AV block has been provided by Ginks et al[17] who described the prognosis of 839 patients who had required pacing for chronic complete AV block over a 14-year period. Using standard mortality tables, the expected mortality was 170 deaths and the observed number of deaths was 288—a mortality ratio of 1.7:1. Of particular interst was the very high mortality ratio of 4.5:1 for the 90 patients in the age group 50 to 59 years. Those people between 80 and 89 years of age with AV block had an average survival rate comparable to those in the same age group without AV heart block.

Wolff-Parkinson-White Syndrome (Pre-Excitation Syndrome)

The presence of the Wolff-Parkinson-White syndrome (WPW) predisposes about 12% of the individuals with WPW to various arrhythmias, particularly paroxysmal supraventricular tachycardia (PAT), paroxysmal atrial fibrillation (PAF), atrial flutter (AF), and/or ventricular fibrillation (VF). Concerning the mortality of WPW, no increase in death rates were observed by White and Donovan.[18] Flensted-Jensen[19] followed 47 people with WPW over a 29-year period and found a mortality ratio of 1.7:1. If WPW is associated with attacks of paroxysmal auricular fibrillation (PAF), the prognosis appears to be less favorable. Dreifus et al[20] reported 26 such people who had a 12% incidence of ventricular fibrillation and Curry and Krikler[21] noted 2 deaths in 10 people with WPW and PAF during a 16-year follow-up. The latter data suggest the need for considerable caution in assessing the prognosis of WPW if complicated by PAF.

VENTRICULAR CONDUCTION DEFECTS

Left Anterior Hemiblock (LAH)

Caird et al[3] followed 36 subjects aged 65 years and over with isolated left anterior hemiblock and observed one death compared with an expected 4.1 deaths in three years. Blackburn et al[4] reported this type of block to have a mortality risk ratio of 1.2:1 (ns). Yano et al[22] reported no increase in mortality over four years in 70 subjects. Concerning left axis deviation (LAD), 441 people with LAD who were followed by Medalie et al,[7] showed no increase in their risk ratio. Ostrander's[23] report on 103 subjects with LAD revealed no increase in risk ratio. Rose et al[2] followed 462 middle-aged men with LAD in nonsymptomatic patients and found no significant increase in their risk of CHD death. No increase in CHD mortality was observed in 58 Busselton subjects with isolated LAD. Thus, there is a reasonable amount of documentation to indicate that when LAH or LAD are found to be isolated in otherwise normal subjects, they will not incur additional risk of CHD mortality.

Left Posterior Hemiblock

The few subjects with this disorder that have been prospectively followed have had no excess mortality due to CHD. Packard et al[10] reported a 10-year follow-up of eight such cases and De Padua et al[24] followed 12 people for seven years. This rather limited evidence suggests that as an isolated disorder in clinically normal people, left posterior hemiblock does not imply an increased risk of death due to CHD.

Right Bundle-Branch Block (RBBB)

RBBB in clinically normal subjects has been the subject of various reports. The following studies reported no increased risk for CHD with RBBB: Blackburn et al[4]; Wood et al[25]; Cullen et al[1]; Reusch and Vivas.[26] These studies had periods of observation ranging from 4 to 13 years. Recently, Schneider et al[27] have published their findings from the Framingham study on 70 people (mean age 60 years) who developed complete RBBB over an 18-year follow-up. Although the initial appearance of RBBB was not accompanied by overt clinical events, the subsequent incidence of CHD and CCF was 2.5 and 4 times greater respectively than matched control subjects without RBBB. The CVD mortality was almost three times greater in those developing RBBB compared with cohorts. Eventually, only 21% of subjects with RBBB remained free from apparent clinical abnormalities. The mean period of study after the onset of RBBB was six years with a mean age of onset of 60 years. However, multivariate analysis revealed that newly acquired RBBB had not contributed independently to increased risk of CVD mortality once other risk factors such as blood pressure, diabetes, CHD, CCF, and age were taken into account. On the other hand, within 10 years of onset of RBBB, in the 50 cases with at least one risk factor, CVD mortality was four times greater than in the 20 cases without antecedent or coincidental abnormalities. Thus the Framingham results support the previous findings on the lack of risk for CVD mortality concerning isolated RBBB without coincidental evidence of heart disease, the CVD risks increasing by 4:1 in those with RBBB and other evidence of heart disease.

Left Bundle-Branch Block (LBBB)

Some reports have failed to show a poor prognosis for LBBB but in each instance the numbers have been small or the follow-up period short. There was no increase in the age-specific mortality for LBBB in Busselton subjects.[1]

Rabkin et al[28] followed 29 cases of complete LBBB without clinical evidence of ischemic or valvular heart disease. Over five years they observed a ten times greater incidence of sudden death in those with LBBB than in those without LBBB. Schneider et al[29] have published their follow-up on 55 people who had newly acquired LBBB (including 7 with transient and 3 with intermittent LBBB). The mean age of onset was 62 years. At the point in time of onset of LBBB, 40

(73%) had coexisting cardiovascular abnormalities and 15 (27%) were free from them. Their general findings were that in men, LBBB contributed to increased risk of CVD mortality. In addition, they concluded that in the general middle-aged population, the development of LBBB most commonly indicates the presence of advanced underlying abnormalities. If occurring in otherwise healthy people, LBBB should not be dismissed as an innocuous phenomenon without search for underlying cardiovascular disease. Within 10 years of the onset of LBBB, 50% of those with LBBB died of CVD compared with 11.6% of controls free from LBBB. To date, the Framingham study has shown the most impressive evidence that LBBB in older patients represents a considerable risk of CVD compared with control-free people.

Bifascicular Blocks

The prognosis of the bifascicular blocks has not been clearly established but their outcomes are frequently related to that of the underlying cardiovascular disease rather than to the specific conduction disturbance. Firstly, concerning RBBB with left atrial hypertrophy (LAH) in otherwise normal subjects, Scanlon et al[30] reported one death and four cases developing complete AV block in 20 subjects over a two-year period. Kulbertus[31] reported a five-year annual incidence of 6% of advanced AV block in 38 subjects with no deaths. Inoue et al[32] have reported a favorable prognosis in 30 Japanese patients aged 64 to 89 years with bifascicular block. Over a three-year period, complete AV block developed in 2.4% of patients per year with a 1.1% mortality rate per year.

McAnulty et al[33] conducted a prospective study (average 42.4 months) on 554 patients with chronic bifascicular and trifascicular block. Complete AV block developed in only 19 patients of whom 17 were successfully treated. There were 160 deaths of which 67 (42%) were sudden. The main risks of death were due to associated coronary artery disease, to tachyarrhythmias, and to congestive heart failure, whereas the risks of death from heart block and bradyarrhythmia were low.

Dhingra et al[34] have published their follow-up on 531 people with either one or another form of bifascicular block. There were 60 subjects under 60 years (mean age 43 years) and 58 over 60 (mean age 73 years) who had been carefully screened to exclude any other evidence of heart disease. In this group over a mean follow-up period of 3 years, no younger patient and only one older patient showed spontaneous progression to complete AV block. Concerning mortality, 11 of the younger group (18%) and 24 of the older group (41%) died. Sudden death occurred in 2 (3%) of the younger group and in 10 (17%) of the older group. By comparison, there were 413 people with bifascicular block and evidence of coexisting organic heart disease. Of these, 170 were under 60 years of age (mean age 48 years) and 263 were in the older groups (mean age 71 years). Spontaneous complete AV block was noted to develop in 6 (3%) of the younger group and 14 (5%) of the older group. Concerning mortality, 54 (32%) of the younger age group died and 118 (45%) of the older group died during a mean 3.3 years and 3.0 years respectively. Sudden death occurred in 29 (17%) of the younger patients and 45 (18%) of the older patients. This three-year study of bifascicular block indicates that the mortality in the younger group was nearly doubled by the coexistence of organic heart disease (18% vs 32%) but this was not so in older patients (41% vs 45%). The death rates in this study appear to be much higher than expected. In the group of people with bifascicular block and otherwise normal hearts, there was an annual risk of death of 6% in those of average age 43 years and 11% in those averaging 70 years of age. In the absence of a quoted control group of subjects, this mortality rate can be compared with the annual risk of death in the 1976 Australian population. The risk of death in unselected people of mean age 43 years was 4/1000 per annum for men and 2.5/1000 per annum for women. For those of mean age 73 years, the annual risk of death was 66/1000 for men and 41/1000 for women. These comparisons suggest more than a tenfold increase in the risk of death for younger people with bifascicular block in otherwise normal hearts. In older people, the risk ratio appeared about twice that of an Australian white population. Finally, regardless of age, the annual risk of developing complete AV block was less than 1% in those with no evidence of associated organic heart disease as compared to those with evidence of CHD.

ARRHYTHMIAS

Atrial Fibrillation and Atrial Flutter

Atrial fibrillation (AF) and flutter have long been known to occur in conjunction with various types of heart disease and in these instances the prognosis is mainly dependent on the coexisting pathologic process. Very few reports have been published about isolated AF in otherwise normal hearts. Blackburn et al[4] found a five-year CHD mortality ratio of 13:1 in 40- to 59-year-old men compared with carefully matched controls. In their five-year study, Rose et al[2] found the age-adjusted CHD mortality in 47 40- to 64-year-old men with isolated AF to have a risk ratio of 3.5:1. In 28 Busselton[1] subjects found with AF, only 4 subjects had AF in isolation of other ECG codes of whom 2 subsequently died over 13 years. Of the remaining 24 found with AF with one or more additional ECG codes, 18 (75%) had died. Wolf et al[35] reported that Framingham subjects with idiopathic AF showed a significant increase in 24-year mortality due to strokes. In 481 person years, the expected rate for stroke was 7.43 compared with an observed rate of 45.45 (observed:expected 5.6:1). Over the ensuing 24 years, in the 45 persons aged 50 to 62 years at entry with idiopathic AF, 33 (73%) developed either CHD or congestive heart failure and 11 (24%) had a stroke. Thus idiopathic AF in Framingham subjects was a strong predictor of eventual vascular pathology. Also Kannel et al[36] observed the development of atrial fibrillation (AF) in 49 men and 49 women over a period of 22 years. Of these, 18 men and 12 women had AF in the absence of CVD. The development of AF was associated with a doubling of overall mortality and of mortality from cardiovascular disease.

Ventricular Extrasystoles

Despite their poor reputation when occurring during a coronary occlusion or myocardial infarction, the risks for ventricular extrasystoles (VE) have usually appeared minimal in otherwise normal subjects. *No increases* in age-adjusted risk ratios for otherwise normal subjects with VE on resting ECGs were revealed by the studies of Chiang et al,[37] Rodstein et al,[38] Fisher and Tyroler,[39] and Kannel et al.[40] Barrett et al[41] agreed with the conclusion that it would be impossible to demonstrate any benefit with long suppressive therapy of VE. In a study of 25 people with complex ventricular ectopy in the resting ECG, Kennedy et al[42] found significant obstruction at angiography in only six subjects. Kennedy et al[43] had previously investigated 18 asymptomatic patients without apparent cardiac disease, incidentally discovered with the aid of a 24-hour ambulatory ECG, to have ventricular ectopic beats of more than a mean 100 b/h. All subjects had normal coronary arteriograms. They found that 72% demonstrated multiform or repetitive patterns with more than half having elevated LV end-systolic volume (56%), elevated LV end-diastolic volume (67%), and LV end-diastolic pressure (56%). They concluded that myocardial dysfunction was present in the majority of people with ambulatory VE in apparently normal hearts.

Rabkin et al[44] reported on the 10.8-year prognosis of 401 persons in the Manitoba study with ventricular ectopic beats in otherwise clinically normal hearts. The relative risk of sudden death was 1.05 for those aged 40 to 49 years, 4.20 for those aged 50 to 59 years, and 3.28 for those aged 60 to 69 years, and an age-adjusted total of 4.18. Age-specific incidence of total ischemic heart disease (IHD) was significantly ($P < .05$) greater for men aged 40 to 59 years compared with controls without ventricular ectopics. Faster basic ventricular rates significantly correlated with greater IHD probability. Crow et al[45] did not agree that the claims by Rabkin et al[44] on the independent risks of VE from the Manitoba follow-up study can be accepted without question. They consider that all other previous studies lacked consistency in the relationship between VE and CHD risk. They point out that Rabkin et al[44] do not address the crucial point as to whether the findings are fortuitous or due to VE associations with predictors other than age, known or unknown, particularly other ECG findings, blood pressure, blood lipids, activity or left ventricular function.

In Busselton subjects followed for 13 years, Cullen et al[1] observed an age-adjusted risk ratio of 2.1:1 for those with isolated infrequent ventricular ectopic beats (less than 1 per 10 beats). Eleven deaths in 46 subjects ($P < .05$) were noted compared with 15 deaths in 61 subjects with all types of VE ($P < .001$)—a mortality ratio of 2.4:1. A later analysis of these subjects in 16-year data with multiple regressions showed a significant independent association in 60- to 74-year-old women between ventricular ectopic beats and both total mortality ($P < .05$) and coronary heart disease ($P < .05$). Factors in this analysis included blood pressure, cholesterol, body weight, uric acid, glucose, forced expiratory volume (FEV), forced vital capacity (FVC), fatfold and hemoglobin.

Supraventricular Extrasystoles (SVE)

Supraventricular extrasystoles were followed up by Chiang et al[37] in 78 subjects and by Rodstein et al[38] in 122 subjects. SVE involved no increase in the risk of sudden death over 6 and 18 years, respectively. Similarly, the Busselton 13-year data on 18 subjects with isolated SVE revealed a mortality ratio for CVD of 1.4:1 (ns). As for those who develop SVE on stress testing, there has been no long-term information published on the mortality for this abnormality.

Paroxysmal Supraventricular Tachycardia

Although paroxysmal supraventricular tachycardia occurs relatively frequently in clinical practice, no information is available on the prognosis with regard to mortality.

Ventricular Tachycardia (VT)

Rahilly et al[46] followed 18 patients of mean age 37 years with repetitive ventricular tachycardia. During the five-month to eight-year follow-up period, there were no deaths or any worsening of symptoms in these subjects.

CONCLUSIONS

There is evidence that the following isolated ECG abnormalities in symptom-free subjects will increase the risks of death from CHD and CVD: large and moderate sized Q waves, intermediate T wave inversion, third-degree AV block, Wolff-Parkinson-White syndrome in those prone to attacks of atrial fibrillation or atrial flutter, left bundle-branch block, bifascicular block, atrial fibrillation or flutter.

Certain isolated ECG abnormalities in symptom-free persons have too few studies published for accurate estimation of prognosis. Past clinical experience suggests that when present there is a need for a careful examination and surveillance of the patient. These include widespread ST depression, Mobitz 11 AV block, and paroxysmal ventricular tachycardia.

There has been good evidence that left ventricular hypertrophy involved an increased risk of death from CVD, but this risk may be lessened by effective treatment for hypertension. The evidence on isolated ventricular ectopic beats in the resting ECG remains inconclusive.

In the final group of isolated ECG abnormalities in otherwise normal hearts, the available evidence fails to show increase in mortality. These include sino-atrial block, first-degree AV block, second-degree Mobitz type 1 block, Wolff-Parkinson-White syndrome without coexisting paroxysmal atrial fibrillation, right bundle-branch block, supraventricular extrasystoles, paroxysmal supraventricular tachycardia.

The evidence presented in this chapter does not provide a general answer to the questions: Does increasing age worsen the prognosis of an abnormality in the resting ECG? Is it merely that with age the development of additional CVD factors usually determine prognosis? Some evidence shows a higher mortality in younger age groups but this could be due to a weeding-out process of those more sensitive to the abnormality. In certain studies, for example, mortality risks for Q waves were reportedly lower in subjects over 65 years of age than in those below this age. In people with third-degree heart block (complete heart block) on pacemakers, there was a report of high risk of death in those 50 to 59 years of age compared with people of similar ages, yet by 80 to 89 years of age the risk of CHD was no worse than controls of 80 to 89 years of age. Left anterior hemiblock (LAH) in people over 65 years of age was reported to have involved similar risks to that for LAH in younger ages. In another study, the incidence of sudden death in those with ventricular ectopics was slightly higher in those aged 50 to 59 years compared with those aged 60 to 69 years. These exceptions suggest the need for caution when assessing the prognosis of a specific finding in elderly people.

REFERENCES

1. Cullen KJ, Stenhouse NS, Wearne KL, et al: Electrocardiograms and thirteen year cardiovascular mortality in Busselton study. *Br Heart J* 1982; 47:209–212.
2. Rose G, Baxter PJ, Reid DD, et al: Prevalence and prognosis of ECG findings in middle-aged men. *Br Heart J* 1978;40:636–643.
3. Caird FI, Campbell A, Jackson TFM: Significance of abnormalities of electrocardiogram in old people. *Br Heart J* 1974;36:1012–1018.
4. Blackburn H, Taylor HL, Keys A: The electrocardiogram in prediction of five year coronary heart disease incidence among men aged 40 through 59. *Circulation* 1970;41(suppl 1):154–161.
5. Kannel WB, Gordon T, Offutt D: Left ventricular hypertrophy by electrocardiogram. *Ann Intern Med* 1969;71:89–105.
6. Cullen KJ, McCall MG, Stenhouse NS: Changing mortality due to strokes in men following treatment of Busselton hypertensives 1967–1977. *Int J Epidemiol* 1969;71:89–105.
7. Medalie JH, Snyder M, Groen JJ: Angina pectoris among 10,000 men. Five year incidence and univariate analysis. *Am J Med* 1973;55:583–594.
8. Froelicher VF, Yanowitz FG, Thompson AJ, et al: The correlation of coronary angiography and the electrocardiographic response to maximal treadmill testing in 76 asymptomatic men. *Circulation* 1973; 48:597–604.
9. Higgins ITT, Kannel WB, Dawber TR: The electrocardiogram in epidemiological studies. Reproducability validity and international comparison. *Br J Prev Soc Med* 1965;19:53–68.
10. Packard JM, Graettinger JS, Graybiel A: Analysis

of electrocardiograms obtained from 1000 young healthy aviators—Ten year follow-up. *Circulation* 1954;10:384–400.
11. Amat-Y-Leon F, Dhingra RC, Denes P, et al: The natural history of chronic second degree AV nodal block. *Am J Cardiol* 1977;39:324.
12. Zepilli P, Fenici R, Sassara M, et al: Wenckebach second degree AV block in top ranking athletes: An old problem revisited. *Am Heart J* 1980;100: 281–294.
13. Cullen KJ, Collin R: Distance running causing Wenckebach heart-block. *Lancet* 1962;1:729–730.
14. Strasberg B, Amat-Y-Leon F, Dhingra RC, et al: Natural history of chronic second degree atrio ventricular nodal block. *Circulation* 1981;63:1043–1049.
15. Hatle L, Saeterhaug A, Rosketh R: Long term conservative therapy of chronic AV block. *Acta Med Scand* 1974;196:411–414.
16. Reid JM, Coleman EN, Doig W: Complete congenital heart block. Report of thirty-five cases. *Br Heart J* 1982;48:236–239.
17. Ginks W, Leatham A, Siddons H: Prognosis of patients paced for chronic atrio ventricular block. *Br Heart J* 1979;41:633–636.
18. White PD, Donovan H: *Hearts—Their Long Term Follow-Up.* Philadelphia, WB Saunders, 1967.
19. Flensted-Jensen E: Wolff–Parkinson–White syndrome. A long term follow-up of forty-seven cases. *Acta Med Scand* 1969;186:65–74.
20. Dreifus LS, Wellens HJJ, Watanabe Y, et al: Sinus bradycardia and atrial fibrillation associated with the Wolff–Parkinson–White syndrome. *Am J Cardiol* 1976;38:149–156.
21. Curry PVL, Krikler DM: Atrial fibrillation in the Wolff–Parkinson–White syndrome. *Br Heart J* 1975;37:779.
22. Yano K, Peskoe SM, Rhoads GG, et al: Left axis deviation and left anterior hemiblock among 8000 Japanese-American men. *Am J Cardiol* 1975;35: 800–815.
23. Ostrander LD: Left axis deviation. Prevalence associated conditions and prognosis. An epidemiologic study. *Ann Intern Med* 1971;75:23–28.
24. De Padua F, Lopes VM, Pereira-Miguel JM: Left posterior hemiblock. Good prognosis. *Adv Cardiol* 1975;14:157–162.
25. Wood FC, Jeffers WA, Wolferth CC: Follow up study of 64 patients with a right bundle branch conduction defect. *Am Heart J* 1935;10:1056–1066.
26. Reusch CS, Vivas JR: Clinical analysis of right bundle branch block. *Am Heart J* 1959;58:543–546.
27. Schneider JF, Thomas HE, Kreger BE, et al: Newly acquired right bundle branch block. The Framingham Study. *Ann Intern Med* 1980;92:37–44.
28. Rabkin SW, Mathewson FA, Tate RB: Natural history of left bundle branch block. *Br Heart J* 1980;43:164–169.
29. Schneider JF, Thomas HE, Kreger BE, et al: Newly acquired left bundle branch block: The Framingham Study. *Ann Intern Med* 1979;90:303–310.
30. Scanlon PJ, Pryor R, Blount SG: Right bundle branch block associated with left superior or inferior intraventricular block. Clinical setting, prognosis and relation to complete heart block. *Circulation* 1970;42:1123–1133.
31. Kulbertus HE: The magnitude of risk of developing complete heart block in patients with LAD-RBBB. *Am Heart J* 1973;86:278–280.
32. Inoue H, Ueda K, Ohkawa S, et al: Electrophysiologic study and prognosis of chronic bifascicular block. *Jpn Heart J* 1979;20:141–151.
33. McAnulty JH, Rahimtoola SH, Murphy E, et al: Natural history of "high risk" bundle branch block: Final report of a prospective study. *N Engl J Med* 1982;307:137–143.
34. Dhingra RC, Wyndham C, Deedwania PC, et al: The effect of age on atrioventricular conduction in patients with chronic bifascicular block. *Am J Cardiol* 1980;45:749–756.
35. Wolf PA, Dawber TR, Thomas HE, et al: Epidemiologic assessment of chronic atrial fibrillation and risk of stroke: The Framingham Study. *Neurology* 1978;28:973–977.
36. Kannel WB, Abbott RD, Savage DD, et al: Epidemiologic features of chronic atrial fibrillation: The Framingham Study. *N Engl J Med* 1982;306:1018–1022.
37. Chiang BN, Perlman LV, Ostrander LD, et al: Relationship of premature systoles to coronary heart disease and sudden death in the Tecumseh epidemiologic study. *Ann Intern Med* 1969;70:1159–1166.
38. Rodstein M, Wolloch L, Gubner RS: Mortality study of the significance of extrasystoles in an insured population. *Circulation* 1971;44:617–625.
39. Fisher FD, Tyroler HA: Relationship between ventricular premature contractions on routine electrocardiography and subsequent sudden deaths from coronary heart disease. *Circulation* 1973;47:712–719.
40. Kannel WB, Doyle JT, McNamara PM, et al: Precursors of sudden death: Factors related to the incidence of sudden death. *Circulation* 1975;57: 606–613.
41. Barrett PA, Peter CT, Swan HJC, et al: The frequency and prognostic significance of electrocardiographic abnormalities in clinically normal individuals. *Prog Cardiovasc Dis* 1981;23:299–319.
42. Kennedy HL, Pescarmona JE, Bouchard RJ, et al: Coronary artery status of apparently healthy subjects with frequent ventricular ectopics. *Ann Intern Med* 1980;92:179–185.
43. Kennedy HL, Pescarmona JE, Bouchard RJ, et al: Objective evidence of occult myocardial dysfunction in patients with frequent ventricular ectopy without clinically apparent heart disease. *Am Heart J* 1982;104:57–65.
44. Rabkin SW, Francis AL, Mathewson MD, et al: Relationship of ventricular ectopy in men without apparent heart disease to occurrence of ischaemic heart disease and sudden death. *Am Heart J* 1981; 101:135–142.
45. Crow R, Prineas R, Blackburn H: The prognostic significance of ventricular ectopic beats among the apparently healthy. *Am Heart J* 1981;101:244–248.
46. Rahilly GT, Prystowsky EN, Zipes DP, et al: Clinical and electrophysiologic findings in patients with repetitive monomorphic ventricular tachycardia and otherwise normal electrocardiogram. *Am J Cardiol* 1982;50:459–468.

CHAPTER 37
Prognosis in Elderly Patients Following Myocardial Infarction

David Hunt
Graeme Sloman

Coronary heart disease (CHD) is the most important cardiovascular cause of disability in the middle-aged and older age group of the population.

Populations in which CHD is common are characterized by severe, often diffuse involvement of the coronary arteries with atherosclerosis, a pathologic change in the coronary arteries produced by fibrous and fatty deposits often associated with thrombosis. CHD may result in unexpected sudden death, or it may lead to an acute myocardial infarction which may be fatal or may leave the patient with chronic disability such as angina pectoris, persistent congestive cardiac failure, or a cardiac arrhythmia. A great deal can be achieved for the survivors of acute infarction with good follow-up management and specific therapy including coronary artery graft surgery when indicated.

Longitudinal studies of mortality in patients with proven acute myocardial infarction admitted to a coronary care unit are limited. We are fortunate in being able to present hospital mortality figures with one-year follow-up figures from patients admitted to the coronary care unit at the Royal Melbourne Hospital commencing in 1963.

Four series of patients each consisting of 300 consecutive patients with diagnosed definite transmural acute myocardial infarction can be compared. The four groups were collected over the periods 1963 to 1967 (group I), 1969 to 1970 (group II), 1974 to 1975 (group III), and 1978 to 1979 (group IV). Data were collected prospectively after admission and included past history, risk factors, onset and duration of chest pain, observations on admission, complications in hospital and follow-up data to one year. Patients who did not attend the one-year follow-up appointment in a special coronary care unit follow-up clinic were assessed by questionnaire or enquiries through their local doctor.

CONCLUSIONS FROM FOLLOW-UP STUDIES

There has been an overall reduction in mortality to 28 days of patients with definite transmural infarction who were admitted to the coronary care unit (Figure 37-1). Thus the overall mortality to 28 days was 28% and 27% in the two early groups and 12% and 15.3% in the later two groups. One year follow-up data were not available for group I, but the improved mortality to 28 days in groups III and IV was maintained through to one year (Figure 37-1).

The reduction in mortality was seen in all age groups (Figure 37-2) including those over the age of 60 years and those over the age of 70 years. It has been suggested that mortality rates in the coronary care unit have fallen over recent years because patients now being admitted are younger and have less severe infarction, but in our experience this has not been the case and, in fact, the opposite has occurred. Figure 37-3 shows the distribution of all patients in the four groups: 38%, 41%, and 51% of each group were aged 60 years or over (Table 37-1). Similarly, Figure 37-4 and Table 37-2 show the severity of infarction in each group. The highest incidence of mild infarction (ie, infarction without evidence of cardiac failure) was highest in the first group studied.

The mortality of patients with and without cardiac failure has fallen over the years (Figure 37-5) while the 28-day mortality from cardiogenic shock remains unchanged and in the order of 85%. Patients admitted to the coronary care unit following resuscitation from cardiac arrest also show a lower mortality in the recent group (Table 37-3).

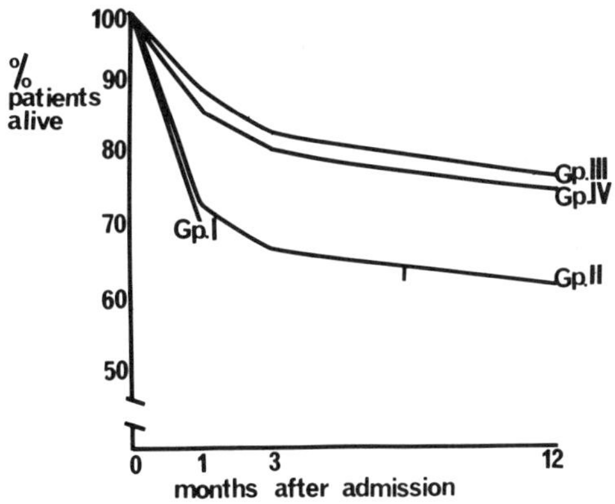

Figure 37-1 Overall mortality for 12 months following acute myocardial infarction in groups I–IV.

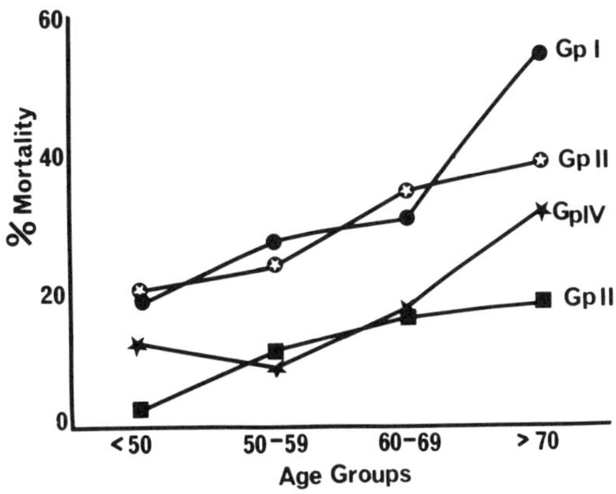

Figure 37-2 Percentage mortality in age groups less than 50 years, 50 to 59 years, and 60 to 69 years, and over 70 years in groups I–IV.

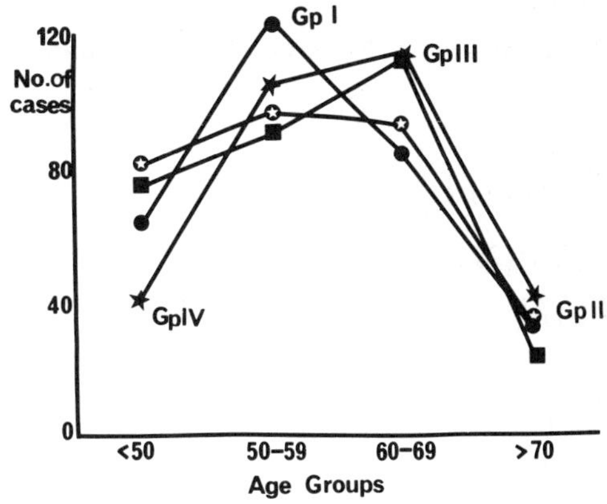

Figure 37-3 Distribution of all patients in four age groups.

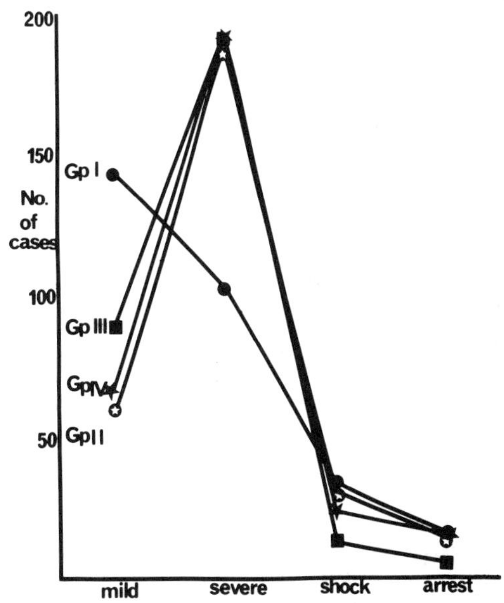

Figure 37-4 Distribution of severity class of patients in each chronological group.

Table 37-1
Age Distribution of Four Groups of Patients

	< 50 yr	50–59 yr	60–69 yr	> 70 yr	Total
Group I (1963–1967)	63 (17.5)*	123 (26.9)	84 (29.8)	30 (53.5)	300 (28)
Group II (1969–1970)	81 (19.7)	97 (23.8)	93 (34.5)	29 (38.0)	300 (27)
Group III (1974–1975)	73 (2.7)	90 (11.2)	114 (16.7)	23 (17.4)	300 (12)
Group IV (1978–1979)	41 (12.2)	105 (8.6)	112 (16.8)	42 (30.9)	300 (15.3)

*Mortality (%) at 28 days is shown in parentheses.

Table 37-2
Clinical Severity of Infarction in Four Groups of Patients Admitted to Coronary Care Unit in 1963–1979

	Mild	Severe	Shock	Previous Cardiac Arrest	Total
Group I (1963–1967)	144 (9.0)*	104 (34.6)	35 (82.9)	17 (41.2)	300 (28)
Group II (1969–1970)	61 (9.8)	189 (21.2)	32 (87.5)	18 (44.4)	300 (27)
Group III (1974–1975)	90 (1.1)	191 (10.5)	14 (85.7)	5 (40.0)	300 (12)
Group IV (1978–1979)	68 (4.4)	191 (9.9)	24 (87.5)	17 (17.6)	300 (15.3)

*Mortality (%) at 28 days is shown in parentheses.

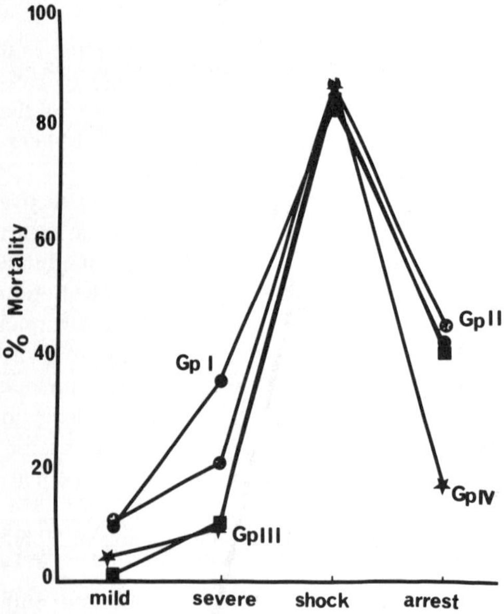

Figure 37-5 Percentage mortality in each clinical class in groups I–IV.

Analysis of the time of arrival of patients with definite transmural cardiac infarction in the coronary care unit has been progressively reduced. In the first series commencing in 1963, 40% of patients were admitted to the coronary care unit within 6 hours of the onset of their pain; in the series commencing in 1978, 53% of patients were admitted to the coronary care unit within 6 hours of onset of symptoms. The study therefore confirms the reduction in mortality in patients over the age of 60 years in the coronary care unit and on 12-month follow-up. This reduction, although not as great as that seen in the younger age groups, is definite and may be due either to a change in the standard of care provided in the coronary care unit or to a change in the natural history of acute myocardial infarction.

CORONARY CARE MANAGEMENT

Over the years there has been a definite change in the management of patients in the coronary care unit. These changes have been related to the management of cardiac failure, cardiac arrhythmias, and the use of anticoagulants. While trends can be identified, dates of commencement have not been documented.

Congestive Cardiac Failure

Following the availability of potent diuretics such as furosemide, there developed a tendency to use intravenous (IV) doses of such agents for evidence of pulmonary venous congestion of any degree of severity. Such therapy has been shown to have a detrimental effect in terms of cardiac output reduction in patients with only mild left ventricular failure (LVF). Over recent years there has been an increase in the use of oral thiazides or even oral furosemide instead of intravenous furosemide.

The use of digitalis has diminished; there are few data to support its use for LVF in acute myocardial infarction (AMI) in patients in sinus rhythm. For atrial arrhythmias, however, it is an excellent drug, but even so verapamil has made inroads in its use in this area.

Vasodilators are now increasingly used for therapy of cardiac failure: one half or one tablet of buccal nitroglycerine, buccal isosorbide, or cutaneous nitroglycerine paste.

Anticoagulants

The fashion with respect to the use of anticoagulants varied in the early series. Full heparinization was used occasionally but *minidose heparin* was not used. In the recent series all patients have minidose heparin and those patients with evidence of large infarcts are given full formal anticoagulation therapy with heparin followed by oral anticoagulants for three months after the acute episode.

Table 37-3
History and Risk Factors

History	Group I	Group II	Group III	Group IV
Myocardial infarction	75 (33)*	89 (37)	75 (16)	85 (22)
Angina	166 (34)	147 (37)	118 (15)	121 (20)
Neither infarct nor angina	108 (18)	131 (16)	158 (7)	146 (8)
Hypertension	39 (26)	53 (26)	100 (10)	130 (14)
Diabetes	10 (40)	14 (43)	27 (11)	28 (25)
Pulmonary disease	27 (41)	16 (31)	16 (6)	13 (15)
Smoking	Unknown	183 (22)	154 (9)	128 (13)

*Mortality (%) is shown in parentheses.

Cardiopulmonary Resuscitation

The policy with respect to cardiopulmonary resuscitation has not altered.

Bradycardia

Nineteen years ago the coronary care protocol advised that any bradycardia less than 60 bpm should be immediately treated with IV atropine. Current practice restricts the use of atropine to patients with hemodynamic complications associated with bradycardia. Similarly, a more conservative attitude now prevails on the use of cardiac pacing, which is reserved for AMI patients with hemodynamic deterioration associated with a slow heart rate or atrioventricular (AV) dissociation. Incidence of arrhythmia is shown in Table 37-4.

Beta-Adrenergic Blocking Drugs

Beta-blockers are used more aggressively in the coronary care unit in the more recent series; however, these have usually been given by the oral route and patients have been admitted to controlled studies where approximately half of the patients have not been receiving an active therapeutic dose of a beta-blocker.

In a recent review of the experience in selective coronary care units in Australia (National Heart Foundation of Australia, 1983) it was found that there had been little change in the sex distribution of patients with cardiac infarction in Australia since 1970 and that the males in the age groups 50 to 59 and 60 to 69 years each accounted for one third of all admissions. There was a tendency in more recent years to admit older men to the coronary care unit and the proportion of patients over 70 years of age increased from 9% to 13.5%, while admissions of those under the age of 50 fell from 24% to 17.5% during the survey period which extended from the first survey in 1970 until the most recent survey carried out in 1980.

Table 37-4
Incidence of Arrhythmias and Conduction Abnormalities

	Group II	Group III	Group IV
Atrial arrhythmias alone	22 (18)	30 (10)	27 (4)
Atrial and ventricular arrhythmias	69 (39)	46 (26)	41 (26)
Ventricular fibrillation in unit	48 (65)	22 (45)	31 (35)
Ventricular tachycardia without ventricular fibrillation	45 (29)	52 (13)	35 (11)
Premature ventricular complexes without ventricular tachycardia or fibrillation	84 (17)	104 (8)	61 (11)
Complete AV block	42 (43)	35 (40)	36 (44)
First- or second-degree atrioventricular block	29 (38)	19 (32)	33 (15)
Intraventricular conduction without AV block	81 (44)	37 (38)	30 (40)
Neither arrhythmic nor conduction defect	60 (0)	66 (3)	73 (4)

SECTION IV
Therapy

CHAPTER 38
Newer Antiarrhythmic Agents and the Elderly Patient

Bramah N. Singh
Ram Kannan
Koonlawee Nademanee
Nagammal Venkatesh

In recent years, numerous antiarrhythmic compounds of varying pharmacologic properties have been developed and characterized.[1] In the past, it has been assumed, that antiarrhythmic compounds exert similar pharmacologic effects during various decades of life. Antiarrhythmic agents are, however, rarely completely selective compounds. A number of them interact with the autonomic nervous system and it is known that adrenergic and cholinergic tissue responsiveness may alter with age.[2] It is also known that disorders of the conducting system of the heart develop more commonly with age and compounds that are essentially without effect in the young may exert a markedly depressant action in the older patient. It is becoming increasingly clear that many of the biologic and physiologic functions of the body that are altered significantly with age may influence pharmacodynamic and pharmacokinetic actions of drugs.[3] Such changes may be reflected in the absorption, distribution, and renal and hepatic metabolism as well as in receptor sensitivity of a variety of drugs in elderly patients when compared to well-matched controls. In this paper, the fundamental mechanisms of action of the newer antiarrhythmic agents are discussed wherever possible with a particular reference to the age-related effects which may bear importantly on the therapeutic role of this emerging group of cardioactive compounds.

EFFECTS OF AGING ON DRUG METABOLISM AND RECEPTOR SENSITIVITY

As indicated above, significant changes occur not only in absorption, distribution, renal clearance, and hepatic metabolism but also in receptor sensitivity of numerous drugs in the elderly.

A number of changes in the gastrointestinal (GI) tract are associated with old age which may influence drug absorption. For example, a reduction in intestinal blood flow occurs in the elderly that could cause a delay in the absorption of drugs. Furthermore, gastric pH increases with age, a change that may alter ionization and solubility of various drugs.[4] Other age-related changes such as decrease in number of absorbing cells and delay in gastric emptying may also be clinically significant.[5] However, although a number of mechanisms exist to explain changes in drug absorption in the elderly, not all are important clinically. For example, the absorption of digoxin is only slightly delayed in the elderly,[6] while a number of other drugs do not show any change in absorption due to age.[7]

In the elderly, drug distribution is affected mainly by changes in body composition, protein binding, volume of distribution, and regional blood flow.

There is a decrease in lean body mass and an increase in adipose tissue in relation to body weight in elderly people.[8] Accordingly, the distribution of drugs is altered depending on the water- or lipid-solubility of the drug.

$$C_{ss} = \frac{\text{dose per interval of time}}{\text{clearance}}$$

Thus, C_{ss} (steady state concentration) will increase as clearance decreases. For many drugs, old age is associated with a decrease in clearance and increased steady state drug concentrations. Thus accentuation of pharmacologic or toxic effects can be expected in the elderly using serum concentrations as an index for pharmacologic activity. Hence either appropriate reduction in dosage or lengthening of the dosage intervals or both have to be considered in clinical therapy of elderly patients. Since the major clearing organs for various drugs are the liver and kidney, the effect of age on hepatic and renal clearance are considered in some detail below.

Old age is associated with a decrease in liver weight and hepatic blood flow, the latter probably due to a drop in cardiac output. Up to 45% reduction in total hepatic blood flow has been observed in elderly people as compared to young adults.[4] The first-pass extraction after oral dosing as well as the steady-state concentrations after an intravenous (IV) bolus will both be affected because of the altered blood flow. There is evidence that the hepatic enzymes of phase I reactions (microsomal hydroxylation and n-dealkylation) may be impaired in old age[9] resulting in reduced plasma clearance and increased steady-state drug levels. The phase II type of reactions (glucorinidation and conjugation) are not greatly affected by old age.[3] Although a decrease in clearance of drugs can be predicted due to altered hepatic function, this has not been a consistent finding with a number of drugs. Thus, serum clearance of propranolol diminishes with age[10,11] but not that of lidocaine although both are flow-dependent and are subject to high hepatic clearance.

Many structural and functional alterations occur in the kidney with age.[12] A reduction of about 35% in glomerular filtration rate has been observed in persons from ages 20 to 90 years.[13] Creatinine production is decreased with age.[13] These changes in renal function will have a significant influence in the elimination of drugs that are removed mainly by the renal route and also of drugs whose metabolites are excreted by the kidney (eg, procainamide, diazepam).

Since patients with advanced age may need multiple drugs daily for various diseases, it is important to consider the drug-to-drug interactions during concomitant therapy. One or all aspects of metabolism, viz, absorption, distribution, and elimination, of one drug can be affected by another, the most significant of these metabolic processes being the influence on drug distribution due to differences in protein binding.[14] The concomitant administration of a second drug could displace the highly protein-bound drug from its tissue-binding sites, as has been documented for the quinidine-digoxin interaction.[15] This effect may be exaggerated in elderly patients in whom there may be a diminution in the number of receptor sites due to hypoalbuminemia.

ELECTROPHYSIOLOGIC MECHANISMS OF ANTIARRHYTHMIC DRUGS

Although there has been controversy regarding the fundamental mechanisms of action of antiarrhythmic compounds,[1,16] there is now increasing agreement that the conventionally available as well as the newer investigational compounds can be classified into four discrete categories.[1]

Class I drugs are those which act by depressing the fast sodium current ("fast response") in cardiac muscle thereby lengthening the effective refractory period; the resting membrane potential is unaffected but phase IV is depressed while the effect on repolarization is variable. For example, in the case of some (now designated as class Ia) such as quinidine, procainamide, and disopyramide, the marked reduction in the fast response (or the fast sodium current) is associated (in an independent way) with a modest lengthening of the action potential (or Q-Tc in vivo), a property that may be both beneficial as well as deleterious under different conditions. For example, in atrial flutter and fibrillation, lengthening of the atrial action potential by these agents may contribute to their tendency to restore and maintain sinus rhythm. In ventricular myocardium the lengthening of the Q-Tc interval in conjunction with a markedly reduced conduction velocity may give rise to atypical ventricular tachycardia (torsade de pointes) in excessive doses or when associated with hypokalemia or hypomagnesemia. In the case of some class I agents, the action potential duration may actually be shortened. With these agents (designated as class Ib), typified by lidocaine, mexiletine, tocainide, diphenylhydantoin, aprindine, and possibly propafenone and ethmozin, the net effect on the effective refractory period is a balance between the time-dependent *increase* due to the inhibition of the fast sodium inward current and the *decrease* due to abbreviation of the time course of repolarization. In recent years, another apparently discrete subcategory (best designated Ic) of class I agents which markedly depress conduction in all parts of the heart and some of which also have a potent suppressant action on premature ventricular contractions ("PVC killers"), has become available. The most prominent compounds in this category are: flecainide, encainide (and its metabolites), lorcainide, cibenzoline, and possibly pirmenol. Another feature that these compounds share is the differential effect that they have on repolarization in ventricular muscle and Purkinje fibers, lengthening it in the former and shortening it in the latter. It is conceivable that the significant arrhythmogenic potential of some of these compounds may relate not only to their markedly depressant effect on conduction but also to the disparity in their actions on cardiac repolarization providing the substrate for focal re-excitation.

Some general features of class I agents merit emphasis. Since these drugs lengthen the effective refractory period and depress the tendency to spontaneous depolarization, they have a wide spectrum of antiarrhythmic action, being effective in arrhythmias due to re-entry as well as in those caused by enhanced automaticity. Another characteristic of class I agents is that they selectively lengthen the effective refractory period of the accessory pathways in the Wolff-Parkinson-White syndrome. Thus, they slow the ventricular response in atrial flutter and fibrillation complicating pre-excitation in which the predominant anterograde AV conduction occurs through the bypass tracts. Another feature of class I antiarrhythmic agents that needs emphasis is the observation that these compounds exert more pronounced effects in partially depolarized myocardial fibers or in those altered so by disease. Thus, in older patients with a higher incidence of multifascicular bundle-branch block and lengthened infranodal AV conduction, complete AV block is more likely to develop than in younger patients. Another feature of class I agents that has emerged recently from clinical studies is that, as a class, the long-term efficacy of these compounds in controlling ventricular tachyarrhythmias may be predictable on the basis of their ability to prevent reinduction of ventricular arrhythmias by programmed electrical stimulation of the heart in the clinical electrophysiology laboratory.[17] These observations suggest that these compounds alter the substrate required for re-entry in patients with organic cardiac disease.

The class II agents have been designated as such by virtue of their common property of reducing sympathetic excitation to the heart. The group in particular includes beta-adrenoceptor blocking drugs. The antiarrhythmic spectrum of these drugs is virtually identical despite the somewhat varying pharmacologic properties in terms of their potencies as local anesthetics, as partial agonists, and as cardioselective or nonselective agents. Their only electrophysiologic action of clinical relevance is the fact that they all block phase-4 depolarization, especially that augmented by endogenous or exogenous catecholamines. Such an effect is exerted through an action on the pacemaker current, at least in Purkinje fibers.[16] It will be apparent that the overall antiarrhythmic spectrum of action of beta-blockers in chronic ventricular arrhythmias will be narrow, an inference that is borne out by clinical observations. However, in recent years, as a class of cardioactive agents, beta-blocking compounds have drawn much attention for their propensity to reduce sudden death in survivors of acute myocardial infarction.[18] It is of interest that this salutary effect is evident in the young as in the old.[18] Furthermore, this effect is related to the beta-blocking property of the compounds and appears to be mediated indirectly through amelioration of ischemia rather than a primary antiarrhythmic action.[19]

Perhaps one of the most significant observations in the last 10 years in the characterization of antiarrhythmic mechanisms has been the demonstration that the uniform lengthening of the action potential duration has a potent effect in preventing the development of arrhythmias.[1,20] This has been suggested by the alterations in the duration of repolarization of intracellularly recorded action potentials in hyperthyroid and hypothyroid atria[21,22] and particularly in relation to the striking effect of the drug amiodarone in prolonging the absolute refractory period in cardiac muscle[20] with little effect on the upstroke velocity of phase 0 of the transmembrane action potential (see below). This effect is exhibited also by bretylium during acute administration, especially in the context of myocardial ischemia[1] and by amiodarone following protracted therapy.[20] Such an effect has been considered to be a distinct mechanism (class III) for the termination of resistant ventricular arrhythmias. For the chronic prophylaxis of resistant life-threatening ventricular arrhythmias amiodarone has recently emerged as perhaps the most potent suppressant. A number of agents which appear to act predominantly by lengthening the action potential duration (with the consequent prolongation of the effective refractory period) are currently under study: sotalol, amiodarone, clofilium, n-acetylprocainamide (Figure 38-1). Other compounds that may also exhibit (at least in part) so-called class III activity are bepridil,[23] and melperone.[24] Some of these agents will be discussed at length below.

Finally, agents which selectively block the slow-channel in the myocardium have been categorized as exhibiting a class IV antiarrhythmic action.[25] Verapamil is a prototype. It has little effect on the upstroke velocity of phase 0; it accelerates phases I and II of repolarization and depresses phase IV especially where it is slow-channel–dependent ("slow response"). Thus, the predominant effect of verapamil is in terminating arrhythmias which use anterograde conduction in the AV node as the essential part of the re-entrant loop. Not all so-called slow-channel blockers lengthen conduction time through the AV node, but those which do (eg, verapamil, diltiazem, gallopamil, bepridil, tiapamil) have antiarrhythmic properties that closely correlate with their ability to prolong the effective and the functional refractory periods of the AV node.

In Table 38-1, various compounds in the different antiarrhythmic classes are presented. It is emphasized, as has been done previously,[26] that

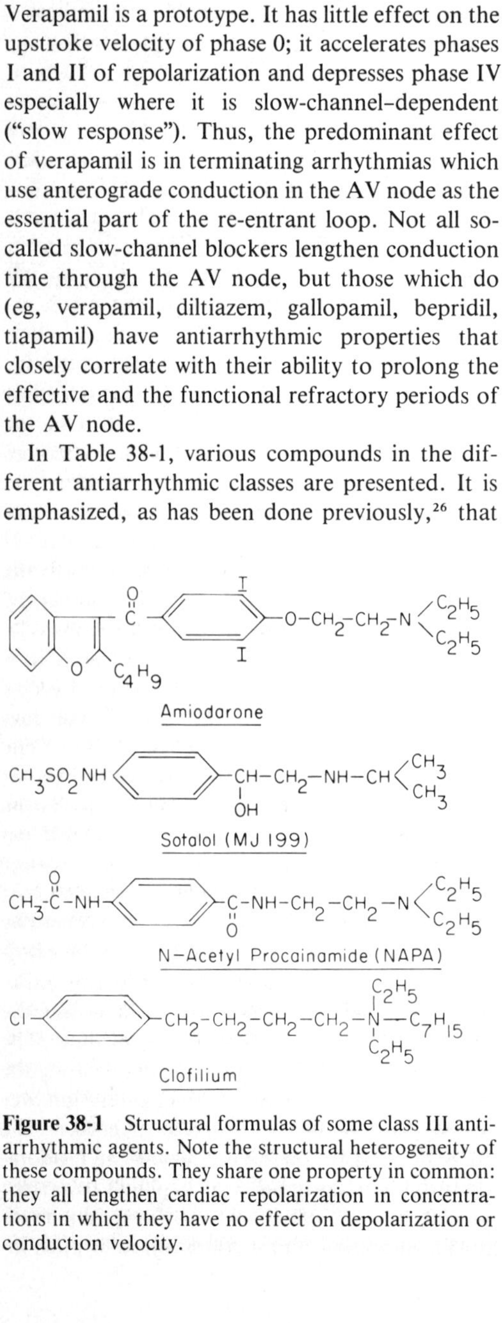

Figure 38-1 Structural formulas of some class III antiarrhythmic agents. Note the structural heterogeneity of these compounds. They share one property in common: they all lengthen cardiac repolarization in concentrations in which they have no effect on depolarization or conduction velocity.

none of the compounds shown is a "pure" member of the stated class. However, the classification is based on the identification of the dominant action that a particular compound has relative to the (1) depression of the fast response, (2) inhibition of sympathetic excitation, (3) uniform prolongation of the action potential duration, and (4) the inhibition of the slow response. It should also be appreciated that the net pharmacologic or therapeutic effects of individual compounds will be determined not only by their overall hemodynamic and electrophysiologic effects relative to their serum and tissue concentrations but also by the presence or absence of associated properties which may indirectly influence their primary fundamental antiarrhythmic actions. This is particularly evident in the case of beta-antagonists (including sotalol), calcium-channel blockers (particularly bepridil), and amiodarone, all of which also have antianginal efficacy while some of them are coronary arterial dilators.

NEWER ANTIARRHYTHMIC DRUGS

Clinicians have long sought an ideal antiarrhythmic agent, one that has a wide spectrum of therapeutic efficacy, is potent, well tolerated by the patient with minimal side-effects while having the necessary pharmacokinetic characteristics for use in the long-term treatment of arrhythmias. Although the development of such a compound still appears to be an elusive goal, a number of new drugs (Table 38-1) has recently been introduced[1] and others are at various stages of characterization and evaluation. The properties of these compounds are encouraging and they merit discussion. The remainder of this chapter will deal with the pharmacologic features and therapeutic applications of these newer compounds with particular reference, wherever possible, to their age-related pharmacodynamic and pharmacokinetic features. Only the most significant agents from the various electrophysiologic classes of antiarrhythmic agents will be discussed. However, only brief mention will be made about calcium antagonists and beta-adrenergic blocking agents as they have a limited role in the control of ventricular tachyarrhythmias—the most important arrhythmias requiring medical therapy in the elderly.

Aprindine

Aprindine is a powerful antiarrhythmic agent for the control of a variety of ventricular as well as supraventricular arrhythmias. It has undergone

Table 38-1
Comparative Mechanisms of Action of Antiarrhythmic Agents

Class I	Class II	Class III	Class IV
a. Quinidine Procainamide Disopryamide	a. Propranolol Oxprenolol Alprenolol Pindolol Timolol Nadolol Acebutolol Atenolol	Sotalol Amiodarone Bretylium Clofilium NAPA Melperone Bepridil	a. Verapamil Diltiazem Tiapamil Gallopamil (D-600)
b. Lidocaine Mexiletine Tocainide Aprinidine Ethimozin Propafenone	b. Sotalol*		b. Bepridil
c. Flecainide Encainide Cibenzoline Indecainide Pirmenol ?			

*Sotalol differs from other beta-antagonists in lengthening cardiac repolarization. Also note that bepridil is a calcium antagonist which differs from other members of the class in lengthening the action potential duration while blocking the slow channel in cardiac muscle. It also blocks the fast channel.

extensive experimental and clinical evaluation, especially in Europe,[27] and is available for IV and oral administration.

Electrophysiologic properties The electrophysiologic effects of aprindine in cardiac muscle relate to changes in both the depolarization and repolarization phases of the action potential. The drug abolishes or depresses phase IV depolarization; its major action is to reduce the upstroke velocity of phase 0, especially at the fast stimulation frequencies and high external potassium concentrations associated with lengthening of the effective refractory period. In intact animals and humans aprindine appears to have a depressant effect at all levels of cardiac conduction, including sino-atrial, atrioventricular, and His-Purkinje, as well as on the anterograde transmission of impulses through the accessory pathways in the preexcitation syndrome. These overall electrophysiologic effects are thus consistent with a wide spectrum of clinical antiarrhythmic action in humans.

Pharmacokinetics The systemic availability of aprindine is high following oral therapy, although 85% to 95% of the drug is protein-bound. Aprindine disposition after single or IV doses may be described in terms of a two-compartment model, but more complex models are required to characterize its kinetics following multiple dosing. In healthy volunteers, $t\frac{1}{2}_a$ was found to be 1.65 hours and the $t\frac{1}{2}_e$ 30.2 hours, whereas in acute myocardial infarction $t\frac{1}{2}_e$ was considerably longer, 59.7 hours. Approximately 85% of the hydroxylated metabolites of aprindine undergoes glucuronidation in the liver; 65% of the drug and its metabolites appear in the urine, the remainder in the feces.[17] The N-desmethyl metabolite of aprindine in small concentrations appears in the plasma of patients receiving long-term therapy and has demonstrated antiarrhythmic actions.[28]

Clinical applications, dosage, side-effects It is of interest that the full antiarrhythmic effect of aprindine may not be manifest for several days despite the administration of a loading dose. The range of therapeutic plasma concentrations of aprindine is narrow (1 to 2 μg/ml), but can be attained with a dose of between 100 and 150 mg daily.[28] Aprindine has been effective in a variety of drug-resistant ventricular arrhythmias and is of particular value in the prophylaxis of potentially lethal dysrhythmias. The drug may also be effective in the circus-movement type of supraventricular arrhythmia, especially those complicating the Wolff-Parkinson-White (WPW) syndrome. The role of aprindine in arrhythmias complicating the late and chronic phases of acute infarction was recently investigated by Hagemeijer et al.[27] The study dealt with a one-year double-blind randomized trial with aprindine (153 patients) compared to placebo (152 patients) following recent myocardial infarction. Entry criteria into the study included the presence of complex premature ventricular contractions (PVCs) demonstrated on Holter recordings. By 12 months, complex PVCs had disappeared in 60% of aprindine-treated patients but in only 25% of those given placebo. The corresponding death rate in the placebo group was 12.5% compared to one of 7.8% in the aprindine group. Although this difference is not statistically significant, the trend indicated that such trials in the high-risk group of survivors of acute infarction may constitute a realistic approach to mortality reduction in this subset of patients.

While the potency of aprindine as an antiarrhythmic agent is no longer in doubt, its narrow toxic/therapeutic ratio should be emphasized. The neurologic side-effects, especially during the initial loading phases, are frequent; as the serum concentration rises to about 2 μg/ml, there is dizziness with ataxia and tremors, and hallucinations become apparent at 3 μg/ml.[28] As indicated above, the drug may reduce the frequency of late postinfarction arrhythmias. This effect needs further critical evaluation relative to the potency of other antiarrhythmic compounds becoming available for investigation.

Mexiletine

Mexiletine, a local anesthetic and anticonvulsant agent, shares close similarities with lidocaine with respect to chemical structure, electrophysiologic effects on nerve and myocardial membranes, and experimental and clinical spectrum of antiarrhythmic actions. However, the drug is orally active since it has a long plasma $t\frac{1}{2}_e$ and is not subject to first-pass hepatic degradation following oral administration. The drug has undergone extensive clinical studies abroad but the evaluation of its efficacy is just beginning in the United States.

Electrophysiologic properties As a class I drug, mexiletine depresses the fast-channel–dependent fibers. The drug has little effect on the normal sinus node automaticity, but it depresses the maximum rate of depolarization (phase 0) in atrial, ventricular, and Purkinje-fiber action potential.[29] As with lidocaine, a marked shortening of the duration of the action potential also occurs, but always to a lesser extent than that of the ERP (effective refractory period).

Clinical pharmacokinetics Mexiletine has high systemic availability following oral ingestion, with peak levels attained in 2 to 4 hours. The t½ in healthy volunteers is about 11.5 hours and ranges between 10 and 26 hours in patients with acute myocardial infarction to whom the concomitant administration of narcotics retards gastric emptying. The metabolism of mexiletine is not completely understood, but occurs largely in the liver, with only 10% of the original dose appearing unchanged in the urine; the renal clearance of the drug is increased by urinary acidosis. About 70% of mexiletine is protein-bound.

Hemodynamic effects As in the case of lidocaine, mexiletine has only mild negative inotropic effects[30] when administered intravenously, with trivial effects on heart rate and blood pressure. The mildly depressant effects on cardiac contractility may, however, be accentuated in patients with myocardial decompensation.

Therapeutic applications The main clinical utility of mexiletine is in the control of ventricular tachyarrhythmias either acutely by use of IV injection or prophylactically following long-term oral administration. However, it is doubtful whether mexiletine has advantages over lidocaine in the acute conversion of ventricular tachycardia except in resistant cases. The main therapeutic role of the drug is in the long-term prophylaxis of recurrent ventricular arrhythmia in the context of ischemic heart disease, especially in the survivors of acute myocardial infarction.

It must be emphasized that the long plasma t½ of mexiletine makes it a desirable agent for testing the possibility that the suppression of ventricular ectopic beats complicating coronary artery disease may significantly reduce mortality from myocardial ischemia.

Dosage and side-effects Therapeutic concentrations of mexiletine (0.5 to 2.0 μg/ml) are usually maintained by daily oral doses of 600 to 1000 mg of the drug administered every 8 to 12 hours in divided dose schedules. For the urgent attainment of therapeutic plasma levels, an oral loading dose of 600 mg may be required; alternatively, an IV loading dose of 150 to 200 mg may be given, followed by either a continuous IV infusion or twice-or-thrice-daily oral doses.

Most of the reported side-effects during the initial administration of the drug persist during maintenance treatment in a small percentage of patients. Neurologic side-effects include tremors, nystagmus, diplopia, dizziness, dysarthria, paresthesia, ataxia, and confusion; GI disorders consist of nausea, vomiting, and dyspepsia. Positive antinuclear factor and thrombocytopenia have been reported, but do not appear to be a common problem. Side-effects appear more often with plasma mexiletine concentrations that exceed 1.5 to 2.0 μg/ml, although the overlap with therapeutic levels is frequent. Cardiac side-effects, including hypotension, bradycardia, and transient AV blocks, occurring with IV administration of mexiletine, have also been reported. Despite these side-effects, mexiletine is well tolerated by most patients and appears to be a suitable antiarrhythmic compound for chronic prophylaxis.[31]

Tocainide is a lidocaine congener which closely resembles mexiletine in its electrophysiologic properties and antiarrhythmic actions. Like mexiletine, it is active following oral ingestion while having excellent bioavailability and prolonged elimination t½. It is still under clinical evaluation as an investigational drug in the United States.

Electrophysiologic and hemodynamic properties There is limited data on the in vitro and in vivo effects of tocainide on cardiac muscle; however, the available data indicate that the electrophysiologic actions of the drug are similar to those of lidocaine and mexiletine.[1] In isolated superfused Purkinje fibers, tocainide decreases the duration of the action potential at 50% repolarization, but more significantly, it depresses the maximal rate of rise of the phase 0 (dV/dt_{max}) of the action potential.

Pharmacokinetics At least 40% of the drug may be exerted unchanged in the urine after oral administration, the actual proportion depending on urinary pH.[32] Because of low hepatic clearance, the hepatic extraction ratio must be small; therefore, tocainide is unlikely to be subject to substantial first-pass effect. Indeed, it is known that in normal volunteers the systemic availability is approximately complete[33]; in patients with cardiac arrhythmias, the drug is rapidly and completely absorbed at dose levels in the therapeutic range.

Peak serum levels occur 60 to 90 minutes after oral ingestion and therapeutic plasma concentrations (6 to 12.0 μg/ml) may be achieved with oral regimens of 400 to 600 mg administered every 8 hours.[33] The elimination t½ of the drug is between 13.5 and 14.7 hours in patients, and a little shorter, 11 hours, in healthy volunteers. Approximately 50% of the drug is bound to plasma proteins at clinical concentrations of the drug, the observed renal clearance of the drug being consistent with the premise that only the free drug is subject to glomerular filtration.[34]

Therapeutic applications, dosage, side-effects The limited available data indicate that tocainide is a potent antiarrhythmic agent for the elective or prophylactic control of ventricular arrhythmias, particularly for long-term suppression.[35] At present, there is no information on the possible role or efficacy of the drug in supraventricular tachyarrhythmias; all the published experience has been in the treatment of ventricular ectopic depolarizations.[35,36] The effective suppression of such arrhythmias was associated with serum levels of the drug above 6.0 μg/ml. The minimum effective range of plasma concentrations is between 3.5 and 7.0 μg/ml, which may be achieved with a total daily dose of between 400 and 1100 mg of tocainide given in two or three divided doses. However, it is often difficult to maintain therapeutic plasma levels on a 12-hour regimen without reaching excessive levels (10 to 15.0 μg/ml) at the peak of the drug absorption, during which central nervous system toxicity may occur. For this reason, an 8-hour dosage regimen might be more appropriate for the maintenance of steady-state plasma drug concentrations throughout the 24 hours.

The patient's tolerance to the drug under these conditions of chronic administration appears satisfactory. Nevertheless, the drug is not totally free of adverse GI and neurologic effects. The most common GI side-effects include anorexia, nausea, vomiting, constipation, and abdominal pain. The neurologic effects are the same as those with mexiletine. However, the drug appears to be generally well tolerated; a number of patients have taken it for many months without significant complaints.

Recently Developed Class I Agents

The newer class I agents (encainide, lorcainide, flecainide, indecainide, propafenone, pirmenol, and cibenzoline), currently under intensive clinical and experimental investigation, are still incompletely characterized. They all share the property of depressing the fast inward sodium current and thereby lengthen the effective refractory period in cardiac muscle. There are differences in the properties of individual agents and undoubtedly in their antiarrhythmic spectrum of activity as well as in their pharmacokinetic properties. As a group they share certain common properties: (1) they have a markedly depressant effect on cardiac conduction; (2) they usually have a potent suppressant effect on ventricular premature contractions; and (3) they have a narrow toxic/therapeutic ratio with a significant potential for arrhythmogenicity, especially in patients with cardiac disease and severely compromised ventricular function. The arrhythmogenicity may relate to the striking propensity to depress conduction and to variably and sometimes differentially (ie, Purkinje fibers vs ventricular muscle) alter myocardial repolarization. At present, there are no data or experience with these compounds in the elderly patient.

Beta-Adrenergic Blocking Agents

An increasing number of new beta-adrenoceptors blocking drugs have recently become available or are awaiting introduction as antiarrhythmic agents. Individual agents will not be discussed because their antiarrhythmic spectra are nearly identical and are apparently not influenced significantly in equipotent beta-blocking doses by their associated properties of cardioselectivity, intrinsic sympathomimetic activity, or membrane-depressant activity, which are present variably in different beta-antagonists (see Table 38-2). The clinician's choice of a particular beta-antagonist for the control of an individual cardiac arrhythmia is thus dictated by the pharmacokinetic characteristics of various beta-blocking compounds (Table 38-3). In the elderly patient, allowance should also be made for the fact that renal and hepatic function decrease as a function of age and that certain beta-antagonists have potentially significant effects on renal blood flow. Perhaps the effect of liver function on beta-blocker kinetics is of more direct clinical relevance in the elderly patient. For example, it has been shown that plasma levels and clearance rate of propranolol, but not of atenolol and sotalol, are related to liver changes. The findings have indicated that the kinetics of beta-blockers eliminated unchanged are independent of the liver and these drugs may be preferable for patients with impaired or reduced hepatic function, as may occur in the elderly patient.

In the case of the elderly patient, it must be emphasized that over and above the issues of altered receptor sensitivity and pharmacokinetics, the exaggerated pharmacologic response to this class of agents may be found in subjects with certain underlying but clinically occult cardiocirculatory disorders. It is known that diseases of the cardiac conduction system increase as a function of age and small doses of beta-blockers may precipitate lapses of conduction in elderly patients with the sick sinus syndrome. Similarly, aggravation of ventricular decompensation is more likely in older patients than in younger for a given degree of beta blockade.

In the last few years a class of antiarrhythmic agents which act by homogeneously prolonging cardiac repolarization has drawn increasing attention as a new approach to the control of a wide spectrum of cardiac arrhythmias. For the present, amiodarone, sotalol, and n-acetylprocainamide (NAPA) appear to be the most promising. Their properties are discussed herein relative to the information available in the literature. The data on other newer class III antiarrhythmic agents is scant.

Amiodarone

Although the antiarrhythmic actions of amiodarone were recognized over 10 years ago,[20] the drug has only recently gained recognition as a potent agent in the control of recalcitrant supraventricular and ventricular arrhythmias.[1] The available data suggest that amiodarone is likely to emerge as the most potent antiarrhythmic agent for the prophylaxis of life-threatening ventricular arrhythmias.[1,37]

Pharmacologic properties Amiodarone is a potent smooth muscle relaxant producing marked coronary and peripheral vasodilation; its initial therapeutic use centered largely on its ability to relieve angina pectoris. Amiodarone produces

Table 38-2
Comparative Pharmacologic Properties of Newer Beta-Adrenoceptor Blocking Drugs

Compound	Beta-blocking Potency (Propranolol = 1)	Cardio-selectivity	Intrinsic Sympathetic Mimetic Activity	Membrane-depressant Activity
Acebutolol	0.3	+	+	+
Atenolol	1.0	+	0	0
Alprenolol	1.0	0	+ +	+
Metoprolol	1.0	+	0	0
Nadolol	3.0	0	0	0
Oxprenolol	0.5	0	+ +	+
Pindolol	6.0	0	+ + +	+
Propranolol	1.0	0	0	+ + +
Sotalol	0.3	0	0	0
Timolol	6.0	0	0	0

0 = absent activity, + = minimal activity, + + = moderate activity, + + + = marked activity.

Table 38-3
Pharmacokinetics of Some Newer Beta-Adrenergic Blocking Drugs Compared to Those of Propranolol

Pharmacokinetic Parameter	Propranolol	Sotalol	Nadolol	Pindolol	Timolol	Atenolol	Acebutolol
Extent of absorption	>90%	>90%	30%	>90%	>90%	50%	>70%
Bioavailability	30%	>60%	30%	90%	75%	40%	20%–60%
Interpatient variations in plasma levels	20-fold	10-fold	7-fold	4-fold	7-fold	4-fold	10-fold
Beta-blocking plasma concentration (ng/ml)	50–100	100–200	50–100	50–100	5–10 ng/ml	0.2–0.5	400–600
Protein-binding	93%	54%	30%	57%	10%	<5%	84%
Lipophilicity	High	Low	Low	Moderate	Low	Low	Moderate
Elimination half-life (h)	3.5–6	7–20	14–24	3–4	3–4	6–9	4–6
Predominant route of elimination	HM	RE	RE	RE (40% unchanged and HM)	RE (20% unchanged and HM)	RE (mostly unchanged)	RE and HE
Active metabolites	Yes	0	0	0	0	0	Yes

HM = hepatic metabolism, RE = renal elimination.
Pharmacokinetic data on some of the newer beta-blockers (eg, acebutolol) are still incomplete and are therefore not discussed.

noncompetitive blockade of α- and β-catecholamine receptors[38] and antagonizes the inotropic and chronotropic actions of glucagon. Chronic oral administration of amiodarone to conscious animals produces bradycardia and reduces myocardial oxygen consumption (as measured by the tension-time index) in a manner analogous to hypothyroidism; the peak effects are not apparent for several weeks following the start of drug therapy.

However, subsequent studies have revealed that the observed changes during chronic therapy are not due to the development of hypothyroidism[39] despite the fact that the compound has almost 40% of its weight as iodine. Transmembrane potentials in the atrial and ventricles of rabbits treated with amiodarone demonstrated homogeneous prolongation of the action potential duration[1] with a trivial reduction in the maximal rate of depolarization and very little effect on isometric contraction. Amiodarone also prolonged the duration of the action potential in the rabbit sinus node preparation[40] while decreasing the slope of the spontaneous diastolic depolarization. These electrophysiologic observations in experimental animals are in general agreement with those in humans.

For example, amiodarone (5 to 10 mg IV) has been found to slow the sinus nodal discharge rate, to lengthen AV nodal conduction time, and to increase atrial and ventricular monophasic action potential duration and refractory periods.[1] The effective refractory period of the accessory pathways in patients with the WPW syndrome is also lengthened by amiodarone—more often in an anterograde than in a retrograde direction.[1] During long-term oral therapy, the drug has produced prolongation of the QT interval in patients with ischemic heart disease[39] and has lengthened the atrial repolarization time as demonstrated by the use of intra-atrial suction electrodes during right ventricular catheterization.[1] Since the uniform lengthening of the repolarization phase in cardiac muscle induced by amiodarone is virtually identical to that produced by hypothyroidism, the question has arisen whether amiodarone might exert its fundamental action by selectively blocking the effects of thyroid hormones on the cardiac muscle, a possibility that was considered over 10 years ago.[20]

It is, however, known that amiodarone invariably increases serum levels of T_4 and of the metabolically inactive deiodination product, reverse T_3 (rT_3), accompanying a small depression in the level of rT_3. The levels of the thyroid-binding proteins are not altered and the alterations in the thyroid hormones are not associated with clinically discernible changes in thyroid state.[41] Particularly intriguing are the consistent increases in the levels of rT_3; serum rT_3 could be related in a remarkably predictable fashion to the antiarrhythmic efficacy and toxicity of the drug. For example, in our laboratory the upper limits of serum rT_3 levels is 50 ng/dl. When the level rises to 55 to 100 ng/dl during chronic amiodarone therapy, there is suppression of the arrhythmia, the level needed for complete suppression varying from patient to patient. Toxicity becomes apparent when serum rT_3 levels exceed 100 to 110 ng/dl. Furthermore, once a steady-state drug administration is reached, and this may take 2 to 5 months, the cessation of therapy is followed by a slow decline of rT_3 levels with an elimination half-life varying between 25 to 55 days. The arrhythmia recurs when the rT_3 level falls below 55 ng/dl; thus the elimination half-life of rT_3 during chronic therapy with amiodarone may be used to monitor therapy with the drug. In our hands, the technic has proved extremely useful in optimizing the full therapeutic potential of amiodarone while avoiding the development of adverse reactions.

Pharmacokinetics Amiodarone has unusual pharmacokinetic characteristics. It has a short $t\frac{1}{2}_e$ after acute administration and its elimination $t\frac{1}{2}$ could vary over a wide range (14 to 120 days) after chronic administration.[42] Tissue uptake studies in humans[43] show that adipose tissue is a major organ of uptake of amiodarone. Since aging is associated with an increased body fat content, one would expect an increased accumulation of the lipophilic drug in elderly patients which might produce toxic effects. Amiodarone is rapidly converted to a metabolite, desethylamiodarone, after a single oral dose and the concentration of the metabolite can approach that of the parent drug during chronic therapy. Preliminary data from our laboratory show that a correlation may exist between the serum desethylamiodarone and clinical efficacy and toxicity while serum amiodarone levels do not seem to be useful in this regard.[44] It is conceivable that the reduced hepatic blood flow accompanying old age will alter the amount and proportion of the metabolite formed and hence the pharmacologic effects. Uptake of the metabolite and the parent drug by the erythrocytes, which has been suggested recently as an index to monitor side-effects,[45] could be altered in the elderly resulting in higher serum concentrations as has been reported for meperidine by Chan et al.[46]

Clinical applications, dose, side-effects Although amiodarone may be administered intravenously, its major utility as an antiarrhythmic agent is in the chronic prophylaxis of recalcitrant arrhythmias. The IV dose is 5 to 10 mg/kg of body weight, administered slowly; the onset of action is in 5 to 10 minutes.

In man, 5 mg/kg of body weight of IV amiodarone has little effect on myocardial contractility, but diminishes peripheral vascular resistance; 10 mg/kg doses reduce left ventricular contractility and elevate the filling pressures, but no serious aggravation of cardiac decompensation has been reported during protracted oral therapy with amiodarone in patients with heart disease.[47] The oral maintenance dose is usually between 200 and 800 mg given once daily, the onset of action following the initial dose being about 4 to 6 hours. The full antiarrhythmic spectrum of amiodarone is still not known, but a number of relatively uncontrolled studies suggest that the drug almost uniformly suppresses all tachyarrhythmias associated with WPW syndrome.[48]

In a recent study, Rosenbaum et al[37] reported "total suppression and control" of supraventricular arrhythmias in 98 of 106 patients (92.4%) and of ventricular arrhythmias in 119 of 145 patients (82%). Further studies involving careful quantitative analysis of Holter recordings before and during drug administration have revealed an extraordinary and sustained potency for the drug to control life-threatening ventricular arrhythmias resistant to conventional antiarrhythmic agents (Figure 38-2). For example, Nademanee et al[49] found that 600 to 1200 mg of amiodarone daily eliminated all complex ventricular ectopic activity and reduced by 95% to 98% all PVCs in 18 patients with symptomatic recurrent ventricular tachycardia or fibrillation, over 50% of whom had histories of one or more cardiac arrests. During a mean follow-up period of about 15 months, episodes of ventricular tachycardia or fibrillation have not recurred and the effects on PVCs have been maintained. These data clearly suggest the need for controlled clinical trials with amiodarone in the high-risk subset of the survivors of acute myocardial infarction.

In the past much emphasis was placed on the side-effects of amiodarone rather than on its extreme potency and long therapeutic half-life. The side-effects cannot, of course, be ignored, but they are reversible. The incidence of GI side-effects, such as nausea, vomiting, and constipation, is small and not particularly troublesome. Of particular significance is the development of a slate gray or bluish skin discoloration, which may regress over many months after amiodarone is stopped. In a very small number of patients, thyroid dysfunction, both hypothyroidism and hyperthyroidism, has been reported.[1]

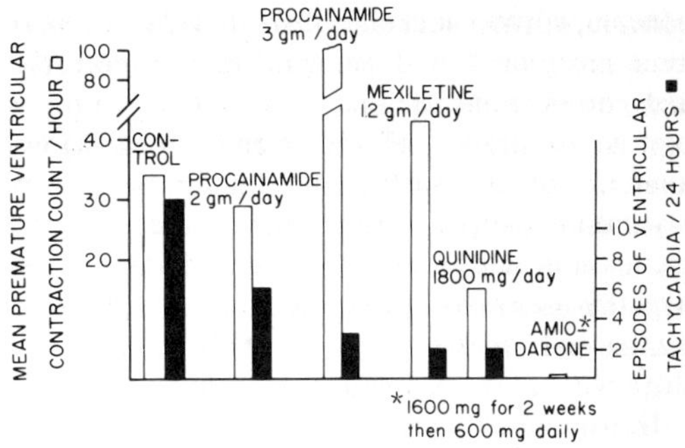

Figure 38-2 Comparative antiarrhythmic effects of amiodarone and conventional antiarrhythmic compounds. Ordinate: mean PVC counts per hour (open bars) and number of episodes per 24 hours of ventricular tachycardia (solid bars). Note the near complete suppression of all PVCs and elimination of episodes of ventricular tachycardia by amiodarone. Conventional agents were less effective.

Perhaps the most consistent and significant complication of oral amiodarone therapy is the development of yellowish-brown granular corneal deposits.[1,50] Such microdeposits do not interfere with vision,[1,50] and are reversible after cessation of therapy. It is also possible to minimize or prevent them either by reducing the dose or by discontinuing drug administration periodically. This also applies to other side-effects such as transient elevations of the serum levels of hepatic enzymes, interstitial pulmonary infiltrates, peripheral neuropathy, and proximal muscular weakness. Despite such side-effects—all of which are usually reversible and have not proved serious—amiodarone clearly has a role in the control of serious ventricular tachyarrhythmias. An appropriate perspective must be developed in the case of a drug that has a clear therapeutic role in malignant ventricular arrhythmias; the incidence of side-effects needs to be balanced against the drug's extraordinary potency not only in recurrent life-threatening ventricular tachycardia and fibrillation but also in most other cardiac arrhythmias.

Sotalol

The antiarrhythmic properties of sotalol need to be distinguished from those of other beta-adrenoceptor blocking drugs. At least in a certain range of dose and plasma concentrations, the drug exerts beta-blocking property and exhibits pharmacodynamic actions characteristic of other beta-antagonists.[51] Thus, one may expect the compound to have an antiarrhythmic spectrum of activity similar to other beta-antagonists. However, unlike other such agents, sotalol consistently and significantly lengthens the action potential duration in all cardiac tissues, especially in doses and concentrations in excess of those producing substantial beta-blockade. This property is associated with a corresponding prolongation in the effective refractory period and hence antiarrhythmic effects over and above those accountable by beta-blockade.

Pharmacodynamic and electrophysiologic properties Both in vitro and in vivo, sotalol exhibits competitive beta-blocking property, with a potency one half to one fifth that of propranolol. It is devoid of sympathomimetic, cardioselective, or membrane-depressant actions.[51] Unlike other beta-antagonists, but in common with other class III antiarrhythmic compounds, in animals as well as in man, hemodynamic studies have indicated that the drug has little or no negative inotropic effect[52,53] even in the presence of advanced chronic heart failure.[54] There is uniform lengthening of the action potential duration with a negligible change induced on depolarization. This action was first demonstrated by Singh and Vaughn Williams[55] and provided the basis for the contention that "isolated" lengthening of the action potential duration constituted a discrete antiarrhythmic mechanism. The clinical electrophysiologic actions are in accord with those demonstrated in the experimental laboratory, representing the summation of effects due to beta-blockade and those induced by the lengthening of the action potential duration and refractoriness.

Pharmacokinetics Sotalol is well observed in man and peak plasma concentrations occur at about 3 hours. The bioavailability of oral sotalol in man is 100% indicating that first-pass hepatic biotransformation does not occur. The apparent elimination half-life of the compound after IV administration is about 7 hours with 80% of the dose appearing unchanged in the urine over a period of 24 hours. In contrast, after oral drug administration, only 55% of the dose is excreted in 24 hours and 73% after 72 hours, with an elimination half-life of about 17 hours.

Sotalol is an ideal drug to study age-related changes because it has very little protein-binding capacity, is excreted unchanged, and does not form metabolites.[56] In a recent study, Ishizaki et al[57] examined the pharmacokinetics and pharmacodynamics of sotalol in young normal and elderly hypertensive patients. They found a prolongation in elimination half-life and a reduction in plasma clearance of sotalol. They attribute the decrease in clearance to impaired renal function in the elderly.[5] Renal insufficiency has been shown to increase the $t\frac{1}{2}_e$ and decrease the clearance of sotalol.[58] Aging is associated with a reduction in cardiac output (30% to 40% between the ages of 25 to 65) and this may also be contributing to the observed decreased clearance of sotalol in the elderly. Ishizaki et al[57] also observed a decrease in volume of distribution while the absorption of sotalol did not change due to age. In comparing the pharmacologic effects, a high correlation between plasma sotalol concentration and beta-blockade was found while the correlation was poor between heart rate and serum sotalol concentrations.

Therapeutic applications, dosage, side-effects The clinical antiarrhythmic effects of sotalol, though predictable on the basis of its electrophysiologic and pharmacologic effects, are still not fully evaluated. However, preliminary data are available establishing the fact that sotalol slows sinus tachycardia, slows the ventricular response in atrial flutter and fibrillation, while converting a significant number of patients to sinus rhythm. Similarly, when given intravenously, the drug converts many cases of paroxysmal re-entrant supraventricular tachycardia to sinus rhythm by inhibiting AV nodal conduction. Furthermore, the drug is effective in terminating or slowing as yet undefined numbers of patients with ventricular tachycardia, and in suppressing premature ventricular contractions after IV as well as after oral administration. Whether the drug also has an arrhythmogenic potential is not known but in cases of overdosage and in association with hypokalemia, atypical ventricular tachycardia (*torsade de pointes*) has been reported in the context of abnormal Q-Tc interval prolongation.[59] The usual IV doses of sotalol range from 1.5 to 2.5 mg/kg. Daily doses have ranged from 360 to 900 mg but side-effects, usually those due to beta-blockade, are frequent and limiting at high doses.

N-Acetylprocainamide (NAPA)

This compound is the major metabolite of procainamide which has been found to have significant antiarrhythmic properties.[60] NAPA has recently attracted much attention because of its unusual and expected pharmacologic features. First, studies in man[61] have revealed that the agent differs significantly from the parent compound in having no class I electrophysiologic effects, its main action being to prolong the action potential duration. This fulfills the definition of a so-called class III agent and as such is expected to have no depressant effect on the myocardium. Second, unlike the parent compound, NAPA has a longer elimination half-life, is excreted essentially by the kidney, and, above all, has little or no propensity to induce systemic lupus erythematosus. Finally, since its dominant pharmacologic property is to produce "isolated" prolongation of the action potential in cardiac muscle, without other associated features (eg, beta-blocking, cholinergic, or membrane-depressant properties), the compound offers unique opportunities for use as a pharmacologic tool to test the significance of action-potential lengthening to control disorders of cardiac rhythm. For these reasons the role of NAPA as an antiarrhythmic compound merits detailed investigation in patients of all ages.

Calcium Antagonists

The spectrum of antiarrhythmic activity of slow-channel inhibitors or calcium antagonists are similar. These compounds are of particular value in the elective and prophylactic control of supraventricular tachyarrhythmias with a limited role in those of a ventricular origin.

Verapamil is the prototype calcium antagonist and has the most clearly defined antiarrhythmic properties. Other agents in the class include gallopamil (D-600 or methoxyderivative of verapamil), tiapamil, nifedipine, and diltiazem. The antiarrhythmic effects of these compounds can be correlated with their electrophysiologic properties which may differ significantly among different compounds and also between isolated tissues in intact animals and man.[62-64] As a class they do not increase the effective refractory period of the atria, ventricle, His-Purkinje fibers, or the accessory tracts in the heart. The dominant action is slowing of conduction in the AV node with the prolongation of the AV nodal refractory period. The most marked changes are produced by verapamil, the least by nifedipine, which is devoid of antiarrhythmic actions.

Verapamil and diltiazem are two calcium antagonists which terminate paroxysmal supraventricular tachycardia and slow the ventricular response in atrial flutter and fibrillation. Both compounds are also of prophylactic value in preventing recurrences of paroxysmal supraventricular tachycardia and controlling the ventricular response in atrial flutter and fibrillation during long-term oral therapy. Their value in ventricular arrhythmias is uncertain but they are unlikely to be effective except in those complicating coronary artery spasm.[64]

In the elderly patient, there are two features of the properties of calcium antagonists which may become of therapeutic significance. First, it is known that these drugs are more depressant on the myocardium and conduction in the setting of pre-existing disease. Thus, the administration of verapamil and diltiazem in the elderly patient with clinically latent myocardial dysfunction or conduction system disease, may lead to the aggravation of cardiac failure or the development of sinus node dysfunction with excessive bradycardia or AV block, complications which are uncommon in younger patients. Second, the alterations in the kinetics of these drugs may produce higher plasma and tissue drug concentrations with longer elimination half-lives.[65] For example, Morelli et al[66] found that the time to peak plasma concentration of diltiazem was longer in the older group of patients than in the younger subjects (5 ± 1 hours vs 3 ± 0.6 hours). They also reported a significantly longer elimination half-life in the older subjects (10.9 ± 0.9 hours vs 6.6 ± 0.1 hours).

The first-pass metabolism of verapamil mainly occurs in the liver and its hepatic clearance is dependent on liver blood flow. Verapamil also has a high hepatic extraction ratio of 0.8. Little information is available on the effects of aging on the pharmacokinetics of verapamil in elderly subjects. One may speculate that aging will exert a significant effect on the metabolism of verapamil by affecting its hepatic clearance and formation of metabolites. In this context it is of interest that Freedman et al[67] studied the kinetics of verapamil in a group of patients with coronary artery spasm whose ages ranged from 32 to 65 years. It was found that the slope of the terminal log-linear portion of the plasma concentration-time curve, determined during a washout after long-term oral administration, correlated significantly with the patients' ages. Older patients demonstrated longer elimination half-lives.

CONCLUSIONS

In recent years, there has been an increase in the number of antiarrhythmic agents synthesized and numerous compounds are currently under experimental and clinical investigation. New compounds have been developed in each of the four known electrophysiologic classes of antiarrhythmic agents. Since the most serious and life-threatening dysarrhythmias occur in patients with organic heart disease, the incidence of which increases with age, it is clearly important to define the age-related effects of antiarrhythmic compounds. Surprisingly, there remains a major hiatus in knowledge about the influence of age on the pharmacodynamics and pharmacokinetics of antiarrhythmic compounds, old and new. An increase in our knowledge in this setting is likely to make antiarrhythmic therapy in the elderly safer and more effective.

ACKNOWLEDGMENTS

This study was supported by grants from the Medical Research Service of the Veterans Administration, and the American Heart Association, Greater Los Angeles Affiliate, Los Angeles, Calif.

REFERENCES

1. Singh BN, Collett JT, Chew CYC: New perspectives in the pharmacologic therapy of cardiac arrhythmias. *Prog Cardiovasc Dis* 1980;22:243–301.
2. Schoken DD, Roth GS: Reduced β-adrenergic receptor activity in man. *Nature* 1977;267:856–858.
3. Greenblatt DJ, Sellers EM, Shader RI: Drug disposition in old age. *N Engl J Med* 1982;306:1081–1095.
4. Geokas MC, Haverback BJ: The aging gastrointestinal tract. *Am J Surg* 1969;117:881.
5. Montgomery R, Haeney MR, Ross IN, et al: The ageing gut: A study of intestinal absorption in relation to nutrition in the elderly. *Q J Med* 1978;47:197.
6. Cusack B, Kelly J, O'Malley K, et al: Digoxin in the elderly: Pharmacokinetic consequences of old age. *Clin Pharmacol Ther* 1979;25:772–776.
7. Divoll M, Ameer B, Abernathy DR, et al: Age does not alter acetaminophen absorption. *J Am Geriatr Soc* 1982;30:240.
8. Norris AH, Lundy T, Shock NW: Trends in elected indices of body composition in men between the ages of 30 and 80 years. *Ann NY Acad Sci* 1963;110:623.
9. Kato R, Vasanetti P, Frontino G, et al: Variation in the activity of liver microsomal drug metabolising enzymes in rats in relation to age. *Biochem Pharmacol* 1964;13:1037–1042.
10. Castelden CM, George CF: The effect of age on the hepatic clearance of propranolol. *Br J Clin Pharmacol* 1979;7:49–54.
11. Vestal RE, Wood AJ, Branch RA, et al: Effects of age and cigarette smoking on propranolol disposition. *Clin Pharmacol Ther* 1979;26:8–15.
12. Epstein M: Effects of aging on the kidney. *Fed Proc* 1979;38:168.
13. Rowe JN, Andres R, Tobin JD, et al: The effect of age on creatinine clearance in man: A cross-sectional and longitudinal study. *J Gerontol* 1976;31:155.
14. Hall MRP: Drug interactions in the elderly. *Gerontology* 1982;28(suppl 1):18–24.
15. Bigger JT: The quinidine–digoxin interaction. *Mod Concepts Cardiovasc Dis* 1982;51:73.
16. Hauswirth O, Singh BN: Ionic mechanisms in heart muscle in relation to the genesis and the pharmacologic control of cardiac arrhythmias. *Pharmacol Rev* 1979;30:5–63.
17. Mason JW, Winkle RA: Accuracy of the ventricular tachycardia induction study for predicting longterm efficacy and inefficacy of antiarrhythmic drugs. *N Engl J Med* 1980;303:1073–1077.
18. The Norwegian Multicenter Study Group: Timolol-induced reduction in mortality and reinfarction in patients surviving acute myocardial infarction. *N Engl J Med* 1981;304:801–807.
19. Singh BN, Venkatesh N: The role of β-adrenergic blockade in the prevention of sudden death and reinfarction in the survivors of acute myocardial infarction. *Am Heart J* 1984;107:189–200.
20. Singh BN, Vaughn-Williams EM: The effect of amiodarone, a new antianginal drug, on cardiac muscle. *Br J Pharmacol* 1970;39:657–668.
21. Singh BN: Amiodarone: Historical Development and Pharmacologic Profile. *Am Heart J* 1983;106:788–797.
22. Freedberg AS, Papp JGY, Vaughn-Williams EM: The effect of altered thyroid state on atrial intracellular potentials. *J Physiol (Lond)* 1970;207:357–370.
23. Kane KA, Winslow E: Antiarrhythmic and electrophysiologic effects of a new antianginal agent, bepridil. *J Cardiovasc Pharmacol* 1980;2:193–203.
24. Platou ES, Refsum H, Myhre ESP, et al: The mode of antiarrhythmic action of melperone. *Adv Pharmacol Toxicol* 1982;50:108–122.
25. Singh BN, Vaughn-Williams EM: A fourth class of antiarrhythmic action? Effect of verapamil on ouabain toxicity, and atrial and ventricular intracellular potentials, and on other features of cardiac function. *Cardiovasc Res* 1972;6:109–119.
26. Singh BN, Hauswirth O: Comparative mechanisms of action of antiarrhythmic drugs. *Am Heart J* 1974;87:367–382.
27. Hagemeijer F, Glaser B, Van Durme JP, et al: Design of a study to evaluate drug therapy of serious ventricular rhythm disturbances after an acute myocardial infarction. *Eur J Cardiol* 1977;614:299–310.
28. Fasola AF, Carmichael R: The pharmacology and clinical evaluation of aprindine—A new antiarrhythmic agent. *Acta Cardiol (Brux)* 1974;107:704–714.
29. Yamaguchi I, Singh BN, Mandel WJ: Electrophysiological actions of mexiletine on isolated rabbit atria and canine ventricular muscle and Purkinje fibers. *Cardiovasc Res* 1979;13:288–296.
30. Saunamaki KI: Hemodynamic effects of a new antiarrhythmic agent, mexiletine (Ko 1173) in ischemic heart disease. *Cardiovasc Res* 1975;9:788–792.
31. Campbell NPS, Partridge JF, Adgey AAJ: Long-term oral antiarrhythmic therapy with mexiletine. *Br Heart J* 1978;40:796–801.
32. Lalka D, Meyer MB, Duce B: Pharmacokinetic studies of 2-amino-2′-6′-propionoxylidide HCl (W-36095) in normal subjects, abstracted. *Pharmacologist* 1974;16:219.
33. Meyer MB, Lalka D, Duce B, et al: Pharmacokinetics of W-36095 in normal volunteers, abstracted. *Clin Pharmacol Ther* 1975;17:240.

34. Lalka D, Meyer MB, Duce BR: Kinetics of oral antiarrhythmic lidocaine congener tocainide. *Clin Pharmacol Ther* 1976;19:757–776.
35. Winkle RA, Meffin PJ, Fitzgerald JW: Clinical efficacy and pharmacokinetics of a new orally effective antiarrhythmic, tocainide. *Circulation* 1976;54:884–889.
36. Woosley RL, McDevitt DG, Nies AS: Suppression of ventricular ectopic depolarizations by tocainide. *Circulation* 1977;56:980–984.
37. Rosenbaum MB, Chiale PA, Halper MS: Clinical efficacy of amiodarone as an antiarrhythmic drug. *Am J Cardiol* 1976;38:934–944.
38. Charlier R: Cardiac actions in the dog of a new antagonist of adrenergic excitation which does not produce competitive blockade of adrenoreceptors. *Br J Pharmacol* 1970;49:668–674.
39. Pritchard DA, Singh BN, Hurley PJ: Effects of amiodarone on thyroid function in patients with ischemic heart disease. *Br Heart J* 1975;37:856–860.
40. Goupil N, Lenfant J: The effects of amiodarone on the sinus node activity of the rabbit heart. *Eur J Pharmacol* 1976;29:23–31.
41. Nademanee K, Melmed S, Hendrickson JA, et al: Role of serum T_4 and reverse T_3 in monitoring antiarrhythmic efficacy and toxicity of amiodarone in resistant arrhythmias. *Am J Cardiol* 1981;47:482.
42. Kannan R, Nademanee K, Hendrickson JA, et al: Amiodarone kinetics after oral doses. *Clin Pharmacol Ther* 1982;31:438–442.
43. Maggioni A, Maggi A, Volpi A, et al: Amiodarone distribution in human tissues after sudden death during Holter recording. *Am J Cardiol* In Press.
44. Nademanee K, Kannan R, Wagner R, et al: Role of amiodarone desethylamiodarone and reverse T_3 serum levels in monitoring antiarrhythmic efficacy and toxicity: Superiority of rT_3 and desethylamiodarone levels. *Circulation* 1983;68:III–278 (abstract).
45. Heger JJ, Prystowsky EN, Zipes DP: Relationships between amiodarone dosage, drug concentrations and adverse side effects. *Am Heart J* 1983;106:887–894.
46. Chan L, Kendall MJ, Mitchard M, et al: The effect of aging on plasma pethidine concentration. *Br J Clin Pharmacol* 1975;2:297–304.
47. Barzin J, Fréson A: Éssais cliniques de l'amiodarone dans les affections coronariennes. *Brux Med* 1969;49:105–109.
48. Rosenbaum MB, Chiale PA, Ryba D, et al: Control of tachyarrhythmias associated with Wolff–Parkinson–White syndrome by amiodarone hydrochloride. *Am J Cardiol* 1974;34:215–223.
49. Nademanee K, Hendrickson JA, Cannom DS, et al: Control of life-threatening ventricular arrhythmias by amiodarone. *Am Heart J* 1981;6:754–768.
50. Geerts ML: Amiodarone pigmentation. An electron microscopic study. *Arch Soc Dermatol Belg* 1971;23:339–351.
51. Opie LH: Drugs and the heart: β-blocking agents. *Lancet* 1980;1:693–698.
52. Frankel WS, Soloff LA: Sotalol: A new safe β-adrenergic receptor blocking agent. *Am J Cardiol* 1968;22:266–272.
53. Lawrie TD, Hutton I, Lorimer AR, et al: Hemodynamic effects of sotalol, in Smart AG (ed): *Advances in Beta Adrenergic Blocking Therapy.* Amsterdam, Excerpta Medica, 1974, vol 1, pp 35–40.
54. Brooks H, Banas J, Meister S, et al: Sotalol induced beta-blockade in cardiac patients. *Circulation* 1970;42:99–109.
55. Singh BN, Vaughn-Williams EM: A third class of antiarrhythmic action. Effects on atrial and ventricular intracellular potentials and other pharmacological actions on cardiac muscle of mJ 1999 and AH 3474. *Br J Pharmacol* 1970;39:675–687.
56. Schnelle B, Garrett ER: Pharmacokinetics of the β-adrenergic blocker sotalol in dogs. *J Pharm Sci* 1974;63:362–367.
57. Ishizaki T, Hirayama H, Tamara K, et al: Pharmacokinetics and pharmacodynamics in young normal and elderly hypertensive subjects: A study using sotalol as a model drug. *J Pharmacol Exp Ther* 1980;212:173.
58. Berglund G, Descamps R, Themis JA: Pharmacokinetics of sotalol after chronic administration to patients with renal insufficiency. *Eur J Clin Pharmacol* 1980;18:321.
59. Laakso M, Pentikainen PJ, Pyorala K, et al: Prolongation of the QT interval caused by sotalol—Possible association with ventricular tachyarrhythmias. *Eur Heart J* 1981;2:353–358.
60. Atkinson A, Lee W, Quinn M, et al: Dose ranging trial of N-acetylprocainamide in patients with premature ventricular contractions. *Clin Pharmacol Ther* 1977;21:575–580.
61. Sung R, Juma Z, Saksena S: Electrophysiologic properties and antiarrhythmic mechanisms of intravenous N-acetylprocainamide in patients with ventricular dysrhythmias. *Am Heart J* 1983;105:811–819.
62. Singh BN, Hecht HS, Nademanee K, et al: Electrophysiologic and hemodynamic actions of slow channel blocking compounds. *Prog Cardiovasc Dis* 1982;25:103–131.
63. Singh BN, Nademanee K: Calcium antagonists and control of cardiac arrhythmias. *Baylor College of Medicine Cardiology Series* 1983;6:6–26.
64. Singh BN, Nademanee K, Baky SH: Calcium antagonists: Clinical use in the treatment of arrhythmias. *Drugs* 1983;25:125–153.
65. Kates RE: Calcium antagonists: Pharmacokinetic properties. *Drugs* 1983;25:113–124.
66. Morelli PL, Rovei V, Mitchard M, et al: Pharmacokinetics and metabolism of diltiazem in man (observations on healthy volunteers and angina pectoris patients), in Bing RJ (ed): *New Drug Therapy with a Calcium Antagonist.* Amsterdam, Excerpta Medica, 1979, pp 152–168.
67. Freedman SB, Richman DR, Ashley JJ, et al: Verapamil kinetics in normal subjects and patients with coronary artery spasm. *Clin Pharmacol Ther* 1981;30:644–652.

CHAPTER 39

The Rational Use of Anticoagulants in the Older Patient: Efficacy vs. Complications

J. Colin Forfar

Although it is over 40 years since Karl Paul Link isolated the hemorrhagic factor from moldy sweet clover hay that was responsible for the hitherto mysterious bleeding disorder in the cattle of Alberta and North Dakota,[1] the place of anticoagulants in the prophylaxis and management of many cardiovascular diseases remains controversial. There is no doubt that their introduction into clinical medicine represented a major therapeutic advance by providing potent agents whose pharmacologic effects could be readily demonstrated and quantified. They offered considerable promise for the prevention and management of many clinical problems, particularly those affecting the elderly, in which thrombosis and/or embolism played a prominent role.

At least three factors have contributed to the controversy. First, anticoagulant therapy has been assessed against a background of change in the natural history and prevalence of many cardiovascular disorders and substantial modifications in their routine clinical management. Both of these factors alter the importance of thromboembolic events in the pathogenesis of disease and hence the value of anticoagulation as a preventive or therapeutic measure. Thus, reports in the 1940s of a 10% mortality rate from pulmonary embolism after myocardial infarction[2] and in the 1960s of a clinical incidence of pulmonary embolism of approximately 5%,[3] are of doubtful relevance to the management of myocardial infarction in the 1980s when early patient mobilization is routine. Second, acceptable evidence for clinical drug efficacy should now be based on prospective, randomized, meticulously controlled and analyzed clinical trials usually using a double-blind design avoiding the recognized pitfalls of data evaluation and interpretation.[4] Few, if any, of the early trials on the use of anticoagulants have fulfilled such criteria.[5] Third, evaluation of the efficacy of anticoagulant therapy has been hampered by lack of uniformity in laboratory evaluation of the clotting defect and recommended therapeutic range. Such variability makes the comparison of reductions in thromboembolic events and hemorrhagic complications of therapy in different series very difficult. It is not widely appreciated that, in general, the coagulation defect for the coumarin anticoagulants recommended in North America (based mainly on the Quick test reagents of animal origin) is significantly greater than that in Europe (based on British Comparative Thromboplastin as a reference thromboplastin).[6] It is, therefore, probable that a component of the variability in drug efficacy and toxicity between different centers will be related to dosage.

Several general theories of aging have been proposed to explain the progressive reduction in absolute organ function associated with a decrease in functional reserve and progressive impairment of homeostatic mechanisms. The rational use of anticoagulants in the older patient requires knowledge of the indications and hazards of drug usage in that patient, coupled with an understanding of the potential influence that age, disease, and concomitant drug therapy may have on the risks and benefits of drug administration. It should be recognized, for example, that although thromboembolic events in the older patient may have profound consequences for the patient and the community, a hemorrhagic complication of anticoagulant therapy resulting in a significant internal or external blood loss is likely to be tolerated much less well in the older patient than in the young.

PHARMACOLOGIC PRINCIPLES IN THE USE OF ANTICOAGULANTS

Heparin

Heparin, the first anticoagulant developed for clinical use, is a highly acidic mucopolysaccharide produced throughout the body but mainly in the lung, liver, and gastrointestinal (GI) tract. Commercial preparations are made from porcine intestine and bovine lung and although they show significantly different properties, this is of little practical significance. The drug is active only when given parenterally, and its major anticoagulant effect is to enhance the activity of antithrombin III (heparin cofactor), a plasma globulin that inhibits a number of serine-active protease enzymes involved in blood coagulation. As many of the enzymes involved in blood coagulation are serine-active proteases, heparin acts to inhibit several steps in the coagulation cascade (Figure 39-1).

Traditionally, this anticoagulant has been administered by intermittent intravenous (IV) injection every 4 to 6 hours or by continuous IV infusion using calibrated infusion pumps. Continuous administration of heparin is widely used and avoids some of the variability in anticoagulant effect resulting from bolus therapy with a short half-life agent (1 to 2 hours). The assumption that continuous administration of heparin improves its antithrombotic effectiveness, however, remains unproven. IV administration of 20,000 to 40,000 units per day (for continuous infusions 5000 to 10,000 units loading dose followed by 10 to 20 units/kg/h for maintenance) is usually required for an established thromboembolism. The low-dose subcutaneous route of administration (5000 units every 6 to 10 hours) may be suitable for primary prophylaxis in high-risk situations, based on accumulating evidence that heparin exerts significant antithrombotic effects in doses that do not significantly modify in vitro blood coagulation.[7] The low-dose regimens tend to minimize hemorrhagic complications and do not require laboratory monitoring. Although evidence for efficacy as a prophylactic agent in this form is varied, they represent a short-term, simple, and safe method of anticoagulant administration that may have particular attractions in the older patient.

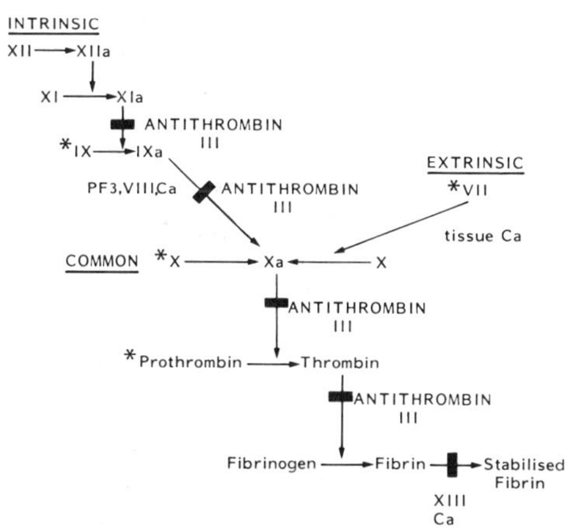

Figure 39-1 Simplified intrinsic, extrinsic, and common coagulation systems. The bars indicate the sites of action of heparin and the asterisks identify factors that are inhibited by coumarin drugs.

For many years, the whole blood coagulation time was used to monitor the in vivo effects of heparin but this has been largely replaced by more reliable and reproducible tests such as the activated partial thromboplastin time or plasma thrombin time.[8] The usual therapeutic range for these tests is two to three times normal. It appears that levels less than 1.5 times the control value are associated with a risk of recurrent thromboembolism. Unfortunately, the risk of bleeding is not clearly predictable, although severe hypertension, invasive procedures, underlying lesions prone to hemorrhage, pre-existing coagulation or platelet defects and prolonged periods of excessive anticoagulation (eg, after intermittent bolus IV therapy) are proposed risk factors for hemorrhage.[9] Testing for the in vivo anticoagulant effect of heparin may be undertaken at any time during continuous infusion but should be done in the hour before the next IV bolus dose. Laboratory control for low-dose subcutaneous heparin is unnecessary as an anticoagulant effect is not usually detectable using conventional coagulation assays.

Coumarins and Indandiones

This group of oral anticoagulants is derived from two basic chemical structures, the 4-hydroxy coumarins and the 1,3-indandiones, and act indirectly on the coagulation system by inhibiting the synthesis of the vitamin K–dependent clotting factors II (prothrombin), VII, IX, and X (Figure 39-1). Although the biochemical basis for their anticoagulant effect is incompletely understood, it involves inhibition of the vitamin K–dependent decarboxylase enzyme system in the hepatocyte, with impaired formation of the normal amino-acid Y-carboxyglutamic acid found at several sites toward the N-terminal end of coagulation factors II, VII, IX, and X.[10] As a result of this inhibition, abnormal analogues are produced that lack calcium-binding sites and are defective in coagulation. The 24- to 48-hour lag period between peak plasma levels of the coumarin-like drugs and peak anticoagulant effect represents the time required for the removal of the preformed coagulation factors from the circulation. The levels of the four factors fall according to their in vivo survival times, being shortest for factor VII, and progressively longer for factors IX, X, and II. The indandione anticoagulants have been largely replaced by coumarin derivatives because of a relatively high incidence of adverse reactions with the former. Warfarin sodium, by far the most commonly prescribed coumarin oral anticoagulant, is well absorbed from the GI tract and an initial dose of 10 to 15 mg provides controlled reduction in the vitamin K–dependent clotting factors over a 36- to 72-hour period. The administration of larger loading doses is unnecessary and may cause rapid reduction of factor VII activity with excessive prolongation of the prothrombin time.[11] Maintenance therapy varies widely between patients, usually in the range of 2 to 10 mg daily and is influenced by complex interactions involving vitamin K availability, hepatic function, plasma-protein binding, co-existing disease and concomitant administration of the drugs. All of these factors may be influenced by age and are discussed in more detail below.

The plasma prothrombin time is used almost universally in North America to monitor oral anticoagulant effect and is sensitive to three of the four vitamin K-dependent clotting factors. Many modified thromboplastins and technical modifications to Quick's original one-stage prothrombin time have been suggested. From the point of view of accurate comparisons between efficacy and risks of therapy between different centers, the most important element in the test is the use of nationally (and preferably internationally) standardized thromboplastins[12] on a blood specimen carefully collected into a polypropylene tube. Thrombotest,[13] based on bovine thromboplastin, is sensitive to depression of factor IX activity but there is no clear evidence that it confers any advantages in monitoring anticoagulant therapy in a routine clinical setting.

The variability in recommended coagulation defect resulting from the use of different thromboplastins is considerable. The optimum therapeutic range commonly recommended in North America for rabbit tissue thromboplastin (eg Simplastin) is 1.5 to 3 times normal. This results in a considerable antithrombotic effect but a relatively high risk of hemorrhagic complications. In view of the reduced therapeutic ratio for anticoagulants in the elderly, a less intensive regime of 1.5 to 2 times normal is recommended. This latter range corresponds to a British Corrected Prothrombin Ratio of 2 to 4 times normal with a similar range using the International Committee on Thrombosis and Haemostasis proposed standardization.[14] It is highly desirable that recommended coagulation defects in different laboratories in Europe and North America are comparable to avoid continuing confusion in the interpretation of trials of drug efficacy and complications.[15]

PHARMACODYNAMIC AND PHARMACOKINETIC CONSIDERATIONS

Age

In 1980, an estimated 11% of the total population of the United Kingdom was over 65 years of age, a proportion that is likely to exceed 15% by the year 2040. The elderly are particularly prone to illness and periods of hospitalization on account of cardiovascular disease and it is therefore appropriate to consider to what extent age per se will influence responses to anticoagulant therapy. This has particular relevance to the interpretation of several studies suggesting that bleeding is a particular problem in the older patient on long-term therapy.[16,17]

Three general mechanisms of altered drug effects in old age have been proposed. First, a change in drug sensitivity with age, ie, a greater response with a given tissue concentration and receptor site occupancy. Second, drug disposition may be influenced by age with altered catabolism and excretion giving a higher concentration at the drug's site of action for a given dose. Finally, some independent change in target organ function, such as increased blood vessel fragility for anticoagulants, may increase the tendency for side-effects (hemorrhage) and therefore reduce the therapeutic ratio of the agent in question. Each of these mechanisms should be considered in assessing anticoagulant usage in the elderly.

In a combined pharmacodynamic and pharmacokinetic study, Shepherd et al[18] suggested that sensitivity to warfarin was increased in the elderly by showing a greater depression of the synthesis of the vitamin K-dependent clotting factors for a given plasma warfarin concentration, compared to younger subjects. The difference was not explicable by a change in clotting factor degradation rate between the young and elderly. Plasma warfarin half-life, volume of distribution, plasma clearance, and protein binding were similar in the two groups. Possible reasons for the age-related increase in sensitivity of the clotting factors to warfarin include a decreased affinity of the system for vitamin K or an increased affinity for warfarin in the elderly. Furthermore, relative deficiency of vitamin K in the older patients could not be excluded. In 177 hospitalized patients, the mean daily dose of warfarin was 40% lower in patients over 70 years of age than for those aged 40 to 50 years.[19] In a cross-sectional study of the influence of age on long-term oral anticoagulant response, Husted and Andreasen[20] showed a greater depression of the vitamin K-dependent clotting factors in elderly patients (61 to 70 years) compared to those under that age. This occurred despite a lower maintenance dose of anticoagulant in the older group. It is thus probable that sensitivity to oral anticoagulants increases with age, necessitating a small reduction in maintenance dosage for a similar coagulation defect. Age per se, however, is a weak determinant of warfarin sensitivity.

The effects of age on heparin sensitivity have not been systematically investigated.

If receptor sensitivity to a drug does not alter with age, changes in drug effect may occur as a consequence of alteration of drug clearance, the major determinant of drug accumulation during multiple dosage. As the clinical effects of the anticoagulant drugs are proportional to their plasma concentration, a reduction in clearance with age would be expected to enhance both therapeutic and toxic effects.

Despite extensive plasma protein binding, the anticoagulant activity of heparin disappears from the apparent first order kinetics, although both clearance and plasma half-life are dependent on dose. This behavior is most readily explained by assuming saturable metabolism with end-product inhibition. A liver heparinase enzyme metabolizes heparin and the inactive metabolites are excreted in the urine. The plasma half-life of heparin is lengthened significantly by renal impairment and hepatic cirrhosis although it may be accelerated in patients with pulmonary embolism because of increased drug clearance. In general, therefore, increased sensitivity to heparin may be anticipated in the elderly as a consequence of reduced plasma-protein binding, reduced hepatic blood flow, or co-existing liver dysfunction, although very few studies have investigated the effects of age per se.

The extent to which the pharmacokinetic consequences of aging alter warfarin absorption, distribution, and elimination remains controversial and incompletely understood. The 40% to 50% reduction in intestinal perfusion and progressive fall in renal perfusion in the elderly[21] are unlikely to be important because the drug is rapidly and completely absorbed from the GI tract and renal excretion of the active drug is negligible. In contrast, however, changes in plasma-protein binding and hepatic metabolism can substantially alter the activity and clearance of warfarin from the body.

Warfarin is extensively protein-bound in plasma and considerable inter-individual differences in binding have been shown. Warfarin binding capacity is reduced in the elderly,[22] probably through an age-related reduction in plasma albumin,[20] and thus an increased anticoagulant effect may be expected through an increase in free drug concentration at the expense of no change or a reduction in total plasma concentration. At the same time, however, and provided hepatic metabolism remains relatively constant, an increase in free plasma warfarin would be expected to enhance warfarin clearance and hence reduce its biological half-life. In a study of the importance of protein binding as a determinant of warfarin clearance and anticoagulant effect, Yacobi et al[23] showed a fourfold variation in protein binding in 31 patients with cardiovascular disease on regular therapy with a corresponding variability in whole body clearance of the drug. The free warfarin concentration did not, however, relate to the concentration of plasma protein, nor did it predict the patients' prothrombin time, highlighting the complexities of the relationship between drug level and biological effect in man.

Although both the function of the hepatic microsomal enzymes responsible for oxidative drug metabolism and hepatic blood flow decrease with age, most studies have failed to show major differences in warfarin clearance between young and older patients.[18] Thus, reduced hepatic clearance of anticoagulants in the elderly makes a minor contribution to the hypoprothrombinemic responses observed. As discussed above, changes in albumin binding and hence free drug concentration are more important determinants of intrinsic hepatic clearance of the coumarin anticoagulants.

On average, lean body mass decreases and adipose tissue mass increases with respect to total body weight in the elderly.[24,25] Although these changes in body composition will alter the distribution of oral anticoagulants, steady-state plasma concentrations during multiple oral dosage should remain constant, since these levels depend only on dose interval and total body clearance. Furthermore, the extensive plasma-protein binding of the coumarins limit the volume of distribution of these agents to that for albumin.[26]

Disease and Drug Interactions

Many reports have detailed interactions between anticoagulants and other drugs,[27,28] and a full discussion of this is beyond the scope of this chapter. Several important principles, however, have particular application to the elderly, because of the increasing prevalence of disease and, presumably as a consequence of this, the increasing frequency of chronic drug administration with age.

A number of diseases are known to be associated with hypoalbuminemia, either as a result of excessive albumin loss or impairment of biosynthesis. In all, an increase in anticoagulant effect for a given dosage may be anticipated.

Coumarin binding to plasma proteins may be impaired by several diseases. Hyperthyroidism, a disease that is prevalent in the elderly[29] and is often associated with cardiovascular consequences requiring anticoagulation, has been associated with an enhanced hypoprothrombinemic response to warfarin.[30] High concentrations of thyroxine can displace warfarin from albumin-binding sites, although protentiation of hypoprothrombinemia may stem predominantly from thyroid hormone–enhanced degradation of clotting factors, rather than changes in warfarin disposition.[31] Hyperbilirubinemia has been associated with an enhanced hypoprothrombinemic response to the coumarins in experimental animals, probably as a consequence of displacement from albumin-binding sites. The importance of this mechanism in the jaundiced patient receiving anticoagulants remains to be determined.

Heart failure is accompanied by an increase in sensitivity to the coumarins.[28] It is unlikely that decreased hepatic perfusion would significantly decrease coumarin clearance because the hepatic extraction ratio for warfarin, for example, is very low (less than 0.5%).[26] Accordingly, changes in hepatic blood flow should not substantially alter its plasma half-life. Indeed, the severity of cardiac decompensation in 19 patients with acute myocardial infarction did not relate to plasma warfarin half-life.[32] It is probable that the increased coumarin responsiveness in heart failure is associated with the redistribution of body water and consequent accumulation of the free anticoagulant at hepatic receptor sites.

Liver dysfunction may increase coumarin responsiveness in several ways. For the reasons discussed above, it is unlikely that diminished hepatic perfusion per se would substantially alter drug clearance. Reduction in hepatic parenchymal function, however, would be expected to exert a more substantial influence, reflecting either a decreased intrinsic coumarin clearance rate, or a diminished capacity of the liver to synthesize coagulation factors, or both. If albumin synthesis was impaired, then a further mechanism for increased responsiveness would exist through increased levels of free coumarin, although clearance rates should also increase. The synthesis of albumin, however, is not markedly decreased until liver damage is extensive and therefore the frequency with which this mechanism is important in determining the overall anticoagulant response is likely to be low.

It has become increasingly apparent in the last few years that patients with poor renal function show higher unbound fractions of highly bound anionic drugs in plasma than patients with normal kidney function.[33] Warfarin binds less extensively to uremic plasma, and the free drug fraction correlates well with the degree of renal impairment and increases as renal function deteriorates. Reduced binding may be due to the presence of endogenous binding inhibitors, or some qualitative alteration in uremic albumin.[34] Although increased coumarin responsiveness has been reported in patients with renal dysfunction,[28] available clinical studies suggest that impaired renal function does not substantially increase the risks of anticoagulant therapy on a pharmacokinetic or pharmacodynamic basis.[35] Nevertheless, further study of the risks of coumarin anticoagulation in the presence of compromised platelet-mediated and capillary homeostasis is required.

There are two major reasons for the relatively high frequency of drug interactions with the coumarin anticoagulants. First, oral anticoagulants are usually administered over prolonged time periods for the consequences or prevention of cardiovascular disease. Concurrent administration of other cardiovascular drugs, diuretics, antibiotics, hypnotics, sedatives, or analgesics is virtually universal at some time during anticoagulant therapy. Second, the coagulation defect can be reliably measured and is of importance for both the therapeutic and toxic effects of this group of drugs. All physicians should be familiar with drug interactions involving anticoagulants as their prediction, avoidance where possible, prompt recognition, and treatment will minimize hemorrhagic complications of therapy.

Three mechanisms of drug interaction have clinical relevance. First, drugs that decrease vitamin K bioavailability will induce hypoprothrombinemia by depression of the synthesis of the vitamin K-dependent clotting factors. Although drugs that bind bile salts or increase intestinal motility should theoretically reduce absorption of dietary vitamin K, there is little evidence that a significant hypoprothrombinemic effect follows their use. Increased sensitivity to oral anticoagulants may also follow the use of several antibiotics, presumably through decreased bacterial synthesis of vitamin K. However, the contribution of bacterial synthesis to vitamin K bioavailability only becomes quantitatively important when dietary intake of the vitamin is poor.

Second, coumarin disposition may be influenced by drug effects on absorption, plasma-protein binding or metabolism. Drug effects on absorption are minor and important only for dicumarol, the only coumarin that is not reliably and completely absorbed from the gut. The most important drug interaction involves displacement of coumarin binding to albumin, with consequent increase in free and therefore biologically active anticoagulant. Such displacement may be competitive, where the drug competes for the same albumin-binding sites as the coumarin, or noncompetitive where a structural change in the albumin molecule is induced such that the affinity or number of coumarin-binding sites is decreased. In general, acidic drugs (ionized at physiologic pH) decrease or displace coumarin binding on a competitive basis, whereas basic drugs interfere with binding on a noncompetitive basis. As only 2% to 3% of plasma coumarins are not albumin-bound, a small increase in their fraction can considerably enhance the anticoagulant effect. Potentiation of the anticoagulant effect is not the only consequence of displacement of coumarins from their binding site as the increase in free coumarin results in its enhanced metabolic clearance from the plasma and therefore shortened plasma half-life. This will cause a decline in total plasma concentration until the free coumarin level returns to that prior to the addition of the displacing drug. Thus the hypoprothrombinemic action is temporary and its magnitude and duration are dependent on the displacing drug, the specific coumarin, and the individual patient. In general, the hypoprothrombinemic effect of warfarin is potentiated within 24 hours, is maximal within 3 to 5 days and returns to the original state within 10 to 14 days, at a lower plasma warfarin concentration. Important drugs displacing warfarin from its binding sites include chloral hydrate, phenylbutazone, ethacrynic acid, and sulfonamides. A schematic representation of the expected changes in anticoagulation with such a drug is shown in Figure 39-2.

Several drugs have been shown to increase the activity of the hepatic microsomal mixed function oxidase enzymes that are responsible for the metabolic inactivation of the coumarins. Induction of enzymes that metabolize coumarins will shorten their plasma half-lives and decrease their total and free concentration in plasma. This has been demonstrated for more than 20 drugs, including most barbiturates, glutethimide, meprobamate, and phenylbutazone.[36] The acceleration of metabolic inactivation will result in an increase in the dose of coumarin required for adequate suppression of clotting factor synthesis with an unpredictable increase in dosage of up to 100% over several days. More importantly, patients whose prothrombin time has been well maintained during administration of an enzyme inducer will develop excessive hypoprothrombinemia and a serious risk of hemorrhage when the inducer is withdrawn. Under such circumstances, an appropriate reduction in maintenance anticoagulant dose must be anticipated. Many enzyme-inducing drugs also modify coumarin binding to plasma proteins and therefore their net effect may be difficult to predict for the individual. A few drugs decrease the rate of metabolism of the coumarins by inhibiting the metabolizing enzymes,[37] but the clinical importance of this type of interaction remains uncertain.

Third, drug interactions may result from drug-induced changes in one or more of the many intravascular, vascular, and extravascular mechanisms responsible for hemostasis other than those dependent on the activity of the vitamin K-dependent clotting factors. Interference with platelet function from the use of aspirin, sulfinpyrazone, dipyridamole, or mefenamic acid and the use of agents causing ulceration of the GI tract directly (aspirin, phenylbutazone, indomethacin) are obvious examples. Such drugs may cause significant bleeding in coumarin-treated patients despite maintenance of the prothrombin time with the desired therapeutic range.

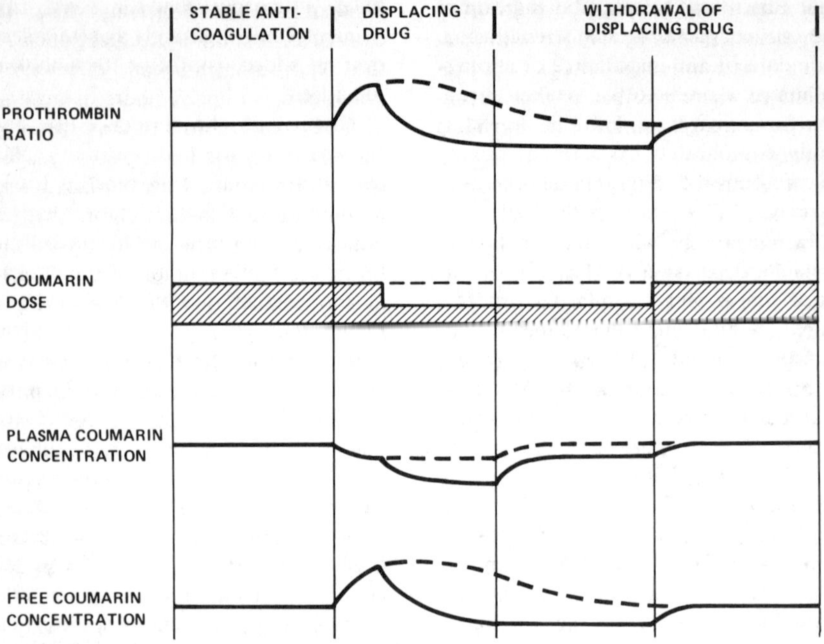

Figure 39-2 Changes in coagulation response and coumarin levels in patients on chronic anticoagulants given a drug that displaces coumarins from albumin. The dotted line shows expected responses when the administered coumarin dose is kept constant.

THERAPEUTIC CONSIDERATIONS

Indications

As discussed earlier, much of the evidence for the use of anticoagulant therapy is based on poorly designed or poorly controlled studies conducted against a background of change in the natural history of many cardiovascular diseases and their management. It must be stressed that the rational use of anticoagulants in the elderly requires careful appraisal of the risks and benefits for the individual and that factors such as severity of disease, coexisting disease, patient understanding, likely drug compliance, and coexisting drug therapy are probably more important considerations than patient age in the decision for anticoagulation.

The effectiveness of anticoagulants in treating deep venous thrombosis and pulmonary embolism has been established for over 20 years.[38] With rare exceptions, patients should receive IV heparin as a bolus followed by continuous infusion for 5 to 10 days. Oral therapy with warfarin can be started concurrently, and heparin discontinued once a stable oral anticoagulant effect has been achieved. The optimum duration of oral anticoagulant therapy has not been determined but most authorities recommend 3 to 6 months if there is no predisposition to thrombosis or history of recurrent disease. Long-term therapy should be considered in such circumstances. Recent evidence has suggested that a less intense oral anticoagulant regime may be equally effective in the prophylaxis of deep venous thrombosis and be associated with fewer hemorrhagic complications. Further evidence of efficacy is, however, required before this recommendation can be routinely recommended.

Patients with congestive heart failure are at increased risk of venous thromboembolism, particularly if thereapy promotes venous stasis through prolonged periods of immobility and bed rest. Early studies have suggested an incidence of pulmonary embolism of up to 16% in patients admitted with heart failure,[39] although at autopsy, pulmonary embolism is even more prevalent.[40] Short-term prophylactic therapy in the hospitalized patient can be achieved by low-dose subcutaneous heparin in a dose of 5000 units every 6 to 12 hours. The effectiveness of this treatment in preventing deep venous thrombosis and pulmonary embolism is established[41] and the risk of hemorrhage seems small. In patients with chronic, recurrent heart failure and cardiomegaly, long-term oral anticoagulant therapy may be justified. With coexisting atrial fibrillation and/or mitral valve disease (discussed below), the indications for chronic anticoagulation are strengthened. There is little data on the importance of etiology of heart failure as a predictor of venous thromboembolism. Severe cardiomyopathies, however, are frequently complicated by both pulmonary and systemic embolism and chronic anticoagulation is indicated.

Thromboembolism is a major cause of morbidity and mortality in chronic rheumatic heart disease, affecting one in five patients.[42] The risk is less in patients with predominant aortic valve disease or mitral regurgitation[43] but both age and coexistent atrial fibrillation are independent risk factors.[44] In patients with mitral stenosis, the incidence of systemic embolism increases from 1% in the third decade to over 30% in the seventh decade.[44] Embolism at the time of mitral valvotomy or valve replacement has been reported in up to 10% of cases.[5] It has been estimated from early series that embolism was the primary cause of death in 16% to 33% of patients who died from rheumatic heart disease. Recurrent embolism occurred frequently in survivors of the first episode with a high mortality within the first year. It has been widely accepted that chronic anticoagulation reduces the risk of thromboembolism in patients with rheumatic heart disease. Long-term therapy is indicated in all patients with mitral stenosis complicated by atrial fibrillation (persistent or paroxysmal), heart failure, or marked left atrial enlargement irrespective of age. Anticoagulation should be considered in all elderly patients with rheumatic heart disease other than mitral stenosis but the risk/benefit ratio is less compelling in this group and the decision for long-term therapy should be based on appraisal of all risks and benefits on an individual basis. As discussed above, age per se should not be considered an important contraindication to chronic therapy.

Atrial fibrillation has long been associated with an increased risk of thromboembolism independent of the severity of any valve lesion. The risk of embolism in patients with nonrheumatic heart disease complicated by atrial fibrillation is less but is increased in the presence of cardiomegaly or coexisting heart failure.[45] Cardioversion is also associated with a risk of systemic embolism which is probably significantly reduced by prior anticoagulation.[46] Atrial fibrillation is a common complication of hyperthyroidism, especially in the older patient, and the risk of a thromboembolic complication may be greater than is generally recognized. Although no controlled studies are available, anticoagulation for atrial fibrillation is prudent (unless strongly contraindicated) whenever an added risk factor for embolism has been identified.

There is no clear evidence that anticoagulant therapy influences early mortality following myocardial infarction, although this is not, perhaps, surprising since death usually occurs as a consequence of the initial infarct rather than of new arterial thrombosis. Systemic embolization from endocardial mural thrombus is a minor contributor to mortality after transmural infarction but is a more important course of morbidity, occurring in some 6% of patients who are not treated with anticoagulants.[47] Autopsy studies suggest that the true incidence of systemic embolization is higher, because some emboli are not recognized and because patients with large infarcts and poor prognosis are at highest risk from thromboembolic complications.[3,5] Venous thromboembolism has been identified using fibrinogen I 125 scanning in over 20% of patients post-myocardial infarction.[48] The incidence is considerably higher where infarction is complicated by heart failure or shock. There is ample evidence that venous thromboembolism is favorably modified by anticoagulation.[5,47] Short-term anticoagulation should be considered in all patients, especially where added risk factors (age, size of infarction, immobility, obesity, previous venous thrombosis) are identified. Like almost every other therapeutic intervention (with the possible exception of beta-adrenoceptor blockade), the place of anticoagulants in secondary prophylaxis after myocardial infarction is controversial. Early trials have been rightly criticized for methodologic inconsistencies.[49] More recently, an important Dutch study from six centers analyzed the effect of discontinuing anticoagulant therapy on mortality and morbidity in ambulant patients over 60 years of age on therapy after a proven infarct at least six months previously.[50] Among protocol compliers, a significant difference in total two-year mortality emerged (placebo 13.4%, anticoagulant 7.5%, $P = 0.02$). Analyzed on an intention-to-treat basis, deaths attributed to recurrent myocardial infarction were also reduced substantially (27 placebo, 11 anticoagulant). Although the incidence of bleeding was higher in the anticoagulant group, none of these events had an adverse effect on mortality. It is of interest that sudden death (defined as death in less than 30 minutes) was not modified by anticoagulation. These results do not necessarily apply to initiation of anticoagulant therapy, rather than its discontinuation, but they underline the need for careful re-evaluation of antithrombotic agents in parallel with those influencing platelets and the vessel wall.

Chronic oral anticoagulation is indicated in all patients following prosthetic valve replacement with the exception of tissue bioprostheses, where the risk of thromboembolism appears to be relatively low. Although no prospective clinical trial has documented the benefit of anticoagulants in patients with prosthetic heart valves, systemic embolism has been documented in up to 50% of patients not on warfarin therapy,[51] and is more likely to occur in patients on anticoagulants when dosage control is inadequate.[52] It is likely that prosthetic valves requiring anticoagulation will be in routine clinical use for the foreseeable future because of doubts over the long-term durability of the biological prostheses.

Hazards

The therapeutic objective of minimizing the risks of thromboembolic complications by anticoagulation must be balanced against the risks of hemorrhage as a complication of therapy. Because of lack of agreement on the desirable coagulation defect and lack of uniformity in assessment and quantification of anticoagulant effect, it is perhaps not surprising that the incidence of hemorrhage has varied widely in reported series from a few to over 40%.[53]

It is probable that the risks of significant hemorrhage in patients receiving IV heparin are greater than for the oral anticoagulants but the consequences are of lesser importance as nearly all of these patients are hospitalized during therapy, the drug has a short half-life, and its anticoagulant action can be readily reversed. It has been estimated that hemorrhage, either major or minor, may be expected once per 100 days of drug administration at a dose greater than 20,000 units per day. Several studies have suggested that the elderly, particularly women, are prone to hemorrhage during heparin administration.[54] As the risk of bleeding is always greater when coagulation is excessively prolonged, particular care is required in monitoring the effect of the drug in this group. Coon and Willis[17] also showed an age-related increase in the frequency of hemorrhage in all anticoagulated patients although the majority (87%) of episodes occurred in hospitalized patients, rather than outpatients (Table 39-1).

In a more recent analysis between 1970 and 1978, age did not appear as a risk factor for hemorrhage in 1362 patient years of out-patient oral anticoagulant treatment. The mean age of 46 patients who suffered a significant hemorrhagic complication of therapy (for which medical advice was sought), 51 ± 10 years, was not significantly different from the group as a whole (541 patients, mean age 55 ± 10 years). Fifty-seven hemorrhagic events were documented with equal frequency in men and women, giving an incidence of hemorrhage of 8.5% among all patients and 4.2% per patient-treatment year. Life-threatening events included fatal intracranial hemorrhage (2 patients), hematemesis and melena (13 patients), and retroperitoneal hemorrhage (7 patients, Table 39-2). In 25/26 life-threatening events, the prothrombin ratio, where known, was prolonged beyond the therapeutic range (Table 39-3). In contrast, however, the prothrombin ratio was known to be prolonged in the minority of patients with less serious bleeding. The risk of life-threatening hemorrhage is therefore minimized by therapeutic levels of anticoagulation, but less serious events are not. The overall success of control of anticoagulant therapy was also a determinant of the likelihood of bleeding. The proportion of patients who bled was significantly higher in those patients with poor overall anticoagulant control (less than 50% of prothrombin ratio estimates within the therapeutic range) than in those where control was more satisfactory (Figure 39-3).[55] No episodes of hemorrhage were recorded in 40 patients followed

Table 39-1
Frequency of Hemorrhage on Anticoagulants in Relation to Patient Age and Sex

	Hemorrhage		Total Sample		Percent	
Age (yr)	*M*	*F*	*M*	*F*	*M*	*F*
0–39	20	30	351	465	5.7	6.5
40–59	60	54	948	824	6.3	6.5
60–69	38	40	479	414	7.9	9.7
70+	22	28	241	216	9.1	13.0

Reproduced with permission from Coon and Willis.[17]

for 193 patient years of treatment where prothrombin estimations were therapeutic on at least 90% of estimations.

An unexpected finding of this study was a durational effect, as far as the risk of hemorrhage was concerned (Figure 39-4). Actuarial analysis[56] of the probability of hemorrhage for each completed year of therapy revealed a significantly increased risk between five and eight years on treatment. The relative risk between five and eight years (0.14 ± 0.03) was over three times greater than the risk in the first three years (0.04 ± 0.01).

A likely causative factor for hemorrhage was identified in just under half of the episodes. Concomitant drug administration was frequently implicated, with aspirin, phenylbutazone, and antibiotics most commonly involved. An intrinsic GI lesion was identified in only four of the 13 episodes of hematemesis and melena, despite routine investigation of all cases by barium studies and/or endoscopy.

Table 39-2
Sites of Hemorrhage During Chronic Oral Anticoagulation

Site	Patients
Life-threatening events	
Intracerebral hemorrhage	1
Subarachnoid hemorrhage	1
Hematemesis and melena	13
Retroperitoneal hematoma	7
Perinephric hematoma	2
Hemoptysis	2
Other serious hemorrhages	
Perinephric hematoma	2
Hemarthrosis	2
Hematuria	7
Muscle/skin hematoma	5
Retinal hemorrhage	2
Epistasis	9
Menorrhagia	3
Mixed	1
Total	57

CONCLUSIONS

The rational use of anticoagulant therapy in the elderly requires careful appraisal of the risks and benefits for the individual, coupled with meticulous attention to maintenance of the coagulation defect within the desired therapeutic range. Patient monitoring should be flexible. Those with

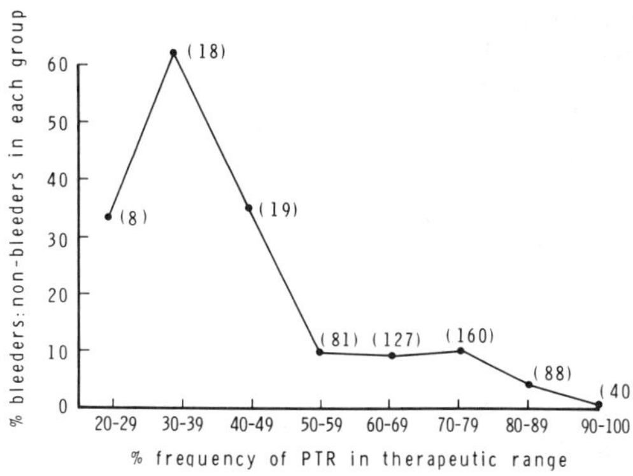

Figure 39-3 Anticoagulant control. Poor control (<50% of prothrombin ratio [PTE] estimations in therapeutic range) is associated with more frequent hemorrhage. The number of patients in each group is shown in parentheses.

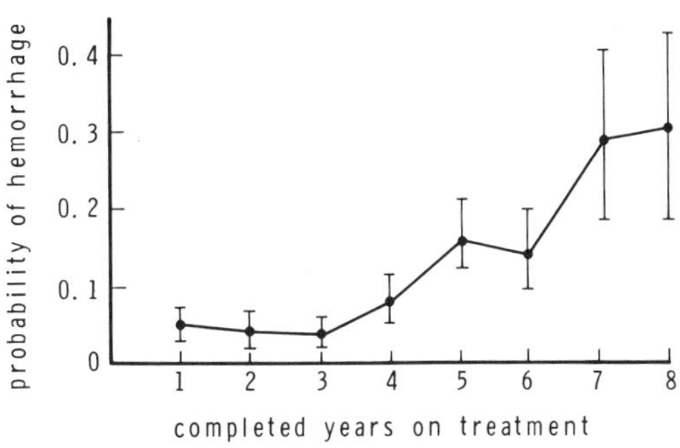

Figure 39-4 Probability of hemorrhage as a function of duration of treatment. The risk of hemorrhage is increased after four years.

Table 39-3
Prothrombin Ratio at Time of Hemorrhage

	Within Therapeutic Range (%)	Beyond Therapeutic Range (%)	Unknown (%)
Life-threatening	1 (2)	25 (44)	0
Not life-threatening	24 (42)	2 (3)	5 (8)
Total	25 (44)	27 (47)	5 (8)

stable coagulation defects and drug dosage have a low risk of hemorrhage and require less frequent estimation of prothrombin activity. Intermittent reinforcement of the precautions required while on anticoagulants, however, should be routine. Patients in whom the coagulation defect has proved difficult to control are at highest risk of hemorrhage and require the closest attention, with, if necessary, hospitalization and intensive pharmacodynamic monitoring. The risks and benefits of treatment may change with time, and periodic reassessment of their value in any individual is required. Much of the usage of these patent agents remains an enigma in that evidence for efficacy is relative and not absolute.

Many of the "grey areas" mentioned above, particularly the use of anticoagulants post-myocardial infarction, require reevaluation using modern, valid trial methodology.

REFERENCES

1. Link KP: The anticoagulant from spoiled sweet clover hay. *Harvey Lect* 1943–44;39:162.
2. Woods RM, Barnes AR: Factors influencing immediate mortality rate following acute coronary occlusion. *Mayo Clin Proc* 1941;16:341.
3. Spain DM, Bradess VA: Sudden death from coronary heart disease. *Chest* 1970;58:107.
4. Mitchell JRA: Anticoagulants in coronary heart disease—Retrospect and prospect. *Br Med J* 1981; 1:257.
5. Rogers PH, Sherry S: Current status of antithrombotic therapy in cardiovascular disease. *Prog Cardiovasc Dis* 1976;19:235.
6. Poller L: Anticoagulants in myocardial infarction. *Lancet* 1981;1:668.
7. Wessler S, Yin ET: Theory and practice of minidose heparin in surgical patients. *Circulation* 1973; 47:671.
8. Wintrobe MM, Lee GR, Boggs DR, et al (eds): Thrombosis and antithrombotic therapy, in *Clinical Haematology*, ed 8. Philadelphia, Lea and Febiger, 1981, chap 52.
9. Martyn DT, James JM: Continuous intravenous administration of heparin. *Mayo Clin Proc* 1971; 46:347.
10. Jackson CM, Nemerson Y: Blood coagulation. *Ann Rev Biochem* 1980;49:765.
11. Deykin D: Warfarin therapy. *N Engl J Med* 1970; 283:691.
12. Loeliger EA: Progress in the control of oral anticoagulation. *Thromb Diath Haemorrh* 1972;28:109.
13. Owren PA: Thrombotest: A new method for controlling anticoagulant therapy. *Lancet* 1959;2:754.
14. International Committee on Thrombosis and Haemostasis (ICSH): Prothrombin time standardisation: Report of the expert panel on oral anticoagulant control. *Thromb Haemost* 1979;42:1073.
15. Poller L: Oral anticoagulants reassessed. *Br Med J* 1982;284:1425.
16. Peyman MA: The significance of haemorrhage during the treatment of patients with the coumarin anticoagulants. *Acta Med Scand* 1958;(suppl 339):1.
17. Coon WW, Willis PW III: Hemorrhagic complications of anticoagulant therapy. *Arch Intern Med* 1974;133:386.
18. Shepherd AMM, Henrick DS, Moreland TA, et al: Age as a determinant of sensitivity to warfarin. *Br J Clin Pharmacol* 1977;4:315.
19. O'Malley K, Stevenson IH, Ward C: Factors influencing anticoagulant control—An epidemiological study in drug interactions, in Morselli PL, Garattini S, Cohen SN (eds): *Drug Interactions.* New York, Raven Press, 1974, p 309.
20. Husted S, Andreasen F: The influence of age on the response to anticoagulants. *Br J Clin Pharmacol* 1977;4:559.
21. Richey DP, Bender AD: Pharmacokinetic consequences of aging. *Ann Rev Pharmacol Toxicol* 1977;17:49.
22. Hayes MJ, Langman MJS, Short AH: Changes in drug metabolism with increasing age: 1. Warfarin-binding and plasma proteins. *Br J Clin Pharmacol* 1975;2:69.
23. Yacobi A, Udall JA, Levy G: Serum protein binding as a determinant of warfarin body clearance and anticoagulant effect. *Clin Pharmacol Ther* 1976;19:552.
24. Bruce A, Andersson M, Arvidsson B, et al: Body composition. Prediction of normal body potassium, body water and body fat in adults on the basis of body height, body weight and age. *Scand J Clin Lab Invest* 1980;40:461.
25. Forbes GB, Reina JC: Adult lean body mass declines with age: Some longitudinal observations. *Metabolism* 1970;19:653.
26. Bachmann K, Shapiro R: Protein binding of coumarin anticoagulants in disease states. *Clin Pharmacokinet* 1977;2:110.
27. Koch-Weser J, Sellers E: Drug interactions with coumarin anticoagulants. *N Engl J Med* 1971;285: 487.
28. O'Reilly R, Aggeler P: Determinants of the response to oral anticoagulants in man. *Pharmacol Rev* 1970;22:35.
29. Ronnov-Jessen V, Kirkegaard C: Hyperthyroidism—A disease of old age? *Br Med J* 1973; 1:41.
30. Self T, Weisburst M, Wooten E, et al: Warfarin-induced hypoprothrombinemia: Potentiation by hyperthyroidism. *JAMA* 1975;231:1165.
31. Weintraub M, Breckenridge R, Griner P: The effects of dextrothyroxine on the kinetics of prothrombin activity: Proposed mechanism of the potentiation of warfarin by D-thyroxine. *J Lab Clin Med* 1973;81:273.
32. Ristola P, Pyorala K: Determinants of the response to coumarin oral anticoagulants in patients with myocardial infarction. *Acta Med Scand* 1972;192: 183.
33. Reidenberg M: The binding of drugs to plasma proteins from patients with poor renal function. *Clin Pharmacokinet* 1976;1:121.
34. Shoeman D, Benjamin D, Azarnoff D: The alteration of plasma proteins in uremia as reflected in the ability to bind diphenylhydantoin. *Ann NY Acad Sci* 1973;226:127.
35. Sachs J, Henderson R: Use of bishydroxycoumarin

in the presence of impaired renal function. *JAMA* 1952;148:839.
36. Conney AH: Pharmacological implications of microsomal enzyme induction. *Pharmacol Rev* 1967; 19:317.
37. Vessell ES, Passananti GT, Greene FE: Impairment of drug metabolism in man by allopurinol and nortriptyline. *N Engl J Med* 1970;283:1484.
38. Barritt DW, Jordan SC: Anticoagulant drugs in the treatment of pulmonary embolism: A controlled trial. *Lancet* 1960;1:1309.
39. Harvey WP, Finch CA: Dicoumarol prophylaxis of thromboembolic disease in congestive heart failure. *N Engl J Med* 1950;242:208.
40. Moran TJ: Autopsy incidence of pulmonary embolism in coronary heart disease. *Ann Intern Med* 1950;32:949.
41. Thomas DP: Heparin in prophylaxis and treatment of venous thromboembolism. *Semin Hematol* 1978; 15:1.
42. Abernathy WS, Willis PW: Thromboembolic complications of rheumatic heart disease. *Cardiovasc Clin* 1973;5:131.
43. Szekely P: Systemic embolization and anticoagulant prophylaxis in rheumatic heart disease. *Br Med J* 1964;1:1209.
44. Casella L, Abelmann WH, Ellis LB: Patients with mitral stenosis and systemic emboli. *Arch Intern Med* 1964;114:773.
45. Askey JM: Embolism and atrial fibrillation, the effect of restoration to normal rhythm with quinidine. *Am J Cardiol* 1962;9:491.
46. Korsgren M, Leskinen E, Peterhoff V: Conversion of atrial arrhythmias with DC shock. *Acta Med Scand* 1965(suppl 431);2.
47. Ebert RV: Anticoagulants in acute myocardial infarction, results of a cooperative clinical trial. *JAMA* 1973;225:724.
48. Wray R, Maurer B, Shillingford S: Prophylactic anticoagulant therapy in the prevention of calf-vein thrombosis after myocardial infarction. *N Engl J Med* 1973;288:815.
49. International Anticoagulant Review Group: Collaborative analysis of long-term anticoagulant administration after acute myocardial infarction. *Lancet* 1970;1:203.
50. Sixty-Plus Reinfarction Group: A double-blind trial to assess long-term anticoagulant therapy in elderly patients after myocardial infarction. *Lancet* 1980;2:989.
51. Duvoisin GE, Brandenburg RO, McGoon DC: Factors affecting thromboembolism associated with prosthetic heart valves. *Circulation* 1967;35(suppl 1):70.
52. Vidne B, Erdman S, Levy MJ: Thromboembolism following heart valve replacement by prosthesis: Survey among 365 consecutive patients. *Chest* 1973; 63:713.
53. Pollard JW, Hamilton HJ, Christensen NA, et al: Problems encountered with long-term anticoagulant therapy. *Circulation* 1962;25:311.
54. Jick H: Efficacy and toxicity of heparin in relation to age and sex. *N Engl J Med* 1968;179:284.
55. Forfar JC: Prediction of hemorrhage during long-term oral coumarin anticoagulation by excessive prothrombin ratio. *Am Heart J* 1982;103:445.
56. Boducer E, Haberman S, Wain WH: Comparative method for actuarial analysis of cardiac valve replacements. *Br Heart J* 1979;42:541.

CHAPTER 40
Thrombolytic Therapy in Myocardial Infarction of the Elderly Patient

Francisco Fuentes
Richard W. Smalling
Charles H. Hicks
Marge Wanta-Matthews
K. Lance Gould

Fifty years have passed since Tillett and Garner discovered the fibrinolytic potential of an extract of hemolytic streptococci.[1] During the last two decades, rapid advances have been made in the elucidation of the structure of plasminogen, plasmin, and some of the activators, particularly streptokinase and urokinase.[2]

The possibility of restoring the patency of vessels occluded by thrombi with streptokinase and urokinase was explored in the late 1960s and 1970s,[3-5] but considerably more progress has been made recently when the thrombolytic agents were administered selectively at the site of the occluding thrombus with angiographic documentation of recanalization before and after the procedure.[6] Although intracoronary infusion of streptokinase in patients with acute myocardial infarction has been found to be the most promising technic for reperfusion and salvage[7-9] of the acutely ischemic myocardium, the role of intracoronary streptokinase infusion has not been defined in elderly patients in whom myocardial infarction is a common problem.

Inherent fibrinolytic activity of patients is subject to great variation. Certain food products,[10] exercise,[11] diabetes mellitus,[12] and atherosclerotic cardiovascular disease[13] all produce some measurable change in the fibrinolytic status of the patient of unclear significance due to inexact analytic methods and their physiologic or practical meaning. Exercise is known to increase thrombolytic activity while diabetes mellitus and atherosclerosis appear to reduce the inherent fibrinolytic activity of the vascular wall. Age has been a factor of controversial importance on fibrinolytic activity of blood. Some authors believe that there is an increase in fibrinolytic activity with age[14] while others have found no changes.[15]

MATERIAL AND METHODS

In order to evaluate the effect of intracoronary thrombolysis in the elderly with acute myocardial infarction and obtain objective data on reperfusion, ventricular function, and mortality, we studied 199 consecutive patients with an acute myocardial infarction after an informed consent was obtained. Patients were excluded from our study only if they had a history of streptokinase allergy, recent cerebrovascular accident, significant valvular disease, recent surgical procedure, chest pain lasting more than 18 hours before admission to our medical facility, or refused this therapy.

The diagnosis of acute myocardial infarction was based on a typical history of myocardial infarction and/or elevation of creatine kinase and/or ST segment elevation in at least two leads. Thallium 201 scintigraphy was obtained prior to coronary arteriography carried out by the Judkin's or Sones technic.

Nitroglycerin 0.1 to 0.5 mg was injected into the stenotic or occluded artery in the distribution of the infarction in order to exclude coronary spasm. If the occlusion or stenosis failed to open after administration of nitroglycerin, a 10,000- to 20,000-unit bolus of streptokinase was injected into the coronary artery followed by a continuous infusion of streptokinase at a rate of 2000 to 4000 units per minute. Coronary angiography was repeated at 15-minute intervals during infusion, or until the artery opened for up to 90 minutes, the maximum infusion time.

After catheterization, the patients were transferred to the coronary care unit. All patients received lidocaine prophylaxis at the time of admission in the emergency room followed by continuous intravenous infusion of lidocaine if there was no contraindication and the drug was well tolerated.[16]

Redistribution images using thallium 201 were obtained 4 hours later, immediately followed by gated cardiac blood pool imaging for determination of left ventricular ejection fraction and qualitative assessment of regional wall motion. In previous studies, we demonstrated that ejection fraction measured by radionuclide technics and by contrast angiography before administration of streptokinase did not change during the 4 hours after infusion of streptokinase,[7] the improvement occurring only days later in patients successfully reperfused. In subsequent studies, therefore, base-line gated blood pool images were obtained immediately after streptokinase therapy in order to reduce delay in reperfusion therapy as much as possible.

All reperfused patients were maintained on dipyridamole, aspirin, propranolol (if tolerated), isosorbide dinitrate, and recently a calcium channel blocker was added. Creatine kinase and isoenzymes, lactate dehydrogenase, and clotting parameters including prothrombin time, partial thromboplastin time, thrombin time, fibrinogen, and fibrin split product were obtained in all patients and repeated every 6 hours for a period of 24 hours. Cardiac enzymes were measured for 2 more days.

Gated blood pool images also were obtained before hospital discharge or before coronary artery bypass surgery 10 days (mean) following admission. We defined elderly for this study as a person who is 65 years old or older.[16] The data are presented as mean values and standard deviations, analyzed for significance by a paired t test for changes between admission and discharge ejection fraction in the same patient, and on unpaired t test for differences between groups of patients.

RESULTS

Our study group comprised 34 elderly patients treated with intracoronary streptokinase. A control group comprised 25 elderly patients with acute myocardial infarction who met exclusion criteria for thrombolytic therapy or refused the protocol and did not undergo coronary angiography. The two groups had identical medical management and radionuclide studies on admission and discharge. A second control group comprised 113 patients younger than 65 years who underwent intracoronary thrombolytic therapy and a subgroup of similar age who did not undergo coronary angiography because of refusal or specific exclusion criteria.

As shown in Table 40-1, the mean age in our elderly study group was 71 ± 5 years old and in the control group 74 ± 6 years old. There were 21 males and 13 females in the study group and 7 males and 18 females in the control group, differences that were not statistically significant. The distribution of anterior and inferior wall myocardial infarction was similar in both groups. In patients younger than 65 years, the mean age was 50 ± 9 in both treated and control groups, with more males than females in the streptokinase group that was significant at $P < 0.005$.

The number of elderly patients with total occlusion was 74% which is similar to the prevalence observed in the group of patients below age 65 with acute myocardial infarction. The number of patients demonstrating reperfusion in the small study group over 65 years old was 56% compared to 76% reperfusion in the younger patients below 65 years old. However, if patients in cardiogenic shock or pulmonary edema were excluded, analysis of the elderly patients in Killip functional class I and II shows that 13 of 17 or 76% were successfully reperfused after thrombolytic therapy, a percentage of success comparable to that in the younger patients.

Sequential changes in left ventricular function using radionuclide ejection fraction (EF) are shown in Table 40-2A and B. The average EF in the elderly was 37 ± 14% on admission and 41 ± 14% at discharge, a change that did not reach statistical significance, however. In the age group below 65 years old with successful reperfusion, a statistically significant improvement in EF was found, 40 ± 13% to 46 ± 12% ($P < .001$).

In nine elderly patients with initial abnormal left ventricular function (EF below 50%), the EF on admission was 31 ± 10% and 36 ± 6% at discharge. Again, those changes indicated some

Table 40-1
Clinical Significance of Intracoronary Thrombolysis

	Patients >65 Years Old				Patients <65 Years Old		
	ICSK		*Control*		*ICSK*		*Control*
Number	34		25		113		27
Age	71 ± 5	ns	74 ± 6		50 ± 9	ns	50 ± 9
Males	21	*P* .01	7		92	*P* .005	15
Females	13		18		21		12
Anterior MI	17	ns	14		21	ns	12
Inferior MI	17		11		61		12
CAO	25 (74%)		–	*P* = ns	84 (74%)		–
Rep	14/25 (56%)		–	*P* = 0.34	64/84 (76%)		–
Rep I–II	13/17 (76% reperfusion)				63/83 (76%)		–
Rep III + IV	1/8 (12.5%)		–		1/1		–
Class III and IV	8/34 (24%)	ns	2/25 (8%)		2/113 (2%)	ns	1/27 (4%)
No. III and IV of total patients (%)		10/59 (17%)		*P* < 0.001		3/140 (2%)	

ICSK = intracoronary streptokinase; CAO = number with total coronary artery occlusion; Rep = number demonstrating reperfusion; Rep I–II = number demonstrating reperfusion in Killip class I and II; Rep III–IV = number demonstrating reperfusion in Killip class III and IV; Class III–IV = number in Killip class III–IV.

Table 40-2A
Left Ventricular Ejection Fraction

	← Admission	*P*	Discharge
Patients >65 years old			
ICSK reperfusion (n = 12)	37 ± 14	ns	41 ± 14
P = ns			
Control (n = 21)	44 ± 12	ns	44 ± 12
Patients <65 years old			
ICSK reperfusion (n = 60)	40 ± 13	.001	46 ± 12
P = ns			
Control (n = 25)	43 ± 14	ns	44 ± 14

ICSK = intracoronary streptokinase.

Table 40-2B
Left Ventricular Ejection Fraction in Patients with Reduced Left Ventricular Function at Admission

	← Admission	*P*	Discharge
Patients >65 years old			
ICSK reperfusion (n = 9)	31 ± 10	ns	36 ± 6
P = ns			
Control (n = 15)	38 ± 8	ns	39 ± 11
Patients <65 years old			
ICSK reperfusion (n = 45)	35 ± 9	.001	43 ± 9
P = ns			
Control (n = 16)	35 ± 10	ns	38 ± 12

ICSK = intracoronary streptokinase.

improvement but were not statistically significant. In 45 younger patients with initial abnormal ventricular function, there was a statistically significant improvement in EF 35 ± 9% to 43 ± 9% ($P < 0.001$).

The cardiac mortality in the elderly was compared between the study group and the control group as well as between patients in Killip's class I and II as shown in Table 40-3. There were 8 deaths out of 34 patients in the study group

Table 40-3
Cardiac Mortality in Elderly Patients

	No. Patients (%)	Benefit Ratio
Cardiac mortality		
Study group	8/34 (24)	
Control	6/25 (24)	1.00:1
Cardiac mortality in class I and II		
Study group	2/27 (7.4)	
Control	4/23 (17.4)	2.63:1

(24%), and 6 deaths out of 25 patients in the control group (24%). However, cardiogenic shock and/or pulmonary edema occurred in 17% of the elderly (10/59) and in 2% of the younger group (3/140), as shown in Table 40-1. When the patients in cardiogenic shock and pulmonary edema were excluded from both streptokinase and control groups, the cardiac mortality in the streptokinase group was 2 of 27 (7.4%) compared to 4 of 23 (17.4%) in the control group. Thus, there was a 2.6 to 1 improvement for survival in elderly patients in Killip's class I and II treated with intracoronary thrombolytic therapy. These differences are not statistically significant, probably due to inadequate numbers as evidenced by comparable changes in the larger group of younger patients where they were significant.

Seven elderly patients who received intracoronary streptokinase subsequently underwent aortocoronary artery bypass graft but none in the control group had bypass surgery. One patient in cardiogenic shock who underwent intra-aortic balloon counterpulsation and intracoronary thrombolytic therapy survived and was discharged from the hospital (Figure 40-1). The rest of the patients in cardiogenic shock could not be reperfused and all died.

DISCUSSION

Over the past several years, it has become increasingly evident that acute myocardial infarction is caused by sudden coronary thrombosis.[9,17]

Intracoronary streptokinase has readily accomplished coronary thrombolysis in younger patients.[6-9] This report is the first time that its use has been investigated in the elderly. Our study indicates that 74% of patients have total occlusion of the coronary arteries. When we exclude patients in cardiogenic shock or severe congestive heart failure, 76% of elderly patients achieve thrombolysis, which is similar to the percentage success in the younger group. Therefore, our data indicate that the patency rate is the same at all ages if patients with pulmonary edema and cardiogenic shock are excluded. We think it is also important to point out that a relatively larger percentage of elderly patients were in shock and pulmonary edema as compared to the younger group where shock and pulmonary edema were uncommon. These findings are comparable to other studies[18] in which fibrinolytic treatment with streptokinase infusion in peripheral arterial occlusion revealed no correlation between success rate and patient's age.

The incidence of bleeding in our group was low with small hematomas identified at the arterial puncture site in only two patients. In order to minimize bleeding the catheter introducers were left in place for approximately 6 hours after the streptokinase infusion and then removed. No anaphylactic or significant allergic reaction were noted in our patients.

DIAGNOSIS OF MYOCARDIAL INFARCTION

In evaluating elderly patients with acute myocardial infarction, a high level of clinical suspicion, elevation of creatine kinase, ST segment changes, and/or presence of new Q waves, and in some patients a resting thallium 201 scan are necessary to make the diagnosis.

Chest pain occurs in 17% to 48% of elderly persons with myocardial infarction.[19] Atypical symptoms such as dyspnea, indigestion, confusion, and restlessness may be the presenting symptoms of acute myocardial infarction. The ECG is useful in demonstrating acute ST-T wave changes. The V_{3R}-V_{4R} and V_7-V_8 leads should be included in patients with suspected myocardial infarction in order to better study the right ventricular and lateral left ventricular walls. In our study, the distribution of inferior and anterior wall myocardial infarction was similar. All patients experienced a significant rise of creatine kinase and its MB fraction.

Previous studies[20] have shown the sensitivity of resting thallium 201 imaging to be 90% to 95% in patients with transmural myocardial infarction imaged within the first 12 hours after onset of symptoms. This is an excellent technic, not only for diagnosis of acute myocardial infarction but to study the residual tissue viability on the 4-hour redistribution images.[21] However, since it shows only perfusion defects it is not specific for recent

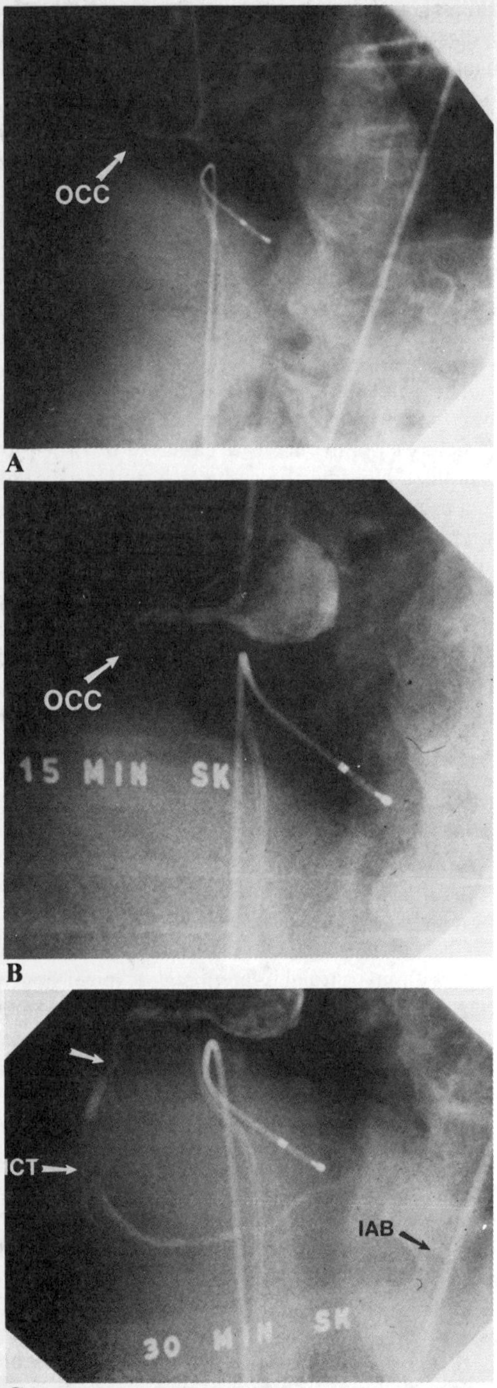

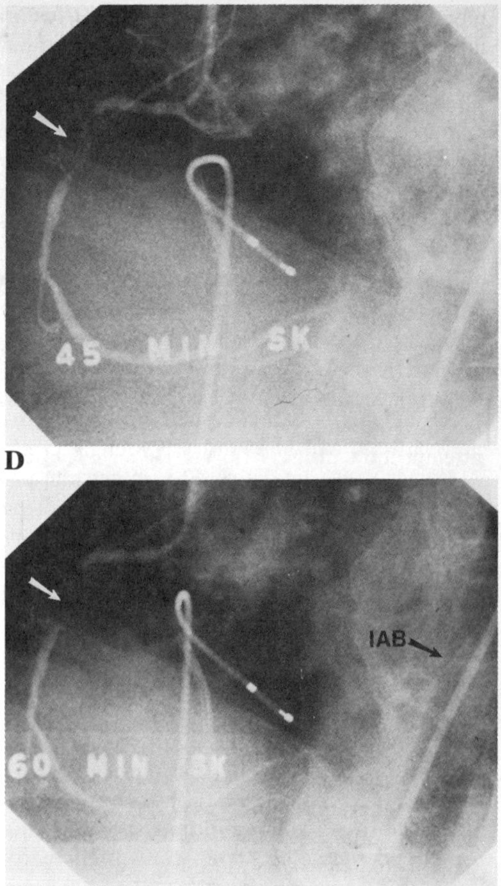

Figure 40-1 Single frames taken from right coronary cineangiogram before (**A**), at 15 minutes (**B**), 30 minutes (**C**), 45 minutes (**D**), and 60 minutes (**E**) post-intracoronary streptokinase infusion in an elderly patient in cardiogenic shock. Arrows designate site of occlusion (OCC), intracoronary thrombi (ICT) and intra-aortic balloon (IAB).

vs old myocardial infarction and may be abnormal with only resting angina, due to low coronary flow without infarction.

CARDIAC CATHETERIZATION

Right and left cardiac catheterization, prophylactic temporary pacemaker placement, and intracoronary fibrinolysis were safely performed in all patients except one who died of stroke while attempting right coronary angiography. A right heart catheterization is necessary to exclude right ventricular infarct and monitor pulmonary diastolic pressure during the procedure. We have routinely positioned a pacemaker catheter in the right ventricle for therapy of arrhythmias.

The risk of intracoronary thrombolytic therapy can be reduced with the above procedure. Our complications rate in all age groups is significantly lower than that reported by other groups.[22]

In elderly patients with associated peripheral vascular disease, the procedure may be technically more difficult requiring either an arm or femoral artery approach. During reperfusion, arrhythmias are primarily premature ventricular beats and rarely nonsustained ventricular tachycardias or complete atrioventricular block. They should be aggressively treated by a pacemaker or with antiarrhythmic therapy as needed.

The procedure should be kept as brief as possible with minimal injection of contrast material and angiographic images reduced to a minimum with left ventriculography avoided if the left ventricular end-diastolic pressure is higher than 30 mmHg. As with most invasive procedures, only well-trained and experienced nurses, radiology technicians, and physician-angiographers should attempt intracoronary fibrinolysis.

Cardiogenic shock has been found to be the most common cause of death in patients hospitalized for acute myocardial infarction.[23,24] When it occurs early, life-sustaining devices such as the intra-aortic balloon counterpulsation should be placed before coronary angiography is performed.[25] Percutaneous intra-aortic balloon placement and subsequent thrombolysis appear to be the most logical therapeutic sequence of steps for treating early cardiogenic shock. In one cardiogenic shock patient in our study (Figure 40-1), intracoronary thrombolysis was successfully achieved after stabilization using intra-aortic balloon counterpulsation. He was discharged from the hospital and remained well and functional 6 months later.

LEFT VENTRICULAR FUNCTION

In the elderly we observed an improvement in left ventricular function that was not statistically significant, probably due to inadequate numbers of patients in the elderly group, since a comparable change in EF in a larger number of patients below age 65 was statistically significant.

In the larger group of younger patients, improvement of left ventricular function at 10 days after lysis of the thrombus was significant at $P < 0.001$, but was not significant in the group without reperfusion.

CORONARY ARTERY BYPASS SURGERY

Although several reports have described aortocoronary artery bypass surgery[26] with a low mortality of 1.6%,[27] there are no reports of early revascularization within approximately 2 to 3 weeks post-myocardial infarction in the elderly. Seven of our patients in the streptokinase group with multivessel disease underwent early aortocoronary bypass without surgical mortality.

The benefits of the surgical procedure should not be denied a vigorous, otherwise well, elderly patient, since the number of vessels involved and the amount of tissue at risk of jeopardy affect the prognosis more than any other factor. When left ventricular function is severely impaired post-myocardial infarction, surgery should be recommended with caution due to the high incidence of complications and deaths.

MORTALITY

The average length of life has risen from 47 to 73 years in this century,[28] with cardiovascular disease being the most frequent cause of death in the elderly. Acute myocardial infarction or one of its complications, congestive heart failure, cardiogenic shock or cardiac arrhythmias, often precipitate the final event.

The prevalence of pulmonary edema and cardiogenic shock due to acute myocardial infarction in the elderly is high. The mortality due to acute myocardial infarction is therefore related to age, ranging from 30% in persons 69 years old to 64% in persons 80 years old.[29]

In our study the prevalence of shock was 17% in the older group but was 2% in the younger group, a fact which explains the higher mortality in the older group. When patients in cardiogenic shock or pulmonary edema were eliminated from our study and only Killip's class I and II were included, the mortality was 7.4% in streptokinase-treated patients with a 2.6 to 1 improvement in survival compared to an untreated elderly control group. This difference is not significant statistically, due most likely to inadequate numbers but, as before, parallels the beneficial effects seen in the larger group of younger patients in whom intracoronary streptokinase significantly improved survival by a comparable and significant amount. The patients in shock or pulmonary edema affect the statistics in this way, because failure to achieve reperfusion is closely linked to shock, pulmonary edema and death.

In this study, acute thrombosis of an atherosclerotic coronary artery was found to be the commonest cause of myocardial infarction in the elderly. The results of our study also suggest that intracoronary thrombolytic therapy may be beneficial for preserving ventricular function and reducing mortality. However, the favorable directional improvements in ventricular function and mortality are not statistically significant probably due to inadequate numbers of patients in our study as compared to equivalent changes in the larger group of younger patients where the beneficial changes are statistically significant. Intracoronary streptokinase therapy does not appear to benefit elderly patients in cardiogenic shock or pulmonary edema.

ACKNOWLEDGMENTS

We are indebted to Greg Freund for technical assistance in carrying out these studies and to Mary Cholakian for manuscript processing.

REFERENCES

1. Tillett WS, Garner RL: Fibrinolytic activity of hemolytic streptococci. *J Exp Med* 1933;58:485–502.
2. Dettori AG: Physiopathological basis of thrombolytic therapy. *J Gerontol* 1971;19:727–742.
3. Boucek RJ, Murphy WP Jr, Sommer LS, et al: Segmental perfusion of the coronary arteries with fibrinolysis in man following a myocardial infarction. *Am J Cardiol* 1960;6:525–533.
4. Boyles PW, Meyer WH, Graff J, et al: Comparative effectiveness of intravenous and intra-arterial fibrinolysis therapy. *Am J Cardiol* 1960;6:439–446.
5. Kordenat RK, Kesdi P, Powley D: Experimental intracoronary thrombosis and selective in situ lysis by catheter technique. *Am J Cardiol* 1972;30:640–645.
6. Rentrop KP, Blanke H, Karsch KR, et al: Initial experience with transluminal recanalization of the recently occluded infarct-related coronary artery in acute myocardial infarction – comparison with conventionally treated patients. *Clin Cardiol* 1979;2: 92–105.
7. Reduto LA, Smalling RW, Freund GC, et al: Intracoronary infusion of streptokinase in patients with acute myocardial infarction: Effects of reperfusion on left ventricular performance. *Am J Cardiol* 1981;48:403–409.
8. Gould KL: New technology for coronary heart disease. *JAMA* 1981;245:689–694.
9. Fuentes F, Smalling RW, Freund GC, et al: New therapy for acute myocardial infarction: Intracoronary thrombolysis. *Texas Med* 1983;79:51–54.
10. Fearnley GR, Ferguson J, Chakrabarti R, et al: Effect of beer on blood fibrinolytic activity. *Lancet* 1970;1:1318.
11. Sherry S, Lindemeyer RI, Fletcher AP, et al: Studies on enhanced fibrinolytic activity in man. *J Clin Invest* 1959;38:810–821.
12. Bogie W, George J, Crane CW: Fibrinolytic activity in treatment of diabetes. *Lancet* 1976;2:312.
13. Peabody RA, Tsapagas MJ, Wu KT, et al: Altered endogenous fibrinolysis and biochemical factors in atherosclerosis. *Arch Surg* 1974;109:309–313.
14. Robertson BR, Pandolfi M, Nilsson IM: "Fibrinolytic capacity" in healthy volunteers at different ages as studied by standardized venous occlusion of arms and legs. *Acta Med Scand* 1972;191:199–202.
15. Hamilton PJ, Douson AA, Ogston D, et al: The effect of age on the fibrinolytic enzyme system. *J Clin Pathol* 1974;27:326–329.
16. Kovar MG: Elderly people: The population 65 years and over, in Health United States 1976–1977, DHEW Pub. HRA 77-1232. Washington DC, Government Printing Office 1977, p 9.
17. DeWood MA, Spores J, Notske, et al: Prevalence of total coronary occlusion during the early hours of transmural myocardial infarction. *N Engl J Med* 1980;303:897–902.
18. Martin D: Age-related problems in the procedure of fibrinolytic treatment with streptokinase. *Aktuel Gerontol* 1978;8:169–176.
19. Harris R: Cardiovascular diseases in the elderly. *Med Clin North Am* 1983;62:379–394.
20. Wackers FJ, Sokole EB, Samson G, et al: Value and limitations of thallium-201 scintigraphy in the acute phase of myocardial infarction. *N Engl J Med* 1976;295:1–5.
21. Pohost GM, Okada RD, O'Keefe DD, et al: Thallium redistribution in dogs with severe coronary artery stenosis of fixed caliber. *Circ Res* 1981;48:439–446.
22. Serruys PW, Van Den Brand M, Hooghoudt TEH, et al: Coronary recanalization in acute myocardial infarction: Immediate results and potential risks. *Eur Heart J* 1982;3:404–415.
23. Scheidt S, Ascheim R, Killip T: Shock after acute myocardial infarction: A clinical and hemodynamic profile. *Am J Cardiol* 1970;26:556–564.
24. Page DL, Caulfield JB, Kastor JA: Myocardial changes associated with cardiogenic shock. *N Engl J Med* 1971;285:133–137.
25. DeWood MA, Notske RN, Hemley ER, et al: Intraaortic balloon counter-pulsation with and without reperfusion for myocardial infarction shock. *Circulation* 1980;61:1105–1112.
26. Gann D, Cohn C, Hildner FJ, et al: Coronary artery bypass surgery in patients seventy years of age and older. *J Thorac Cardiovasc Surg* 1977; 73:237–241.
27. Knapp WS, Douglas S, Craver JM, et al: Efficacy of coronary artery bypass grafting in elderly patients with coronary artery disease. *Am J Cardiol* 1981;47:923–930.
28. Fries JF: Aging, natural death and the compression of morbidity. *N Engl J Med* 1980;303:130–135.
29. Goodman J: *Geriatric: Cardiovascular System, in MKSAP VI. Selected Topic in Internal Medicine.* Philadelphia, American College of Physicians, 1983, pp 300.

CHAPTER 41
Coronary Artery Surgery in Patients Over 65 Years of Age

Bernard J. Gersh
Richard A. Kronmal
Hartzell V. Schaff
Michael B. Mock
Robert L. Frye

Older patients constitute a growing segment of our population with coronary artery disease, and this is the commonest cause of death in the elderly. Many of these patients lead productive lives and enjoy relatively good health apart from severe angina pectoris. Figure 41-1 illustrates the prodigious increase in the numbers of older patients undergoing coronary artery surgery in the United States. Improved surgical technics have reduced morbidity and mortality of coronary artery bypass thus expanding the role of coronary artery surgery to patients at higher risk, including the elderly. At the Cleveland Clinic, patients aged ≥65 years of age constituted 1% of the bypass surgery population between 1967 and 1970 but 12% of those undergoing surgery in 1978.[1] In a large series reported by Rahimtoola et al[2] patients aged ≥66 years constituted 7% of the bypass surgical population between 1969 and 1973, increasing to 17% between 1974 and 1979.

"Tiberius Caesar once said that a man over 60 who holds out his hand [pulse] to a physician is ridiculous" (Plutarch, *Moralia*[3]). Despite this advice, it is clear that attitudes toward coronary bypass surgery in the elderly have changed. It is no longer a question of "can it be done?" but rather "should it be done and if so, in which subgroups of patients?"[3]

This chapter will review the base-line characteristics, perioperative mortality, and long-term results of coronary artery bypass surgery in patients aged ≥65 years, with particular emphasis on the comparison with younger patients. The relative contribution to perioperative mortality and long-term survival of advanced age *alone* and other circumstances *associated* with age will be addressed.

Much of the data to be presented arises from the registry of the National Heart, Lung and Blood Institute Coronary Artery Surgery Study (CASS) of 24,179 patients with suspected or proven coronary artery disease who were admitted to 15 cooperating centers between 1974 and 1979.[4–6] The reader is referred to previous descriptions of the study design, methods, definitions of terms, and base-line data.[4–6] For a list of cooperating clinical sites in the CASS study, see Appendix to Chapter 35, this volume.

In a previous chapter, data on survival of medically treated patients ≥65 years from the CASS study have been presented. It should be emphasized that comparison between medically and surgically treated elderly patients made on the basis of the data presented in these two chapters are not valid because of different base-line characteristics, the time periods of analysis, exclusion criteria, and methods of survival analysis. We believe that comparison of survival with medical or surgical treatment requires, at a minimum, use of the same data base and mathematical adjustment of multiple base-line variables.

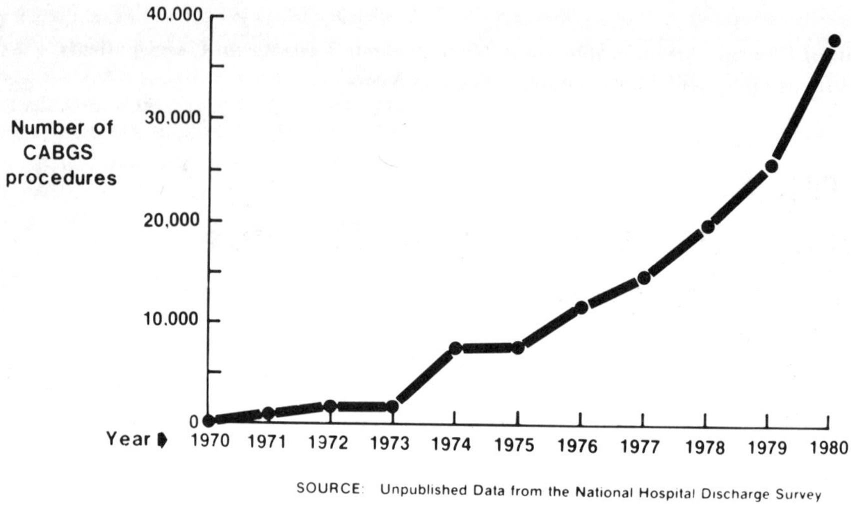

Figure 41-1 The number of coronary revascularization procedures performed in US short-stay hospitals on patients aged over 65 years. (Unpublished data from the National Hospital Discharge Survey.)

BASE-LINE CHARACTERISTICS OF PATIENTS AGED ≥65 YEARS UNDERGOING CORONARY ARTERY SURGERY

Differences in base-line characteristics could influence the results of coronary artery bypass surgery in varying age groups. Direct comparisons of base-line variables in older and younger patients undergoing coronary artery surgery are scanty.[4,7] Table 41-1 compares the preoperative clinical, arteriographic, and hemodynamic status of CASS patients aged ≥65 years undergoing *isolated* coronary bypass surgery with those younger than age 65. Differences between the groups are small, yet highly significant statistically. Older patients are clearly more symptomatic and "sicker" than their younger counterparts; perhaps this is a reflection of a reluctance to select older patients for bypass surgery unless they are severely symptomatic with extensive disease. Others have remarked upon the greater severity of angina and functional disability in older patients.[7-9] The propensity for the elderly to have other medical diseases is obvious and 55% of patients had one or more of the listed medical conditions. Older patients had a greater incidence of unstable angina (69% had rest angina) and features of congestive heart failure. The higher occurrence of triple-vessel disease and of left main coronary artery disease in CASS patients aged ≥65 years is consonant with the severity of their symptoms and with other features reflecting left ventricular dysfunction and cardiomegaly. It is intriguing that far fewer older patients are cigarette smokers (11% vs 34%), probably reflecting the prominent role of cigarette smoking as a risk factor for *premature* death from coronary artery disease.

Knapp et al[7] compared base-line characteristics in patients above and below the age of 70 years undergoing bypass surgery. Older patients had a higher incidence of unstable angina (83% vs 69%), a lower incidence of single-vessel disease, and more left ventricular dysfunction, as evidenced by cardiomegaly and a history of heart failure. The incidence of diabetes and hypertension was equal in the two groups but there were strikingly fewer cigarette smokers among the elderly.

A study of 200 patients ≥65 years of age undergoing arteriography but not necessarily surgery by Boucek et al[10] revealed a 20% incidence of single-vessel disease, almost twice that in the CASS series.[4,10] Discrepancies are likely the result of patient selection since the CASS series was confined to patients undergoing surgery.

Other analyses of coronary bypass surgery in older patients do provide some basis for comparison with the CASS data, despite a nonuniformity of definitions and a lack of comparative information in younger patients within the same institution. In all series associated medical conditions are common, with an incidence of diabetes ranging from 9% to 15%,[7,11-13] hypertension from 14% to 39%,[7,12-14] cerebrovascular disease from 5% to 7%,[11,14] and peripheral vascular disease from 15% to 19%.[8,12,14] In most reports patients

Table 41-1
Comparison of Clinical, Arteriographic, and Hemodynamic Variables in CASS Patients Aged 65 Years or Older and Those Younger Than 65 Years

	Patients <65 yr		Patients ≥65 yr		
Variable	*No.*	*Total (%)*	*No.*	*Total (%)*	*P*
Clinical					
Diabetes mellitus	864	7827 (11)	161	1086 (15)	<0.001
Cerebrovascular disease	187	7827 (2)	37	1086 (3)	<0.05
Peripheral vascular disease	698	7827 (9)	105	1086 (10)	ns
Hypertension	2724	7827 (35)	401	1086 (37)	ns
Chronic pulmonary disease	642	7827 (8)	106	1086 (10)	ns
One or more of the above associated diseases	3945	7827 (50)	595	1086 (55)	<0.01
Present cigarette smoking	2669	7827 (34)	118	1086 (11)	<0.001
Unstable angina	3038	7208 (42)	597	1086 (55)	<0.001
Congestive cardiac failure score ≥3*	234	7827 (3)	86	1085 (8)	<0.001
Basilar rales on auscultation	176	7825 (2)	67	1085 (6)	<0.001
Serum cholesterol >300 mg/dl	579	5965 (10)	58	756 (8)	ns
Hemodynamic and arteriographic					
Cardiothoracic ratio ≥0.50	1192	4850 (25)	235	656 (36)	<0.001
Triple-vessel disease	3619	7818 (46)	660	1086 (61)	<0.001
Left main coronary artery stenosis ≥70%	673	7814 (9)	143	1086 (13)	<0.001
Left main coronary artery stenosis ≥70% and left dominant circulation	48	7827 (0.6)	19	1086 (1.7)	<0.001
Left ventricular end-diastolic pressure ≥20 mmHg	1255	7667 (16)	240	1047 (23)	<0.001
Ejection fraction <50%	1292	5815 (22)	173	788 (22)	ns
Left ventricular wall motion score >10	1529	7549 (20)	250	1033 (24)	<0.005

Reproduced with permission from Gersh et al.[4]
*Score includes the number of positive responses to a history of cardiac failure, the use of diuretics, the use of digitalis, and the presence of pulmonary rales and an S_3 gallop on the admission physical examination (possible score 0 to 5).

with triple-vessel disease predominate, with an incidence ranging from 35% to 67%.[7,12,15] Single-vessel disease was present in a minority (9% to 20%) of surgically treated patients.[7,12,15]

Direct comparison with other large surgical populations is difficult since these contain patients in all age groups. Nonetheless since older patients (aged ≥65 years) account for a *minority* of these series,[1,2] these data may be used as a guide to the preoperative status of a younger population. Severe anginal symptoms and unstable angina are commoner in older patients undergoing coronary artery bypass than in younger coronary surgical patients. The distribution of disease, including left main coronary artery disease, in two large surgical series is not markedly different from that described in elderly patients.[1,2]

If cardiomegaly is used as a guide to left ventricular dysfunction, older patients fare poorly with cardiomegaly present in 36% of the CASS patients aged ≥65 years as opposed to 14% in the series of Rahimtoola et al.[2]

In summary, the *preoperative* status of older patients aged ≥65 years undergoing coronary artery bypass surgery is similar to that in younger patients, but there are distinctions. The older patient is likely to be more symptomatic with angina (including rest pain). Coronary anatomy is not markedly different but triple-vessel disease and left ventricular dysfunction are commoner in the older patient. The differences are presumably related to attitudes toward selection of elderly patients for coronary artery surgery and are subject to change. Attention should be drawn to the frequency of associated medical diseases in older patients since these may strongly influence their early and late postoperative course. These differences in base-line characteristics in older patients undergoing bypass surgery may account for some of the increased mortality reported after coronary artery surgery in the elderly and are addressed later in this chapter.

PERIOPERATIVE MORTALITY

Most cardiologists and surgeons accept the notion that risk of coronary artery surgery increases with age. Perioperative (30-day) mortality was

5.2% in 1086 CASS patients aged ≥65 years, which is significantly greater than the perioperative mortality of 1.9% in patients younger than 65 years entered into CASS during the same time period ($P < .001$).[4] Perioperative mortality was 4.6% in patients aged 65 to 69 years; 6.6% in those aged 70 to 74 years; and 9.5% in 42 patients aged ≥75 years.[4] Nearly all these series cited in Table 41-2 confirm that the mortality of coronary artery bypass surgery is considerably higher in older patients, particularly in those in the 70 years and older age group. The wide range in reported mortality (illustrated in Table 41-2) is likely a reflection of different patient populations, the small size of some series, and the major changes in operating technics and methods of myocardial protection during the last decade.

Analysis of the overall CASS experience showed an impressive relationship between operative mortality and advanced age, particularly in men (Figure 41-2).[24] Similarly, Kirklin et al[20] have emphasized the marked effect of age ≥70 years on operative risk. In contrast, a multivariate analysis by Loop et al demonstrated no independent effect of age on operative mortality.[25]

Operative mortality has progressively declined over the last 10 years[1,2] and in older patients a similar trend is seen, particularly when results during the early "learning phase" of coronary artery bypass surgery are compared with those currently attainable.[2,15,16,18,23]

Complications and Causes of Death

In the CASS series, the commonest cause of death was cardiogenic shock or heart failure (31/57 patients) and approximately one half of these were associated with a definite perioperative myocardial infarction. This corresponds to the experience of others.[9,13,14,16,23,25] Primary arrhythmias accounted for approximately 10% of perioperative deaths and although 16% of patients who died had a cerebrovascular episode during the perioperative period, this was the *sole* cause of death in only two patients. Garcia et al noted a significant incidence of postoperative cerebrovascular accidents in patients aged ≥65 years of 6% with stroke accounting for 1% of early postoperative deaths.[14] Calcification of the ascending aorta may be more severe in older patients and operative trauma producing atherosclerotic cerebral emboli may be a cause of perioperative stroke.[7] Fortunately, most cerebrovascular episodes do not cause a permanent neurologic deficit.

Most observers believe that the incidence of postoperative complications is higher in the elderly.

Table 41-2
Perioperative Mortality in Patients Aged >65 Years Undergoing Isolated Coronary Bypass Surgery

Reference	Dates of Surgery	No. of Patients	Age (yrs)	Perioperative Mortality (%)	Patients Undergoing Other Cardiac Surgical Procedures (%)
Rahimtoola et al[2]	1969–1979	333	≥66	2.1	0
Gersh et al[4]	1974–1979	1086	≥65	5.2	0
Knapp et al[7]	1974–1979	121	≥70	1.6	0
Hamby et al[8]	1973*	17	≥65	5.9	0
Hochberg et al[9]	1971–1979	75	≥70	12.0	0
Berry et al[11]	1975–1979	65	≥70	3.1	9.2
Meyer et al[12]	1969–1974	67	≥70	18.5	0
Gann et al[13]	1969–1975	30	≥70	6.7	0
Garcia et al[14]	1970–1973	265	≥65	3.0	9.8
Du Cailar et al[15]	1970–1978	85	≥65	12.0	0
Ashor et al[16]	1969–1972	78	≥65	2.6	0
McCallister et al[17]	1975*	48	≥70	6.3	unknown
Stephenson et al[18]	1978*	25	≥70	0	0
Berman et al[19]	1976–1978	17	≥70	17.6	0
Kirklin et al[20]	1977	19	≥70	21.1	0
Stringer et al[21]	1969–1975	207	≥65	4.3	unknown
Smith et al[22]	1970–1976	47	≥65	19.1	0
Jolly et al[23]	1973–1979	330	≥65	9.1	0
Tucker et al[26]	1969–1975	67	≥70	4.5	0
Barnhorst et al[43]	1968–1973	27	≥66	3.7	0

Unless otherwise stated, series are confined to patients with *isolated* coronary artery bypass grafting.
*Date of report.

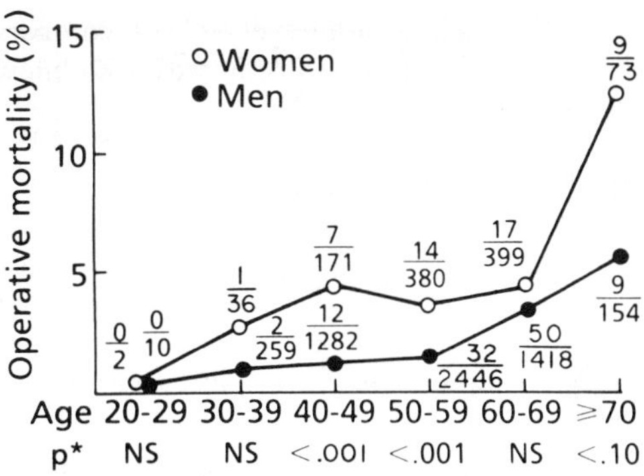

Figure 41-2 Operative mortality by age and sex for 1061 women and 5569 men. Chi-square for trend with increasing age (years); men, $P < 0.001$; women, NS. (Reproduced with permission from Kennedy et al.[24])

In a large series of 119 hospital survivors aged ≥70 years, nonfatal postoperative complications were more frequent than that in younger patients; including stroke (3 patients), supraventricular tachycardia (28 patients), transient psychosis (9 patients), heart block requiring a permanent pacemaker (2 patients), intra-aortic balloon counterpulsation (5 patients), and pulmonary embolism (4 patients).[7] The greater morbidity following coronary artery surgery in older patients is illustrated by the longer duration of hospital stay after operation in comparison with younger patients[4] (Table 41-3).

Predictors of Perioperative Mortality

Estimates of perioperative mortality for an overall group tell us little about those patients who are likely to fare differently from the group as a whole. The CASS analysis attempted to identify subgroups of patients (within the older age group) with favorable benefit-to-risk ratios.[4] Perioperative mortality was strongly influenced by the severity of preoperative angina pectoris. In patients with angina strictly related to exertion, mortality was only 1.7% as opposed to 6.6% in those with rest angina. Patients with stable angina had an operative mortality of 2.9% but this was 7% in those with unstable angina. In contrast to the overall CASS data which incorporated mainly younger patients, mortality of those aged ≥65 years did not differ between the sexes. This was 4.7% in men vs 6.9% in women (ns). Other variables obtained from the clinical history and base-line examination which were associated with an increased operative mortality were the presence of intercurrent medical diseases, current cigarette smoking, and features of congestive heart failure. The presence of one or more associated medical conditions (Table 41-1) increased perioperative mortality to 6.6% in comparison to 3.5% in those without any of these diseases.

Tables 41-4 and 41-5 illustrate the influence of the preoperative hemodynamic and arteriographic status on operative mortality in older patients.[4] Those with relatively well-preserved ventricular function without cardiomegaly or marked elevation of left ventricular end-diastolic pressure enjoy a relatively low operative risk. This conforms with other studies of large surgical populations which emphasized the potent influence of left ventricular dysfunction on survival.[1,2,25,27,28] Not surprisingly the extent of coronary disease does influence perioperative mortality (Table 41-5) but is overshadowed by the consequences of severe stenosis of the left main coronary artery and in particular, the uncommon but lethal combination of left main coronary artery disease in a left dominant circulation. The potential hazard of coronary surgery in patients with left main coronary artery disease has been stressed by others[29,30,32] and it is likely that these lesions or combination of

Table 41-3
Duration of Hospital Stay After Coronary Artery Bypass Surgery in Survivors According to Age

Age (yr)	Days (mean) ± SEM	P
65–69	12.9 ± 0.2	
70–74	14.0 ± 0.5	< 0.005
75–84	16.5 ± 1.8	
≥65	13.3 ± 0.2	<0.001
<65	11.4 ± 0.9	

Reproduced with permission from Gersh et al.[4]

Table 41-4
Perioperative Mortality: Associated Hemodynamic Variables

Variable	No. Patients (%)	P
Cardiothoracic ratio		
<0.50	14/421 (3.3)	<0.04
≥0.50	16/235 (6.8)	
Left ventricular end-diastolic pressure		
<20 mmHg	34/807 (4.2)	<0.02
≥20 mmHg	20/240 (8.3)	
Ejection fraction		
≥50%	25/615 (4.1	<0.02
<50%	15/173 (8.7)	

Reproduced with permission from Gersh et al.[4]

Table 41-5
Perioperative Mortality: Associated Arteriographic Variables

Variable	No. Patients (%)	*P*
Gensini score		
<200	18/509 (3.5)	<0.03
≥200	39/569 (6.9)	
Left main coronary artery stenosis		
<70%	43/943 (4.6)	<0.03
≥70%	17/143 (11.9)	
≥70% and left dominant circulation	8/19 (42.1)	<0.01
≥70% and right dominant or balanced circulation	9/124 (7.3)	

Reproduced with permission from Gersh et al.[4]

lesions are commoner in the elderly (see Table 41-1).

Understandably the priority of surgery is related to outcome. In patients aged ≥65 years undergoing *elective* surgery operative mortality was 3.9% but mortality for emergency surgery was 13.7%.[4] Operative mortality was not influenced by the number of grafts inserted nor by the number of distal anastomoses per patient. In summary the determinants of perioperative mortality in the elderly are similar to those previously shown to be influential in large surgical populations consisting of mainly younger patients.[2,24,25,27,31] Ventricular dysfunction and heart failure, left main coronary artery disease, the severity of symptoms, the priority of the procedure, and intercurrent medical diseases exert their toll in *all* age groups.[4] Yet, the operative risks remain higher in the older patient, even in low-risk categories.[24,31]

LONG-TERM RESULTS OF CORONARY ARTERY BYPASS SURGERY

The cumulative five-year survival of 1086 CASS patients ≥65 years of age undergoing coronary artery surgery is compared to 7827 patients aged <65 years in Figure 41-3.[5] Five-year survival was 91% and 83%, respectively, in the two groups. The greatest difference in mortality is early in the first year reflecting perioperative deaths, and the subsequent rate of attrition remains slightly greater in the older group. Figure 41-4 demonstrates that five-year survival is related to age (even within the older age group) with the major impact again on perioperative mortality. In

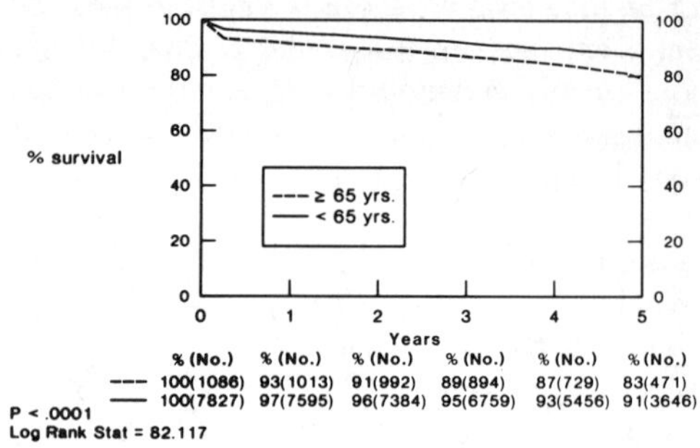

Figure 41-3 Comparison of cumulative five-year survival of patients aged 65 years or older and those younger than 65 years. (Reproduced with permission from Gersh et al.[5])

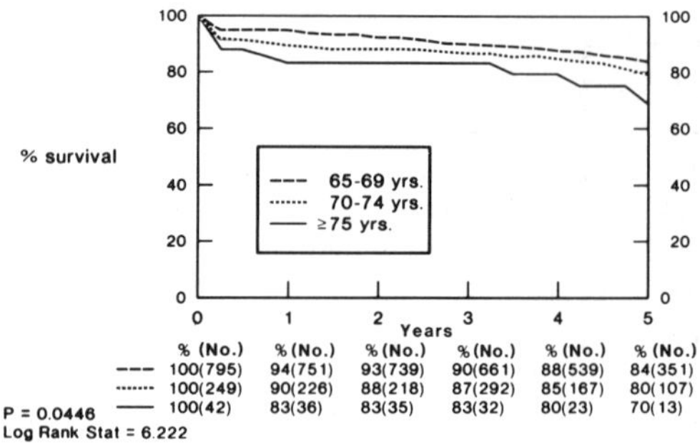

Figure 41-4 Cumulative five-year survival of patients aged 65 years or older. Three groups are shown on the basis of age: 65 to 69 years, 70 to 74 years, and 75 years or older. (Reproduced with permission from Gersh et al.[5])

30-day surgical survivors, subsequent five-year survival was 88%, 85%, and 77%, respectively, in the three age groups: 65 to 69 years, 70 to 74 years, and age ≥75 years.[5] Survival was similar in men and women, being 82% and 85% respectively.

Comparison with other surgical populations of older patients is limited by the short duration of follow-up and a lack of actuarially determined survivorship in many studies.[11-14,16,17,19] Du Cailar et al reported an 80% five-year survival in patients aged 65 years or older.[15] Hochberg et al reported a five-year survival of 85% in patients aged 70 years or older.[9] Better survival rates in older patients are attainable. Survival was 95% for patients above and below the age of 70 years in one series,[7] and 93% at two years in another.[18] Five-year survival in 260 patients reported by Rahimtoola et al[33] in patients aged 66 years or older with unstable angina was 84%, remarkably similar to the CASS data. Subsequent attrition was low with the probability of survival at 10 years being 79%.[33]

That long-term prognosis is related to age is evident from the bulk of available data. What is more surprising but welcome are the excellent long-term results reported in several series of coronary bypass surgery in older patients.

Causes of Death

Table 41-6 lists the causes of death in 30-day surgical survivors in the CASS series.[5] There are statistically significant differences between the causes of death in the two age groups which may be explained in part by the increased incidence of intercurrent medical diseases in the elderly and their vulnerability to the subsequent development of other illnesses. Noncardiac deaths related to atherosclerotic disease and other noncardiac causes of death accounted for 45% of deaths in older patients but only 28% in the younger group. Cardiac deaths including sudden death, accounted for 53% and 69% of deaths in the respective groups. At least 37% of deaths in *all* age groups were noncardiac.

Preoperative Determinants of Late Survival (Patients <65 years)

Intercurrent medical diseases Figure 41-5 illustrates the pronounced impact of other medical conditions on both preoperative and late mortality. Five-year survival was 89% in older patients without any associated medical disease, falling to 71% in those with two or more diseases. The influence of intercurrent illnesses on the long-term results of coronary artery surgery has previously received little emphasis. One look at the causes of death after coronary artery surgery (Table 41-3) draws attention to this oversight, particularly in older patients. Hypertension had no effect on perioperative mortality but strongly influenced the subsequent attrition rate.[5] Hypertensive elderly individuals have a substantially greater incidence of stroke, coronary artery disease, and congestive heart failure than their normotensive counterparts, and longevity after bypass surgery is reduced.[5,34] Treatment of hypertension in this postsurgical population (in whom drug control is often more difficult) would appear to be prudent.[35]

Number of vessels diseased Neither the number of vessels diseased (Figure 41-6) nor the number of grafts significantly influenced five-year survival in this series of older patients. However, there is a trend suggesting diminished survival in

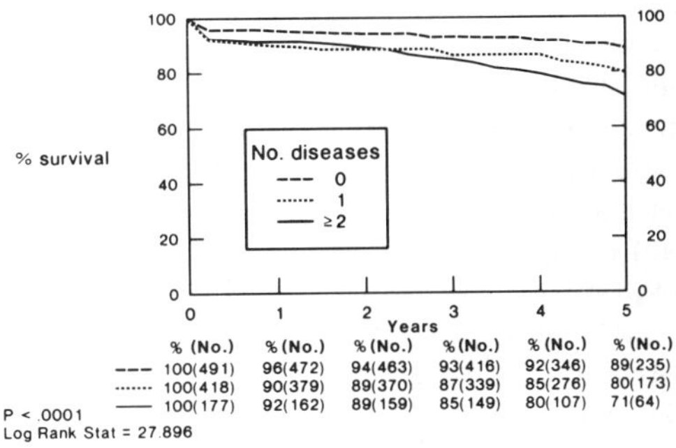

Figure 41-5 Cumulative five-year survival of patients aged 65 years or older. Three groups are shown on the basis of the number of associated medical diseases: none, one, and two or more associated medical diseases. Diseases included are diabetes mellitus, cerebrovascular disease, peripheral vascular disease, hypertension, and chronic pulmonary disease. (Reproduced with permission from Gersh et al.[5])

Table 41-6
Causes of Late Death in 30-Day Surgical Survivors

Cause of Death*	Age <65 yr *No. of Patients (%)*	Age >65 yr *No. of Patients (%)*
Cardiac direct	279 (51)	53 (40)
Cardiac contributory	45 (8)	11 (8)
Sudden unexplained	58 (10)	6 (5)
Noncardiac but related to arteriosclerotic vascular disease	26 (5)	18 (14)
Noncardiac *not* related to arteriosclerotic vascular disease	131 (23)	41 (31)
Suicide	4 (1)	0 (0)
Unknown	9 (2)	2 (2)
Total late deaths	552	131

*For definitions, see Principal Investigators of CASS and Their Associates.[6]
Reproduced with permission from Gersh et al.[5]

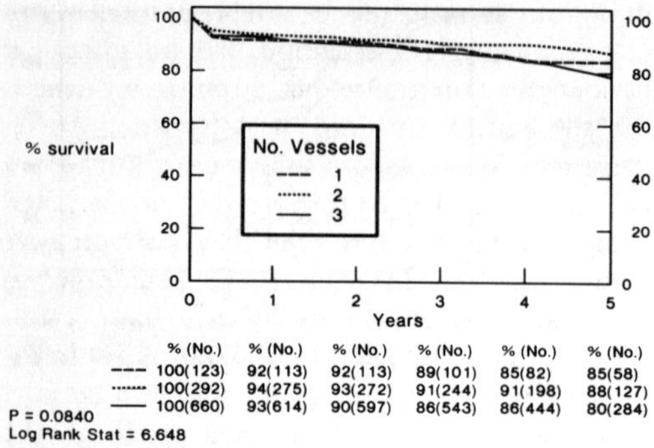

Figure 41-6 Cumulative five-year survival in patients aged 65 years or older categorized by the number of vessels diseased. (Reproduced with permission from Gersh et al.[5])

patients with triple-vessel disease. It is likely that the trend toward more extensive revascularization minimizes the independent effect of multivessel disease on long-term survival, at least over a 5- to 10-year period.[33,36,37] Adequate vascularization is certainly achievable in older patients and the 2.6 grafts inserted per patient compares with other large series.[5]

Left ventricular dysfunction The profound effect of ventricular dysfunction on survival is shown in Figures 41-7A and B. Five-year survival was 88% in those with an ejection fraction of ≥50%; 79% in those with an ejection fraction of 36% to 50%; and only 47% in patients with an ejection fraction of <35%. In Figure 41-7B, ventricular function is characterized by a wall motion score in which the left ventricle is divided into five segments. (For definition see reference 6.) The profound effect of left ventricular dysfunction on long-term survival after coronary artery bypass surgery has been extensively documented and this applies to all age groups.[1,2,36–38]

In summary, older patients undergoing coronary artery surgery have a poorer long-term outlook than similarly analyzed younger patients. Nonetheless, it is reassuring to note that overall survival at five years is in excess of 80%. The late results are determined in part by variables which exert their influence on *perioperative* mortality and by others that are *independent* of the perioperative period. Using the stepwise Cox Proportional Hazards model on all patients ≥65 years of age undergoing isolated coronary artery surgery in the CASS series, the best predictors of *late* survival were: indices of ventricular dysfunction, the number of associated medical diseases, and a combination of left main coronary artery stenosis of ≥70% plus a left dominant circulation.[5] With the analysis *confined* to 30-day surgical survivors, the influence of left main coronary artery disease on late outcome was eliminated.[5] Thus, while there are quantitative differences in late outcome between older and younger patients, the most important determinants of a successful surgical result are similar in both age groups. Elderly patients with good ventricular function and those without intercurrent medical diseases have a five-year survival approaching 90%.

Independent Effect of Age on Mortality

We might well ask whether the higher perioperative mortality and poorer long-term survival in older patients arises from differences in measured preoperative variables or whether this is an inevitable consequence of age per se. Table 41-1 underscores the less favorable base-line characteristics of the older patients. Stepwise linear discriminant analyses have been used to assess the

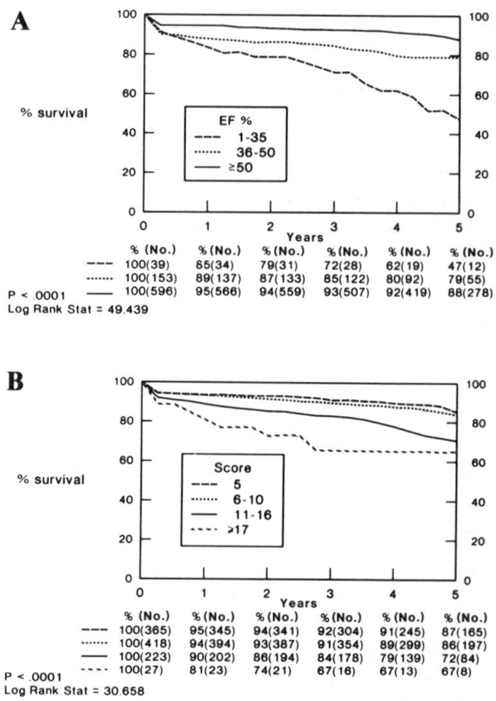

Figure 41-7 Five-year survival data categorized on the basis of ventricular function. **A** Ventricular function was assessed by measurement of the ejection fraction; the analysis incorporates 788 patients in whom this was measured. **B** Effect of ventricular wall motion score on 5-year survival. (Reproduced with permission from Gersh et al.[5])

independent predictive power of age on perioperative mortality and on five-year survivorship in a large series of CASS patients undergoing isolated coronary artery bypass surgery, irrespective of age[4] (and unpublished data). Using these statistical technics, advanced age does appear to be an independent (but by no means the most significant) predictor of perioperative and longer term mortality. The most potent predictors of *perioperative* mortality were indices of ventricular dysfunction and the association between left main coronary artery stenosis of ≥70% and left dominance. With regard to long-term (five-year) mortality, ventricular dysfunction and the presence of associated medical diseases had the most prognostic significance.

This leads to the conclusion that the adverse effect of age on the mortality of coronary artery surgery is due in part to differences in preoperative status. Older patients are "sicker" and can be characterized preoperatively as a group at higher risk on the basis of their clinical, arteriographic, and hemodynamic features. This, however, is not the sole explanation. Since advanced age is an *independent* predictor of an adverse outcome, there must be other "unmeasured" characteristics intrinsic to old age which influence survival after coronary artery surgery. Although results of coronary artery bypass in older patients are good, it is clear that advanced age inherently increases the risks of surgical intervention. Isolated reports to the contrary should not alter this basic premise. Technical expertise may further reduce the risk of bypass surgery in the elderly, but it would be unrealistic to expect this to equal that in younger patients.

> "My diseases are an asthma and a dropsy, and what is less curable, seventy-five."
>
> SAMUEL JOHNSON

FUNCTIONAL OUTCOME AFTER CORONARY BYPASS SURGERY

The emphasis on randomized trials of coronary artery surgery has been on survival. Unfortunately, the large randomized trials comparing coronary artery bypass surgery with medical therapy have excluded patients over age 65. Since even the longest survival in the patient over age 65 is of abbreviated duration, that elusive and indefinable goal, namely the "quality of life," assumes equal if not greater importance than survival for the older patient. Figure 41-8 illustrates the actuarial recurrence of angina in CASS survivors in two age

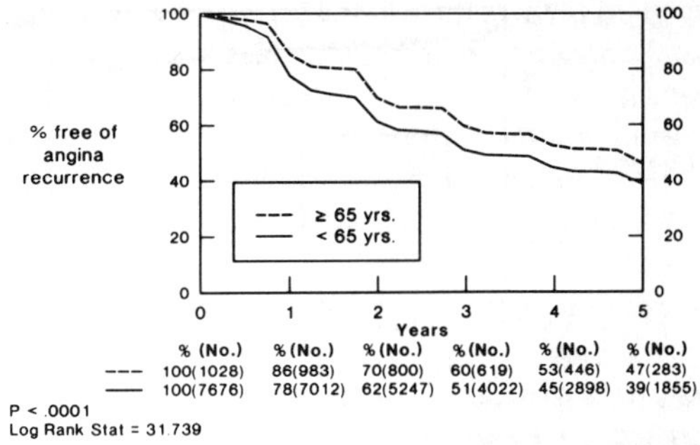

Figure 41-8 Comparison of the actuarially determined recurrence of angina in 30-day hospital survivors in patients aged 65 years or older and those younger than 65 years. (Reproduced with permission from Gersh et al.[5])

groups: aged ≥65 years and <65 years.[5] Recurrence of angina in both age groups is higher than that previously reported[38,39] and may relate to the actuarial method of analysis in which the first occurrence of angina is taken as an end point, irrespective of the patient's symptomatic status at the time of last follow-up. Angina-free survival was actually better in patients over the age of 65 and suggests that older patients derive similar symptomatic benefits from coronary bypass surgery, as do a younger population. This may also relate in part to lower levels of activity in the elderly and also to their poorer survival, thus reducing the number at risk of developing angina.

Demonstration that coronary bypass surgery effectively improves symptoms in older patients is provided by others.[7,13–15,26] Knapp et al[7] reported that 95% of their patients improved or were angina-free at follow-up and similar results were obtained by Garcia et al.[14] In another series of patients aged ≥70 years after an average follow-up duration of 22.2 months, 94% were free of angina.[9] "Excellent or good" results were noted in 70% of patients followed for a mean of 16 months by Gann et al.[13] Du Cailar et al noted that 68% of patients aged ≥65 years of age were asymptomatic 30 months post-bypass surgery with 94% improved by at least one class of the New York Heart Association functional classification.[15]

Although survival in the CASS series did not differ between the sexes,[4,5] there was a striking difference in the symptomatic benefits of the operation.[4,5] Freedom from recurrence of angina (actuarially determined) was 67% in men but only 48% in women at five years. That women fare less well than men with regard to the long-term functional outcome of coronary bypass surgery, even though survival rates are comparable, has been emphasized by others.[40-42] This is probably related to the smaller size in body surface area of women which correlates with small hearts and reduced coronary artery caliber.[41,42] Less complete revascularization increases the likelihood of the recurrence of angina but this applies to all age groups.

VALVE REPLACEMENT COMBINED WITH MYOCARDIAL REVASCULARIZATION

The combined procedure of valve replacement and coronary artery bypass surgery substantially increases the mortality compared to either procedure alone. In an earlier study from the Mayo Clinic this was particularly noticeable in patients older than 65 years of age.[43] Jolly and associates analyzed their experience with combined valve replacement and coronary artery surgery between the years 1973 and 1979.[23] For combined aortic valve replacement and bypass surgery, the mortality was 39% in patients 70 years and older, 21% in those aged 65 to 69 years, and 9% in all age groups. An improvement in results during the last three years of their experience is evident. For combined mitral valve replacement and coronary artery surgery, mortality was 42% in those aged 70 years and older, 26% in the group aged 65 to 69 years, and 25% in all age groups.[23]

CONCLUSIONS

We must accept that coronary artery surgery in the elderly entails a higher operative risk and poorer long-term survival than in younger people. The major impact of age appears in the 70-year and older age group. Results have improved markedly in recent years and the mortality reported in the early experience with coronary surgery does not apply to the 1980s. Overall, long-term survival is excellent and in specific subgroups of patients, namely those with relatively good left ventricular function and without intercurrent medical diseases, it approaches 90% at five years. Factors influencing early and late results are qualitatively similar to those which affect the surgical outcome in younger patients. The symptomatic benefits of the procedure are similar in both age groups but relief of angina is less impressive in women.

The greater the risk the more stringent should be the grounds for implementation of any procedure. The essential issue of coronary bypass surgery in the management of ischemic heart disease in older patients is the same as in a younger population but the *emphasis* is different. In the elderly the ability of a procedure to enhance the quality of life may supersede or at least be of equal importance to its effects on survival. When it comes to the individual elderly patient, the decision is basic—are the risks worth the potential benefits?

This philosophy requires careful attention to the medical and also to the social circumstances of the patient. By dividing patients into subgroups according to specific clinical, hemodynamic, and arteriographic characteristics, we can obtain an indication of perioperative risk and the chances of long-term survival and symptomatic improvement. Recognition of other medical conditions, which are in many cases an integral part of the frailty of advanced age, is an essential step in the decision to perform surgery. Furthermore, this knowledge may be crucial to both early and late postoperative management.

Inasmuch as estimation of these *measurable* variables will influence therapeutic strategies, they do not take into account other equally important features of the elderly that are less amenable to quantitation. Gann et al[13] stressed the importance of "physiological age" as opposed to "chronological age." Assessment of physiological age requires a clear picture of the patient's activities, aspirations, and social circumstances. This information is essential to any assessment of disability due to angina pectoris in an older patient. These factors *in conjunction* with a clinical and invasive evaluation of the patient's cardiovascular and overall medical status are indispensable to the decision to perform coronary bypass surgery in older patients.

There is no doubt that elderly patients with severely symptomatic coronary artery disease can be substantially helped by coronary revascularization. The current state of coronary artery surgery is such, that advanced age alone should no longer be considered a contraindication to coronary bypass surgery but rather a stimulus to exercise clinical judgment.

REFERENCES

1. Loop FD, Cosgrove DM, Lytle BW, et al: An 11 year evolution of coronary arterial surgery (1967–1978). *Ann Surg* 1979;190:444–455.
2. Rahimtoola SH, Grunkemeier GL, Teply JF, et al: Changes in coronary bypass surgery leading to improved survival. *JAMA* 1981;246:1912–1916.
3. McIntosh HD: Aortocoronary bypass grafting: An internist's perspective. *Circulation* 1982;65(suppl 2):77–80.

4. Gersh BJ, Kronmal RA, Frye RL, et al: Coronary arteriography and coronary artery bypass surgery: Morbidity and mortality in patients ages 65 years or older. A report from the Coronary Artery Surgery Study. *Circulation* 1983;67:483-491.
5. Gersh BJ, Kronmal RA, Schaff HV, et al: Long-term (5 year) results of coronary bypass surgery in patients aged 65 years or older (A report from the Coronary Artery Surgery Study—CASS). *Circulation* 1983;68(suppl 17):II-190–II-199.
6. Principal Investigators of CASS and Their Associates: National Heart, Lung and Blood Institute Coronary Artery Surgery Study (CASS). *Circulation* 1981;63(suppl 1):1.
7. Knapp WS, Douglas JS Jr, Craver JM, et al: Efficacy of coronary artery bypass grafting in elderly patients with coronary artery disease. *Am J Cardiol* 1981;47:923-927.
8. Hamby RL, Wisoff BG, Kolker P, et al: Intractable angina pectoris in 65 to 79 year age group: A surgical approach. *Chest* 1973;64:46-50.
9. Hochberg MS, Levine FH, Daggett WM, et al: Isolated coronary artery bypass grafting in patients seventy years of age and older. *J Thorac Cardiovasc Surg* 1982;84:219-223.
10. Boucek RJ, Romanelli R, Willis WH Jr, et al: Sex differences in obstructive coronary artery disease in patients 65 years of age or older with angina pectoris. *Circulation* 1982;66:926-929.
11. Berry BE, Acree PW, Davis DJ, et al: Coronary artery bypass operation in septuagenarians. *Ann Thorac Surg* 1980;31:310-313.
12. Meyer J, Wukosch DC, Seybold-Epting W, et al: Coronary artery bypass in patients over 70 years of age: Indications and results. *Am J Cardiol* 1975; 36:342-345.
13. Gann D, Colin C, Hildner FJ, et al: Coronary artery bypass surgery in patients seventy years of age and older. *J Thorac Cardiovasc Surg* 1977;73: 237-241.
14. Garcia JM, Cheanvechai C, Effler DB: Myocardial revascularization in patients aged 65 years and older. *Cardiovasc Clin* 1975;7:83-91.
15. Du Cailer C, Chaitman BR, Castonguay Y: Risks and benefits of aortocoronary bypass surgery in patients aged 65 years or more. *Can Med Assoc J* 1980;122:771-774.
16. Ashor GW, Meyer BW, Lindesmith GG, et al: Coronary artery disease. Surgery in 100 patients 65 years of age and older. *Arch Surg* 1973;107:30-33.
17. McCallister BD, Schmeidt M, Reed WA, et al: Coronary artery bypass in patients over the age of 70: Initial and late results, abstracted. *Circulation* 1975;51/52(suppl 2):91.
18. Stephenson LW, MacVaugh H, Edmunds LH: Surgery using cardiopulmonary bypass in the elderly. *Circulation* 1978;58:250-254.
19. Berman ND, David TE, Lipton IH, et al: Surgical procedures involving cardiopulmonary bypass in patients aged 70 or older. *J Am Geriatr Soc* 1980; 28:29-32.
20. Kirklin JW, Kouchoukos NT, Blackstone EH, et al: Research related to surgical treatment of coronary artery disease. *Circulation* 1979;60:1613-1618.
21. Stringer RJ, Tucker BL, Stefanik G, et al: Coronary bypass grafting in the older age group. *Circulation* 1975;51/52(suppl 2):245.
22. Smith JM, Lindsay WG, Lillehei RC, et al: Cardiac surgery in geriatric patients. *Surgery* 1976;80: 443-448.
23. Jolly WW, Isch JH, Shumacker HB Jr: Cardiac surgery in the elderly, in Noble RJ, Rothbaum DA (eds): *Geriatric Cardiology.* Philadelphia, FA Davis, 1981.
24. Kennedy JW, Kaiser GC, Fisher LD, et al: Clinical and angiographic predictors of operative mortality from the Collaborative Study in Coronary Artery Surgery (CASS). *Circulation* 1981;63:793-802.
25. Loop FD, Berrettoni JH, Pichard A, et al: Selection of the candidate for myocardial revascularization: A profile of high risk based on multivariate analysis. *J Thorac Cardiovasc Surg* 1975;69:40-45.
26. Tucker BL, Lindesmith GG, Stiles QR, et al: Myocardial revascularization in patients 70 years of age and older. *West J Med* 1977;126:179-183.
27. Hammermeister KE, Kennedy JW: Predictors of surgical mortality in patients undergoing direct myocardial revascularization. *Circulation* 1974; 59(suppl 2):112.
28. National Cooperative Study Group: Unstable angina pectoris: National Cooperative Study Group to compare surgical and medical therapy. II. In-hospital experience and initial follow-up results in patients with one, two and three vessel disease. *Am J Cardiol* 1978;42:839-843.
29. Chaitman BR, Rogers WJ, Davis K, et al: Operative risk factors in patients with left main coronary artery disease. *N Engl J Med* 1980;303:953-957.
30. Jones EL, King SB III, Craver JM, et al: The spectrium of left main coronary artery disease; variables affecting patient selection, management, and death. *J Thorac Cardiovasc Surg* 1980;79:109-115.
31. Kennedy JW, Kaiser GC, Fisher LD, et al: Multivariate discriminant analysis of the clinical and angiographic predictors of operative mortality from the Collaborative Study in Coronary Artery Surgery (CASS). *J Thorac Cardiovasc Surg* 1980;80:876-883.
32. Takaro T, Hultgren HN, Lipton MJ, et al: The VA cooperative randomized study of surgery for coronary arterial occlusive disease. II. Subgroup with significant left main lesions. *Circulation* 1976; 54(suppl 3):107.
33. Rahimtoola SH, Nunley D, Grunkemeier G, et al: Ten-year survival after coronary bypass surgery for unstable angina. *N Engl J Med* 1983;308:676-680.
34. Kannel WB, Gordon T: Evaluation of the cardiovascular risk in the elderly: The Framingham study. *Bull NY Acad Med* 1978;54:573-578.
35. Connolly DC, Elveback L, Oxman HA: Coronary heart disease in residents of Rochester, Minnesota 1950-1975. III. Effect of hypertension and its treatment on survival of patients with coronary artery disease. *Mayo Clin Proc* 1984;59:247-250.
36. Hammermeister KE, DeRouen TA, Dodge HT: Variables predictive of survival in patients with coronary disease: Selection by univariate and multivariate analyses from the clinical, electrocardiographic, exercise, arteriographic, and quantitative angiographic evaluations. *Circulation* 1979;59: 421-428.
37. Cox DR: Regression models and life-tables. *J R Stat Soc* 1972;34:187-192.
38. Cameron A, Kemp HG Jr, Shimomura S, et al:

Aortocoronary bypass surgery: A 7-year follow-up. *Circulation* 1979;60(suppl 1):9.

39. Campeau L, Lespérance J, Hermann J, et al: Loss of the improvement of angina between 1 and 7 years after aortocoronary bypass surgery: Correlations with changes in vein grafts and in coronary arteries. *Circulation* 1979;60(suppl 1):1.
40. Douglas JS Jr, King SB III, Jones EL, et al: Reduced efficacy of coronary bypass surgery in women. *Circulation* 1981;64(suppl 2):11.
41. Fisher LD, Kennedy JW, Davis KB, et al: Association of sex, physical size, and operative mortality after coronary artery bypass in the Coronary Artery Surgery Study (CASS). *J Thorac Cardiovasc Surg* 1982;84:334–39.
42. Loop FD, Golding LR, MacMillan JP, et al: Coronary artery surgery in women compared with men: Analyses of risk and long-term results. *J Am Coll Cardiol* 1983;1(2):391–400.
43. Barnhorst DA, Giuliani ER, Pluth JR, et al: Open-heart surgery in patients more than 65 years old. *Ann Thorac Surg* 1974;18:81–89.

CHAPTER 42
Coronary Revascularization in the Elderly Patient

Tetsuo Ishimori
T. Anthony Don Michael
Elias Hanna

It is agreed that coronary artery bypass surgery improves the quality of life and long-term outlook of patients under 65 with mild to moderate angina pectoris, especially in the presence of significant left main coronary artery disease and/or disease affecting three or more coronary arteries.[1-3] However, the long-term effects of coronary revascularization surgery in the elderly have not been well established. In this chapter, current indications for coronary revascularization surgery, the management of pre- and postoperative problems, special precautions during surgical procedures, and results of surgery in elderly patients are discussed.

Ischemic heart disease is the major cause of morbidity and mortality in the elderly.[4,5] This is compounded by the inherent difficulties and limitations of detecting the disease in this age group. Clinical presentation of ischemic heart disease is distinctively different in comparison with younger patients; the activity of the elderly patient is often limited and angina pectoris may not be a significant symptom while dyspnea on exertion as a clinical manifestation of coronary artery disease is rather common and often ascribed to chronic obstructive pulmonary disease. Moreover, symptoms of angina pectoris mimic other problems commonly seen in the elderly, such as degenerative arthropathy or gastrointestinal disorders. Thus, these patients are not infrequently overlooked because of their age. An additional consideration is the fact that there is a sparsity of literature on the subject of the symptom complexes of ischemic heart disease in the elderly. All these factors appear to be the major reasons why it is difficult to establish the diagnosis of atherosclerotic disease in the elderly, despite it being one of the most common causes of death. Even though the diagnosis is established and appropriate treatment given, there may be difficulties in compliance due to social factors. However, it is important to recognize that there is a significant subset of highly symptomatic patients who complain of disabling angina in spite of currently available "maximal medical management." Although coronary revascularization surgery has been considered as a therapeutic alternative for this particular group of patients, it has hitherto been believed that morbidity and mortality is exceptionally high,[6-8] and this excludes the therapeutic modality. Recent reports,[9-13] however, indicate substantial improvement in mortality and morbidity of coronary artery revascularization surgery for selected elderly individuals who have otherwise good physical and mental health.

INDICATIONS FOR SURGERY

It is well established that the prognosis of coronary artery disease is clearly dependent upon the extent of the vessel involvement and the left ventricular function,[14-17] but it is not clear that this prognostic implication holds true in the geriatric patient. Unfortunately, the natural history of this specific group of geriatric patients who require coronary artery bypass surgery is not known and will not be available in the near future. As such, improvement of longevity after successful myocardial revascularization surgery will be an important future issue to evaluate. Despite this, as the geriatric mortality from coronary artery disease is quite high and survivorship after coronary revascularization from severe atherosclerotic heart disease is clearly an advantage for certain subsets of young patients, it can be argued that it may be useful for a similar elderly population. Analyzing symptoms and ensuring good general health appears to be the most important consideration, prior to referral for coronary artery bypass surgery. Hence coronary revascularization surgery is justified under the following circumstances:

1. *Stable angina pectoris with three-vessel coronary artery disease not controlled by maximal medical therapy.* Medical management may not be possible in the elderly due to the side-effects of therapy such as hypotension and bradycardia. In this group the main goals of myocardial revascularization are to relieve severe and often disabling chest pain and to help the patient maintain or improve the quality of his life. In addition, coronary revascularization surgery may well improve longevity in elderly patients in certain subsets.

2. *Left main coronary artery disease.* Over the past decade, significant left main coronary artery stenosis has been found to be, prognostically, the most important single lesion involving the coronary arteries. Long-term mortality for medically treated patients with left main stenosis of 70% or greater has proved to be grave.[18] This appears to hold true for the elderly patient, too. As indicated by previous authors, left main coronary artery disease of 50% or more has also been demonstrated to have a grave prognosis.[19] It has not been shown that survivorship has been altered by the advent of modern medical treatment. Thus, there is a well-established indication for coronary artery revascularization in these patients to improve symptoms as well as to prolong life.

3. *In conjunction with other clinically dictated procedures, such as valve replacement, ventricular aneurysmectomy, etc.* In patients with advanced valvlular heart disease, severe coronary atherosclerosis has been frequently observed.[20,21] Additionally, in patients in whom left ventricular aneurysmectomy is indicated, coronary artery bypass surgery should be considered.[22]

4. *Preinfarctional (unstable) angina.* Recent reports[9,13] disclose a higher incidence of severe refractory angina pectoris of unstable nature with significant myocardium at risk in the elderly patients with advanced coronary atherosclerosis, refractory to medical management. Coronary artery revascularization surgery is accepted as an indication in this subset because of poor prognosis.[23] Patients with unstable angina who cannot be adequately treated by the currently available maximal medical management would be the logical candidates for coronary bypass surgery, regardless of their age. The operative mortality of patients with unstable angina has been low[24,25] and postoperative symptomatic relief is dramatic.[26,27]

5. *Postinfarction angina.* This seems to be a reasonable indication as postinfarction angina is a predictor of a high incidence of multivessel disease.[28-30] Thus, persistent or recurrent angina should be interpreted as incomplete myocardial infarction and/or compromised collateral blood supply. Coronary bypass surgery is indicated under these circumstances irrespective of age, especially if "angina at a distance" occurs. This relates to the dismal prognosis of this condition if treated medically.

6. *Variant angina with critical obstruction in addition to spasm (Prinzmetal's angina).* This disease is notorious for the malignant nature of its clinical presentation and prognosis.[31] Although the role of percutaneous transluminal coronary angioplasty in this subset is unknown, coronary artery revascularization surgery should be considered in patients who show critical occlusive atherosclerotic disease with failure of medical therapy. Excellent symptomatic relief is expected.[31,32] On the contrary, coronary bypass surgery has not been as successful in patients with variant angina who do not have critical occlusive atherosclerotic coronary artery disease.[32-34]

7. *Postcardiac arrest with severe coronary artery disease.* These patients have a high mortality rate subsequent to discharge.[35] In most instances there is a background of severe multivessel coronary artery disease, predicting the need for surgical intervention and appropriate drug therapy after electrophysiological testing. (Ishimori and Don Michael: unpublished data, January 1983).

It should be restated that all elderly patients who are considered for coronary revascularization surgery should have acceptable general health, other than their cardiac status. As such, the same indications would apply as in young individuals for coronary revascularization.

PREPARATION FOR CORONARY ARTERY BYPASS SURGERY

In accordance with the prerequisite of good general health, patients who are considered for coronary revascularization surgery should be carefully evaluated for disorders of the elderly, including latent stroke. The presence or absence of neurologic problems by history is vital. Carotid bruits with or without symptoms should be evaluated. Recent literature indicates a high incidence of asymptomatic lesions in the carotid arteries in the neck which may harbor advanced disease.[36] For this reason, noninvasive prescreening evaluations, such as Doppler ultrasound study and/or digital subtraction angiography,[36–38] should be considered for patients prior to surgical intervention regardless of whether carotid bruits are present or absent. Depending upon the findings, aortic arch studies and carotid angiograms may need to be performed. The appropriate management of this condition at the time of coronary artery revascularization surgery[39] may diminish morbidity and mortality. Other atherosclerotic vascular problems should also be looked for. Chronic obstructive pulmonary disease and benign prostatic hypertrophy are other common concomitant disorders of the elderly. Appropriate evaluation and management of these problems may prevent unnecessary problems in the postoperative period.

TECHNICS OF CORONARY REVASCULARIZATION SURGERY IN THE ELDERLY

There are no special technical differences; the shorter the procedure during cardioplegia the better the overall immediate postoperative results, in the elderly patients. The following rules can be stated.

1. It is believed that the saphenous vein graft is preferred to the internal mammary artery in view of technical difficulty with fragile ribs, the need to conserve time, the relatively limited life expectancy in the elderly, and pulmonary complications. On the other hand, as the natural history of this particular group of patients is not well known, it appears to be more logical to utilize surgical technics similar to those used in younger patients. In this context, left internal mammary coronary artery bypass surgery may be considered for selected elderly patients, especially in view of its higher patency rate.

2. Special care should be taken at the time of surgery in view of frequent observations of the following findings: (*a*) Calcification of the ascending aorta is quite common and special care should be taken at the site of the anastomosis of the proximal segment of the saphenous vein graft. Femoral artery cannulation is preferred to arch cannulation because of fragility of the aorta. By the same token, peripheral vascular disease is common and femoral artery cannulation sites for perfusion should be cautiously utilized and previously evaluated, angiographically, if indicated. (*b*) Calcification of the coronary arteries is quite common and calcification of the distal coronary artery is frequently observed, which may create technical difficulties with the distal anastomosis of the saphenous vein graft. (*c*) Because of the likelihood of generalized atherosclerosis, the maintenance of adequate perfusion pressure to prevent postoperative neurologic and renal complications is vital. Fluid and electrolyte management during and immediately after the operation is especially important.

POSTOPERATIVE MANAGEMENT

Immediate Care

Essentially the same care is required in this particular group of patients as in others. As indicated, fluid and electrolyte maintenance to conserve renal function is vital. An important consideration in the elderly patient is the neurologic problem. Cerebrovascular accidents are occasionally seen. Postoperative mental confusion is frequently pronounced and prolonged. The pathophysiologic mechanisms for these neurologic problems are poorly understood. Recovery is somewhat slow and unpredictable. Sternal infections tend to be observed more frequently. Special postoperative care for chronic obstructive lung disease is frequently required. In addition, conduction disturbances, such as bradyarrhythmia, as well as atrioventricular (AV) block, are much more frequently observed in older than in younger patients and may require temporary and/or permanent pacemakers. Sternal dehiscence can be seen more frequently in the elderly because chronic obstructive pulmonary disease and degenerative osteoarthropathy may be present.

Long-Term Care

Essentially the same follow-up protocols are used as in other patients. Patients are evaluated periodically by the attending cardiologist 3 weeks after surgery, then in 2 months or sooner, as needed. Re-evaluation serves to detect complications, as well as determine the patient's ability to return to regular activities. Patients are followed at 3- to 6-month intervals or sooner depending upon progress. Either a cardiovascular exercise test, a thallium 201 stress scintigram, or multigated wall motion study may be performed, depending on the preoperative and surgical anatomy. Unless the patient is compromised by disabling angina with maximal medical therapy after coronary artery bypass surgery, redo surgery is not recommended. Depending upon the findings of the coronary arteriograms, coronary angioplasty may be considered.[40,41] Antiplatelet therapy is given routinely to patients who have had coronary artery bypass surgery. An attempt is made to reduce risk factors as recommended for young patients. Suitable patients may be referred for cardiac rehabilitation.

RESULTS OF SURGERY

Operative Mortality

Operative mortality is defined as death occurring within 30 days following operation. Reported results of coronary revascularization surgery in the elderly are summarized in Table 42-1. As the table shows, the morality rate has been acceptable, although still much higher than that reported in younger patients.

Operative Morbidity

The possible postoperative complications of coronary revascularization include: pulmonary embolism, bleeding requiring re-exploration, myocardial infarction, hepatitis, cerebrovascular accident, sepsis, congestive heart failure, pneumonia, pericarditis, Dressler's syndrome, renal failure, gastrointestinal bleeding. These are also observed postoperatively in younger patients. In the immediate postoperative period, mental confusion may be frequent and prolonged. In addition, recovery is generally slower with an average hospital stay of 18 days for those patients older than 70 years of age.[9]

Table 42-1
Operative Mortality in Patients Aged 70 Years or Older

Series	No. of Patients	Operative Mortality (%)
Ashor et al (1973)[6]	22	2 (9.1)
Meyer et al (1975)[7]	67	9 (13.4)
McCallister et al (1975)[12]	48	3 (6.2)
Gann et al (1977)[10]	30	2 (6.6)
Stephenson et al (1978)[14]	25	None
Berman et al (1980)[8]	17	3 (17.6)
Gersh et al (1981)[11]	262	18 (6.8)
Akins (1982)[9]	53	2 (3.8)
Ishimori et al (1982)[13]	39*	3 (7.7)*

*Patients with left main coronary artery disease.

Late Symptomatic Results

There is presently little doubt about the value of coronary artery bypass surgery grafting for relief of angina pectoris.[42] The average number of patients who are painfree in the early postoperative period has been high in numerous reported series. This holds true for the elderly patient.[9,17] The functional capacity also showed significant improvement.

Longevity

It has been well documented that coronary revascularization surgery is quite effective in prolonging life in patients under the age of 65 with three-vessel and left main coronary disease.[1-3,42] Long-term follow-up results are, however, not available for elderly patients. In these patients, the average 2-year follow-up of cumulative survival after coronary bypass surgery is reported to be 93% for patients who are suffering from severe coronary artery disease.[9] For patients who have left main coronary artery disease, a cumulative survival of 97% is reported after coronary revascularization.[13] However, the number of patients in these series is limited, and further detailed reports are awaited.

SUMMARY

In the United States the average life expectancy for females aged 70 is 14.8 years, while that for males is 11.1.[43] With this in mind, the main purpose of myocardial revascularization should be not only to relieve severe disabling angina but also to help the patient maintain or improve the quality and duration of life. Medical management alone may fail to accomplish these aims. Thus, patients in older age groups should have the benefit of angioplasty or surgical treatment. Although surgical procedures carry a somewhat higher risk in patients 70 years of age or older, careful selection of patients for coronary revascularization is justified. At present, coronary revascularization is not considered for asymptomatic patients. In recent reports, mortality rates for patients in their seventh decade who underwent coronary revascularization surgery have been found to be acceptably low. Technical advances and greater experience in performing the procedures have, presumably, led to the decline. Unfortunately, surgical morbidity in the elderly is still quite high in spite of technical advancement in the perioperative period. To avoid excessive morbidity in the elderly patient, careful evaluation and management of systemic disease prior to surgery, particularly in the central nervous system, should be carried out. Intraoperatively, shortening the procedure during cardioplegia would be expected to yield better postoperative results. For those patients who have incurable and progressive disabling disorders, such as malignant tumors, cerebrovascular accidents or ischemia with permanent neurologic deficit, and other disorders which of themselves limit life and its quality, coronary revascularization surgery is not indicated. However, despite the fact that the natural history of this group of patients is not well documented as yet, it is emphasized that, where indicated, coronary revascularization surgery should be carried out prudently, conscientiously, and without hesitation.

ACKNOWLEDGMENT

Darlene Durham, CMA, assisted in the typing of this chapter.

REFERENCES

1. Varnaukas E, Olsson SB, Carlstrom E, et al: Long-term results of prospective randomized study of coronary artery bypass surgery in stable angina pectoris. *Lancet* 1982;2:1173–1180.
2. Lawrie GM, Morris GC, Howell JF, et al: Improved survival after 5 years in 1144 patients after coronary artery bypass surgery. *Am J Cardiol* 1978;42: 709–715.
3. Sheldon WC, Rincon G, Pichard AD, et al: Surgical treatment of coronary artery disease: Pure graft operations with a study of 741 patients followed 3–7 years. *Prog Cardiovasc Dis* 1975;18(3):237–253.
4. Kennedy RD, Andrew GR, Caid FI: Ischemic heart disease in the elderly. *Br Heart J* 1977;39:1121–1127.
5. Kitchin AH, Lowthers CP, Milne JS: Prevalence of clinical and electrocardiographic evidence of ischemic heart disease in the older population. *Br Heart J* 1973;35:946–953.
6. Ashor GW, Meyer BW, Lindesmith GG, et al: Coronary artery disease. Surgery in 100 patients 65 years of age and older. *Arch Surg* 1974;107:30–33.
7. Meyer J, Wukasch DJ, Deybold-Epting W, et al: Coronary artery bypass in patients over 70 years of age: Indications and results. *Am J Cardiol* 1975; 36:343–345.
8. Berman ND, David TE, Lipton IH, et al: Surgical procedures involving cardiopulmonary bypass in patients aged 70 or older. *J Am Geriatr Soc* 1980;28:29–32.
9. Akins GH: Can your elderly patients benefit from coronary artery surgery? *J Cardiovasc Med* 1982;7: 1226–1229.
10. Gann D, Colin C, Hildner FJ, et al: Coronary artery bypass surgery in patients seventy years of age and older. *J Thorac Cardiovasc Surg* 1977; 73:237–241.
11. Gersh B, Frye RL, Kronmal RK, et al: Coronary angiography and coronary artery bypass surgery in elderly patients. *Am J Cardiol* 1981;47:494.
12. McCallister BD, Schmeidt M, Reed WA, et al: Coronary artery bypass in patients over age of 70 initial and late results. *Circulation* 1975(suppl 2);52:11.
13. Ishimori T, Don Michael TA, Hanna E: Surgical management of left main coronary artery disease in the elderly patient. *Am J Cardiol* 1982;49:919.
14. Stephenson LW, MacVaugh HI, Edmunds LH Jr: Surgery using cardiopulmonary bypass in the elderly. *Circulation* 1978;58:250–254.
15. Proudfit WL, Bruschke AVG, Sones FM Jr: Natural history of obstructive coronary artery disease: Ten-year study of 601 nonsurgical cases. *Prog Cardiovasc Dis* 1978;21:53–78.
16. Burggraf GW, Parker TO: Prognosis in coronary artery disease. *Circulation* 1975;51:146–156.
17. Webster JS, Moberg C, Rincon G: Natural history of severe proximal coronary artery disease as documented by coronary cineangiography. *Am J Cardiol* 1974;33:195–200.
18. Conley MJ, Ely RL, et al: The prognostic spectrum of left main stenosis. *Circulation* 1978;57:947.
19. Takaro T, Hultgren HN, Lipton MJ, et al: The VA cooperative randomized study of surgery of coronary arterial occlusive disease. II. Subgroup with significant left main lesions. *Circulation* 1976; 54(suppl 2):107–117.
20. Bonchek LI, Anderson RP, Rosch JK: Should arteriography be performed routinely before valve replacement. *Am J Cardiol* 1973;30:462–469.
21. Ishimori T, Heupler F, Shirey EK, et al: Angina pectoris and coronary atherosclerosis in patients with mitral stenosis. *Chest* 1976;70:430.
22. Mullen DC, Posey LP, Gabriel R, et al: Prognostic considerations in the management of ventricular aneurysm. *Ann Thorac Surg* 1977;23:455–460.
23. Gazes PC, Mobley EM Jr, Faris HM Jr, et al: Preinfarctional (unstable) angina—A prospective study—Ten year followup. *Circulation* 1973; 48:331–337.
24. Cheanvechai C, Effler DB, Loop FO, et al: Emergency myocardial revascularization. *Am J Cardiol* 1973;32:901.
25. Langou RA, Wiles JC, Cohen LS: Coronary surgery for unstable angina pectoris; Incidence and mortality of perioperative myocardial infarction. *Br Heart J* 1978;40:767–772.
26. Hatcher CR, Jones EL, King SB III, et al: The surgical treatment of unstable angina pectoris. *Ann Surg* 1975;181:754–759.
27. Boreheok LJ, Rahimtoola SH, Anderson RP, et al: Late results following emergency saphenous vein bypass grafting for unstable angina. *Circulation* 1974;50:972–977.
28. Moss AJ, DeCamilla J, Davis H, et al: The early posthospital phase of myocardial infarction: Prognostic stratification. *Circulation* 1976;54:58–64.
29. Chaitman BR, Waters DD, Cobard F, et al: Prediction of multivessel disease after inferior myocardial infarction. *Circulation* 1978;57:1085–1090.
30. Stenson RE, Flamm MD Jr, Zaret BL, et al: Transient ST segment elevation with postmyocardial infarction angina: Prognostic significance. *Am Heart J* 1975;89:449–454.
31. Bentivoglio LG, Ablaza SGG, Greenberg LF: By-

pass surgery for prinzmetal angina. *Arch Intern Med* 1974;134:313–316.
32. Johnson AD, Stroud HA, Vieweg VR, et al: Variant angina pectoris: Clinical presentations, coronary angiographic patterns, and the results of medical and surgical management in 42 consecutive patients. *Chest* 1978;73:786–794.
33. Gaasch WH, Lufschanowski R, Leachman RD, et al: Surgical management of prinzmetal variant angina. *Chest* 1974;66:614–621.
34. Hart NJ, Silverman ME, King SB: Variant angina pectoris caused by coronary artery spasm. *Am J Med* 1974;56:269–274.
35. Roy D, Waxman HL, Kienzle MG, et al: Clinical characteristics and long term follow-up in survivors of cardiac arrest: Relation to inducibility at electrophysiologic evaluation. *Circulation* 1982(suppl 2); 66:25.
36. Hennerici M, Aulich A, Sandmann W, et al: Incidence of asymptomatic extracranial arterial disease. *Stroke* 1981;12:750–758.
37. Fell G, Breslau P, Knox RA, et al: Importance of non-invasive ultrasonic-Doppler testing in the evaluation of patients with asymptomatic carotid bruits. *Am Heart J* 1981;102:221–226.
38. Coffey CE, Massey EW, Robert KB, et al: Occurrence of stroke following coronary artery bypass graft surgery. *Circulation* 1982(suppl 2);66:45.
39. Ennis CL, Lowrie GM, Morris GC Jr, et al: Improved results of carotid endarterectomy in patients with symptomatic coronary disease: An analysis of 1546 consecutive carotid operations. *Stroke* 1979;10:122–125.
40. Gruntzig AR, Senning A, Siegenthaler WE: Nonoperative dilatation of coronary artery stenosis: Percutaneous transluminal coronary angioplasty. *N Engl J Med* 1978;30:61.
41. Hamby RI, Katz S: Percutaneous transluminal coronary angioplasty: Its potential impact on surgery for coronary artery disease. *Am J Cardiol* 1980;45: 1161.
42. Hurst JW, King SB, Logue RB, et al: Value of coronary bypass surgery. *Am J Cardiol* 1978;42:443.
43. Statistical abstract of the United States. US Department of Commerce, Washington DC, 1979, p 17.

CHAPTER 43

Surgical vs Nonsurgical Management of the Elderly Patient Following Myocardial Infarction

William J. Rogers

Acute myocardial infarction remains the leading cause of death in the United States, and affects approximately 1.5 million persons yearly, of whom approximately one-third die of causes related to the acute event.[1] Longitudinal studies have demonstrated that, in addition to the significant morbitidy (heart failure, angina) following myocardial infarction, there is also an increased risk of death during the months and years following myocardial infarction, calculated at 10% to 15% during the first year, and 20% to 30% by the third year postinfarction.[2-8] Most deaths following acute myocardial infarction are cardiac-related and over half of them are sudden deaths.

Angiographic studies from our institution and elsewhere have documented that a majority of patients undergoing angiography postinfarction have multivessel coronary artery disease.[9-11] Because there is evidence that patients with symptomatic multivessel coronary artery disease tend to have a better prognosis when treated with coronary revascularization surgery than when treated medically,[12] it is conceivable that "prophylactic" coronary revascularization surgery in selected patients following acute myocardial infarction might improve longevity as well as "quality of life." We have recently studied this hypothesis in a group of selected patients who underwent coronary arteriography during the convalescent period following their acute myocardial infarction.[13] Additionally, we have extended the analysis to determine whether the potential benefits of surgery might apply equally to both elderly and younger patients following acute myocardial infarction.

METHODS

Patient Population

Our study population was drawn from a group of 281 patients with acute myocardial infarction admitted to our coronary care unit within 48 hours of first symptoms of infarction during a three-year time interval (Figure 43-1). Of the 232 infarct survivors, coronary arteriograms were advised on two thirds (156). Among the patients in whom coronary arteriograms were not advised, 44 patients were age 65 or older, 15 had incapacitating noncardiac illnesses, 13 had undergone recent prior coronary angiography, and 4 patients had been transferred to other hospitals during the early phase of their postinfarction convalescence. Of the 232 infarct survivors, 56% (129) underwent coronary angiography within 60 days of infarction. These 129 patients were retrospectively divided into three groups (Figure 43-1): (1) a surgical group comprising 43 patients who had CABG; (2) a medical group comprising 51 patients who were "surgical candidates" defined by left ventricular ejection fraction exceeding 25% and two or more "jeopardized" myocardial segments as defined below; and (3) nonsurgical candidates, a group comprising 35 patients having either ejection fraction less than or equal to 25% or less than two jeopardized segments, or both. The groups were further stratified by age (< age 60, ≥ age 60).

Method of Identifying Jeopardized Ventricular Segments

We performed biplane cine left ventricular angiograms in the anteropostero/lateral or in the 45° right anterior oblique/60° left anterior oblique/25° cranial projections.[14] Left ventricular end-diastolic and end-systolic silhouettes were superimposed (Figure 43-2) and ten regions of segmental wall motion were identified. These regions were assumed to be supplied by the vessel segments listed in Figure 43-2, based on the known distribution of the coronary arteries.[15]

"Jeopardized" ventricular segments were defined as ventricular segments having preservation of inward systolic wall motion with their "supply artery" having 70% or greater stenosis. Akinetic or dyskinetic segments were assumed in this post-infarction group to represent irreversibly damaged tissue and were not designated as jeopardized, regardless of the patency of their supply vessel. Thus, a person with preserved inward wall motion of all ten ventricular segments but proximal three-vessel coronary artery disease would have a total of ten jeopardized segments. On the other hand, a patient with a 100% mid-right coronary artery stenosis, otherwise normal coronary anatomy, and akinesis of ventricular segments 4, 5, and 8, would have no residual jeopardized segments, since this patient would have no viable segments supplied by stenotic arteries.

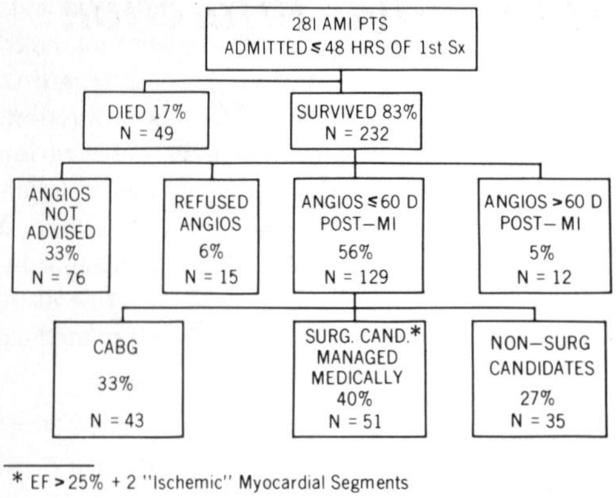

Figure 43-1 Derivation of the study population. AMI = acute myocardial infarction, Sx = symptoms, ANGIOS = coronary and left ventricular angiography, CABG = coronary artery bypass graft surgery, Cand = candidates, EF = ejection fraction, D = days. (Reproduced with permission from Rogers et al.[13])

Surgery and Follow-up

Coronary artery bypass graft surgery was performed utilizing individual or sequential saphenous vein grafts. Either hypothermic ischemic arrest or cold cardioplegia was utilized for myocardial preservation. A trained interviewer conducted follow-up by telephone at a mean of

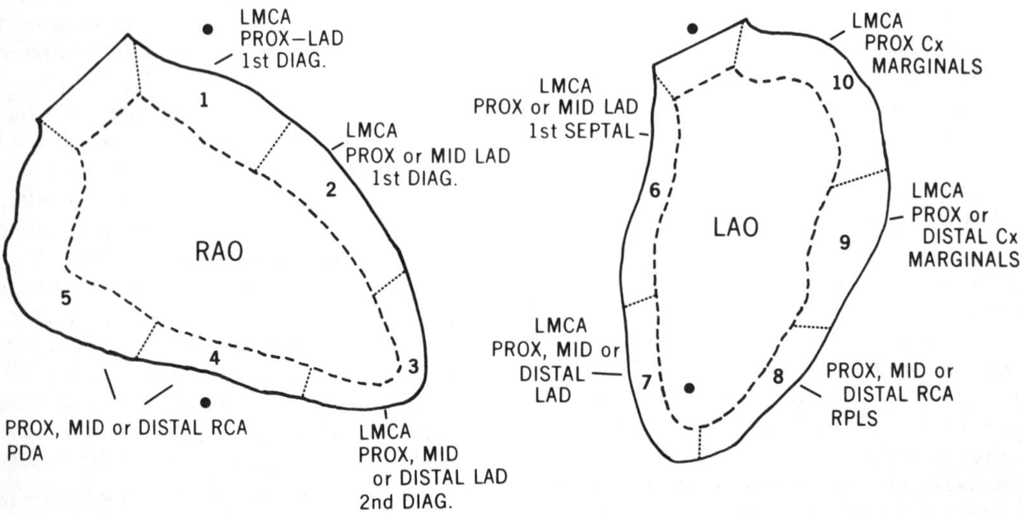

Figure 43-2 Identification of jeopardized left ventricular segments. Left ventricular end-diastolic and end-systolic silhouettes in biplane projections were superimposed. Left ventricular perimeter was divided into ten regions and the segment thought to supply each region is indicated. For example, a greater than 70% stenosis of the middle left anterior descending coronary artery (LAD) could jeopardize any of ventriculographic segments 2, 3, 6, or 7 showing preserved inward systolic wall motion. RAO = right anterior oblique, LAO = left anterior oblique, LMCA = left main coronary artery, PROX = proximal, DIAG = diagonal, RCA = right coronary artery, PDA = posterior descending coronary artery, Cx = circumflex coronary artery, RPLS = right posterior lateral segment. (Reproduced with permission from Rogers et al.[13])

23 ± 2 months after infarction. Severity of heart failure and angina were graded as classes I–IV according to the criteria of the New York Heart Association.[16] Asymptomatic patients were designated as class I.

Statistical Analysis

Data are expressed as mean ± SEM. Differences between continuous variables were assessed by the nonpaired t test and differences between dichotomous variables were assessed by the chi-square test.

The Kaplan-Meier life table method[17] was utilized to construct survival curves, plotted from the date of myocardial infarction. In the analysis only cardiac deaths, including sudden deaths and operative deaths, were utilized; noncardiac deaths were treated as censored observations. Differences between survival curves were determined using Gehan's technic.[18]

RESULTS

Comparison of Surgical Candidate Subsets

Of the 94 surgical candidates, the 43 patients managed surgically and the 51 patients managed medically were remarkably similar with regard to age, sex, location of prior myocardial infarction, admission hemodynamics, precatheterization symptoms, and hemodynamic status at catheterization (Table 43-1). Surgical patients had a greater prevalence of prior myocardial infarction, and at catheterization, surgical patients had more significantly (≥70%) stenotic vessels than medical

Table 43-1
Characteristics of Surgical Candidates

	Surgical Group (n=43)	Medical Group (n=51)	*P*	Aged <60 yr (n=69)	Aged ≥60 yr (n=25)	*P*
Age (years)	54 ± 1	54 ± 1	ns	50 ± 1	65 ± 1	
(Range)	(34–71)	(34–73)		(34–59)	(60–73)	
Sex (% males)	84%	90%	ns	84%	96%	ns
Prior MI by ECG	13 (30%)	5(10%)	0.01	12 (17%)	6 (24%)	ns
Location and extent of MI						
Anterior transmural	21 (49%)	17 (33%)		25 (36%)	13 (52%)	ns
Posterior transmural	9 (21%)	22 (43%)	ns	23 (33%)	8 (32%)	
Nontransmural	5 (12%)	2 (4%)		5 (7%)	2 (8%)	
Undetermined	8 (19%)	10 (20%)		16 (23%)	2 (8%)	
Admission systolic BP (mmHg)	131 ± 4	131 ± 3	ns	130 ± 2	134 ± 5	ns
Admission heart rate (bpm)	81 ± 3	78 ± 2	ns	77 ± 2	85 ± 4	ns
Days from MI to catheterization	26 ± 1	24 ± 1	ns	25 ± 1	24 ± 2	ns
Symptoms preceding catheterization						
Angina class						
1	27 (63%)	43 (84%)		51 (74%)	19 (76%)	
2	10 (23%)	5 (10%)	ns	13 (19%)	2 (8%)	ns
3	3 (7%)	1 (2%)		3 (4%)	1 (4%)	
4	3 (7%)	2 (4%)		2 (3%)	3 (12%)	
CHF class						
1	37 (86%)	49 (96%)		63 (91%)	23 (92%)	
2	4 (9%)	1 (2%)	ns	4 (6%)	1 (4%)	ns
3	2 (5%)	1 (2%)		2 (3%)	1 (4%)	
4	0 (0%)	0 (0%)		0	0	
Catheterization data						
CI (L/min/m²)	3.0 ± 0.1	3.3 ± 0.1	ns	3.2 ± 0.1	3.0 ± 0.2	ns
PAEDP (mmHg)	11 ± 1	11 ± 1	ns	11 ± 1	10 ± 1	ns
Ejection fraction (%)	42 ± 2	45 ± 2	ns	45 ± 1	39 ± 3	.03
Number vessels ≥70% stenotic						
1	3 (7%)	16 (31%)		14 (20%)	5 (20%)	
2	15 (35%)	23 (45%)	<.0005	30 (43%)	8 (32%)	ns
3	25 (58%)	12 (23%)		25 (36%)	12 (48%)	
Jeopardized segments/patient	4.9 ± 0.3	3.9 ± 0.2	<.01	4.3 ± 0.2	4.4 ± 0.3	ns
Days from catheterization to surgery	73 ± 8	—	—	142 ± 26 (34 pts)	53 ± 16 (11 pts)	.05

MI = myocardial infarction, BP = blood pressure, CHF = heart failure, CI = cardiac index, PAEDP = pulmonary arterial end-diastolic pressure.

patients. There were more jeopardized ventricular segments among the surgical group as well.

Analysis of the surgical candidates by age groupings (Table 43-1) showed no differences between patients age <60 and age ≥60 with respect to sex, prevalence of prior myocardial infarction, location or extent of infarction, admission hemodynamics, symptoms preceding catheterization, or hemodynamic or angiographic findings at catheterization. However, the older patients did have a lower left ventricular ejection fraction at catheterization. When surgery was performed, it was performed significantly earlier in the older patients than it was in the younger patients (Table 43-1).

Further analysis of the surgical candidates according to both surgical group and age group showed no significant differences between the older and younger patients within the surgical or medical group (Table 43-2).

Operative Data

Coronary revascularization was performed at a mean of 73 ± 8 days (range 25 to 262 days) after infarction. There was one perioperative death among the 43 patients (2%), and definite evidence of perioperative myocardial infarction was identified in that patient but in no other patients in this series. There were 2.1 ± 0.1 proximal anastomoses and 3.1 ± 0.2 distal anastomoses. Fourteen ancillary surgical procedures were performed in 13 patients, including 8 coronary endarterectomies, 2 scar resections, 2 intra-aortic balloon insertions, 1 mitral valve replacement, and 1 true aneurysm resection.

Table 43-2
Surgical Candidate Subgroups

	Surgical Group			Medical Group		
	Aged <60 yr (n=32)	*Aged ≥60 yr (n=11)*	*P*	*Aged <60 yr (n=37)*	*Aged ≥60 yr (n=14)*	*P*
Age (years)	50 ± 1	64 ± 1	—	50 ± 1	65 ± 1	—
(Range)	(34–59)	(60–71)	—	(34–59)	(60–73)	—
Sex (% males)	81%	91%	ns	86%	100%	ns
Prior MI by ECG	12 (38%)	6 (55%)	ns	22%	7%	ns
Location and extent of MI						
Anterior transmural	15 (47%)	6 (55%)		10 (27%)	7 (50%)	
Posterior transmural	7 (22%)	2 (18%)	ns	16 (43%)	6 (43%)	ns
Nontransmural	3 (9%)	2 (18%)		2 (5%)	0 (0%)	
Undetermined	7 (22%)	1 (9%)		9 (24%)	1 (7%)	
Admission systolic BP (mmHg)	132 ± 4	129 ± 7	ns	129 ± 3	138 ± 7	ns
Admission heart rate (bpm)	76 ± 3	93 ± 8	ns	78 ± 3	79 ± 3	ns
Days from MI to catheterization	27 ± 2	24 ± 2	ns	24 ± 1	25 ± 4	ns
Symptoms preceding catherization						
Angina class						
1	20 (63%)	7 (64%)		31 (84%)	12 (86%)	
2	9 (28%)	1 (9%)	ns	4 (11%)	1 (7%)	ns
3	2 (6%)	1 (9%)		1 (3%)	0 (0%)	
4	1 (3%)	2 (18%)		1 (3%)	1 (7%)	
CHF class						
1	28 (88%)	9 (82%)		35 (95%)	14 (100%)	
2	3 (9%)	1 (9%)	ns	1 (3%)	0 (0%)	ns
3	1 (3%)	1 (9%)		1 (3%)	0 (0%)	
4	0 (0%)	0 (0%)		0 (0%)	0 (0%)	
Catheterization data						
CI (L/min/m²)	3.1 ± 1	2.7 ± 0.2	ns	3.3 ± 0.2	3.2 ± 0.2	ns
PAEDP (mmHg)	11 ± 1	10 ± 1	ns	11 ± 1	10 ± 2	ns
Ejection fraction (%)	44 ± 2	38 ± 5	ns	47 ± 2	40 ± 3	ns
Number vessels ≥70% stenotic						
1	2 (6%)	1 (9%)		12 (32%)	4 (29%)	
2	12 (38%)	3 (27%)	ns	18 (49%)	5 (36%)	ns
3	18 (56%)	7 (64%)		7 (19%)	5 (36%)	
Jeopardized segments/patients	5.0 ± 0.3	4.6 ± 0.6	ns	3.8 ± 0.3	4.1 ± 0.4	ns
Days from catheterization to surgery	80 ± 9	53 ± 16	ns	—	—	—

MI = myocardial infarction, BP = blood pressure, CHF = heart failure, CI = cardiac index, PAEDP = pulmonary arterial end-diastolic pressure.

Survival in Surgical vs Nonsurgical Candidates

Among the 129 patients undergoing angiography within 60 days of infarction, survival at three years postinfarction was not significantly different in the 94 surgical candidates compared to the 35 nonsurgical candidates (Figure 43-3). However, the nonsurgical candidates were a heterogeneous group comprising 24 patients with single-vessel disease whose long-term survival was excellent (100%) and 11 patients with multivessel disease and poor left ventricular function whose three-year survival was poor (58% ± 16%) (Figure 43-3).

Survival Stratified by Age

Among the 129 infarct survivors undergoing coronary arteriography within 60 days of infarction, overall survival was not significantly different among the 34 patients age ⩾60 years in comparison to the 95 patients age <60 years (Figure 43-4).

Survival Among Surgical Candidate Subgroups

Among the 94 surgical candidates, survival was not significantly different between the patients managed with coronary artery bypass graft (CABG) surgery and those managed medically (Figure 43-5) though there was a trend toward improved survival among the surgically managed patients.

Further stratification into four subgroups based on age and CABG (Figure 43-6) showed no significant differences between the four subgroups, although again the trend toward improved survival among surgically managed patients was noted. Interestingly, a trend toward improved survival in the "elderly" patients, both in the medical and surgical groups, was also noted, though not statistically significant.

The 94 surgical candidates were further examined according to extent of coronary disease (single vessel vs multivessel), left ventricular ejection fraction (⩽40% vs >40%), and number of jeopardized segments (⩽3 vs >3) (Table 43-3). Improved survival was noted in patients with multivessel disease and in patients with ejection fraction >40% treated surgically, and this trend approached statistical significance ($P = .11$) (Table 43-3). Among patients having three or more jeopardized left ventricular segments, survival was significantly improved in surgically compared to medically managed patients (3-year survival of 93 ± 5% vs 64 ± 11%, $P < .05$). The older patients (aged ⩾60 years) have ejection

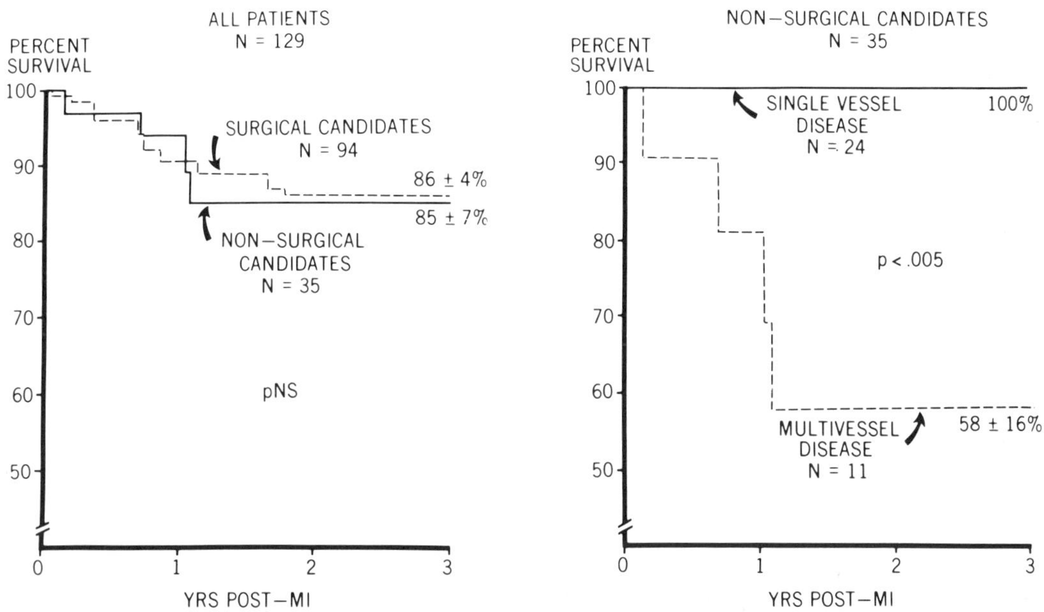

Figure 43-3 Survival among patients having angiography early post-myocardial infarction (MI). Survival was similar in surgical and nonsurgical candidates (left), but the nonsurgical candidates had remarkably different survival rates when grouped according to the extent of coronary artery disease (right). (Reproduced with permission from Rogers et al.[13])

fraction ≥40% had a significantly (P = .09) improved survival compared to the younger patients (aged <60 years). However, survival did not differ between older and younger patients with regard to extent of coronary artery disease or extent of jeopardized myocardium. Further subdividing the population according to medical vs surgical therapy within the older and younger age groupings showed no significant differences in three-year survival between age groupings (Table 43-4).

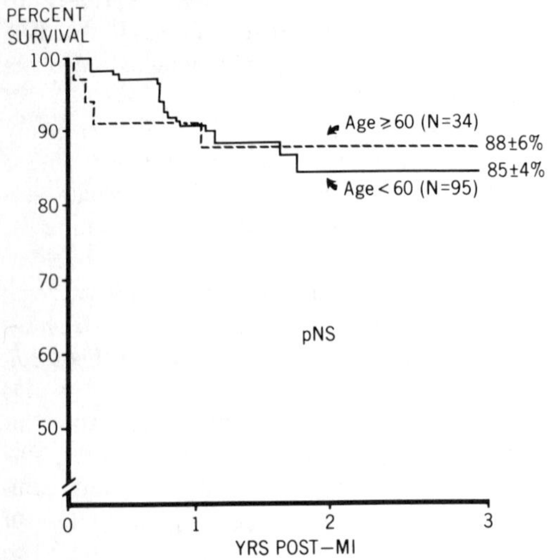

Figure 43-4 Survival in 129 patients stratified by age having angiography early after myocardial infarction. Survival was not significantly different overall in patients ≥ age 60 vs those patients age < 60. MI = myocardial infarction.

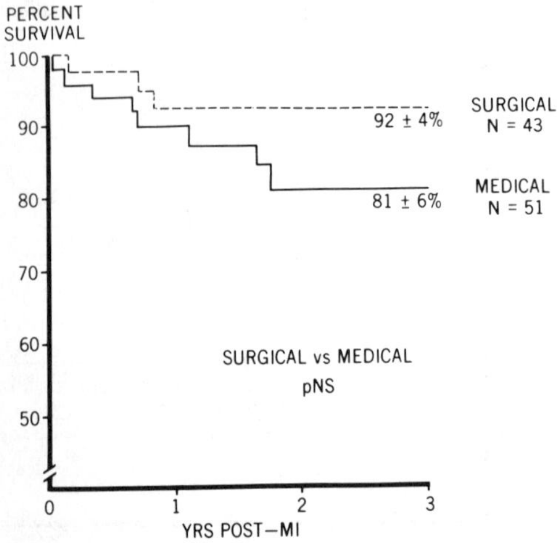

Figure 43-5 Survival in surgical candidates according to surgical or medical management. There was a trend toward improved survival among the surgical group, though this trend did not reach statistical significance. MI = myocardial infarction. (Reproduced with permission from Rogers et al.[13])

Functional Status at Follow-up

No significant differences were noted at follow-up relative to angina or heart failure class, employment status, or incidence of recurrent myocardial infarction. Likewise, these parameters did not differ between patients aged >60 and those aged ≤60 years, although there were significantly more younger than older patients employed preoperatively.

DISCUSSION

In this retrospective study of survivors of acute myocardial infarction who underwent coronary and left ventricular angiography within 60 days of acute myocardial infarction, we found that most such patients are surgical candidates, that coronary artery bypass surgery can be done with a low operative mortality and morbidity, and that there are significant trends toward enhanced long-term survival among surgically managed patients having multivessel disease and ejection fraction exceeding 40% and four or more residual jeopardized ventricular segments. Finally, in this highly selected series, patients aged 60 or older appeared to fare as well or better than their counterparts (aged <60), whether managed surgically or medically.

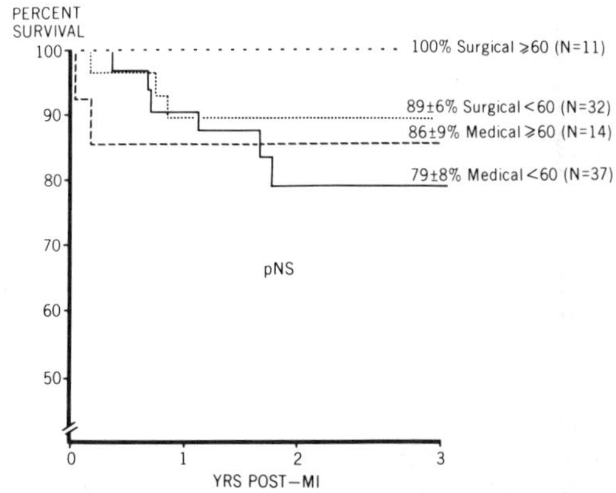

Figure 43-6 Survival in surgical candidates stratified according to age and treatment received. There was a trend toward improved survival in patients managed surgically as well as in patients ≥ age 60, but these trends did not reach statistical significance. MI = myocardial infarction.

Table 43-3
Survival in Surgical Candidates

	Three-Year Survival					Three-Year Survival				
	Medical		*Surgical*			*Aged <60 yr*		*Aged ≥60 yr*		
	%	(n)	%	(n)	*P*	%	(n)	%	(n)	*P*
All patients	81 ± 6	(51)	92 ± 4	(43)	ns	84 ± 5	(69)	92 ± 5	(25)	ns
Single-vessel disease	100	(16)	100	(3)	ns	100	(14)	100	(5)	ns
Multivessel disease	75 ± 8	(35)	92 ± 5	(40)	.11	80 ± 6	(55)	90 ± 7	(20)	ns
Ejection fraction ≤40%	70 ± 12	(22)	81 ± 10	(18)	ns	60 ± 12	(23)	94 ± 6	(17)	.09
Ejection fraction >40%	89 ± 6	(29)	100	(25)	.11	95 ± 3	(46)	88 ± 12	(8)	ns
≤3 Jeopardized segments	100	(24)	90 ± 9	(13)	ns	96 ± 4	(28)	100	(9)	ns
>3 Jeopardized segments	64 ± 11	(27)	93 ± 5	(30)	<.05	75 ± 8	(41)	88 ± 8	(16)	ns

Table 43-4
Survival in Surgical Candidates Subgroups Three-Year Survival

	Surgical Group					Medical Group				
	Aged <60 yr		*Aged ≥60 yr*			*Aged <60 yr*		*Aged ≥60 yr*		
Subgroup	%	(n)	%	(n)	*P*	%	(n)	%	(n)	*P*
All surgical candidates	89 ± 6	(32)	100	(11)	ns	79 ± 8	(37)	86 ± 9	(14)	ns
Single-vessel disease	100	(2)	100	(1)	ns	100	(12)	100	(4)	ns
Multivessel disease	89 ± 6	(30)	100	(10)	ns	71 ± 10	(25)	80 ± 13	(10)	ns
Ejection fraction ≤40%	71 ± 14	(12)	100	(16)	ns	46 ± 19	(11)	91 ± 9	(11)	ns
Ejection fraction >40%	100	(20)	100	(5)	ns	92 ± 5	(26)	67 ± 27	(3)	ns
≤3 Jeopardized segments	89 ± 10	(10)	100	(3)	ns	100	(18)	100	(6)	ns
>3 Jeopardized segments	90 ± 7	(22)	100	(8)	ns	59 ± 13	(19)	75 ± 15	(8)	ns

Coronary Artery Bypass Surgery in Elderly Patients

Coronary artery bypass surgery is often recommended to the patient as a means of improving either the *quantity* or *quality* of his life, or both. In the case of the elderly patient who may have already attained or surpassed his expected life span, physicians have traditionally reserved coronary revascularization surgery for those having incapacitating symptoms and thus whose quality of life would be potentially improved by surgery. Hesitancy to recommed coronary revascularization surgery in the aged patient stems from the widespread assumption that, in general, such patients may have either overt or latent multisystem disease and are thus likely to have a higher perioperative mortality than younger patients. Indeed, information that this belief is correct is provided by analysis of perioperative mortality by age. At the University of Alabama Medical Center the hospital mortality of isolated coronary artery bypass grafting approaches 0% in patients aged 60 years or less, but thereafter with advancing age the perioperative mortality rate rises steeply (Figure 43-7).[19]

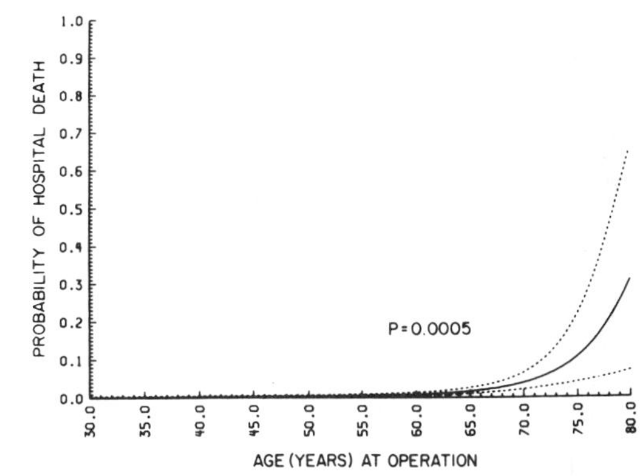

Figure 43-7 Probability of hospital death expressed as a function of age in 757 patients undergoing isolated coronary artery bypass grafting in 1977 at the University of Alabama Medical Center. Dotted lines represent 70% confidence limits about the solid line. (Reproduced with permission from Kirklin et al.[19])

Although a number of studies have addressed the issue of coronary revascularization surgery in the elderly patient,[20-31] the largest reported experience is that of the registry of the Coronary Artery Surgery Study (CASS).[32] This experience included 1086 patients aged 65 years or older who underwent isolated coronary artery bypass graft surgery. The operative mortality of these patients was 5.2%, significantly greater than the perioperative mortality of 1.9% in patients younger than age 65 entered into the same registry. Variables predictive of perioperative mortality among elderly patients were ≥70% left main coronary artery stenosis and a left dominant circulation, elevated left ventricular end-diastolic pressure, cigarette smoking, pulmonary rales, and presence of one or more associated medical diseases.

Coronary Artery Bypass Surgery Post–Myocardial Infarction

The present study tested the hypothesis that early coronary arteriography and coronary revascularization surgery in selected patients post–myocardial infarction might improve longevity and quality of life compared to conventional medical therapy. Obvious limitations of this study include its retrospective, nonrandomized design and the fact that the patients who eventually received surgical therapy had more extensive coronary artery disease than the medically managed surgical candidate goup. A major strength of the study is that coronary arteriograms were obtained in a substantial proportion (83%:129/156) of the infarct population who were deemed "eligible" for intervention. Of these 129 patients studied angiographically, a significant percentage (73%:94/129) were felt to be surgical candidates on the basis of their coronary anatomy and their left ventricular function. Operative mortality was 2% (1/43) and the perioperative infarction rate was 5% (2/43). Long-term (3-year) survival in the surgically managed patients exceeded that of the medically managed patients (92% ± 4% vs 81% ± 6%) but the difference did not reach statistical significance (Figure 43-5). However, when the groups were further subdivided according to the number of coronary vessels diseased, ejection fraction, or number of jeopardized ventriculographic segments, significant differences were found between the surgically managed patients (Table 43-3). Improved survival was noted in the surgically managed patients having multivessel disease, ejection fraction exceeing 40%, or three or more jeopardized ventriculographic segments.

The functional status or "quality of life" at follow-up did not differ significantly between medical and surgical groups (Table 43-5). However, symptom analysis in this study is undoubtedly

Table 43-5
Follow-up Status of Surgical Candidates

	Surgical Groups (n = 43)	Medical Groups (n = 51)	*P*	Aged <60 yr (n = 69)	Aged ≥60 yr (n = 25)	*P*
Days from MI to follow-up	673 ± 61	692 ± 55	ns	662 ± 46	743 ± 86	ns
Alive at follow-up	38 (88%)	42 (82%)	ns	59 (86%)	25 (84%)	ns
Angina class*						
1	28 (78%)	26 (67%)		37 (68%)	17 (81%)	
2	3 (8%)	9 (23%)	ns	8 (15%)	4 (19%)	ns
3	3 (8%)	0		3 (6%)	0 (0%)	
4	2 (6%)	4 (10%)		4 (11%)	0 (0%)	
CHF class*						
1	23 (64%)	31 (79%)		41 (72%)	13 (62%)	
2	8 (22%)	2 (5%)	ns	6 (11%)	4 (19%)	ns
3	4 (11%)	3 (8%)		6 (11%)	1 (5%)	
4	1 (3%)	3 (8%)		4 (7%)	3 (14%)	
Employment status pre-MI*						
Full time	23 (64%)	27 (69%)		42 (78%)	8 (38%)	
Part time	1 (3%)	1 (3%)	ns	1 (2%)	1 (5%)	.02
Unemployed	12 (33%)	11 (28%)		11 (20%)	12 (57%)	
Employment status post-MI						
Full time	15 (42%)	20 (51%)		29 (54%)	6 (29%)	
Part time	2 (6%)	2 (5%)	ns	3 (6%)	1 (5%)	ns
Unemployed	19 (53%)	17 (44%)		22 (40%)	14 (67%)	
Recurrent MI	5 (12%)	3 (6%)	ns	6 (11%)	2 (10%)	ns

*Includes only 75 patients whose functional class and employment status could be ascertained at follow-up. MI = myocardial infarction, CHF = heart failure.

somewhat misleading because most patients had been at limited activity prior to catheterization, while convalescing from their myocardial infarction. It is important to note, however, that at follow-up a substantial proportion of surgically managed patients were essentially asymptomatic.

Coronary Artery Bypass Surgery in the Elderly Patient Postinfarction

Although the present study was not designed to specifically address the issue of coronary revascularization surgery in the elderly patient postinfarction, it is nevertheless informative to compare the outcome of the "elderly" (≥ age 60) patients with their counterparts who are 60 years of age or younger. It should be stressed that our study by no means included all postinfarction patients in the elderly category. Indeed, one of the major reasons for not recommending angiography in our study was advanced age. The elderly patients who were included in our study, however, were generally those whose "physiological age" was appreciably less than their "chronological age" and in whom the clinicians considered that further intervention would not be inappropriate. Thus, although our study does not have applicability to the entire spectrum of elderly patients postinfarction, it does have definite applicability to those patients appearing "physiologically young." In general, we utilized criteria outline by Gann et al[24] to assess physiological age: (1) the patient's activity level preinfarction; (2) the patient's motivation to return to an active life style; (3) the patient's mental status or alertness; (4) the presence or absence of severe associated medical diseases.

The most interesting finding in our analysis of the elderly population was that they differed very little from their younger counterparts either in terms of base-line characteristics (Table 43-1 and Table 43-2), three-year survival (Table 43-3), or follow-up functional status (Table 43-4). Although the numbers of patients in our analytical subgroups are small, it is apparent that the elderly patients selected for coronary revascularization surgery in our series not only tolerated the surgery itself well, but had an excellent long-term survival. Indeed, of the 11 patients aged ≥60 years undergoing coronary revascularization surgery, there were no early or late deaths. Likewise, among the medical group, survival in the elderly patients was in general not significantly lower than that of the younger patients.

These findings suggest that our "elderly patients" were not truly elderly in terms of their physiologic age and thus had not reached their expected life span. Indeed, the average life expectancy in 1979 in the United States for persons having reached the age of 70 was 14.8 years for women and 11.1 years for men.[33] In our study, survival was 100% at three years among the 11 patients aged ≥60 years undergoing coronary revascularization surgery and was substantially (though not statistically significantly) lower among patients aged ≥60 years having multivessel disease, ejection fraction ≥40%, and three or more jeopardized ventriculographic segments (Table 43-4).

Though our patient numbers are small, making valid statistical conclusions impossible, our data raise important issues concerning the possible relevance of coronary revascularization surgery postinfarction in selected elderly patients as a means of prolonging life. The life expectancy of 11 to 15 years for patients aged 70 years mentioned above would certainly justify surgical attempts at prolonging life if the surgery could be done at relatively low risk. Our data suggest that in selected elderly patients surgery can indeed be done with low risk postinfarction and may be the treatment of choice.

ACKNOWLEDGMENT

This work was supported in part by the National Heart, Lung and Blood Institute (Specialized Center of Research for Ischemic Heart Disease, Contract No. 5P 50HL 17667-09) of the National Institutes of Health, Bethesda, Md.

REFERENCES

1. American Heart Association: *Heart Facts 1983*. Dallas, Texas, American Heart Association's Office of Communications, 1983, p 2.
2. Cooperative study: Death rate among 795 patients in first year after myocardial infarction. *JAMA* 1966;197:906,908–911.
3. Weinblatt E, Shapiro S, Frank CW, et al: Prognosis of men after first myocardial infarction: Mortality and first recurrence in relation to selected parameters. *Am J Public Health* 1968;58:1329–1343.
4. Norris RM, Caughey DE, Mercer CJ, et al: Coronary prognostic index for predicting survival after recovery from acute myocardial infarction. *Lancet* 1970;2:485–488.
5. Vismara LA, Amsterdam EA, Mason DT: Relation of ventricular arrhythmias in the late hospital phase of acute myocardial infarction to sudden death after hospital discharge. *Am J Med* 1975;59:6–10.
6. Schulze RA Jr, Strauss HW, Pitt B: Sudden death in the year following myocardial infarction: Relation to ventricular premature contractions in the late hospital phase and left ventricular ejection fraction. *Am J Med* 1977;62:192–194.

7. Kannel WB, Sorlie P, McNamara PM: Prognosis after initial myocardial infarction: The Framingham Study. *Am J Cardiol* 1979;44:52–55.
8. Bigger JT, Heller CA, Wenger TL, et al: Risk stratification after acute myocardial infarction. *Am J Cardiol* 1978;42:202–205.
9. Schulze RA, Pitt B, Griffith LSC, et al: Coronary angiography and left ventriculography in survivors of transmural and nontransmural myocardial infarction. *Am J Med* 1978;64:108–110.
10. Bertrand ME, Lefebvre JM, Laisne CL, et al: Coronary arteriography in acute transmural myocardial infarction. *Am Heart J* 1979;97:61–63.
11. Turner JD, Rogers WJ, Mantle JA, et al: Coronary angiography soon after myocardial infarction. *Chest* 1980;77:58–60.
12. Hurst JW, King SB III, Logue RB, et al: Value of coronary bypass surgery. *Am J Cardiol* 1978;42: 308–311.
13. Rogers WJ, Smith LR, Oberman A, et al: Surgical vs nonsurgical management of patients after myocardial infarction. *Circulation* 1980;62(suppl 1): 1-67.
14. Rogers WJ, Smith LR, Bream PR, et al: Quantitative axial oblique contrast ventriculography: Validation of the method by demonstrating improved visualization of regional wall motion and mitral valve function with accurate volume determinations. *Am Heart J* 1982;103:185–187.
15. James TN: *Anatomy of the Coronary Arteries.* Hagerstown, Harper and Row, 1961.
16. The Criteria Committee of the New York Heart Association Inc: Diseases of the heart and blood vessels: Nomenclature and criteria for diagnosis, Boston, Little, Brown and Co, ed 6, 1964.
17. Kaplan EL, Meier P: Non-parametric estimation from incomplete observations. *J Am Stat Assoc* 1958;53:457–460.
18. Gehan EA: A generalized Wilcoxon test for comparing arbitrarily singly censored samples. *Biometrika* 1965;52:203–206.
19. Kirklin JW, Kouchoukos NT, Blackstone EH, et al: Research related to surgical treatment of coronary artery disease. *Circulation* 1979;60:1613–1617.
20. Ashor GW, Meyer BW, Lindesmith GG, et al: Coronary artery disease: Surgery in 100 patients 65 years of age and older. *Arch Surg* 1973;107:30–32.
21. Garcia JM, Cheanvechai C, Effler DB: Myocardial revascularization in patients aged 65 and older. *Cardiovasc Clin* 1975;7:83–85.
22. Quinlan R, Cohn LH, Collins JJ: Determinants of survival following cardiac operations in elderly patients. *Chest* 1975;68:498–500.
23. Meyer J, Wukasch DC, Seybold-Epting W, et al: Coronary artery bypass in patients over 70 years of age: Indications and results. *Am J Cardiol* 1975; 36:342–344.
24. Gann D, Cohn C, Hildner FJ, et al: Coronary artery bypass surgery in patients seventy years of age and older. *J Thorac Cardiovasc Surg* 1977;73: 237–239.
25. Stephenson LW, MacVaugh HM III, Edmunds LH: Surgery using cardiopulmonary bypass in the elderly. *Circulation* 1978;58:250–253.
26. Berman ND, David TE, Lipton IH, et al: Surgical procedures involving cardiopulmonary bypass in patients aged 70 or older. *J Am Geriatr Soc* 1980; 28:29–31.
27. DuCailar C, Chaitman BR, Castonguay Y: Risks and benefits of aortocoronary bypass surgery in patients aged 65 years or more. *Can Med Assoc J* 1980;122:771–775.
28. Higginbotham M, Hunt D, White A, et al: Surgical treatment of angina pectoris in the elderly. *Med J Aust* 1981;2:664–667.
29. Knapp WS, Douglas JS, Craver JM, et al: Efficacy of coronary artery bypass grafting in elderly patients with coronary artery disease. *Am J Cardiol* 1981;47:923–925.
30. Berry BE, Acree PW, Davis DJ, et al: Coronary artery bypass operations in septuagenarians. *Ann Thorac Surg* 1981;31:310.
31. Hochberg MS, Levine FH, Daggett WM, et al: Isolated coronary artery bypass grafting in patients seventy years of age and older. *J Thorac Cardiovasc Surg* 1982;84:219–223.
32. Gersh BJ, Kronmal RA, Frye RL, et al: Coronary arteriography and coronary artery bypass surgery: Morbidity and mortality in patients ages 65 years or older. A report from the Coronary Artery Surgery Study. *Circulation* 1983;67:483–485.
33. Statistical abstract of the United States. US Department of Commerce, Washington DC, 1979, p 17.

CHAPTER 44
Percutaneous Transluminal Coronary Angioplasty

David R. Holmes, Jr

The modern application of the concept of transluminal angioplasty of arterial stenoses dates back to Charles Dotter.[1] Development of the concept was stimulated during a case in which an angiography catheter was inadvertently passed through an occluded iliac artery into the abdominal aorta.[2] From this beginning, the "Dotter technic" evolved. With this technic, a small guiding catheter is positioned across an arterial stenosis and then dilating catheters are introduced over the guide. After application of this technic, interest in the procedure gradually increased, mainly in Europe, and an inflatable balloon of polyvinyl chloride was eventually developed. This was used initially in patients with peripheral arterial stenoses and then was modified for cardiac applications.

In 1977, Andreas Grüntzig[3,4] performed the first percutaneous transluminal coronary angioplasty (PTCA) and 1 year later reported on his initial series of patients. In the five years since, there has been explosive growth in the field, a National Heart, Lung, and Blood Institute (NHLBI) PTCA Registry has been formed with approximately 3000 patients enrolled, and an increasing number of coronary dilatations are performed each year.[5,6] The rapid increase in the number of procedures has resulted from (1) continued interest in less invasive means of revascularization, compared with surgical technics, (2) improvements in catheter design, and (3) continued reports on the efficacy and safety of the technic in larger subsets of patients with coronary artery disease.[7-9]

MECHANISM OF DILATATION

The mechanism of dilatation has been studied both in laboratory models and in postmortem human studies.[10-18] In addition, there is a limited amount of pathologic material from patients who died after PTCA.[19]

In laboratory models, balloon inflation results in prompt endothelial damage followed by platelet aggregation and adhesion and fibrin deposition.[12,14,15] With increased inflation, the superficial portion of atherosclerotic plaques is disrupted and there may be intimal splitting and the development of intimal flaps. In addition, in eccentric lesions, the normal wall may be thinned without intimal fracture.[10] Block et al[15] have commented on the important relationship between the size of the stenosis and the expanded balloon. They have demonstrated that if the inflated balloon is larger than the artery, both the plaque and the intima may be split. If the balloon and arterial segment are similar in size, there is endothelial denudation and splitting of the atheroma but not the intima.

Information on the effects of dilatation in diseased human arterial segments remains limited. Castaneda-Zuniga et al[16] have documented stretching of the intima, media, and adventitia, which is associated with intimal rupture and fragmentation. In heart specimens at autopsy, Lee et al[13] documented endothelial disruption, derangement of collagen and elastic fibers, stretching and disruption of the tunica media, and atheromatous compression. In addition, dissecting hematomas have been documented in patients who died after PTCA.[19] Following the initial controlled injury of dilatation, healing takes place, which can result in further retraction of the separated plaque elements and then re-endothelialization.

These variable histopathologic findings in dilated arterial segments result in a wide spectrum of angiographic findings.[20] The most common findings are intraluminal haziness, smooth-walled dilatation, and an intimal flap (Figure 44-1). The intraluminal haziness has been attributed to contrast medium in multiple linear fissures of the dilated segment.[15,16] An intimal flap results from splitting and fragmentation of the atheromatous plaque.[12,15,16]

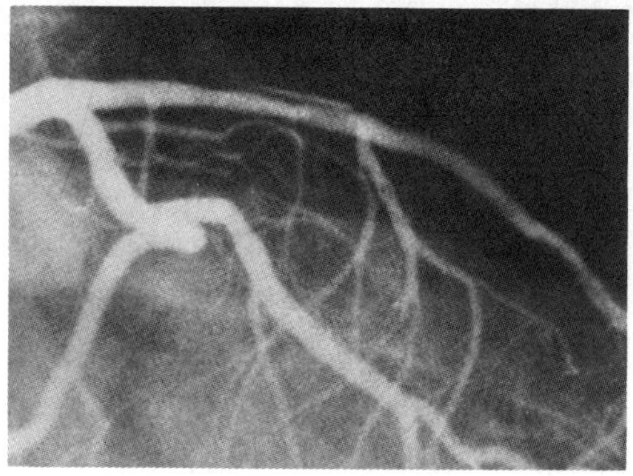

Figure 44-1 Right anterior oblique view of left coronary artery after successful dilatation of stenosis in middle left anterior descending artery. There is a discrete linear density and an intimal flap. (Reproduced with permission from Holmes et al.[20])

EQUIPMENT

Coronary angioplasty catheter systems consist of two major parts: a guiding catheter and the balloon-tipped dilating catheter. In addition, an inflation device is required. Several devices are available, some of which are hand-driven, while others use compressed air or CO_2. In either case, the devices must facilitate the accurate stepwise delivery and maintenance of up to 10 atm of pressure.

Guiding Catheter

Several types of guiding catheters which facilitate intubation of the appropriate coronary artery are available. Although the percutaneous transfemoral approach is most commonly used with preformed Judkins or Amplatz shapes, catheters also are available for use with a brachial approach. The catheters are manufactured in different sizes to accommodate individual variations in size of the aortic root and take-off of the coronary artery. In addition, out-of-plane catheters are available for more selective intubation of the circumflex or left anterior descending coronary arteries. Initially, the size of the guiding system was 9-F; subsequently, the size has been reduced to 8-F, although with the smaller sizes, catheter manipulation may be more of a problem.

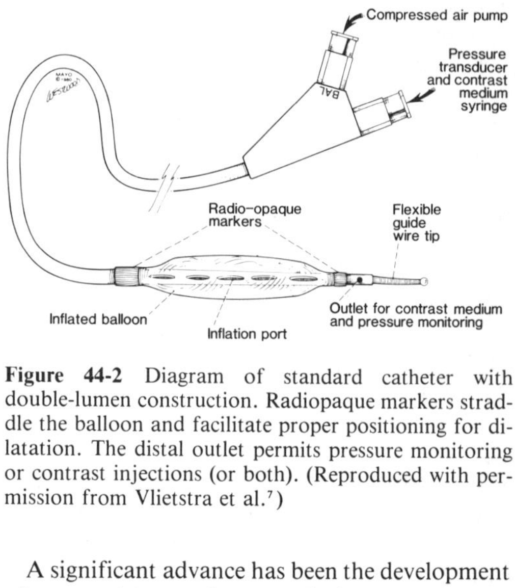

Figure 44-2 Diagram of standard catheter with double-lumen construction. Radiopaque markers straddle the balloon and facilitate proper positioning for dilatation. The distal outlet permits pressure monitoring or contrast injections (or both). (Reproduced with permission from Vlietstra et al.[7])

Balloon-Tipped Dilating Catheter

There have been rapid and continuing advances in the design of the dilating catheter (Figure 44-2). The catheter itself is double-lumen in construction, with a balloon tip that is bracketed by radiopaque markers. These markers facilitate the correct and optimal positioning of the balloon across the stenosis. The balloon is made of polyvinyl chloride or polyethylene.[21] These materials are nonelastic, a feature that is essential to ensure the uniform radial application of the dilating force. Although each catheter varies, most are constructed to withstand up to 10 atm of pressure. Beyond 10 atm, the catheter may weaken and rupture. Several balloon sizes are available, ranging in outside diameter from 2 to 3.7 mm, which allows selection and matching of the catheter to the diseased coronary artery.

A significant advance has been the development of some degree of external tip control. The original systems had a fixed distal wire tip. Subsequent modifications have resulted in a movable distal wire tip that can be shaped and formed (Figure 44-3). These "steerable" systems facilitate passage of the catheters through the coronary artery and the stenosis and allow dilatation of lesions that were previously inaccessible.

TECHNIC

The selection of the approach (brachial vs femoral) and of the guiding and dilating catheters is based on the size and location of the coronary artery to be dilated, the severity of the stenosis, and its location within the coronary artery. Other

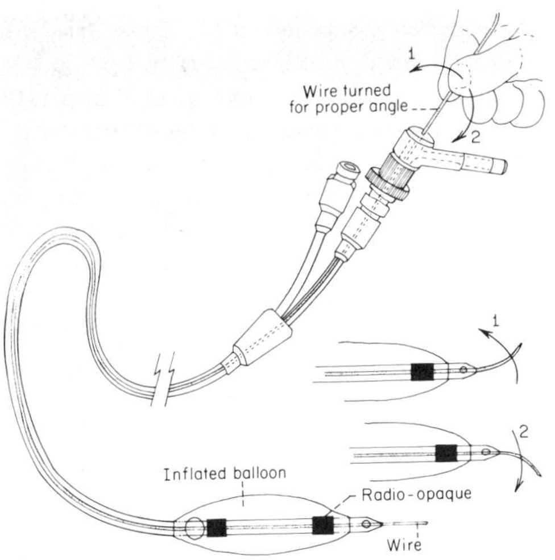

Figure 44-3 Diagram of a "steerable" catheter system. Radiopaque markers facilitate proper positioning for dilatation. Movable central guide wire can be shaped and then externally rotated to facilitate passage of the catheter into more distal or tortuous coronary arteries.

important factors involved in this selection include details of the coronary anatomy, such as the presence of branch vessels or a tortuous proximal coronary artery, the size of the aortic root and take-off of the coronary artery, and the presence of associated cardiovascular diseases, such as arteriosclerosis obliterans.

By the use of standard technics, the coronary ostium is intubated. Five thousand units of heparin sodium are administered. In addition, nitrates and a calcium antagonist are given to prevent coronary artery spasm. The appropriate dilating catheter is selected. If the stenosis is very severe, the smallest catheter with a 2.0-mm balloon is selected. More commonly, however, a 3.0-mm balloon is selected. After being flushed and filled with a solution of 50% contrast medium (Renografin) and 50% normal saline, the balloon catheter is advanced through the guiding catheter into the ostium of the coronary artery. Pressures are recorded simultaneously through the guiding catheter and the balloon-dilating catheter. Under careful fluoroscopic control, the dilating catheter is then advanced through the stenosis, and the downstream pressure is measured (Figures 44-4 and 44-5). Frequent test injections of contrast medium are used to document the proper position. High-quality video playback and x-ray systems are essential during PTCA. These permit detailed assessment of the position of the dilating catheter within the coronary artery and facilitate safe passage of the dilating catheter through the stenosis. After the dilating catheter crosses the stenosis, there is usually a significant gradient of >40 mmHg. This gradient varies, however, depending on the size of the vessel and dilating catheter, the severity of the stenosis, and the collateral vessels.

After proper placement of the balloon, inflations are performed. The number of inflations, duration of inflation, and inflation pressure vary among institutions. Inflation is performed in a stepwise fashion, with the pressure being increased approximately 1 atm at a time, until the lesion is seen to yield and the dumbbell deformity of the stenosis disappears. In general, three to five inflations of 4 to 10 atm, each lasting approximately 15 to 30 seconds, are performed. During inflation, patients may experience angina pectoris and have significant ST segment depression. This is promptly relieved by deflation. Successful dilatation is accompanied by disappearance of the dumbbell deformity of stenosis on the balloon, an increase in distal pressure, and the rapid washout of contrast medium downstream. After maximal

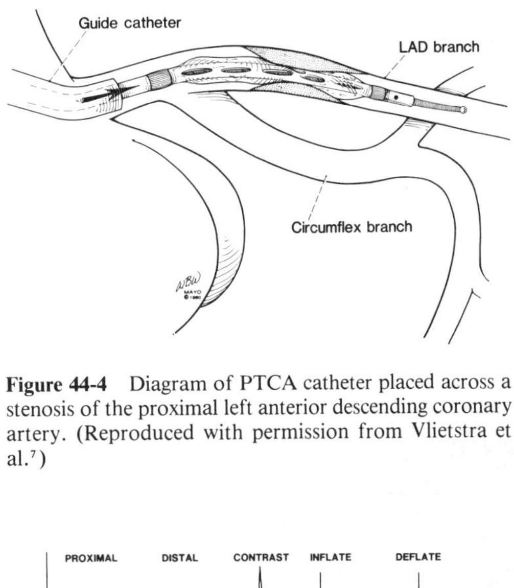

Figure 44-4 Diagram of PTCA catheter placed across a stenosis of the proximal left anterior descending coronary artery. (Reproduced with permission from Vlietstra et al.[7])

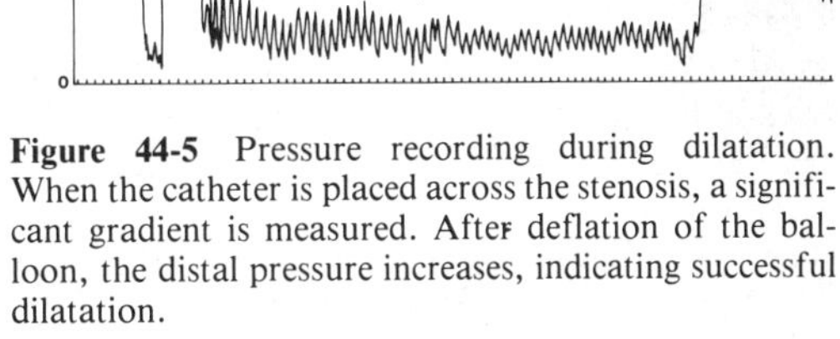

Figure 44-5 Pressure recording during dilatation. When the catheter is placed across the stenosis, a significant gradient is measured. After deflation of the balloon, the distal pressure increases, indicating successful dilatation.

luminal enlargement and gradient reduction, the dilating catheter is withdrawn and angiography is repeated. If repeat angiography documents a significant residual stenosis, a larger dilating catheter is selected and PTCA is again performed. Care must be taken at this time to avoid subintimal passage of the catheter during crossing of the previously dilated segment.

After the procedure, the catheters are removed, and an arterial sheath is left in place to facilitate prompt repeat angiography during the first several hours after PTCA, if clinically indicated. The patient is then sent to the coronary care unit for 24 hours of observation. During this time, routine analysis of cardiac enzymes is done, and electrocardiography is performed. When PTCA is unsuccessful, patients are usually transferred directly to the operating room for surgical revascularization.

PATIENT SELECTION

The criteria for selection of patients have expanded since the original use of PTCA. Initially, the technic was recommended for patients with recent onset of angina pectoris and proximal noncalcified single coronary artery stenoses in whom medical treatment had failed and who were candidates for surgical revascularization.[4,6–8] These selection criteria still identify ideal patients with a high likelihood of success, although adhering to these criteria limits the number of patients who may benefit from the procedure (Figure 44-6). Initially, only from 1% to 10% of patients undergoing saphenous vein bypass graft or cardiac catheterization were considered suitable.[7,8,22–25]

As experience has increased, the criteria for angioplasty have broadened, and PTCA is now being utilized in other patient groups. Recently, there has been increased application in patients with multivessel disease.[26,27] This has the obvious potential of increasing the pool of patients suitable for PTCA. PTCA also has been used in selected patients with total coronary occlusion (Figure 44-7).[28–31] In patients with acute myocardial infarction, PTCA is combined with intracoronary use of streptokinase. In patients with recent coronary occlusion but without associated myocardial infarction, PTCA alone may be used. In these patients, the dilating catheter may be passed through the occlusion and dilatation performed. Finally, patients with bypass graft stenoses may be suitable for PTCA.[32–34] This has been particularly useful in patients with stenoses at the site of distal anastomoses rather than in the graft body itself.

Current selection criteria vary among institutions. This variability depends in major part on the experience and clinical philosophy of the physicians involved. In some institutions, selection criteria remain rigid in order to identify ideal patients and to ensure high success rates. In other institutions, PTCA is attempted in multiple patient subsets, particularly those already scheduled for coronary artery bypass surgery, in order to expand the number of patients who could potentially benefit from a less invasive procedure. It must be remembered when analyzing results that PTCA performed in less-than-ideal patients may result in lower success rates. Selection criteria should evolve as experience with the continued safety and efficacy of the procedure increases. Our current

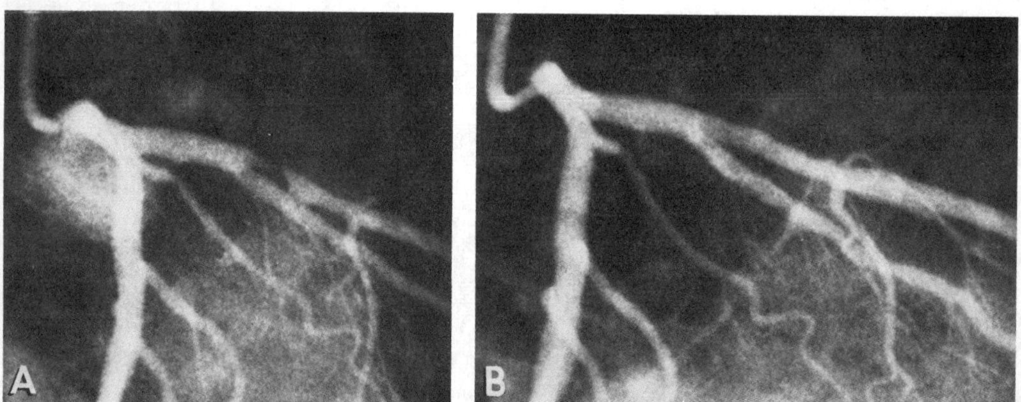

Figure 44-6 Right anterior oblique view of left coronary artery. **A**, Documenting ideal angiographic anatomy for PTCA with a high-grade but subtotal stenosis of the middle left anterior descending artery. (Reproduced with permission from Hartzler et al.[38]) **B**, After dilatation, there is an excellent improvement in the stenosis.

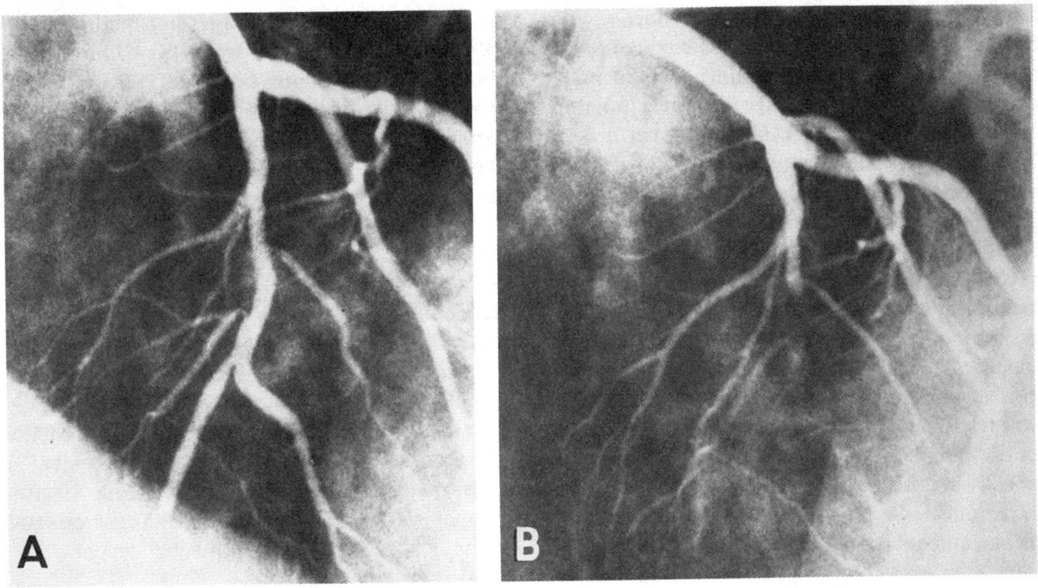

Figure 44-7 Left anterior oblique view of left coronary artery. **A**, Documentation of complete occlusion of the left anterior descending artery prior to PTCA. **B**, After dilatation, there is minimal residual stenosis only.

practice is to the offer PTCA to symptomatic patients with myocardial ischemia who have one or more lesions accessible to the dilating catheter and who are surgical candidates, in the event that either PTCA is unsuccessful or complications occur during dilatation.

ADJUVANT TREATMENT

Various agents are commonly used before, during, and after PTCA. The most frequently used agents are antiplatelet drugs with or without anticoagulants, nitrates to prevent coronary spasm, and calcium antagonists. Our group initiates treatment with aspirin, 1 grain three times a day, and dipyridamole, 75 mg three times a day, 24 to 48 hours before PTCA. Calcium antagonists and nitrates are administered during the procedure. After PTCA, the use of aspirin and dipyridamole is continued for at least 6 months. The use of calcium antagonists also is continued after dilatation.

RESULTS

Early Success

Success rates for PTCA vary, depending on patient selection, operator experience, and definition of success. The NHLBI PTCA Registry defines success as ≥20% improvement in luminal diameter stenosis.[6] At our institution, we use an increase in luminal diameter stenosis of ≥40% as the definition of success. In the most recent information on 1898 patients from the NHLBI PTCA Registry, PTCA was successful in 64%.[5] This registry includes the early experience with PTCA, which may represent the learning curve of the procedure. In ideal patients, particularly those with lesions of the proximal left anterior descending coronary artery, and with the use of new catheters that give some degree of external control, an overall success rate of 80% to 90% is probably attainable. In other patient subsets, including those with multivessel coronary artery disease, recent coronary artery occlusion, saphenous vein bypass grafts, and evolving acute myocardial infarction, excellent success rates are also obtainable.[26-34]

Complications

PTCA results in a wide spectrum of angiographic findings that reflect underlying anatomic pathologic changes in the coronary artery. Although some of these can be considered as indirect consequences of PTCA, others reflect direct complications.[20]

Clinically significant complications have been documented in as many as 8% of cases in the NHLBI PTCA Registry.[35] In that series, myocardial infarction was the most frequent complication (3.5%). Infarction may result from complete occlusion of the dilated vessel. In these patients, the extent of myocardial infarction depends on the presence or absence of adequate collateral vessels and the timing and completeness of myocardial revascularization. Myocardial infarction may also result from occlusion of a small branch vessel arising in close proximity to the dilated vessel (Figure 44-8).

Coronary artery occlusion was documented during PTCA in 2.7% of patients in the NHLBI PTCA Registry.[35] In these patients, coronary occlusion is the most common indication for urgent coronary artery surgery.[36] The occlusion may be secondary to plaque hemorrhage, acute thrombosis, spasm, coronary dissection with luminal compression, or, more rarely, plaque dislodgment or displacement. The treatment of occlusion depends on the clinical setting. When occlusion occurs during PTCA, supplemental nitrates and calcium antagonists should be administered if coronary artery spasm is suspected. In addition, patients with acute occlusion have been successfully redilated and attempts may be made to probe the occlusion and restore flow.[20] Care must be taken to avoid delay in prompt surgical intervention and reperfusion when indicated clinically. Even when prompt surgery is performed, some myocardial necrosis may develop.

In the NHLBI PTCA Registry, in-hospital deaths were documented in 0.9% of cases.[35] Within that group were smaller subsets with higher rates. These subgroups included older patients with multivessel disease and patients with previous saphenous vein bypass graft surgery.[6,37] Continued experience with the procedure and prompt recognition and early treatment of serious complications should reduce the mortality rates. The potential for these serious complications continues to make it appropriate to have cardiovascular surgery standby support for prompt consultation and treatment if needed.

Other complications have been documented and include coronary artery spasm, aneurysmal dilatation, coronary artery dissection, coronary rupture, and distal embolization. Noncardiac complications also are seen. These include vascular injury and systemic embolization. Meticulous attention to details and prompt treatment in these patients are essential in reducing the frequency with which these complications occur and in reducing their adverse consequences.

FOLLOW-UP

Functional Results

Successful PTCA results not only in angiographic improvement and a reduction in the transstenotic gradient but also in improvement of perfusion and in the reduction or abolition of ischemia. Increases in coronary sinus blood flow and normalization of myocardial metabolism have been documented after successful PTCA.[38,39]

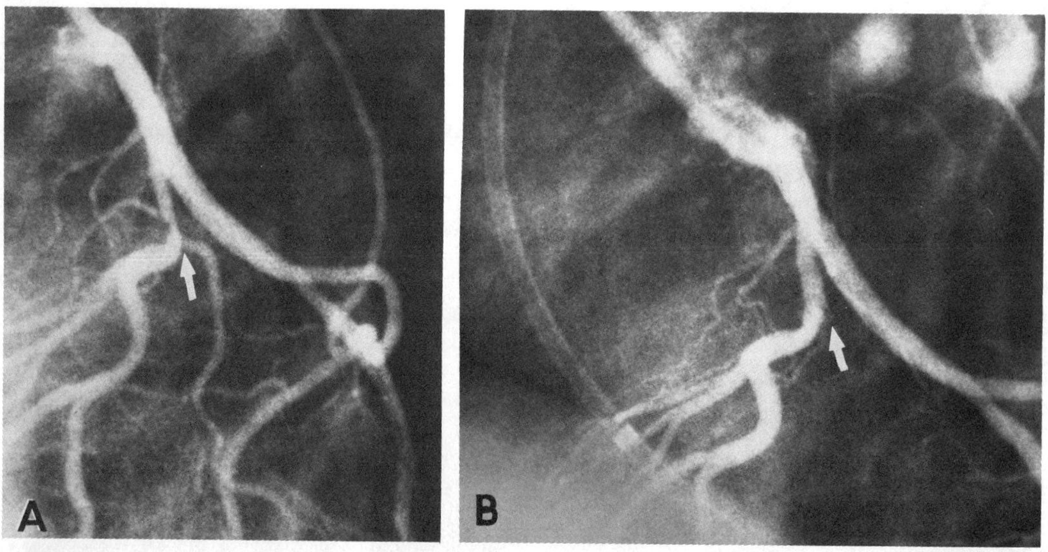

Figure 44-8 **A**, Before PTCA, there is significant stenosis in the proximal left anterior descending artery. A small diagonal vessel (arrow) arises immediately distal to the left anterior descending stenosis. **B**, Immediately after PTCA, there is an excellent result with successful dilatation of left anterior descending coronary artery. However, diagonal vessel is now occluded (arrow).

Similarly, improvements in exercise tolerance with normalization of ischemic treadmill exercise tests, increases in perfusion documented by thallium 201 testing, and improvements in regional wall motion abnormality have been documented.[40,41]

At the present time, the follow-up of patients undergoing PTCA remains limited.[42] We previously analyzed follow-up data from the NHLBI PTCA Registry on 584 patients who underwent PTCA at selected clinical centers before January 1, 1981. These 584 patients represent 76% of the total number of patients who underwent angioplasty at the selected centers during that time. The mean follow-up for these patients was 480 days. PTCA was successful in 68% of the patients and unsuccessful in 30%. In 2%, PTCA was partially successful (one of two lesions dilated successfully) or the details were unknown. Most of the patients with unsuccessful PTCA (81%) underwent surgery either during the hospitalization in which PTCA was attempted or at follow-up. At follow-up, mortality rates were low for both successful and unsuccessful PTCA groups, 2.3% and 2.2%, respectively. And 90% of the patients with successful PTCA were either asymptomatic or were in Canadian Heart functional class I or II. Eighty-eight percent of the patients with unsuccessful PTCA also were asymptomatic or in functional class I or II at follow-up. However, it is important to remember that most of the patients with unsuccessful PTCA had undergone saphenous vein bypass graft surgery.

Restenosis

A major unresolved problem with PTCA is restenosis (Figure 44-9).[42-46] As is true with the follow-up information previously discussed, data on restenosis are also limited because of the selection process that results in patients returning for follow-up angiography. Patients with recurrence of symptoms are most likely to return for follow-up angiography. This may result in a bias toward increased frequency of restenosis. Restenosis rates vary from 20% to approximately 35%.[42-47] When it occurs, restenosis usually does so within the first 6 months after PTCA and is most commonly associated with the recurrence of angina pectoris. However, as many as 25% of patients with angiographically documented restenosis are asymptomatic and undergo angiography only as part of a clinical evaluation protocol.[47]

Risk factors for the development of restenosis have been analyzed. In the NHLBI PTCA Registry, restenosis has been documented in 33% of 440 patients who underwent follow-up angiography.[47] As previously mentioned, the indication for follow-up angiography is very important and may affect this rate of restenosis. In this group, univariate analysis revealed that three factors were associated with restenosis: (1) functional class at entry ($P = 0.007$), (2) sex of the patient ($P = 0.012$), and (3) location of the dilated stenosis ($P = 0.03$). Patients in Canadian Heart class III or IV at entry had a higher incidence of restenosis than did patients in class I or II (37% vs 24%). Male patients had a higher restenosis rate than females (36% vs 21%). Circumflex and bypass graft lesions also had significantly higher restenosis rates. Multivariate analysis revealed the same three factors, although the order of significance varied: sex ($P = 0.001$), coronary artery segment dilated ($P = 0.006$), and Canadian Heart functional class at entry ($P = 0.01$). Age was also selected, with older patients having a

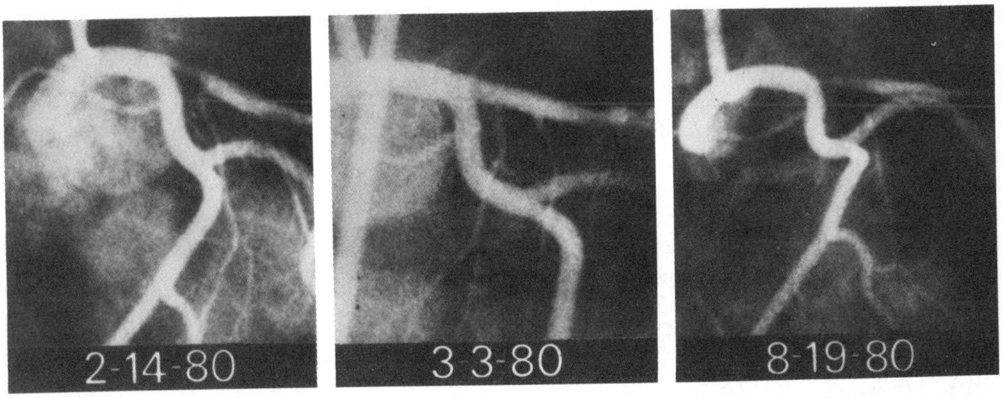

Figure 44-9 Base-line angiogram (2-14-80), documenting high-grade proximal left anterior descending coronary stenosis. After PTCA (3-3-80), showing excellent angiographic result. Subsequently (8-19-80), angina returned and repeat angiography documents restenosis with high-grade stenosis of left anterior descending artery.

higher restenosis rate than younger patients ($P = 0.01$). David et al[48] documented a significantly increased incidence of restenosis in patients with variant angina. In patients with restenosis, however, repeat PTCA can be performed and the success rates have been excellent.[49]

The cause of restenosis remains unknown. Various therapeutic regimens have been designed to prevent recurrence, including anticoagulation, and antiplatelet and calcium antagonist medications, either singly or in combination. As yet, no one treatment regimen has been found to prevent restenosis.[47]

APPROACH IN OLDER PATIENTS

Patients 65 years old or older make up an increasing percentage of our population. Some of these patients may enjoy relatively good health, apart from symptomatic coronary artery disease, although coexistent diseases such as diabetes mellitus and hypertension are relatively common.[50] Older patients are at increased risk during coronary angiography.[51] Gersh et al[52] evaluated major complications related to angiography in 2144 patients 65 years old or older and found that they had a significantly higher incidence of death, myocardial infarction, arterial embolism, and neurologic events than did 17,165 patients who were less than 65 years of age. Despite the relative increase, the absolute rates of mortality and nonfatal infarction were low, being 1.9 and 7.9 per 1000 cases, respectively.

Older patients also are at increased risk during coronary artery surgery.[52–61] Previous reports have documented increased mortality with increasing age in patients more than 65 years of age.[57] Some of this may relate to a higher incidence of associated chronic medical diseases. The actual surgical mortality rates have varied widely in the past, being as high as 20%.[53–56,59,60] More recent studies, however, have shown the rate to be less than approximately 5%.[52,61–63] During a five-year period, however, the symptomatic benefits of bypass surgery in patients 65 years old or older may be similar to those experienced by younger patients.[61] These data indicate that, in selected patients, the decision to proceed with myocardial revascularization should be based on the severity of angina and its effect on the patient's life style rather than on age alone.

Because of the increased morbidity and mortality in older patients undergoing coronary artery bypass graft surgery, PTCA has some important potential applications in older patients. The procedure is less invasive and is associated with less convalescence than surgical revascularization, and the outcome in terms of relief of angina is similar. After successful PTCA, patients are dismissed and often can return to full activity or work within a short time. This more rapid return to full activity after PTCA may result in decreased morbidity, particularly in older patients with associated medical problems, when compared with the longer convalescence after surgical revascularization.

In the NHLBI PTCA Registry, 786 patients 60 years old or older have undergone PTCA.[37] Of these 786 patients, 140 were 70 years old or older. Seventy-four percent had angina pectoris Canadian Heart Association functional class III or IV. The base-line characteristics of these patients can be seen in Table 44-1. Single-vessel disease was present in 70% of these patients and multivessel disease in 26%. An additional 4% had significant stenoses of the left main coronary artery.

PTCA was successful, with an increase in luminal stenosis of $\geqslant 20\%$ without the development of myocardial infarction or need for coronary artery bypass graft surgery in 56.2% of the patients less than 60 years of age (Table 44-2). This success rate compares with the 62.5% for patients 60 years old or older. The incidence of myocardial infarction was similar in patients 60 years of age or younger and those more than 60 years of age. In the group of 786 patients, the overall mortality rate was 2.2%, compared with 0.8% in the group less than 60 years of age. This overall mortality rate is comparable to that seen after surgical revascularization in this group of patients. Thus, in these patients the results of PTCA are comparable to those seen after surgical revascularization and provide an acceptable form of therapy.

CONCLUSIONS

The technic and application of PTCA continue to expand. New and innovative technical advances, such as the development of external con-

Table 44-1
Base-line Characteristics of 786 Patients 60 Years Old or Older

Male sex	66.7%
Class III or IV angina	74.0%
Duration of present level of angina	3.6 months
Time from onset of angina	23.0 months
Prior coronary artery surgery	12.0%
Prior myocardial infarction	26.8%

Table 44-2
Comparison of Coronary Anatomy and Results of PTCA

	Percentage of Patients	
	Aged <60 yr	*Aged ≥60 yr*
Coronary anatomy		
SVD	77	70
Success*	56.2	62.5
Complications		
MI	1.9	2.8
MI and CABG	2.9	2.8
CABG without MI	3.8	3.3
Death		
SVD	0.6	1.8
MVD	0.9	2.4

SVD = single-vessel disease; MI = myocardial infarction; CABG = coronary artery bypass graft; MVD = multivessel disease.
*Defined as angiographic improvement in luminal diameter stenosis ≥20% and no myocardial infarction or coronary artery bypass surgery.

trol of the catheter, should facilitate catheter placement and dilatation of previously inaccessible lesions and should increase the number of patients who may benefit from the procedure. Significant problems continue to exist with PTCA, including acute occlusion, the need for emergency coronary surgery during the procedure, and restenosis during follow-up. In addition, the role of PTCA in patients with multivessel coronary artery disease and during acute myocardial infarction needs continued evaluation. The eventual role of PTCA will depend on our ability to solve the clinical problems associated with the procedure and on the development of a reliable data base to permit comparison of PTCA results with those of current surgical and medical treatment regimens. It is anticipated that as experience increases, the role of PTCA in the treatment of cardiovascular disease will continue to broaden.

REFERENCES

1. Dotter CT, Judkins MP: Transluminal treatment of arteriosclerotic obstruction: Description of a new technic and a preliminary report of its application. *Circulation* 1964;30:654–670.
2. Dotter CT: Transluminal angioplasty: A long view. *Radiology* 1980;135:561–564.
3. Grüntzig A: Transluminal dilatation of coronary-artery stenoses (letter to the editor). *Lancet* 1978; 1:263.
4. Grüntzig AR: Senning Å, Siegenthaler WE: Nonoperative dilatation of coronary-artery stenosis: Percutaneous transluminal coronary angioplasty. *N Engl J Med* 1979;301:61–68.
5. Kent KM, Bentivoglio LG, Block PC, et al: NHLBI percutaneous transluminal coronary angioplasty (PTCA) registry: Four years experience, abstracted. *Am J Cardiol* 1982;49:904.
6. Kent KM, Bentivoglio LG, Block PC, et al: Percutaneous transluminal coronary angioplasty: Report from the Registry of the National Heart, Lung, and Blood Institute. *Am J Cardiol* 1982;49: 2011–2020.
7. Vlietstra RE, Holmes DR Jr, Smith HC, et al: Percutaneous transluminal coronary angioplasty: Initial Mayo Clinic experience. *Mayo Clin Proc* 1981; 56:287–293.
8. Cowley MJ, Vetrovec GW, Wolfgang TC: Efficacy of percutaneous transluminal coronary angioplasty: Technique, patient selection, salutary results, limitations and complications. *Am Heart J* 1981; 101:272–280.
9. Williams DO, Riley RS, Singh A, et al: Evaluation of role of coronary angioplasty in patients with unstable angina pectoris. *Am Heart J* 1981;102:1–9.
10. Sanborn TA, Faxon DP, Waugh D, et al: Transluminal angioplasty in experimental atherosclerosis: Analysis for embolization using an in vivo perfusion system. *Circulation* 1982;66:917–922.
11. Faxon DP, Weber VJ, Haudenschild C, et al: Acute effects of transluminal angioplasty in three experimental models of atherosclerosis. *Arteriosclerosis* 1982;2:125–133.
12. Block PC, Baughman KL, Pasternak RC, et al: Transluminal angioplasty: Correlation of morphologic and angiographic findings in an experimental model. *Circulation* 1980;61:778–785.
13. Lee G, Ikeda RM, Joye JA, et al: Evaluation of transluminal angioplasty of chronic coronary artery stenosis: Value and limitations assessed in fresh human cadaver hearts. *Circulation* 1980;61:77–83.
14. Pasternak RC, Baughman KL, Fallon JT, et al: Scanning electron microscopy after coronary transluminal angioplasty of normal canine coronary arteries. *Am J Cardiol* 1980;45:591–598.
15. Block PC, Fallon JT, Elmer D: Experimental angioplasty: Lessons from the laboratory. *AJR* 1980;135:907–912.
16. Castaneda-Zuniga WR, Formanek A, Tadavarthy M, et al: The mechanism of balloon angioplasty. *Radiology* 1980;135:565–571.
17. Baughman KL, Pasternak RC, Fallon JT, et al: Transluminal coronary angioplasty of postmortem human hearts. *Am J Cardiol* 1981;48:1044–1047.
18. Freudenberg H, Wefing H, Lichtlen PR: Risks of transluminal coronary angioplasty. A postmortal study, abstracted. *Circulation* 1978;58(suppl)2:80.
19. Block PC, Myler RK, Stertzer S, et al: Morphology after transluminal angioplasty in human beings. *N Engl J Med* 1981;305:382–385.
20. Holmes DR Jr, Vlietstra RE, Mock MB, et al: Angiographic changes produced by percutaneous transluminal coronary angioplasty. *Am J Cardiol* 1983;51:676–683.
21. Abele JE: Balloon catheters and transluminal dilatation: Technical considerations. *AJR* 1980;135: 901–906.
22. Holmes DR Jr, Vlietstra RE, Fisher LD, et al: Follow-up of patients from the Coronary Artery Surgery

Study (CASS) potentially suitable for percutaneous transluminal coronary angioplasty. *Am Heart J* 1983;106:981–988.
23. Hamby RI, Katz S: Percutaneous transluminal coronary angioplasty: Its potential impact on surgery for coronary artery disease. *Am J Cardiol* 1980; 45:1161–1166.
24. Berger SM, Gorfinkel HJ: Candidates for transluminal coronary angioplasty, letter to the editor. *Am J Cardiol* 1981;48:810.
25. Hamby RI: Reply. *Am J Cardiol* 1981;48:810.
26. Stertzer S, Dorros G, Myler R, et al: Complex transluminal angioplasty in multivessel coronary artery disease, abstracted. *Am J Cardiol* 1982; 49:904.
27. Hartzler GO, Rutherford BD, McConahay DR, et al: Simultaneous multiple lesion coronary angioplasty—A preferred therapy for patients with multiple vessel disease, abstracted. *Circulation* 1982;66(suppl)2:5.
28. Holmes DR Jr, Vlietstra RE, Reeder GS, et al: Elective percutaneous transluminal coronary angioplasty of total coronary arterial occlusions not associated with acute infarction, abstracted. *J Am Coll Cardiol* 1983;1:656.
29. Meyer J, Merx W, Schmitz H, et al: Percutaneous transluminal coronary angioplasty immediately after intracoronary streptolysis of transmural myocardial infarction. *Circulation* 1982;66:905–913.
30. Meyer J, Merx W, Dörr R, et al: Successful treatment of acute myocardial infarction shock by combined percutaneous transluminal coronary recanalization (PTCR) and percutaneous transluminal coronary angioplasty (PTCA). *Am Heart J* 1982;103:132–134.
31. Gold HK, Leinbach RC, Palacios IF, et al: Effect of immediate angioplasty on coronary patency following infarct therapy with streptokinase, abstracted. *Am J Cardiol* 1982;49:1033.
32. Ford WB, Wholey MH, Zikria EA, et al: Percutaneous transluminal dilatation of aortocoronary saphenous vein bypass grafts. *Chest* 1981;79:529–535.
33. Block PC, Palacios IF, Wholey MH, et al: Percutaneous transluminal angioplasty of stenotic coronary artery bypass grafts, abstracted. *Circulation* 1981;64(suppl 4):109.
34. Douglas JS Jr, Gruentzig AR, King SB III, et al: Long-term results of percutaneous transluminal angioplasty for aorto-coronary saphenous vein graft stenosis, abstracted. *Circulation* 1982; 66(suppl 2):124.
35. Dorros G, Cowley M, Simpson J: National Heart, Lung and Blood Institute Registry report of complications of percutaneous transluminal coronary angioplasty, abstracted. *Am J Cardiol* 1981;47:396.
36. Cowley M, Bentivoglio L, Block P, et al: Emergency coronary artery bypass surgery for complications of coronary angioplasty: NHLBI PTCA Registry experience, abstracted. *Circulation* 1981;64(suppl 4): 193.
37. Mock M, Holmes D Jr, Vlietstra R, et al: Percutaneous transluminal coronary angioplasty (PTCA) in patients ≥60 years of age registered in the NHLBI PTCA Registry, abstracted. *Circulation* 1982;66(suppl 2):329.
38. Hartzler GO, Smith HC, Vlietstra RE, et al: Coronary blood-flow responses during successful percutaneous transluminal coronary angioplasty. *Mayo Clin Proc* 1980;55:45–49.
39. Williams DO, Riley RS, Singh AK, et al: Restoration of normal coronary hemodynamics and myocardial metabolism after percutaneous transluminal coronary angioplasty. *Circulation* 1980;62: 653–656.
40. Hirzel HO, Nuesch K, Gruentzig AR, et al: Short- and long-term changes in myocardial perfusion after percutaneous transluminal coronary angioplasty assessed by thallium-201 exercise scintigraphy. *Circulation* 1981;63:1001–1007.
41. Kent KM, Bonow RO, Rosing DR, et al: Improved myocardial function during exercise after successful percutaneous transluminal coronary angioplasty. *N Engl J Med* 1982;306:441–446.
42. Holmes DR Jr, Vlietstra RE, Mock MB, et al: Follow-up of patients undergoing percutaneous transluminal coronary angioplasty (PTCA): A report from the NHLBI PTCA Registry, abstracted. *Am J Cardiol* 1982;49:916.
43. Dangoisse V, Guiteras Val P, David PR, et al: Recurrence of stenosis after successful percutaneous transluminal coronary angioplasty (PTCA), abstracted. *Circulation* 1982;66(suppl 2):331.
44. Thornton MA, Gruentzig AR, Hollman J, et al: Coumadin vs. aspirin in prevention of recurrence after transluminal coronary angioplasty—A randomized study, abstracted. *Circulation* 1982; 66(suppl 2):262.
45. Jutzy KR, Berte LE, Alderman EL, et al: Coronary restenosis rates in a consecutive patient series one year post successful angioplasty, abstracted. *Circulation* 1982;66(suppl 2):331.
46. Scholl JM, David PR, Chaitman BR, et al: Recurrence of stenosis following percutaneous transluminal coronary angioplasty, abstracted. *Circulation* 1981;64(suppl 4):193.
47. Holmes DR Jr, Vlietstra RE, Smith HC, et al: Restenosis following percutaneous transluminal coronary angioplasty (PTCA): A report from the NHLBI PTCA Registry, abstracted. *Am J Cardiol* 1982;49:905.
48. David PR, Waters DD, Scholl J-M, et al: Percutaneous transluminal coronary angioplasty in patients with variant angina. *Circulation* 1982;66: 695–702.
49. King SB III, Gruentzig AR, Douglas JS Jr, et al: Percutaneous transluminal coronary angioplasty for restenosis following initial successful procedure, abstracted. *Am J Cardiol* 1982;49:904.
50. Kovar MG: Elderly people: The population 65 years and over, in *Health: US 1976–1977.* DHEW Publication No. HRA 77-1232. Washington DC, Government Printing Office. 1977.
51. Davis K, Kennedy JW, Kemp HG Jr, et al: Complications of coronary arteriography from the Collaborative Study of Coronary Artery Surgery (CASS). *Circulation* 1979;59:1105–1112.
52. Gersh BJ, Kronmal RA, Frye RL, et al: Coronary arteriography and coronary artery bypass surgery: Morbidity and mortality in patients ages 65 years or older; a report from the Coronary Artery Surgery Study. *Circulation* 1983;67:483–491.

53. Barnhorst DA, Giuliani ER, Pluth JR, et al: Open-heart surgery in patients more than 65 years old. *Ann Thorac Surg* 1974;18:81–88.
54. Gann D, Colin C, Hildner FJ, et al: Coronary artery bypass surgery in patients seventy years of age and older. *J Thorac Cardiovasc Surg* 1977;73: 237–241.
55. Meyer J, Wukasch DC, Seybold-Epting W, et al: Coronary artery bypass in patients over 70 years of age: Indications and results. *Am J Cardiol* 1975;36: 342–345.
56. Ashor GW, Meyer BW, Lindesmith GG, et al: Coronary artery disease: Surgery in 100 patients 65 years of age and older. *Arch Surg* 1973;107:30–33.
57. Kirklin JW, Kouchoukos NT, Blackstone EH, et al: Research related to surgical treatment of coronary artery disease. *Circulation* 1979;60:1613–1618.
58. Kennedy JW, Kaiser GC, Fisher LD, et al: Clinical and angiographic predictors of operative mortality from the Collaborative Study in Coronary Artery Surgery (CASS). *Circulation* 1981;63:793–802.
59. Smith JM, Lindsay WG, Lillehei RC, et al: Cardiac surgery in geriatric patients. *Surgery* 1976;80:443–448.
60. McCallister BD, Schmeidt M, Reed WA, et al: Coronary artery bypass in patients over the age of 70: Initial and late results, abstracted. *Circulation* 1975;52(suppl 2):91.
61. Gersh BJ, Kronmal RA, Schaff HV, et al: Long-term (5-year) results of coronary bypass surgery in patients 65 years old or older: A report from the Coronary Artery Surgery Study—CASS. *Circulation* 1983;68(suppl 2):190–199.
62. Stephenson LW, MacVaugh H III, Edmunds LH Jr: Surgery using cardiopulmonary bypass in the elderly. *Circulation* 1978;58:250–254.
63. Knapp WS, Douglas JS Jr, Craver JM, et al: Efficacy of coronary artery bypass grafting in elderly patients with coronary artery disease. *Am J Cardiol* 1981;47:923–930.

CHAPTER 45

Diseases of the Arterial Wall: Management of Abdominal Aortic and Peripheral Aneurysms

Sandor A. Friedman
Mohandas Shenoy

Arterial aneurysms are an important source of morbidity and mortality in the elderly. This chapter deals with the approach to these lesions in a few of the most critical locations.

ABDOMINAL AORTIC ANEURYSMS

The distal abdominal aorta is the site of the most common aneurysm because of the turbulence created by the sharp bifurcation of the aorta into the common iliac arteries. Aneurysms in this area are almost always arteriosclerotic in nature, and hypertension is a major risk factor. They are located entirely distal to the renal arteries in more than 95% of cases and often involve the proximal portions of the common iliacs. This lesion is much more common in men than women and usually appears after the sixth decade. There is clearly a statistical association between abdominal aneurysms and other cardiovascular diseases. In one series, 88% of patients had other cardiovascular disease, including 47% with coronary artery, 8% with cerebrovascular and 34% with peripheral arterial disease.[1]

Aneurysms of the abdominal aorta represent a major public health problem. Retrospective autopsy studies suggest that abdominal aortic rupture accounts for one of every 250 natural deaths in people over the age of 50.[2] Unfortunately, the great majority of these aneurysms are not diagnosed during life, and when one is discovered, it is often incidental to a radiographic evaluation of the abdomen performed for another reason.

Symptoms are unusual. These aneurysms are retroperitoneal and have sufficient room for expansion without causing compressive syndromes. Pain is extremely rare until the aneurysm expands to the point of rupture. Even with rupture, there may be little or no pain. When it does occur, it is usually located in the lower back or upper abdomen and is of a sharp, tearing nature, but it may appear in other areas of the abdomen and be quite nonspecific in quality. Some patients complain of abdominal palpitation.

The key to diagnosis is careful physical examination. In most normal individuals, one can palpate an aortic pulsation in the epigastric area. The strength of this pulse depends greatly on body habitus. One must distinguish this normal pulse from the hard, globular pulsatile mass of an aneurysm. The anterior width of this mass can be roughly estimated by finding the lateral borders, and lateral as well as anterior pulsation can usually be appreciated. Often the mass is deviated from the midline, particularly to the left. In about half the cases, a systolic bruit can be heard. The pulsation is often visible and appreciable even with light palpation. This differentiates an aneurysm from an aortic pulse transmitted through some other retroperitoneal mass.

In many cases, one feels a strong pulsation without a definite mass and has difficulty in differentiating between an aneurysm and generalized tortuosity and ectasia of the aorta. This kind of pulsation is more likely to represent an aneurysm if it is localized, deviated to the left or right of the midline, or palpable at or below the periumbilical area. In an obese individual, even a weak pulsation can suggest the possible presence of an aneurysm.

Approximately two thirds of the lesions are sufficiently calcified to appear on plain abdominal roentgenograms, but the procedure of choice in looking for an abdominal aneurysm is ultrasonography. With this noninvasive technic, one can identify an aneurysm in almost every case, judge its precise location and accurately measure its length, width and depth (Figure 45-1). Mural thrombus is also seen quite easily.

The advent of sonography has made aortography obsolete as a diagnostic modality for aortic aneurysm.[3,4] Not only does the former offer the advantage of complete safety, but it is also more accurate than arteriography. Using aortography, one may seriously underestimate the size of an aneurysm and occasionally even miss the diagnosis because it does not distinguish clot from arterial wall.[4]

Prognosis and Treatment

Once the diagnosis is made, one must consider the issue of surgical repair. Statistics from many studies indicate that longevity of untreated patients with significant abdominal aortic aneurysms is less than that associated with several neoplasms, including carcinoma of the breast. The five-year survival from diagnosis of this aneurysm varies in the literature from about 17.2% to 36.4%, with most reports in the lower part of this range.[5,6] In the absence of significant heart disease, the overwhelming majority of deaths result from aneurysmal rupture. When heart disease is present, approximately 50% die of rupture. The wider the aneurysm, the more likely rupture is to occur. Aneurysms below 5 cm rarely rupture before further expansion, and those over 8 cm are particularly dangerous.

In view of these statistics, an aggressive approach to treatment is appropriate. With relatively few exceptions, aneurysms located below the renal arteries should be repaired once they reach 5 to 6 cm in diameter. Several groups have shown a prolongation of life after aneurysm repair. In one series, survival rate was 72% three years after surgery and 58% after five years.[7] Of course, the magnitude of increased longevity depends on the age of the patient at the time of surgery and the presence or absence of serious heart disease. The major contraindications involve serious cardiopulmonary disease. Patients with severe chronic obstructive lung disease, unstable angina, uncompensated congestive heart failure and recent transient ischemic attacks have a significant risk of succumbing to major abdominal surgery and often die of coronary artery or cerebrovascular disease. However, stable cardiac patients with adequate cardiac and pulmonary

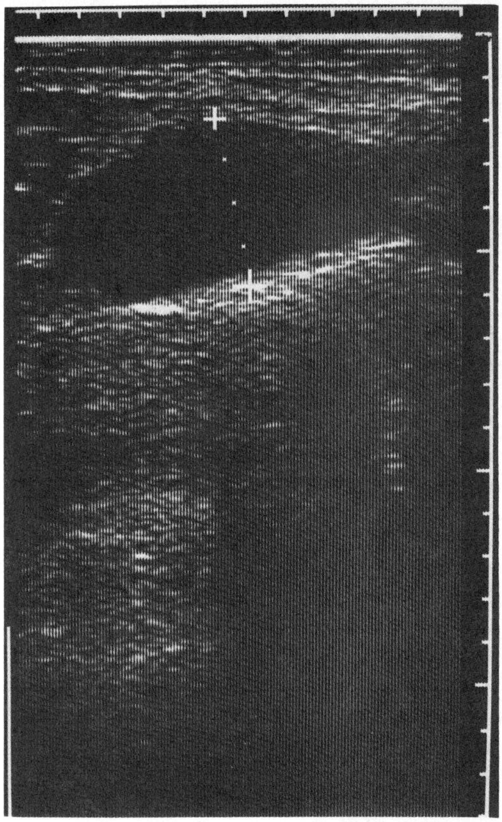

Figure 45-1A An abdominal sonogram reveals an aortic aneurysm without thrombus.

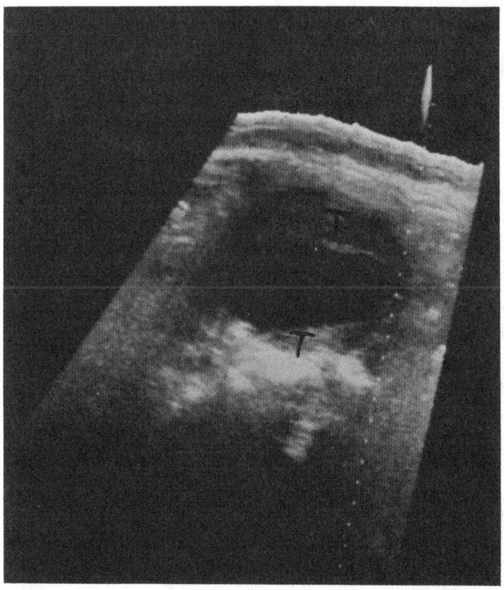

Figure 45-1B Sonography demonstrates an abdominal aortic aneurysm with mural thrombus adherent to both the anterior and posterior walls (T = thrombus).

function can certainly tolerate this surgery. In fact, previously unstable patients may become candidates for aneurysm repair after coronary bypass or carotid endarterectomy procedures. Age is certainly not an absolute contraindication. If patients are chosen with these guidelines and operated on by experienced vascular surgeons, the mortality rate should be less than 4%. If surgery cannot be performed, the patient should be followed with serial sonography every three to four months, instructed not to strain during bowel movements, and warned to seek immediate medical attention if any unusual abdominal or lower back pain occurs.

Complications of surgery include postoperative myocardial infarction, emboli from the aneurysmal sac to the arteries of the lower extremities, and strokes, particularly if there is significant hypotension during surgery. Blood pressure must be carefully controlled especially during aortic clamping, which can produce reflex hypotension. Monitoring of central venous or pulmonary capillary wedge pressure during surgery is advisable. Many surgeons do not require preoperative aortography, but others wish to see the distal run-off in order to plan the location of the distal anastamosis. In addition, some surgeons prefer to visualize the mesenteric vessels before surgery. Of concern is the theoretical possibility of bowel infarction during or after surgery if there is significant obstruction in the superior mesenteric artery or celiac axis, since the inferior mesenteric artery is usually sacrificed during aneurysmal repair. In practice, however, bowel ischemia is rarely a problem, although prolonged ileus of the lower colon and sigmoid occasionally occurs after surgery.

Other complications of abdominal aortic aneurysms, although much less frequent, also merit consideration. Emboli into the large and small arteries of the lower extremities have been noted in a small percentage of cases. It is possible that this process occurs silently in many other cases since femoropopliteal occlusion is more common than aorto-iliac occlusion in patients with aortic aneurysms. Embolization may account for some of this difference. Clotting within the aneurysmal sac has occasionally produced a hemorrhagic disorder secondary to consumption of clotting factors and formation of fibrin split products, which act as anticoagulants.[8] Heparin administration can reverse this process. A third and rare complication is superimposed infection. The most common offender is *Salmonella*[9] which becomes sequestered in thrombus and acts as a nidus for septicemia.

Ruptured Aneurysms

Although most ruptured aneurysms result in death, a small group of patients can be salvaged through immediate surgical intervention. Initial perforation through the posterior wall may be tamponaded by blood clot for several hours before massive intraperitoneal hemorrhage occurs. In this situation, every minute counts. The clinician must always consider the strong possibility of a ruptured aneurysm in any older individual with acute abdominal pain and palpate carefully for a pulsatile mass. The constellation of unexplained abdominal or low back pain and a palpable aneurysm warrants immediate laparotomy without any further evaluation. In most cases, a ruptured or necrotic aneurysm will be found, and surgery is life-saving. Hypotension and pain in older individuals should make one think of aneurysmal rupture even if a prominent pulsation is not felt. The combination of a low blood pressure and surrounding hematoma may dampen the pulsation particularly in a heavy-set individual. If the central venous pressure is low and an electrocardiogram shows no evidence of acute myocardial infarction, these patients should also be taken to the operating room immediately for a small laparotomy incision. It is safer to presume the presence of an aneurysm than to wait for late signs such as a dropping hematocrit and abdominal swelling. At worst, a small incision can be closed if no aneurysm is found.

It is best not to try to restore blood volume to normal until the surgeon has clamped the aorta proximal to the ruptured area because a high perfusing pressure may dislodge the thrombus covering the perforation. The postoperative course of patients with ruptured aneurysms is often quite stormy. Renal failure, usually of the non-oliguric type, is common because of hypotension and volume depletion. The use of mannitol intraoperatively is probably useful in decreasing the severity of this complication. In addition, massive amounts of intravenous fluid are often required during the first two days to maintain blood volume because of sequestration in the inflamed retroperitoneal space, and constant monitoring of pulmonary artery and wedge pressures is advisable. When sequestered fluid is later reabsorbed into the vascular space, pulmonary edema may occur particularly if the patient has underlying heart disease and renal function is impaired. Early institution of dialysis and prophylactic use of digitalis may be helpful in averting this complication.

Other complications include strokes, postoperative pneumonia and adult respiratory distress syndrome, requiring continued intubation and mechanical ventilation. Finally, wound dehiscence can occur secondary to the pressures of abdominal distention and mechanical ventilation. If the patient, despite these potential problems, survives to the fifth day and is still alert, his chances of recovery become good.

POPLITEAL ANEURYSMS

The popliteal artery is the second most common site of aneurysm formation because the vessel is subject to muscular compression proximally as it emerges from Hunter's canal in the lower thigh and more distally by the arcuate popliteal ligament. This compression leads to turbulence and trauma that is compounded by frequent motion of the knee. Popliteal aneurysms occur in association with other aneurysms.[10] In more than half the cases, they are bilateral, and they are associated with abdominal aortic aneurysms in about 35% of cases.[11]

The diagnosis of a patent popliteal aneurysm is easily made by palpation. Sonography is extremely useful for confirming the diagnosis, estimating the size and outlining mural thrombus.[12] An occluded aneurysm is more difficult to appreciate. It appears as a firm or cystic mass under the knee and may be mistaken for synovitis or a popliteal cyst. Sonography should be performed to rule out an aneurysm before any popliteal mass is aspirated.

Complications

Most of these lesions produce no symptoms, but some aneurysms cause pain or numbness along the calf secondary to compression of the posterior tibial nerve. Rupture occurs in only about 10% of patent aneurysms and never occurs after the sac has become occluded with mural thrombus. Occasionally, the aneurysm compresses the adjacent popliteal vein, leading to leg edema and even deep vein thrombosis and pulmonary embolism.

The major complication of popliteal aneurysms is thromboembolism, which can present clinically in several different ways. Rapid occlusion of the aneurysmal sac can cause acute leg ischemia and lead quickly to gangrene, while gradual occlusion may produce intermittent claudication and chronic signs of ischemia. In addition, embolic episodes from the mural thrombus may occur singly or in showers, producing regional ischemia of a foot, a toe or even smaller area of the limb. Popliteal aneurysm is the first diagnosis to consider in a patient who has one or more episodes of limited infarction in a foot especially if the dorsalis pedis or posterior tibial pulse is still palpable. Finally, thrombus within the aneurysmal lumen may change position from time to time so that the popliteal pulse is alternately palpable and imperceptible.

Prognosis and Treatment

Unfortunately, loss of limb secondary to thromboembolism is quite common in patients with popliteal aneurysms. In one series of 70 consecutive patients managed conservatively, thromboembolism occurred in 11, venous compression in 5 and rupture in 4 during a 44-month period.[13] Eighteen patients required amputation including 5 of the 45 with previously uncomplicated lesions. In another series of previously asymptomatic popliteal aneurysms, 29% had complications and 3% lost their legs.[11] On the other hand, surgical repair of a popliteal aneurysm is a relatively easy procedure, which can even be performed under spinal or local anesthesia if there is a contraindication to general anesthesia. Femoral arteriography is performed first in order to assess the distal arterial run-off. The aneurysm does not have to be removed. It can be ligated proximally and replaced by a by-pass graft. Results are excellent, and the mortality rate of the procedure, when performed by competent vascular surgeons, is under 1%.[14]

On the basis of these data, it seems prudent to recommend surgical repair of almost all patent popliteal aneurysms. Only very debilitated patients or those with limited longevity should be excluded. Patients with already occluded aneurysms should be treated like all others with arterial occlusive disease. Femoral artery aneurysms should be handled in a similar fashion.

CAROTID ARTERY ANEURYSMS

Aneurysmal dilatation of a carotid artery is a rare disorder. One surgical group reported three cases over a ten-year period during which 300 aneurysms of major arteries were discovered.[15] True carotid aneurysms must be distinguished from the much more common kinking of the carotid artery, which can also present as a palpable mass. In one series, this kinking was found in almost 80% of carotid arteriograms performed in elderly individuals. Aneurysms almost always develop in the upper neck under the angle of the jaw, while kinking occurs at the base of the neck, particularly on the right side where the carotid artery originates from the innominate artery.

The danger of carotid aneurysms is embolization into cerebral vessels, producing strokes and transient ischemic attacks. Perhaps 50% of these lesions eventually cause cerebral complications. The diagnosis depends on finding a pulsatile neck mass under the angle of the jaw and is corroborated by cerebral angiography. Surgical repair is almost always indicated.

REFERENCES

1. Friedman SA, Hufnagel CA, Conrad PW, et al: Abdominal aortic aneurysms: Clinical status and results of surgery in 100 consecutive cases. *JAMA* 1967;200:1147.
2. Moore HD: Diagnosis of rupture of abdominal aortic aneurysms. *Lancet* 1967;2:184–186.
3. Wheeler WE, Beachley MC, Ranniger K: Angiography and ultrasonography: A comparative study of abdominal aortic aneurysms. *AJR* 1976;126:95–100.
4. Karp W, Eklof BO: Ultrasonography and angiography in the diagnosis of abdominal aortic aneurysm. *Acta Radiol Diagnosis* 1978;19:955–966.
5. Bernstein EF, Fisher JC, Varco RL: Is excision the optimum treatment for all abdominal aortic aneurysms? *Surgery* 1967;61:83–86.
6. Schatz IJ, Fairbairn JF II, Juergens JL: Abdominal aortic aneurysms: A reappraisal. *Circulation* 1962;26:200–204.
7. DeBakey ME, Crawford ES, Cooley DA, et al: Aneurysm of abdominal aorta: Analysis of results of graft replacement therapy 1 to 11 years after operation. *Ann Surg* 1964;160:622–624.
8. Satiani B, Savrin R, Evans WE: Consumption coagulopathy associated with arterial aneurysms. *J Cardiovasc Surg* 1979;20:273–276.
9. Sommerville RL, Allen EV, Edwards JE: Bland and infected arteriosclerotic abdominal aortic aneurysms. *Medicine* 1959;38:207–210.
10. Edmunds LH Jr, Darling RC, Linton RR: Surgical management of popliteal aneurysms. *Circulation* 1965;32:517–520.
11. Wychulis AR, Spittell JA, Wallace RB: Popliteal aneurysms. *Surgery* 1970;68:942–945.
12. Neiman HL, Yao JST, Silver TM: Gray-scale ultrasound diagnosis of peripheral arterial aneurysms. *Radiology* 1979;130:413–416.
13. Gifford RW Jr, Hines EA Jr, Janes JM: An analysis and follow-up study of 100 popliteal aneurysms. *Surgery* 1953;33:284–288.
14. Crichlow RW, Roberts B: Treatment of popliteal aneurysms by restoration of continuity: Review of 48 cases. *Ann Surg* 1966;163:417–421.
15. Carrascal L, Marshiah A, Charlesworth D: Aneurysms of the extracranial carotid arteries. *Br J Surg* 1978;65:590–593.

Index